Bethesda Handbook
of Clinical Oncology

THIRD EDITION

Bethesda Handbook
of Clinical Oncology

THIRD EDITION

Editors

Jame Abraham, MD FACP

Bonnie Wells Wilson Eminent Scholar and Distinguished Professor
Chief, Section of Hematology/Oncology
Director, Comprehensive Breast Cancer Program
Medical Director, Mary Babb Randolph Cancer Center
West Virginia University
Morgantown, West Virginia

James L. Gulley, MD PhD FACP

Director, Clinical Trials Group
Laboratory of Tumor Immunology and Biology
Senior Clinician, Medical Oncology Branch
Center for Cancer Research
National Cancer Institute
National Institutes of Health
Bethesda, Maryland

Carmen J. Allegra, MD

Professor and Chief, Division of Hematology and Oncology
Associate Director for Clinical and Translational Research
Shands/University of Florida Cancer Center
University of Florida
Gainesville, Florida

 Wolters Kluwer | Lippincott Williams & Wilkins
Health

Philadelphia · Baltimore · New York · London
Buenos Aires · Hong Kong · Sydney · Tokyo

Senior Executive Editor: Jonathan W. Pine
Senior Managing Editors: Anne Jacobs/Joyce Murphy
Senior Product Manager: Emilie Moyer
Senior Marketing Manager: Angela Panetta
Manufacturing Manager: Benjamin Rivera
Senior Designer: Stephen Druding
Production Service: Spearhead Global, Inc.
Printer: R.R. Donnelley

3rd Edition
© **2010 by Lippincott Williams & Wilkins**
530 Walnut Street
Philadelphia, PA 19106
LWW.com

1/e Published 2000; 2/e Published 2005

Printed in China

Library of Congress Cataloging-in-Publication Data
Bethesda handbook of clinical oncology / editors, Jame Abraham, James L. Gulley, Carmen J. Allegra. — 3rd ed.
    p. ; cm.
    Includes bibliographical references and index.
    ISBN-13: 978-0-7817-9558-6
    ISBN-10: 0-7817-9558-3
    1. Cancer—Handbooks, manuals, etc.   I.   Abraham, Jame.   II. Gulley, James L. (James Leonard), 1964-   III. Allegra, Carmen J.   IV. Title: Handbook of clinical oncology.
    [DNLM: 1. Neoplasms—therapy—Handbooks. QZ 39 B562 2010]
    RC262.5.B485 2010
    616.99′4—dc22

2009015306

RRS1003

We dedicate this book to those lives that are touched by cancer and to their caregivers who spend endless hours taking care of them.

"May I never forget that the patient is a fellow creature in pain. May I never consider him merely a vessel of disease."

—Maimonides

(*Twelfth-century philosopher and physician*)

Contents

Contributing Authors

Jame Abraham, MD FACP *Bonnie Wells Wilson Eminent Scholar and Distinguished Professor; Chief, Section of Hematology/Oncology; Director, Comprehensive Breast Cancer Program; Medical Director, Mary Babb Randolph Cancer Center, West Virginia University, Morgantown, West Virginia*

David Adelberg, MD *Medical Oncology Branch, Center for Cancer Research, National Cancer Institute, National Institutes of Health, Bethesda, Maryland*

Carmen J. Allegra, MD *Professor and Chief, Division of Hematology and Oncology; Associate Director for Clinical and Translational Research, Shands/ University of Florida Cancer Center, University of Florida, Gainesville, Florida*

Wendy L. Allen, BSc PhD *Research Fellow, Drug Resistance Laboratory, Centre for Cancer Research and Cell Biology, Queen's University Belfast, Belfast, Ireland*

Christina M. Annunziata, MD PhD *Medical Oncology Branch, National Cancer Institute, National Institutes of Health, Bethesda, Maryland*

Jeanny B. Aragon-Ching, MD *Assistant Professor of Medicine, Department of Medicine, Division of Hematology and Oncology, George Washington University Medical Center, Washington DC*

Philip M. Arlen, MD *Director, Clinical Research Group, Laboratory of Tumor Immunology and Biology, National Cancer Institute, National Institutes of Health, Bethesda, Maryland*

Syed J. Asghar, MD *Department of Medical Oncology, Waterford Regional Hospital, Waterford, Ireland*

Nilofer S. Azad, MD *Assistant Professor of Oncology, Johns Hopkins Sidney Kimmel Comprehensive Cancer Center, Baltimore, Maryland*

Ann Berger, MSN, MD *Pain and Palliative Care Service, Warren Grant Magnuson Clinical Center, Bethesda, Maryland*

Susan L. Bever, RN BSN *Clinical Program Manager, Endocyte Incorporated, West Lafayette, Indiana*

Michael J. Birrer, MD PhD *Department of Cell and Cancer Biology, National Cancer Institute, National Institutes of Health, Bethesda, Maryland*

Oscar S. Breathnach, MB FRCPI *Consultant, Department of Medical Oncology, Beaumont Hospital Cancer Centre, Dublin, Ireland*

Eric Bush, Rph MBA MD *Medical Director, Capital Palliative Care Consultants, Georgetown University Hospital, Washington DC*

George Carter, MMS PA-C　*Medical Oncology Branch, National Cancer Institute, National Institutes of Health, Bethesda, Maryland*

Bryan W. Chang, MD　*Department of Therapeutic Radiology, Yale University School of Medicine, New Haven, Connecticut*

Bruce D. Cheson, MD　*Chief of Hematology, Professor of Medicine, Division of Hematology-Oncology, Georgetown University Hospital, Lombardi Comprehensive Cancer Center, Washington DC*

Richard W. Childs, MD　*Senior Investigator, Hematology Branch, National Heart, Lung, and Blood Institute, National Institutes of Health, Bethesda, Maryland*

Linda E. Coate, MD　*Department of Medical Oncology, Waterford Regional Hospital, Waterford, Ireland*

Barbara A. Conley, MD　*Professor and Chief, Division of Hematology and Oncology, Department of Medicine, Michigan State University College of Human Medicine, East Lansing, Michigan*

Vicky M. Coyle, MD　*Drug Resistance Laboratory, Centre for Cancer Research and Cell Biology, Queen's University Belfast, Belfast, Ireland*

Michael Craig, MD　*Assistant Professor of Medicine, Director of Hematologic Malignancy and Transplantation, Division of Hematology/Oncology, Mary Babb Randolph Cancer Center, West Virginia University, Morgantown, West Virginia*

Aaron Cumpston, PharmD　*Pharmacy Clinical Specialist, Pharmacy Department, West Virginia University Hospitals, Morgantown, West Virginia*

William L. Dahut, MD　*Chief, Genitourinary/Gynecologic Clinical Research Unit and Principal Investigator, Medical Oncology Branch, National Cancer Institute, National Institutes of Health, Bethesda, Maryland*

Suzanne G. Demko, PA-C　*Senior Clinical Analyst, Division of Biologic Oncology Products, U.S. Food and Drug Administration, Silver Spring, Maryland*

Marcel P. Devetten, MD　*Associate Professor, Director, Hematopoietic Cell Transplantation Program, University of Nebraska Medical Center, Omaha, Nebraska*

Marnie Dobbin, MS RD　*Clinical Research Dietitian, National Institutes of Health Clinical Center, Department of Nutrition, Bethesda, Maryland*

Cynthia E. Dunbar, MD　*Hematology Branch, National Heart, Lung, and Blood Institute, National Institutes of Health, Bethesda, Maryland*

Kieron Dunleavy, MD　*Investigator and Attending Physician, Lymphoid Malignancies Section, Metabolism Branch, Center for Cancer Research, National Cancer Institute, National Institutes of Health, Bethesda, Maryland*

Daniel E. Elswick, MD *Assistant Professor, Behavioral Medicine and Psychiatry, Mary Babb Randolph Cancer Center, West Virginia University School of Medicine, Morgantown, West Virginia*

Dexter T. Estrada, MD *Assistant Clinical Professor, Department of Medicine; Chief, Hematology/Oncology Section, VA Central California Health Care System, University of California–San Francisco, Fresno, California*

Tito Fojo, MD *Senior Investigator, Medical Oncology Branch, National Cancer Institute, National Institutes of Health, Bethesda, Maryland*

Juan C. Gea-Banacloche, MD *Chief, Infectious Diseases, Experimental Transplantation and Immunology Branch, National Cancer Institute, National Institutes of Health, Bethesda, Maryland*

Thomas J. George, Jr., MD FACP *Assistant Professor, Division of Hematology and Oncology; Director, Gastrointestinal Oncology Program, Shands/University of Florida Cancer Center, University of Florida, Gainesville, Florida*

Giuseppe Giaccone, MD PhD *Chief, Medical Oncology Branch, National Cancer Institute, National Institutes of Health, Bethesda, Maryland*

James L. Gulley, MD PhD FACP *Director, Clinical Trials Group, Laboratory of Tumor Immunology and Biology; Senior Clinician, Medical Oncology Branch, Center for Cancer Research, National Cancer Institute, National Institutes of Health, Bethesda, Maryland*

Martin E. Gutierrez, MD *Medical Director, Michael and Diane Comprehensive Cancer Center, Holy Cross Hospital, Fort Lauderdale, Florida*

Syed I. Haidar, MD *Department of Medical Oncology, Waterford Regional Hospital, Waterford, Ireland*

Upendra P. Hegde, MD *Assistant Professor of Medicine, Division of Hematology/Oncology, Neag Comprehensive Cancer Center, University of Connecticut Health Center, Farmington, Connecticut*

Lee J. Helman, MD *Scientific Director, Clinical Research Department, Center for Cancer Research, National Cancer Institute, National Institutes of Health, Bethesda, Maryland*

Akm Hossain *Mary Babb Randolph Cancer Center, Section of Hematology/ Oncology, Department of Medicine, West Virginia University, Morgantown, West Virginia*

Thomas E. Hughes, PharmD BCOP *Clinical Pharmacy Specialist, Pharmacy Department, National Institutes of Health, Clinical Center, Bethesda, Maryland*

Saad Jamshed, MD *Division of Hematology-Oncology, Georgetown University Hospital, Lombardi Comprehensive Cancer Center, Washington DC*

Puthen V. Jithesh, MSc *Drug Resistance Laboratory, Centre for Cancer Research and Cell Biology, Queen's University Belfast, Belfast, Ireland*

Patrick G. Johnston, MD PhD FRCP FRCPI   *Professor of Oncology and Dean of Medicine, Dentistry and Biomedical Sciences, School of Medicine, Dentistry and Biomedical Sciences, Centre for Cancer Research and Cell Biology, Queen's University Belfast, Belfast, Ireland*

Ronan Kelly, MD   *Clinical Fellow, Medical Oncology Branch, National Cancer Institute, National Institutes of Health, Bethesda, Maryland*

Hung T. Khong, MD   *Associate Professor and Chief of Gastrointestinal Malignancies, Clinical Immunotherapeutics Research Laboratory; Assistant Professor of Oncologic Sciences and Pharmacology, Mitchell Cancer Institute, Mobile, Alabama*

George P. Kim, MD   *Associate Professor, Department of Hematology/Oncology, Mayo Clinic, Jacksonville, Florida*

Ebru Koca, MD   *Fellow, Department of Stem Cell Transplantation and Cellular Therapy, MD Anderson Cancer Center, University of Texas, Houston, Texas*

David R. Kohler, PharmD   *Pharmacy Department, National Institutes of Health Clinical Center, Bethesda, Maryland*

Elise C. Kohn, MD   *Medical Oncology Branch, Center for Cancer Research, National Cancer Institute, National Institutes of Health, Bethesda, Maryland*

Herbert L. Kotz, MD   *Medical Oncology Branch, National Cancer Institute, National Institutes of Health, Bethesda, Maryland*

Barnett S. Kramer, MD MPH   *Office of Disease Prevention, National Institutes of Health, Bethesda, Maryland*

Sewa S. Legha, MD FACP   *Clinical Professor of Medicine, Department of Hematology/Oncology, Baylor College of Medicine, Houston, Texas Director of Melanoma Care at St. Luke's Episcopal Hospital, Houston, Texas*

Gregory D. Leonard, MD   *Department of Medical Oncology, Waterford Regional Hospital, Waterford, Ireland*

W. Marston Linehan, MD   *Chief, Urologic Oncology Branch, National Cancer Institute, National Institutes of Health, Bethesda, Maryland*

Ravi A. Madan, MD   *Associate Clinical Investigator, Medical Oncology Branch and Laboratory of Tumor Immunology and Biology, Center for Cancer Research, National Cancer Institute, National Institutes of Health, Bethesda, Maryland*

Patrick J. Mansky, MD   *Medical Director, Medical Research and Medical Oncologist, The Cancer Team at Bellin Health, Green Bay, Wisconsin*

Michael E. Menefee, MD   *Assistant Professor, Division of Hematology and Oncology, Mayo Clinic, Jacksonville, Florida*

Richard A. Messmann, MD MHS MSc   *Vice President, Medical Affairs, Endocyte Incorporated, West Lafayette, Indiana*

Scott Miller, MD *Division of Intramural Research, National Center for Complementary and Alternative Medicine, National Institutes of Health, Bethesda, Maryland*

Mahsa Mohebtash, MD *Clinical Fellow, Medical Oncology Branch, Center for Cancer Research, National Cancer Institute, National Institutes of Health, Bethesda, Maryland*

Manish Monga, MD *Schiffler Cancer Center, Medical Oncology Division, Wheeling Hospital, Wheeling, West Virginia*

Janaki Moni, MD *Associate Professor, Department of Radiation Oncology, University of Massachusetts Medical School, Worcester, Massachusetts*

Sattva S. Neelapu, MD *Assistant Professor, Department of Lymphoma and Myeloma, MD Anderson Cancer Center, Houston, Texas*

Maryland Pao, MD *Clinical Director, Department of Health and Human Services, National Institute of Mental Health, National Institutes of Health, Washington DC*

Alyssa C. Perroy, MD *Department of Hematology-Oncology, Medical Corps, US Air Force, Wright-Patterson Medical Center, Ohio*

Richard L. Piekarz, MD PhD *Staff Clinician, National Cancer Institute, National Institutes of Health, Bethesda, Maryland*

Jondavid Pollock, MD PhD *Radiation Oncologist, The Schiffler Cancer Center, Division of Radiation Oncology, Wheeling Hospital, Wheeling, West Virginia*

Muzaffar H. Qazilbash, MD *Associate Professor of Medicine, University of Texas; Co-Director, Stem Cell Transplantation Fellowship Program; Associate Director, Hematology-Oncology Fellowship Program, Department of Stem Cell Transplantation and Cellular Therapy, MD Anderson Cancer Center, Houston, Texas*

Sarah W. Read, MD *Medical Officer, Division of AIDS, National Institute of Allergy and Infectious Diseases, National Institutes of Health, Bethesda, Maryland*

June L. Remick *Nurse Practitioner, West Virginia University Hospital, Morgantown, West Virginia*

Donald L. Rosenstein, MD *Director, Comprehensive Cancer Support Program; Professor of Psychiatry, University of North Carolina at Chapel Hill, Chapel Hill, North Carolina*

Inger L. Rosner, MD *Clinical Fellow, Urologic Oncology Branch, National Cancer Institute, National Institutes of Health, Bethesda, Maryland*

Kerry Ryan, MPH MSHS PA-C   *Medical Oncology Branch, National Cancer Institute, National Institutes of Health, Bethesda, Maryland*

Ayman Saad, MD   *Assistant Professor, Section of Neoplastic Diseases and Related Disorders, Department of Internal Medicine, Medical College of Wisconsin, Milwaukee, Wisconsin*

M. Wasif Saif, MD MBBS   *Associate Professor and Director, Gastrointestinal Cancers Program, Yale Cancer Center, Yale University School of Medicine, New Haven, Connecticut*

Manish Sharma   *Section of Hematology/Oncology, Mary Babb Randolph Cancer Center, West Virginia University, Morgantown, West Virginia*

Elizabeth Smyth, MB MRCPI   *Fellow, Medical Oncology, Department of Medical Oncology, Beaumont Hospital Cancer Centre, Dublin, Ireland*

Ramaprasad Srinivasan, MD PhD   *Senior Investigator, Urologic Oncology Branch, National Cancer Institute, National Institutes of Health, Bethesda, Maryland*

Jamie Stagl, MD   *Division of Intramural Research, National Center for Complementary and Alternative Medicine, National Institutes of Health, Bethesda, Maryland*

Magesh Sundaram, MD MBA FACS   *Chief, Division of Surgical Oncology, Department of Surgery, West Virginia University School of Medicine, Morgantown, West Virginia*

Kevin K. Tay, MD   *Clinical Fellow, Lymphoid Malignancies Section, Medical Oncology Branch, Center for Cancer Research, National Cancer Institute, National Institutes of Health, Bethesda, Maryland*

Carter VanWaes, MD PhD   *Chief, Head and Neck Surgery Branch; Clinical Director, National Institute for Deafness and Other Communicative Disorders, National Institutes of Health, Bethesda, Maryland*

Sakar M. Wahby, PharmD   *Oncology Clinical Pharmacist, Pharmacy Department, National Institutes of Health Clinical Center, Bethesda, Maryland*

Dawn B. Wallerstedt, MSN CRNP   *Scientific Program Manager, Military Medical Research, Samueli Institute, Alexandria, Virginia*

Wyndham H. Wilson, MD PhD   *Senior Investigator and Chief, Lymphoma Therapeutics Section, Metabolism Branch, Center for Cancer Research, National Cancer Institute, National Institutes of Health, Bethesda, Maryland*

Preface

The *Bethesda Handbook of Clinical Oncology* is a clear, concise, and comprehensive reference book for the busy clinician to use in his or her daily patient encounters. The book has been compiled by clinicians who are working or have been trained at the National Cancer Institute and National Institutes of Health as well as scholars from other academic institutions. To limit the size of the book, less space is dedicated to etiology, pathophysiology, and epidemiology and greater emphasis is placed on practical clinical information. For easy accessibility to the pertinent information, long descriptions are avoided, and more tables, pictures, algorithms, and phrases are included.

The *Bethesda Handbook of Clinical Oncology* is not intended as a substitute for the many excellent oncology reference textbooks available that are essential for a more complete understanding of the pathophysiology and management of complicated oncology patients. We hope that the reader-friendly format with its comprehensive review of the management of each disease with treatment regimens including dosing and schedule, make this book unique and useful for oncologists, oncology fellows, residents, students, oncology nurses, and allied health professionals.

The field of oncology has changed substantially since the first edition of this book was published ten years ago. For the third edition, we have updated all chapters and added two completely new chapters–Basic Genomics for Practicing Oncologists and Basic Principles of Radiation Oncology. We have worked to capture the advances in the field and listened to the feedback from readers to improve this edition. We hope that anyone needing a comprehensive review of oncology will find the *Bethesda Handbook of Clinical Oncology* to be an indispensable resource.

Jame Abraham
James L. Gulley
Carmen J. Allegra

Acknowledgments

Our sincere thanks to all our esteemed colleagues and friends who contributed to this book.

We thank our publishers, Lippincott Williams and Wilkins, and dedicated staff members at the company who have been supporting this book for the past ten years. We would like to thank Ms. Bonnie Casey for carefully editing many chapters and offering suggestions.

This book would not be possible without the strong and continued support of Mr. Jonathan Pine, Senior Executive Editor at Lippincott Williams and Wilkins. We thank our wives, Shyla, Trenise and Linda, for their encouragement and support in this endeavor.

SECTION 1

Head and Neck

1

Head and Neck Cancer

Dexter T. Estrada, Carter VanWaes, Janaki Moni,
and Barbara A. Conley

EPIDEMIOLOGY

The incidence of head and neck squamous cancer is more than 500,000 cases per year worldwide, and 40,000 to 50,000 cases per year in the United States, where it comprises approximately 3% to 5% of all new cancers and 2% of all cancer deaths (1). Most patients are older than 50 years, and incidence increases with age; the male-to-female ratio is 2.5:1. The age-adjusted incidence is higher among black men, and, stage-for-stage, survival among African Americans is lower overall than in whites (1 and references therein). Death rates have been decreasing since at least 1975, with rates declining more rapidly in the last decade (1). Ninety percent of these cancers involves squamous cell histology. The most common sites are the oral cavity, pharynx, larynx, and hypopharynx. Nasal cavity and paranasal sinus cancers, salivary gland malignancies, and various sarcomas, lymphomas, and melanoma are less common.

RISK FACTORS

Heavy alcohol consumption increases the risk of developing squamous head and neck cancer twofold to sixfold, whereas smoking increases the risk 5- to 25-fold, depending on gender, race, and the amount of smoking. Both factors together increase the risk 15- to 40-fold. Smokeless tobacco and snuff are associated with oral cavity cancers. Case-control studies show that the relative risk for developing erythroplasia or cancer in tissues in contact with snuff powder (cheek and gum) is nearly 50-fold (2). In many parts of Asia and some parts of Africa, chewing betel with or without tobacco and slaked lime is associated with premalignant lesions and oral squamous cancers (3,4).

Multifocal mucosal abnormalities have been described in patients with head and neck cancer ("field cancerization") (5). There is a 2% to 6% risk per year for a second head and neck, lung, or esophageal cancer in patients with a history of cancer in this area. Those who continue to smoke have the highest risk. Second primary cancers represent a major risk factor for death among survivors of an initial squamous carcinoma of the head and neck (6–8).

Epstein-Barr virus (EBV) has been detected in virtually all nonkeratinizing and undifferentiated nasopharyngeal cancers but less consistently in squamous nasopharyngeal cancers (9). Cancers of the oropharynx and tonsil can be associated with human papillomavirus (HPV) infection (10–12). The incidence of HPV-associated cancers is more common in nonsmokers and seems to be increasing in several countries.

Disorders of DNA repair (e.g., Fanconi anemia) as well as organ transplantation with immunosuppression are associated with increased risk of squamous head and neck cancer (13).

PREVENTION AND CHEMOPREVENTION

The most important recommendation for prevention of head and neck cancer is to avoid smoking and to limit alcohol intake. Premalignant lesions occurring in the oral cavity, pharynx, and larynx may manifest as leukoplakia (a white patch that does not scrape off and that has no other obvious cause)

TABLE 1.1. *Premalignant lesions*

	Leukoplakia	Erythroplakia	Dysplasia
Clinical features	White patch or plaque occurring in surface of mucous membrane that does not rub off, once other oral diseases are ruled out	Bright red velvety plaques that cannot be characterized clinically or pathologically as being due to any other condition	Can present as leukoplakia, erythroplakia, or without obvious macroscopic findings
Probability of progression to malignant lesions	4%	15%–30% of dysplastic lesions	15%–30%
Histopathology	Hyperkeratosis associated with variable histologic findings; rarely contain dysplasia or carcinoma (invasive or in situ carcinoma found in only 6% of cases)	Mild to moderate dysplasia in 10% of patients; severe dysplasia, in situ or invasive carcinoma in 90% of cases	True histologic diagnosis: pleomorphic changes, increased number of nucleoli, prominent nucleoli

Source: From McFarland M, Abaza NA, El-Mofty S. In: Damjanov I, Linder J, eds. *Anderson's pathology.* St. Louis: Mosby, 1996, with permission.

or erythroplakia (friable reddish or specked lesions) (Table 1.1). The risk of leukoplakias without dysplasia progressing to cancer is about 4%. However, up to 40% of severe dysplasias or erythroplasias progress to cancer. Retinoids can reversibly improve premalignant histology. However, randomized, placebo-controlled clinical trials in patients with curatively treated head and neck squamous cell carcinoma failed to find any benefit for 13-*cis*-retinoic acid, retinyl palmitate, *N*-acetyl-cysteine (NAC), or the combination of retinyl palmitate and NAC in preventing second primary cancers or in improving survival (14,15).

Presently, there is no effective chemoprevention for patients at risk for head and neck squamous cancer. An NCI study of PPAR agonists for prevention of oral premalignant lesions is underway at this writing, but final results are pending. Other avenues of research are also being pursued (16). Chemoprevention outside a clinical trial is not recommended and is potentially harmful (17–19).

ANATOMY

A simplified depiction of extracranial head and neck anatomy is presented in Fig. 1.1.

The patterns of lymphatic drainage divide the neck into several levels (Fig. 1.2). Level I comprises the submental or submandibular nodes; level II (upper jugular lymph nodes) extends from the skull base to the hyoid bone; level III (middle jugular lymph nodes) is the area between the hyoid bone and the lower border of the cricoid cartilage; level IV (lower jugular lymph nodes) is the area between the cricoid cartilage and the clavicle; level V is the posterior triangle; level VI is the anterior compartment from the hyoid bone to the suprasternal notch, bounded on each side by the medial carotid sheath; and level VII is the area of the superior mediastinum. Masses more than 3 cm in greatest dimension can be groups of nodes or a single node, with the tumor extending into the soft tissues (20). Knowledge of the lymphatic drainage of the neck assists in locating a primary tumor when a palpable lymph node is the initial presentation, enabling the surgeon or radiation oncologist to plan appropriate treatment of both primary and neck diseases.

STAGING

Clinical staging is based on physical examination and imaging tests. The staging systems put forth by the American Joint Committee for Cancer (AJCC) (Table 1.2) and the Union Internationale Contre

(text continues on page 8)

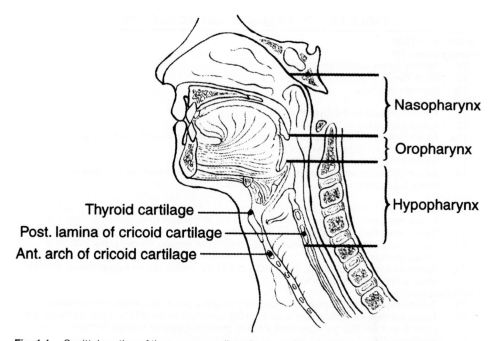

Fig. 1.1. Sagittal section of the upper aerodigestive tract. [Used with the permission of the American Joint Committee on Cancer (AJCC), Chicago, Illinois. The original source for this material is the *AJCC Cancer Staging Manual, sixth edition* (2002) published by Springer-Verlag, New York.]

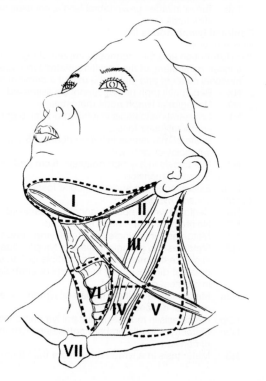

Fig. 1.2. Diagram of the neck showing levels of lymph nodes. Level I, submandibular; level II, high jugular; level III, midjugular; level IV, low jugular; level V, posterior jugular; level VI, tracheoesophageal; level VIII, superior mediastinal, is not shown. [Used with the permission of the American Joint Committee on Cancer (AJCC), Chicago, Illinois. The original source for this material is the *AJCC Cancer Staging Manual, sixth edition* (2002) published by Springer-Verlag, New York.]

TABLE 1.2. *TNM staging of head and neck tumors*

Definition of TNM

Primary tumor (T)

TX	Primary tumor cannot be assessed
T0	No evidence of primary tumor
Tis	Carcinoma in situ

Nasopharynx

T1	Tumor confined to the nasopharynx
T2	Tumor extends to soft tissue
T2a	Tumor extends to the oropharynx and/or nasal cavity without parapharyngeal extension[a]
T2b	Any tumor with parapharyngeal extension[a]
T3	Tumor involves bony structures and/or paranasal sinuses
T4	Tumor with intracranial extension and/or involvement of cranial nerves, infratemporal fossa, hypopharynx, orbit, or masticator space

Oropharynx

T1	Tumor 2 cm or less in greatest dimension
T2	Tumor more than 2 cm but not more than 4 cm in greatest dimension
T3	Tumor more than 4 cm in greatest dimension
T4a	Tumor invades the larynx, deep/extrinsic muscle of tongue, medial pterygoid, hard palate, or mandible
T4b	Tumor invades lateral pterygoid muscle, pterygoid plates, lateral nasopharynx, or skull base or encases carotid artery

Hypopharynx

T1	Tumor limited to one subsite of hypopharynx and 2 cm or less in greatest dimension
T2	Tumor invades more than one subsite of hypopharynx or an adjacent site, or measures more than 2 cm but not more than 4 cm in greatest diameter without fixation of hemilarynx
T3	Tumor more than 4 cm in greatest dimension or with fixation of hemilarynx
T4a	Tumor invades thyroid/cricoid cartilage, hyoid bone, thyroid gland, esophagus, or central compartment soft tissue[b]
T4b	Tumor invades prevertebral fascia, encases carotid artery, or involves mediastinal structures

Regional lymph nodes (N)

Nasopharynx

The distribution and the prognostic impact of regional lymph node spread from nasopharynx cancer, particularly of the undifferentiated type, are different from those of other head and neck mucosal cancers and justify the use of a different N classification scheme.

NX	Regional lymph nodes cannot be assessed
N0	No regional lymph node metastasis
N1	Unilateral metastasis in lymph node(s), 6 cm or less in greatest dimension, above the supraclavicular fossa[c]
N2	Bilateral metastasis in lymph node(s), 6 cm or less in greatest dimension, above the supraclavicular fossa[c]
N3	Metastasis in a lymph node(s):[c] 6 cm and/or to supraclavicular fossa N3a Greater than 6 cm in dimension
N3b	Extension to the supraclavicular fossa[d]

Oropharynx and hypopharynx

NX	Regional lymph nodes cannot be assessed
N0	No regional lymph node metastasis
N1	Metastasis in a single ipsilateral lymph node, 3 cm or less in greatest dimension
N2	Metastasis in a single ipsilateral lymph node, more than 3 cm but not more than 6 cm in greatest dimension, or in multiple ipsilateral lymph nodes, none more than 6 cm in greatest dimension, or in bilateral or contralateral lymph nodes, none more than 6 cm in greatest dimension.
N2a	Metastasis in a single ipsilateral lymph node more than 3 cm but not more than 6 cm in greatest dimension
N2b	Metastasis in multiple ipsilateral lymph nodes, none more than 6 cm in greatest dimension
N2c	Metastasis in bilateral or contralateral lymph nodes, none more than 6 cm in greatest dimension
N3	Metastasis in a lymph node more than 6 cm in greatest dimension

(Continued)

TABLE 1.2. *(Continued)*

Distant metastasis (M)

MX	Distant metastasis cannot be assessed
M0	No distant metastasis
M1	Distant metastasis

Stage grouping: Nasopharynx

Stage 0	Tis	N0	M0
Stage I	T1	N0	M0
Stage IIA	T2a	N0	M0
Stage IIB	T1	N1	M0
	T2	N1	M0
	T2a	N1	M0
	T2b	N0	M0
	T2b	N1	M0
Stage III	T1	N2	M0
	T2a	N2	M0
	T2b	N2	M0
	T3	N0	M0
	T3	N1	M0
	T3	N2	M0
Stage IVA	T4	N0	M0
	T4	N1	M0
	T4	N2	M0
Stage IVB	Any T	N3	M0
Stage IVC	Any T	Any N	M1

Stage grouping: Oropharynx, hypopharynx

Stage 0	Tis	N0	M0
Stage I	T1	N0	M0
Stage II	T2	N0	M0
Stage III	T3	N0	M0
	T1	N1	M0
	T2	N1	M0
	T3	N1	M0
Stage IVA	T4a	N0	M0
	T4a	N1	M0
	T1	N2	M0
	T2	N2	M0
	T3	N2	M0
	T4a	N2	M0
Stage IVB	T4b	Any N	M0
	Any T	N3	M0
State IVC	Any T	Any N	M1

[a]Parapharyngeal extension denotes posterolateral infiltration of tumor beyond the pharyngobasilar fascia.

[b]Central compartment of soft tissues includes prelaryngeal strap muscles and subcutaneous fat.

[c]Midline nodes are considered ipsilateral nodes.

[d]Supraclavicular zone or fossa is relevant to the staging of nasopharyngeal carcinoma and is the triangular region originally described by Ho. It is defined by three points: (a) the superior margin of the sternal end of the clavicle, (b) the superior margin of the lateral end of the clavicle, (c) the point where the neck meets the shoulder. Note that this would include the caudal portions of levels IV and V. All cases with lymph nodes (whole or part) in the fossa are considered N3b.

Source: Used with permission of the American Joint Committee on Cancer (AJCC), Chicago, Illinois. The original source for this material is the *AJCC Cancer Staging Manual, sixth edition* (2002) published by Springer-Verlag, New York.

TABLE 1.3. *Common presenting signs and symptoms of head and neck cancer*

Painless neck mass
Odynophagia
Dysphagia
Hoarseness
Hemoptysis
Trismus
Otalgia
Otitis media
Loose teeth
Ill-fitting dentures
Cranial nerve deficits
Nonhealing oral ulcers

le Cancer (UICC) (tumor, node, metastasis [TNM]) are used. The AJCC classification (20) emphasizes resectability status by dividing advanced disease stages into stage IVA (resectable), stage IVB (unresectable), and stage IVC (distant metastatic disease).

The T classification indicates the extent of the primary tumor. It differs for each site. For primary tumors of the oral cavity, hypopharynx, and oropharynx, lesions greater than 4 cm are classified as T3. Vocal cord paralysis with a larynx or hypopharynx primary indicates at least T3. Lesions with local invasion of adjacent structures indicate T4.

The N classification is uniform for all primary sites, except nasopharynx. For all primary sites except nasopharynx, any clinical lymph node involvement indicates at least stage III, and nodes larger than a single 3-cm ipsilateral node are classified as stage IV regardless of T stage.

The presence of distant metastasis (M1) indicates stage IVC disease. Mediastinal lymph node involvement is considered distant metastasis.

Tumor grade has not shown significant association with outcome and is not considered when staging head and neck cancers.

PRESENTATION

Signs and symptoms are usually secondary to mass effect and/or pain from primary tumor or involved lymph nodes and invasion of adjacent structures or nerves (Table 1.3). Adult patients with any of these symptoms for more than 4 weeks should be referred to an otolaryngologist. Delay in diagnosis is common for reasons such as patient delay or repeated courses of antibiotics for otitis media or sore throat. A lateralized firm cervical mass in an elderly smoker is highly suggestive of squamous cell carcinoma. For nasopharyngeal cancers, the most common presenting symptom is a neck mass, sometimes in the posterior triangle. In advanced lesions, cranial nerve abnormalities may be present.

With the exception of hypopharyngeal and nasopharyngeal cancers, distant metastases are uncommon at presentation. The most common sites of distant metastases are lung and bone; liver involvement is less common.

DIAGNOSIS

The history should include:

1. Tobacco exposure (pack years; amount chewed; and duration of habit, current or former)
2. Alcohol exposure (number of drinks per day)
3. Other risk factors mentioned earlier
4. Cancer history of patient and family
5. Signs and symptoms listed in Table 1.3
6. Thorough review of systems

The head and neck physical examination should include the following:

1. Careful inspection of the scalp, ears, nose, and mouth
2. Palpation of the neck and mouth, assessment of tongue mobility, determination of restrictions in the ability to open the mouth (trismus), and bimanual palpation of the base of the tongue and floor of the mouth
3. Mirror or flexible endoscopic examination of the nasal passages, nasopharynx, oropharynx, hypopharynx, and larynx
4. Special attention to the examination of cranial nerves

Abnormalities are suggested by asymmetry in the physical examination. Direct or indirect laryngoscopy should be strongly considered for symptoms of hoarseness or sore throat not cured by a single course of antibiotics.

Friability (easy bleeding), an indicator of an early malignant process or erythroplakia (see Table 1.1), is frequently associated with severe dysplasia or carcinoma in situ and the site should be biopsied. When neck mass is the first presentation, the primary site can be located and biopsied in approximately 80% of cases. If no primary site is obvious, tissue diagnosis can be obtained by fine needle aspiration (FNA) biopsy of the node, with sensitivity and specificity approaching 99%. A nondiagnostic FNA does not rule out the presence of tumor.

Computerized tomography (CT) scan remains the primary imaging study for evaluation of bone involvement and metastatic adenopathy. Magnetic resonance imaging (MRI) may complement the CT scan with greater resolution of soft tissue. Positron emission tomography (PET) scans combined with CT (PET/CT) are being used more frequently to detect tumors or nodes that are not obvious on other scans and for monitoring for disease recurrence in patients with advanced locoregional disease treated with concurrent chemotherapy and radiotherapy who have residual anatomical abnormalities on CT or MRI (21).

Diagnostic and staging laryngoscopy and nasopharyngoscopy should be performed to identify site of origin and extent of primary tumor and to obtain biopsies. With occult primary tumors, directed biopsies of the nasopharynx, tonsil, base of tongue, and pyriform sinus should be performed (Fig. 1.3). Bilateral tonsillectomy will sometimes reveal the source of an occult cancer. Esophagoscopy and bronchoscopy may be indicated for symptoms such as dysphagia, hoarseness, cough, or to search for occult primary.

Surgical biopsy of a neck mass before endoscopy is contraindicated if a squamous cell carcinoma is suspected. Studies show that open biopsy may worsen local control, increase the rate of distant metastases, and decrease overall survival rate, possibly by spreading the disease at the time of the biopsy. Finally, an open biopsy does not provide any information additional to that obtained from FNA, and laryngoscopy is still necessary for treatment planning.

WORKUP AND STAGING EVALUATION

After the diagnosis of cancer is established, the patient should be clinically staged by physical examination and radiologic studies, usually by CT scan and/or MRI of the primary tumor, neck, and chest. CT scan better defines the cortical bone and is better than MRI for evaluating metastatic adenopathy. MRI has superior soft tissue contrast, does not involve radiation, and may be better than CT scan for primary tumor staging. PET/CT scanning is indicated for staging patients with advanced head and neck cancers (21). A chest radiograph, chest CT scan, or PET/CT is indicated for all patients because of the risk of a second lung malignancy. Additional studies vary according to the clinical stage, symptoms, and primary site.

PROGNOSIS

The most important determinant of prognosis is stage at diagnosis. The 5-year survival for stage I patients exceeds 80% but is less than 40% in stages III and IV disease. Most patients have locally advanced disease involving one or several lymph nodes on one or both sides of the neck. The presence

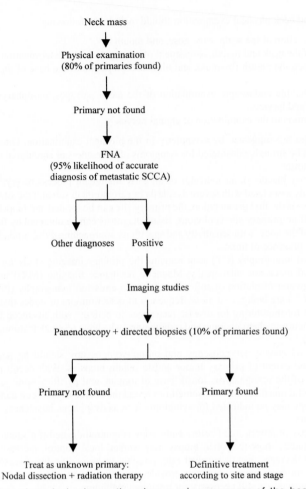

Fig. 1.3. Evaluation of cervical adenopathy when a primary cancer of the head and neck is suspected.

of a palpable lymph node in the neck generally decreases the survival rate by 50% compared to the same T stage without node involvement.

Most relapses occur locoregionally. Distant metastases are more commonly seen later in the course of the disease or as part of relapse after successful initial treatment, and predominantly involve lung, bone, and liver. The lifetime risk of developing a new cancer for a patient with head and neck cancer is 20% to 40% (6,8). After 3 years, development of a new cancer represents the greatest survival risk (Tables 1.4–1.6).

SCREENING

Careful examination of the head and neck is warranted in individuals with risk factors or suggestive symptoms. Mucosal abnormalities and palpable neck masses should be biopsied (see the section on diagnosis).

The U.S. Preventive Task Force (http://www.ahrq.gov/clinic/uspstfix.htm) does not recommend regular screening for oral cancer in the general population but recommends counseling for cessation

(text continues on page 14)

TABLE 1.4. *Head and neck cancer: Oral cavity*

Site	Epidemiology	Natural history and common presenting symptoms	Nodal involvement	Prognosis (5-yr survival)
Lip	Risk factors are sun exposure and tobacco; 3,600 new cases a year; 10 to 40 times more common in white men than in black men or women (black or white)	Exophytic mass or ulcerative lesion; more common in lower lip (92%); slow-growing tumors; pain and bleeding	5%–10% Midline tumors spread bilaterally Level I more common (subman-dibular and submental); upper lip lesions metastasize earlier: level I and also preauricular	T1, 90% T2, 84% With lymph node involvement, 50%
Alveolar ridge and retromolar trigone	10% of all oral cancers; M:F, 4:1	Exophytic mass or infiltrating tumor, may invade bone; bleeding, pain exacerbated by chewing, loose teeth, and ill-fitting dentures	30% (70% if T4) Levels I and II more common	T1, 85% T2, 80% T3, 60% T4, 20%
Floor of mouth	10%–15% of oral cancers, (occurrence 0.6/100,000); M:F, 3:1; median age, 60 yr	Painful infiltrative lesions, may invade bone, muscles of floor of mouth and tongue	T1, 12%; T2, 30%; T3, 47%; and T4, 53% Levels I and II more common	By stage: I, 85%–90% II, 80% III, 66% IV, 32% Advanced stage, 30%
Hard palate	0.4 cases/100,000 (5% of oral cavity); M:F, 8:1; 50% cases squamous, 50% salivary glands	Deeply infiltrating or superficially spreading pain	Less frequently: 6%–29%	By stage: I, 75% II, 46% III, 36% IV, 11%
Buccal mucosa	8% of oral cavity cancers in United States; women > men	Exophytic more often, silent presen-tation; pain, bleeding, difficulty in chewing	10% at diagnosis	18%–77% all stages

M:F, male-to-female ratio.

TABLE 1.5. *Head and neck cancer: Oropharynx and larynx*

Site	Epidemiology	Natural history and common presenting symptoms	Nodal involvement	Prognosis (5-yr survival)
Base of tongue	4,000 new cases annually in the United States; M:F ratio, 3 to 5:1. May be HPV-associated	Advanced at presentation (silent location, aggressive behavior); pain, dysphagia, weight loss, and otalgia (from cranial nerve involvement); neck massis a frequent presentation	All stages: 70% (T1) to 80% (T4) Levels II and III more common, also IV, V, and VI	By stage: I, 60% II, 40% III, 30% IV, 15%
Tonsil, tonsillar pillar, and soft palate	Tobacco and alcohol are the most significant risk factors. HPV common	Tonsillar fossa: more advanced at presentation: 75% stage III or IV; pain, dysphagia, weight loss, and neck mass Soft palate: more indolent, may present as erythroplakia	Tonsillar pillar T2, 38% Tonsillar fossa T2, 68% (55% present with N2 or N3 disease)	Tonsillar fossa, 93% (stage I) to 17% (stage IV) Soft palate, 85% (stage I) to 21% (stage IV)
Posterior pharyngeal wall		Advanced at diagnosis (silent location); pain, bleeding, and weight loss; neck mass is common initial symptom	Clinically palpable nodes T1, 25% T2, 30% T3, 66% T4, 75% Bilateral involvement is common	By stage: I, 75% II, 70% III, 42% IV, 27%
Supraglottis	35% of laryngeal cancers	Most arise in epiglottis; early lymph node involvement due to extensive lymphatic drainage; two-thirds of patients have nodal metastases at diagnosis	Overall rate: T1, 63%; T2, 70%; T3, 79%; T4, 73% Levels II, III, and IV more common	By stage: I, 70–100% II, 50–90% III, 45–70% IV, 20–60%
Glottis	Most common laryngeal cancer	Most favorable prognosis; late lymph node involvement; usually well differentiated, but with infiltrative growth pattern; hoarseness is an early symptom; 70% have localized disease at diagnosis	Sparse lymphatic drainage, early lesions rarely metastasize to lymph nodes. Clinically positive: T1, T2 Levels II, III, and IV more common T3, T4, 20%–25% 2%	T1, 74–86% T2, 67–75% T3, 55 T4, 50
Subglottis	Rare, 1%–8% of laryngeal cancers	Poorly differentiated, infiltrative growth pattern unrestricted by tissue barriers; rarely causes hoarseness, may cause dyspnea from airway involvement; two-thirds of patients have metastatic disease at presentation	20%–30% overall Pretracheal and paratracheal nodes more commonly involved	26% overall

M:F, male-to-female ratio.

TABLE 1.6. *Head and neck cancer: Hypopharynx, nasal cavity, paranasal sinuses, and nasopharynx*

Site	Epidemiology	Natural history and common presenting symptoms	Nodal involvement	Prognosis (5-yr survival)
Hypopharynx	2,500 new cases yearly in United States; etiology: tobacco, alcohol, and nutritional abnormalities	Aggressive, diffuse local spread, early lymph node involvement; occult metastases to thyroid and paratracheal node chain; pain, neck stiffness (retropharyngeal nodes), otalgia (cranial nerve X), irritation, and mucus retention 50% present as neck mass; high risk of distant metastases	Abundant lymphatic drainage Up to 60% have clinically positive lymph nodes at diagnosis	Survival varies between sites within hypopharynx T1, T2, 40% T3–T4, 16%–37%
Nasal cavity and paranasal sinuses	Rare, 0.75/100,000 occurrence in United States Nasal cavity and maxillary sinus, four-fifths of all cases M:F, 2:1 Increased risk with exposure to furniture, shoe, textile industries; nickel, chromium, mustard gas, isopropyl alcohol, and radium	Nonhealing ulcer, occasional bleeding, unilateral nasal obstruction, dental pain, loose teeth, ill-fitting dentures, trismus, diplopia, proptosis, epiphora, anosmia, and headache, depending on site of invasion Usually advanced at presentation	10%–20% clinically positive nodes Levels I and II more common	60% for all sites all stages, 30% for T4
Nasopharynx	Rare (1/100,000) except in North Africa, Southeast Asia, and China, far northern hemisphere Associated with EBV, diet, genetic factors	Most common initial presentation: neck mass Other presentations: otitis media, nasal obstruction, tinnitus, pain, and cranial nerve involvement	Clinically positive: WHO I, 60% WHO II and III, 80%–90%	T1, 37%–60% T2, 46%–68% T3, 16%–25% T4, 11%–40%

M:F, male-to-female ratio; EBV, Epstein-Barr virus.

of tobacco use and limitation of alcohol intake. The American Cancer Society (www.cancer.org) recommends oral examination during physician or dental appointments. The oral examination should include inspection of all mucosal areas, assessment of range of motion of tongue, bimanual palpation of floor of mouth, palpation of the tongue, and assessment of dental health. Any of the complaints described earlier require evaluation, especially if symptoms persist for more than 4 weeks or after treatment for presumed infection.

TREATMENT

The management of patients with head and neck cancer is complex. The choice of treatment modality depends on the stage and site of disease. Patients with locally advanced disease should be evaluated by a multidisciplinary team including an otolaryngologist or head and neck surgical oncologist, radiation oncologist, medical oncologist, dentist, prosthodontist, nutritionist, speech and swallowing pathologist, and personnel involved in rehabilitation before treatment is initiated.

In general, either surgery or radiation is effective as single-modality therapy for patients with early-stage disease (stage I or II) for most sites. The choice of modality depends on local expertise, patient preference, and functional result. For 60% of patients with locally advanced disease (stages III, IV, and M0), combined-modality therapy is indicated.

Surgery

The nature of the surgical procedure is determined primarily by the size of the tumor and the structures involved.

Resectability depends on the experience of the surgeon and the rehabilitation team. In general, a tumor is unresectable if the surgeon believes that all gross tumor cannot be removed or that local and distant control will not be achieved after surgery even with adjuvant radiation therapy. Generally, involvement of the skull base, pterygoid, and deep neck musculature and of the major vessels portends a poor outcome with surgery as a primary modality.

T1 and T2 lesions of the oral cavity, oropharynx, and hypopharynx may be amenable to wide local excision with a 2 cm margin, and closed by primary or secondary intention, skin graft, or local tissue flap reconstruction. Carcinoma in situ, T1 and T2 lesions of the larynx may be treated by microlaryngoscopic mucosal excision, cordectomy, or one of the various external hemilaryngectomy or partial laryngectomy procedures that have been developed. Newer technology for transoral and transnasal endoscopic surgical approaches have been recently investigated for resection of T1, T2, and selected T3 carcinomas involving the larynx, paranasal, and skull base region. Extensive surgeries and those involving function of the tongue frequently require myocutaneous flaps or microvascular free flaps to achieve a more functional reconstruction. However, as will be discussed below, with the advent of primary therapy with concurrent chemoradiotherapy for advanced cancers of the larynx, nasopharynx, oropharynx, and hypopharynx, surgery is increasingly being used for treatment of advanced neck disease (N2, N3) and for salvage of nonresponding or recurrent tumors of the primary site.

Cervical lymph node dissections may be elective or therapeutic. Elective neck dissections are done at the time of surgery in patients with necks that are clinically negative when the risk of a positive lymph node is at least 30%. Therapeutic neck dissections are done for clinically obvious masses. Cervical lymph node dissections are classified as radical, modified radical, or selective. The radical dissection includes removal of all lymph nodes in the neck from levels I to V (see Fig. 1.2), including removal of the internal jugular vein, spinal accessory nerve, and sternocleidomastoid muscle. This surgery is now rarely performed because of excessive morbidity, especially loss of shoulder function. The modified radical dissection preserves one or more of the nonlymphatic structures. In selective neck dissections, only certain levels of lymph nodes are removed based on the specific lymphatic drainage from the primary site. With no palpable or CT scan evidence of clinical nodal involvement, nodal metastases will be present beyond the confines of an appropriate selective neck dissection less than 10% of the time. Sentinel lymph node dissection and PET scanning are currently being evaluated for use in diagnosing positive lymph nodes in patients with necks that are clinically negative.

Radiation Therapy

Over the past two decades, radiation therapy has evolved from a primitive modality fraught with toxicity to a fine art that demands a keen appreciation of both tumor biology and radiation physics. The use of computed tomography for simulation and three-dimensional techniques for treatment planning facilitated greater accuracy in portal design based on an improved understanding of the radiographic extent of the tumor. Intensity-modulated radiation therapy techniques helped to reduce normal tissue toxicity while maintaining high doses to the target volume. The advantages of these advances have been demonstrated very eloquently in the management of head and neck cancer by an improvement in loco-regional control (22–24) and a decrease in normal tissue toxicity (25–28). Brachytherapy offers similar advantages when performed by experienced physicians (29,30).

Early-stage (T1, T2, N0) disease responds well to single-modality treatment with either surgery or radiation therapy. Radiation therapy allows organ preservation—as evidenced by its role in the management of early-stage cancers of the glottis larynx and pharynx (31–37).

More advanced disease requires the integration of radiation therapy with other modalities. When surgery is the primary modality, as in the case of paranasal sinus or salivary gland tumors, postoperative radiation therapy or chemoradiation is generally preferred to the preoperative setting and is recommended for close or positive margins, T4 disease, perineural or lymphovascular invasion, large and/or multiple positive lymph nodes, extracapsular extension, and recurrent disease after an initial surgical procedure (38). Radiation therapy has been effectively combined with chemotherapy to allow organ preservation and improved survival in the management of advanced laryngeal and pharyngeal cancers.

Concomitant chemotherapy and radiation has proven more efficacious than sequential treatment, although there is some evidence that neoadjuvant chemotherapy followed by concomitant chemoradiation may be effective as well. There is now a growing body of evidence demonstrating an improvement in outcome by adding EGFR receptor inhibition to radiation with or without chemotherapy (39). Cooperative group multicenter trials are underway to study this concept.

Advances in diagnostic imaging have contributed to improvements in radiation therapy planning. Both PET and MRI allow better tumor delineation (40–42). Current technology allows fusion of the images from various imaging techniques on each patient so that the radiation oncologist may outline the tumor more accurately (43,44). Although target delineation for IMRT is currently time consuming and labor intensive, algorithms are being developed to automate this process (45).

Traditionally, radiation therapy has been delivered at 1.8 to 2 Gy once daily for a total of 50 to 70 Gy with successive field reductions based on risk assessment. IMRT allows the integration of all sites into a single plan with lower-risk areas receiving lower doses per fraction while higher-risk areas receive higher doses per fraction (46). Altered fractionation schemes have had mixed success (47,48). These include hyperfractionation (1.2–1.5 Gy twice or thrice daily) and the concomitant boost technique (1.8 Gy in the morning to the entire field followed by 1.5 Gy in the evening to a smaller field encompassing high-risk disease). With either schedule, it is essential to maintain 4 to 6 hours between fractions to allow normal tissue repair (47). Although altered fractionation improves outcome, this is offset by an increase in acute toxicity without any increase in long-term complications (47,48). The integration of chemotherapy with altered fraction schedules is under investigation (48,49).

Reirradiation without and with chemotherapy has been studied in patients with recurrent local and regional disease. Reirradiation has usually been studied in selected patients with relatively limited recurrent disease allowing conformal treatment. Response and short-term local control rates of 15% to 30% are observed, and longer term control of 1 to 2 years is observed in 10% to 20% (50,51).

Common severe acute radiation toxicity includes dermatitis, mucositis, loss of taste, xerostomia, dysphagia, and hair loss. Decreased hearing occurs less commonly. Dental evaluation and necessary extractions should be performed before radiation because dental extractions in a radiated mandible can lead to osteonecrosis (52). Dentulous patients should be given prophylactic fluoride. Patients receiving radiation are at high risk for tooth decay due to the xerostomia caused by injury to the salivary glands as well as mucosal damage. Radioprotectors such as amifostine and pilocarpine have not demonstrated a consistent ability to decrease xerostomia (53). IMRT techniques enabling the reduction of dose to the parotid glands have had more success (26,54). Similarly, permanent swallowing dysfunction can be avoided by decreasing the dose to the pharyngeal musculature (55–57). Prophylactic, pretreatment and posttreatment evaluations by a speech therapist also help in preventing and alleviating dysphagia in these patients.

Chemotherapy

Historically, chemotherapy was used for palliation without proven survival advantage in patients with locally recurrent or disseminated disease. Combination chemotherapy yields higher response rates but has increased toxicity when compared with single agents. The choice of single-agent or combination chemotherapy depends on the patient's performance status. Single agents with more than 10% response activity are listed in Table 1.7 (58–72). Combination regimens have been developed to improve response rates (Table 1.8) (73,74). Prior to the use of taxane combinations, meta-analyses and randomized trials demonstrated improved response for cisplatin compared with methotrexate, improved response for cisplatin and 5-fluorouracil (5-FU) combination compared with single drugs, and improved response for cisplatin and 5-FU combination when compared with other regimens for treatment of recurrent or metastatic head and neck squamous cancer. In the metastatic or recurrent setting, the combination of cisplatin and infusional 5-FU produces a 70% response rate and a 27% complete remission (CR) rate in chemotherapy-naive patients (75), but the response rate is 30% to 35% in patients who have relapsed after radiation therapy (see Table 1.8) with less than 10% complete responses. A randomized trial of cisplatin and 5-FU versus carboplatin (300 mg/m²) and 5-FU versus weekly methotrexate in patients with recurrent or metastatic head and neck squamous cancer demonstrated response rates of 32%, 21%, and 10%, respectively. Median survival was not improved by combination chemotherapy (6.6, 5.0, and 5.6 months, respectively) (76).

TABLE 1.7. *Active chemotherapeutic agents for metastatic/recurrent squamous cancer of the head and neck*

Drug	Dose	Response rate	Median survival	Reference	Comments
Methotrexate	40–60 mg/m²/wk	16%–23.5%	6 mo	58–60	Better response rates reported in patients not exposed to chemoradiation or platinum
Cisplatin	50 mg/m² d1 and 8 or 80–100 mg/m² q21–28d	8%–28.6%	6 mo	58, 60	
Paclitaxel	250 mg/m² over 24 h, with G-CSF (NOT recommended)	36%–40%	9.2 mo	61	
	80 mg/m²/wk	9.3%	235 d		
Docetaxel	80–100 mg/m² OR q21d 30 mg/m²/wk	11%–42% 42%	8.4 mo	62–65	11% in platinum-refractory patients
Pemetrexed	500 mg/m² q21d	26%	7.3 mo	67	
Irinotecan	75 mg/m²/wk × 2 q3wk or	14.2%	214 d	68	
	75–125 mg/m²/wk × 4 q5wk	26.3%			
Gemcitabine	800–1,250 mg/m² weekly × 3 q4wk	13%		69	
Vinorelbine	30 mg/m²/wk	7.5%–16%	32 wk	70, 71	
Cetuximab	400 mg/m² week 1250 mg/m² weekly	10%	5–6 mo	72	
Erlotinib	150–250 mg daily	4%	20% 1-year survival	72	

TABLE 1.8. *Active combination chemotherapeutic regimens for recurrent/metastatic squamous cancer of the head and neck*

Regimen	Response rate	Median survival	Reference	Comments
Cisplatin 100 mg/m² 5-FU 1,000 mg/m²/ d Cl × 96 h q21d	32%	6.6 mo	73,74	277 patients No prior chemotherapy Doses modified <25% toxicity or lack of toxicity
Cisplatin 75 mg/m² Paclitaxel 175 mg/m² (3 h infusion) q21d	28%	9 mo 30% 1-yr survival	74	No significant difference from cisplatin–5-FU in efficacy or quality of life; cisplatin and pacli-taxel may have fewer toxicities compared to cisplatin and 5-FU

Carboplatin may be slightly less active than cisplatin for head and neck squamous cancer, but is preferred in patients at high risk for cisplatin toxicity, that is, those with renal dysfunction, neuropathy, or hearing loss (76).

Both docetaxel and paclitaxel have shown antitumor activity (61–65). For paclitaxel regimens given every 3 weeks, 3-hour infusions are probably the best balance between theoretically optimum exposure and tolerable toxicity (66). Docetaxel is usually administered at doses of 60 to 100 mg/m² every 3 to 4 weeks. Weekly schedules are being evaluated (64). Taxane combinations, including paclitaxel with ifosfamide and cisplatin or carboplatin, and docetaxel with cisplatin and 5-FU (77–79), show promising response rates. Epidermal growth factor inhibitors, combined with chemotherapy, have also shown intriguing results (80,81).

The role of chemotherapy has expanded significantly because of the results of clinical trials incorporating chemotherapy in multimodality regimens for previously untreated disease.

Studies have evaluated the use of chemotherapy administered before (i.e., neoadjuvant or induction chemotherapy), during (i.e., concomitant chemotherapy), or after (i.e., adjuvant chemotherapy) radiation therapy or surgery.

Combined modality (chemoradiation) is indicated for patients with locally advanced disease that would require total laryngectomy if treated by surgery and who wish to preserve the larynx, for patients who are technically resectable but who are not medically fit enough for surgery, and for patients with technically unresectable locally advanced cancer. In the patient who presents with locally advanced tumor concomitant with distant metastasis, local control of the disease may prevent infectious and necrotic complications.

Induction Chemotherapy

Induction chemotherapy followed by definitive radiation therapy in patients responding to chemotherapy has been studied for organ preservation in patients with locally advanced cancers of the larynx and of the hypopharynx. The advantages of induction chemotherapy include reduction of tumor burden potentially allowing more effective local control with surgery or radiation, as well as organ preservation, though at the price of increased toxicity, cost, and length of treatment.

In stages III and IV larynx cancer, and hypopharynx cancer, no significant survival difference was demonstrated for chemotherapy followed by radiotherapy compared to surgery followed by radiotherapy (82,83), though two-thirds of surviving patients had larynx preservation. Surgical salvage was eventually necessary for about one-third of the patients with larynx cancer treated with chemotherapy and radiation, and therefore close follow-up is required in the event that salvage surgery is needed. For laryngeal cancer, concomitant cisplatin and radiation therapy has since been shown to lead to better local control and organ preservation, but not survival, compared to neoadjuvant chemotherapy followed by radiation or radiation alone (84).

Recently, several investigators have studied combinations of taxanes, platinums, and fluorouracil as induction chemotherapy prior to radiation or to concomitant chemoradiation. A phase III study in stages III and IV cancers of the oral cavity, oropharynx, hypopharynx, and larynx demonstrated improved disease-free and overall survival after follow-up of 32.5 months, for patients receiving the triplet chemotherapy compared to cisplatin and fluorouracil for up to four courses prior to radiation alone (85). A second study used cisplatin and fluorouracil with or without paclitaxel for three courses, followed by chemoradiation with high-dose cisplatin on days 1, 22, and 43 if response was at least 80%. This trial also showed that complete response rate (the primary end point of the trial) was improved (33% vs. 14%) in the triplet arm. With a median follow-up of 23 months, survival data had not yet matured (86). A third phase 3 trial randomized unresectable or organ preservation patients to induction therapy with cisplatin and fluorouracil with or without docetaxel, followed by radiation with weekly carboplatin at AUC 1.5. With a median follow-up time of 42 months, treatment with the triple drug neoadjuvant therapy showed a 30% improvement in survival (79).

Presently, induction chemotherapy with a taxane, cisplatin, and 5-fluorouracil combination followed by radiation therapy can be considered as a reasonable treatment strategy, particularly in patients with unresectable cancers and good performance status. Data are awaited on trials that randomized patients to concomitant chemoradiation treatment with or without induction chemotherapy.

CONCOMITANT CHEMORADIATION

The rationale for concomitant chemoradiation is based on experimental evidence of synergism between chemotherapy and radiation that is theoretically mediated by interference of chemotherapy with multiple intracellular radiation-induced stress-response pathways involved in apoptosis, proliferation, and DNA repair (87). The finding that certain chemotherapeutic agents (e.g., cisplatin, 5-FU, taxanes, and hydroxyurea) can induce radiosensitivity and increase log cell kill from radiation supports this treatment strategy. Cisplatin, the most extensively evaluated drug in recent large randomized trials, has the advantage of not having mucositis as toxicity; although as a radiation enhancer, it does increase radiation-induced mucositis.

Recent meta-analyses and randomized clinical trials published before 2001 show that for locally advanced head and neck squamous cell carcinoma, concomitant chemoradiation produces a small but significant survival advantage of about 8% compared to radiation therapy alone (88–90). The U.S. intergroup compared concomitant cisplatin and radiation to split-course radiation with cisplatin and 5-FU to standard radiation alone in patients with unresectable head and neck squamous cancer and showed that concurrent cisplatin at 100 mg/m^2 every 21 days with daily radiation significantly improved survival rates (91). A randomized trial of neoadjuvant cisplatin and 5-FU followed by radiation versus concurrent cisplatin and 5-FU with radiation in patients with unresectable head and neck cancer showed similar survival rates but improved locoregional control for the concomitant arm. This early study highlighted the importance of aggressive supportive care for concomitant regimens, including adequate fluid and electrolyte support (92). Concomitant platinum-based chemoradiation has become a standard therapy for patients with unresectable advanced head and neck cancer with good performance status.

Although no randomized phase 3 trial has been reported, results using taxanes with 5-FU and/or cisplatin show promising results as do regimens containing 5-FU and hydroxyurea with concomitant twice-daily radiation, with both chemotherapy and radiation administered together every other week (93). Agents that inhibit epidermal growth factor receptor (EGFR) signaling have been evaluated as radiation enhancers in head and neck squamous cancer. More than 90% of head and neck squamous cancers express EGFR (94), and increased expression has been correlated with poorer survival rates after radiation therapy (95,96). The EGFR inhibitory monoclonal antibody cetuximab has been shown to result in an enhancement of response and survival over radiation therapy (RT) alone, although more than 50% of the trial participants had oropharyngeal primary tumors, a type previously associated with greater responsiveness to RT (39). In contrast to trials comparing radiotherapy with or without chemotherapy, there was no reduction in distant metastases in the cetuximab arm. Clinical studies are ongoing with combinations of EGFR inhibitors, with radiation and with standard chemotherapy agents. Recent studies suggest that additional molecular alterations, in addition to EGFR, are likely to be important for response.

These include activation of the prosurvival signal-activated transcription factors nuclear factor-kappaB, signal transduction and transcription-3 (STAT-3), and inactivation or mutation of tumor suppressor p53 (97), as well as epithelial-to-mesenchymal transition (98,99). Agents targeting some of these pathways such as bortezomib and quinacrine (NF-κB, p53) and STAT decoy are under investigation as a result of combinatorial activity observed with EGFR or standard chemotherapy agents in preclinical studies (100–103).

Elective lymph node dissection is often carried out after chemoradiation in patients with N2, N3, or multiple nodes at diagnosis, regardless of nodal response to chemoradiation, when complete response is obtained at the primary site. N2 or greater nodes often (about 20%) harbor tumor even if a clinically complete response is obtained in the neck with chemoradiation (104). Surgical salvage may be attempted if complete control is not achieved at the primary or locoregional site. Major complications with surgical salvage are found in about 52% of patients previously treated with organ-preserving regimens (105).

Because concomitant regimens are associated with increased toxicity compared with sequential chemoradiation, patients should be followed closely for dehydration, electrolyte abnormalities, and adequacy of nutritional intake. In some patients, placement of an enteral feeding tube during or prior to the start of concomitant chemoradiation is performed because the incidence of grade 3 or greater mucositis is 70% to 80%.

Adjuvant Chemotherapy

A large randomized study in resected patients with stage III or IV disease compared adjuvant radiation therapy with adjuvant chemotherapy followed by radiation. This trial showed improved local control and overall survival rates approaching statistical significance for a subset of patients treated with chemotherapy who were at high risk for local recurrence. Patients with low-risk disease (negative resection margins, one or no positive nodes, and no extracapsular spread of tumor) did not benefit from adjuvant chemotherapy (106).

Adjuvant concomitant cisplatin and radiation in patients at high risk for recurrence after surgery has been studied both in Europe and in the United States. Both studies found a possible benefit in disease-free and overall survival for patients receiving concomitant cisplatin and radiation, particularly in patients with positive margins or extracapsular extension of tumor (107).

SITE-SPECIFIC HEAD AND NECK TUMORS

Oral Cavity

The oral cavity includes the lip, anterior two-thirds of the tongue, floor of the mouth, buccal mucosa, gingiva, hard palate, and retromolar trigone. Approximately 20,000 new cases are diagnosed annually in the United States. Squamous cell carcinoma is the histologic type observed in most cases.

The epidemiology, natural history, common presenting symptoms, risk of nodal involvement, and prognosis for specific subsites are shown in Table 1.4. Early lesions (stages I and II) are treated with surgery or radiation therapy as single-modality therapy. For resectable locally advanced disease (stages III and IV, and M0), surgery followed by radiation therapy is indicated (Fig. 1.4). Definitive radiation therapy with or without chemotherapy is an option for patients with resectable disease at any stage who have high medical or surgical risk, or according to patients' preference (based on discussions about quality of life, functional outcome, and toxicity profile of each treatment). Treatment for locally advanced and metastatic disease is discussed in subsequent text.

Oropharynx

The oropharynx includes the base of the tongue, tonsils, posterior pharyngeal wall, and the soft palate.

The epidemiology, natural history, common presenting symptoms, risk of nodal involvement, and prognosis for specific subsites of the oropharynx are shown in Table 1.5. Treatment may include primary

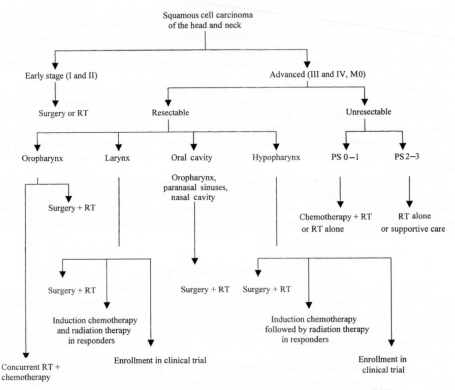

Fig. 1.4.   Treatment for head and neck squamous cell carcinomas (M0).

surgery and postoperative radiotherapy. Increasingly, primary radiation therapy with chemotherapy is being used for stage III or IV disease as a result of superior organ preservation and swallowing when compared to surgical resection and reconstruction of the tongue base, reserving surgery for management of regional node metastases or for salvage of persistent disease. Randomized trials show that concurrent chemotherapy and radiotherapy significantly improve locoregional control and survival compared with radiotherapy (108). Increased complexity, toxicity, and need for close follow-up of this combined-modality approach mandates that the patient has adequate performance status and psychosocial resources.

Larynx

Risk factors are a history of tobacco and/or alcohol intake. In addition, certain dietary factors and exposure to wood dust, nitrogen mustard, asbestos, and nickel have been implicated as etiologic factors. The male-to-female ratio for laryngeal cancer is 4.5:1, with a peak incidence in the sixth decade of life. This disease is 50% more common in African Americans than in whites and 100% more common in whites than in Hispanics and Asians. More than 95% of laryngeal cancers are squamous cell carcinomas.

Laryngeal cancers can be supraglottic, glottic, and/or subglottic. The epidemiology, natural history, common presenting symptoms, risk of nodal involvement, and prognosis for specific subsites of the larynx are shown in Table 1.5.

Early cancers not requiring laryngectomy (T1–T2 N0) are usually treated with radiation or micro-endoscopic surgery. If lymph nodes are involved, neck dissection and/or neck radiation is indicated.

Locally advanced resectable tumors (T3–T4 or T2 N+) may be treated with surgery and adjuvant radiation if locoregional risk factors are present (i.e., close or positive margins, T4 tumor involving laryngeal-cricoid cartilage or hyoid bone, lymphatic or vascular or perineural involvement, vascular invasion, multiple positive nodes, extracapsular invasion, subglottic extension, or prior tracheostomy). An alternative is the use of combined radiation and chemotherapy. In 1991, the Veterans Administration Laryngeal Study Group trial established (82) that sequential chemotherapy with cisplatin and infusional 5-FU followed by radiation therapy in highly responsive patients resulted in equivalent survival and a larynx preservation rate of about 66% compared to treatment with surgery followed by radiation. A subsequent randomized phase 3 trial conducted in the United States comparing radiation therapy alone, sequential chemotherapy and radiation therapy, and concomitant cisplatin and radiation therapy for organ preservation in patients with locally advanced laryngeal cancer demonstrated that concurrent cisplatin (100 mg/m^2 on days 1, 22, and 43) and radiation therapy resulted in better laryngectomy-free survival, larynx preservation rate, and local–regional control rate than either sequential (induction) cisplatin and 5-FU followed by radiation therapy or radiation therapy alone. Induction chemotherapy followed by radiotherapy was shown to have no advantage over radiotherapy alone. Survival rate was not significantly different for the three treatments, in part reflecting the ability to surgically salvage laryngeal cancer patients treated for organ preservation. It is of interest to note that patients who received any chemotherapy regardless of receiving radiotherapy or not had a lower metastatic rate at 2 years than did patients who received radiation alone (84). Patients with high-volume T4 disease (with destruction of larynx or massive extension of supraglottic laryngeal cancer to the base of tongue) are not likely to obtain functional laryngeal and swallowing preservation without aspiration, and should be treated with surgery followed by radiation therapy rather than by organ preservation therapy, if possible.

Speech rehabilitation is critically important for patients with advanced laryngeal cancer who are undergoing total laryngectomy. Phonation options include a mechanical electrolarynx, esophageal speech, and tracheoesophageal puncture. Most patients can obtain satisfactory communication through one of these techniques.

Patients whose lesions are unresectable or patients who are considered to have high surgical risks are candidates for definitive radiation therapy with chemotherapy if performance status is good. The treatment for a patient with metastatic disease is discussed later.

Hypopharynx

The epidemiology, natural history, common presenting symptoms, risk of nodal involvement, and prognosis for specific subsites of the hypopharynx are shown in Table 1.6.

Early cancers not requiring laryngectomy (most T1 N0–N1; small T2 N0) can be treated with surgery or radiation. Locally advanced resectable tumors (T3–T4 any N) may be treated with surgery followed by radiation or sequential or concomitant chemoradiation. In these cases, surgery involves total laryngectomy and partial or total pharyngectomy and neck dissection. Even with this radical surgery and the consequent functional impairment of the tumor, the survival prognosis is poor.

Combined-modality treatment with chemotherapy and radiation allows organ function preservation with chances of survival being equivalent to that after surgery. Patients who achieve a complete response at the primary site after two to three cycles of induction chemotherapy (see Table 1.6) receive definitive radiation, whereas those achieving less than complete response at the primary site undergo surgery. A large randomized trial is in progress comparing induction chemotherapy followed by radiation therapy to concomitant chemoradiation in patients with hypopharyngeal cancer. The outcome of this trial will provide more definitive information on the most efficacious therapy.

Patients who are prone to high surgical or medical risks can be treated with radiation. The management of metastatic disease is discussed later.

Nasal Cavity and Paranasal Sinuses

The epidemiology, natural history, common presenting symptoms, risk of nodal involvement, and prognosis for carcinomas of the nasal cavity and paranasal sinuses are shown in Table 1.6.

Most tumors are squamous cell carcinomas and are usually slow growing with low incidence of metastasis.

Carcinomas of the nasal cavity and paranasal sinuses are usually detected in patients in advanced stages because of the relatively silent tumor location. Treatment follows the same general guidelines as those for oral cancer. If feasible, surgery is the preferred primary management since response to radiation is often incomplete when bone is involved.

Nasopharynx

The epidemiology, natural history, common presenting symptoms, risk of nodal involvement, and prognosis for nasopharyngeal cancer are shown in Table 1.6. It is rare in most parts of the world, with an incidence of less than 1 case per 100,000 population. However, it is endemic in certain areas, including North Africa, Southeast Asia, China, and the far northern hemisphere. EBV is strongly associated with nasopharyngeal carcinoma. This association has been demonstrated by serologic studies and by the detection of the viral genome in tumor samples. Diet (salt-cured fish and meat) and genetic susceptibility are other probable risk factors; tobacco and alcohol are not risk factors, except in a minority of cases.

The World Health Organization (WHO) classification divides nasopharyngeal carcinoma into three types: type I, keratinizing squamous cell carcinoma; type II, nonkeratinizing squamous cell carcinoma; and type III, undifferentiated carcinoma (20). Type II, the most common, is also sometimes referred to as *lymphoepithelioma* because of the characteristic exuberant lymphoid infiltrate accompanying malignant epithelial cells.

The most common initial presentation is a neck mass. Other presenting signs and symptoms are related to tumor growth, with resulting compression or infiltration of neighboring organs. These include serous otitis media, nasal obstruction, tinnitus, pain, and involvement of one or multiple cranial nerves.

Nasopharyngeal carcinoma has a high metastatic potential to regional nodes and distant sites. WHO type I has the greatest propensity for uncontrolled local tumor growth and the lowest propensity for metastatic spread (60% clinically positive nodes) compared with WHO type II and type III cancers (80–90% clinically positive nodes). Even though WHO type I cancer is associated with a lower incidence of lymphatic and distant metastases than are types II and III, its prognosis is worse because of a higher incidence of deaths from uncontrolled primary tumors and nodal metastases.

The prognoses for different stages of nasopharyngeal carcinoma are shown in Table 1.6.

General treatment guidelines are shown in Fig. 1.5. Surgery is usually not recommended because of anatomic considerations and the pattern of spread of the cancer via the retropharyngeal lymphatics. Radiation has been the standard treatment, with good results (local control rates: T1–T2, 70–90%; T3–T4, 30–65%), and remains the standard of care for early (stages I and II) cancer.

In a randomized trial in the United States, concurrent cisplatin (cisplatin 100 mg/m^2 every 21–28 days) and daily radiation followed by three courses of adjuvant cisplatin and 5-FU was shown to improve overall survival (76% for concurrent chemoradiation vs. 46% for radiation therapy alone) (109). On the basis of this study, concurrent chemoradiation followed by adjuvant chemotherapy is considered standard treatment for locally advanced nonmetastatic (stages III and IV) nasopharyngeal cancer in the United States. Other drugs, such as taxanes, appear to have activity but have not been evaluated extensively.

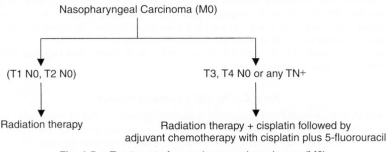

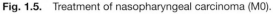

Fig. 1.5.   Treatment of nasopharyngeal carcinoma (M0).

ADVANCED HEAD AND NECK TUMORS: UNRESECTABLE, RECURRENT, AND METASTATIC DISEASE

In patients with good performance status (ECOG 0-1), concurrent radiation and chemotherapy is considered standard treatment for patients with newly diagnosed locally advanced unresectable disease. In several recent trials, chemoradiation therapy was shown to improve the overall survival, disease-free survival, and/or local control when compared with radiation therapy alone. Several cisplatin or carboplatin-containing regimens and several standard and altered fractionation-radiation regimens have been evaluated. In patients with poor performance status, radiation alone is a reasonable option.

Local or regional recurrences can sometimes be salvaged by radiation therapy or surgery. In patients unable to undergo resection, reirradiation with a dose of 60 Gy with or without concomitant chemotherapy can achieve prolonged survivals in about 15% to 20% of highly selected patients (110). In nasopharyngeal carcinoma, a second course of radiation may be delivered. If salvage is not possible, palliative treatment will be guided by the performance status of the patient.

Single-agent or combination chemotherapy is indicated for palliation of patients with good performance status with local or distant recurrence and of those patients presenting with distant metastasis. Combination chemotherapy achieves higher response rates at the cost of increased toxicity when compared with single-agent chemotherapy. The most active agents are listed in Table 1.7. Cisplatin plus infusional 5-FU (see Table 1.8) or cisplatin with a taxane are the most commonly used combination-chemotherapy regimens. Weekly methotrexate or taxanes have also shown some activity in patients with advanced head and neck tumors. Targeted agents, such as erlotinib and cetuximab, may have some palliative effect (72) as single agents, and appear to be promising in combination with platinum-based regimens (111). The choice of single-agent or combination chemotherapy depends on preference and performance status of patients. Patients with good performance status, no prior chemotherapy for treatment of recurrent disease, and minimal tumor burden may benefit most from combination chemotherapy. A small subset of these patients may achieve durable complete response and prolonged survival. However, the median response duration to combination or single-agent chemotherapy is about 3 to 4 months.

The median survival for patients with locally recurrent or disseminated disease is 6 to 9 months, and only 20% to 30% are alive at 1 year. No therapy has been shown to affect survival rate. Therefore, whenever possible, patients should be encouraged to enroll in clinical trials that evaluate new agents or new combination regimens.

Cancer of Unknown Primary Site (of the Head and Neck)

The workup of a patient with a neck mass is shown in Fig. 1.3. Nasopharyngeal, oropharyngeal, and hypopharyngeal origins are most common. In 10% of cases, a primary tumor is not found, and the term "cancer of unknown primary site" is used.

Cervical lymph node involvement (except supraclavicular) by squamous carcinoma indicates a head and neck primary tumor. Unknown primary tumors of the head and neck are usually treated with neck dissection and radiation. The prognosis is roughly equivalent to cancers with the same N (nodal) status. Five-year survival ranges from 30% to 50% in patients treated definitively.

Salivary Gland Cancer

Salivary gland cancers make up about 3% of all head and neck cancers diagnosed in the United States yearly. Tobacco and alcohol consumption are not risk factors, except possibly in women. Ionizing radiation and certain occupational exposures (e.g., in workers in rubber and automotive industries, wood workers, and farm workers) have been associated with the development of salivary gland cancer.

The salivary glands are classified as major (parotid, submandibular, and sublingual) and minor (distributed along upper aerodigestive tract, predominantly in the oral and nasal cavities and the paranasal sinuses). About 75% of parotid gland neoplasms are benign, whereas about 75% of submandibular, sublingual, and minor salivary gland tumors are malignant.

Most salivary gland tumors are benign, and the most common histology is pleomorphic adenoma, which is characterized by slow growth and few symptoms, and is most frequently seen in the parotid

TABLE 1.9. *Salivary gland benign tumors*

Pleomorphic adenoma (benign mixed tumor)
Warthin tumor (papillary cystadenoma lymphomatosum)
Monomorphic adenoma
Benign lymphoepithelial lesion
Oncocytoma
Ductal papilloma
Sebaceous lymphadenoma

gland. The most common presentation of benign salivary gland tumors is asymptomatic swelling of the lip, the parotid, or the submandibular or the sublingual gland. Persistent pain or neurologic involvement (mucosal or tongue numbness and facial nerve weakness) suggests malignant disease. The benign salivary gland tumors are listed in Table 1.9.

The clinical characteristics and prognosis of specific malignant salivary gland tumors are shown in Table 1.10.

TABLE 1.10. *Salivary gland malignant tumors:*
Clinical characteristics and prognosis

Histology	Clinical characteristics	Prognosis
Mucoepidermoid carcinoma	Most common malignant tumor in major salivary glands; most common in parotid glands (32%) Low grade: local problems, long history, cure with aggressive resection; rarely metastasizes High grade: locally aggressive, invades nerves and vessels, and metastasizes early	Low grade: 76%–95% 5-yr survival High grade: 30%–50% 5-yr survival
Adenocarcinoma	16% of parotid and 9% of submandibular malignant tumors Grade correlates with survival	76%–85% 5-yr survival 34%–71% 10-yr survival
Squamous cell carcinoma	Uncommon: 7% of parotid gland and 10% of submandibular gland malignant tumors Grade correlates with survival Squamous cell carcinoma of temple, auricular, and facial skin can metastasize to parotid nodes and can be confused with primary parotid tumor	24% 5-yr survival 18% 10-yr survival
Acinic cell carcinoma	<10% of all salivary gland malignant tumors Low grade with slow growth, infrequent facial nerve involvement, infrequent and late metastases (lungs) Regional metastasis in 5%–10% of patients	82% 5-yr survival 68% 10-yr survival
Adenoid cystic carcinoma	Most common malignant tumor in submandibular gland (41%), 11% of parotid gland High incidence of nerve invasion, which compromises local control 40% of patients develop metastases; most common site of metastases is the lung. Patients may live many years with lung metastasis, but visceral or bone metastases indicate poor prognosis	5-yr survival: 50%–90% 10-yr survival: 30%–67% 15-yr survival: 25%
Malignant mixed tumor	14% of parotid gland and 12% of submandibular gland cancers May originate in previous pleomorphic adenoma Lymph node involvement in 25% of cases; 26%–32% of patients develop metastases	5-yr survival: 31%–65% 10 yr; 23%–30%

Surgery is the mainstay of treatment for all localized stages of salivary gland tumors. Postoperative radiation is indicated for localized tumors of high-grade histology that are large, with close or positive margins, and/or positive regional lymph nodes. Radiation is the primary treatment for unresectable tumors. The role of chemotherapy is limited to the management of locally recurrent, unresectable disease or distant metastatic disease. There is no established standard chemotherapy for salivary gland cancer. Regimens employing cisplatin, carboplatin, anthracyclines, taxanes, cyclophosphamide, and 5-FU result in transient responses in 14% to 30% of patients with adenocarcinoma or mucoepidermoid carcinoma (112), but the effect on survival is unknown.

Molecular characterization of salivary gland tumors has included EGFR-dependent pathways, angiogenesis, cell cycle inhibition, and apoptosis that may eventually provide prognostic information and predict response to conventional chemotherapy as well as newer targeted treatments (113–118). Targeted therapies, particularly inhibitors of EGFR, VEGF or its receptors, and Her-2/neu, have been tested in phase 2 clinical trials (119,120). Larger trials are needed to confirm the activity of these new agents against salivary gland cancers either alone, or in combination with conventional chemotherapeutic agents that have previously been shown to be active in this disease. Patients with good performance status should be encouraged to enter clinical trials.

Follow-up

Curative treatment of patients with head and neck cancer should be followed by a comprehensive head and neck physical examination every 1 to 3 months during the first year after treatment, every 2 to 4 months during the second year, every 3 to 6 months from years 3 to 5, and every 6 to 12 months after year 5. The thyroid-stimulating hormone (TSH) level should be checked every 3 to 6 months if the thyroid is irradiated. Generally, thyroid hormone replacement therapy should begin when, and if, TSH remains stably elevated, before symptoms of hypothyroidism appear. Up to 50% of patients will develop hypothyroidism by 5 years after radiation therapy to the head and neck. Patients with nasopharyngeal tumors who were treated with radiation are at risk for pituitary failure (121,122).

The highest risk of relapse is during the first 3 years after treatment. After 3 years, a second primary tumor in the lung or head and neck is the most important cause of morbidity or mortality. Because of this risk, a semiannual chest radiograph is recommended. Some recurrences, as well as second primaries, can be treated with curative intent.

OTHER HEAD AND NECK TUMORS

Sarcoma

Soft tissue sarcomas of the head and neck are relatively rare. Of head and neck sarcomas, 80% are seen in adults and 20% are in children. These tumors are heterogeneous and can present in any head and neck site, commonly as a submucosal or subcutaneous painless mass. In the hypopharynx and nasopharynx, the presenting symptoms may be cranial nerve abnormalities or airway or swallowing difficulties. As in sarcomas at other sites, grade is an important prognostic indicator. High-grade, aggressive tumors such as malignant fibrous histiocytoma, angiosarcoma, osteogenic sarcoma, neurofibrosarcoma, and soft part sarcomas tend to be locally aggressive and spread along neurovascular structures, fascia, and bone. In addition to aggressive local behavior, there is a high risk for metastatic disease, particularly in lung, bone, central nervous system, and liver. Metastatic disease may occur without local lymph node involvement. Sarcomas may arise after radiation therapy, but this is very uncommon in the head and neck region. The prognosis for these secondary sarcomas may be worse than for primary sarcomas.

Treatment depends on stage, age of the patient, tumor type, location, and size. Wide margin en bloc resection is the goal, but may not be possible because of the proximity of vital structures. Adjuvant postoperative radiation and/or brachytherapy can improve local control in aggressive sarcomas. The major indications for adjuvant radiation are high-grade sarcomas or positive margins, lesions greater than 5 cm, and recurrent sarcoma. Elective neck radiation is not necessary because the incidence of occult positive lymph nodes is low. Soft tissue and possibly osteogenic sarcomas may benefit from adjuvant or neoadjuvant chemoradiation. Such patients should be referred to clinical trials when possible. Overall survival rate approaches 60% for patients with sarcomas of the head and neck (123,124).

Melanoma

Mucosal melanomas represent less than 1.5% of all melanomas. About 50% of mucosal melanomas occur in the head and neck, and more than 20% of melanomas that occur in the head and neck region are mucosal. The age of diagnosis is 60 to 80 years. The hard palate is the most common site. Nearly one-third of these tumors are amelanotic. The proportion of mucosal melanomas is higher in African American and Hispanic populations than in white populations. Although rare in the United States, mucosal melanomas are more frequent in Japan and in some parts of Africa. Mucosal melanomas may be multiple, may have satellite lesions, may invade angiolymphatics, and can metastasize. They behave more aggressively than skin melanomas. Lymph node metastasis is observed at presentation in up to 48% of patients. Surgery is the mainstay of treatment for local or locoregional disease. Prophylactic lymph node dissection is not recommended. Radiation, when used, is usually employed adjuvantly for positive margins or used palliatively for local recurrence or unresectability. Adjuvant use of radiation has not been shown to improve survival. Prophylactic nodal radiation is not recommended. Chemotherapy and immunotherapy have been studied, but the effect of these interventions on survival when used as palliation or as adjuvant therapy has not been defined. Patients should be encouraged to enter clinical trials where available. Mean overall 5-year survival is 17% (range 0–48%) (125).

Novel Targeted Therapies and Future Directions

EGFR is overexpressed in most head and neck squamous cancers, and therapies targeting this receptor and its downstream pathways are currently under investigation. Increased expression of EGFR correlates with poorer prognosis in this cancer. Mechanisms of resistance to EGFR-targeted agents have been described in other tumors. In squamous cancers of the head and neck, there is a small incidence of ras mutations or the EGFR mutations described for colon and lung cancers. However, the EGFRvIII mutations, which lack the extracellular domain, seem to be present on a substantial number of squamous head and neck cancers, in conjunction with wild-type EGFR receptors. The presence of EGFRvIII mutants correlates with decreased response to EGFR inhibitors as well as to cisplatin in vitro (126). As in other cancers, angiogenesis may be a good target, and studies are underway with angiogenesis inhibitors in squamous cancers, as well as differentiated and medullary thyroid cancers. Other promising targets under investigation as single agents and in combination with chemotherapy or radiation include mTOR, Akt, c-met, STAT-3, NF-κB, and IGF-1R. Treatments that ameliorate the toxicities of chemoradiation such as xerostomia and dysphagia are also under study. Better discernment of the optimal curative treatment for an individual patient as well as individualized therapy for recurrent or metastatic disease awaits improved diagnostics. Molecular characterization of tumors is a promising field that will likely lead to individualized treatment and prevention approaches.

ACKNOWLEDGMENTS

The authors would like to acknowledge Arlene Forastiere, MD, and David Gius, MD.

REFERENCES

1. Jemal A, Siegel R, Ward E, et al. Cancer statistics, 2008. *CA Cancer J Clin* 2008;58:71–96.
2. Rodu B, Jansson C. Smokeless tobacco and oral cancer: a review of the risks and determinants. *Crit Rev Oral Biol Med* 2004;15:252–263.
3. Sankaranarayanan R, Duffy SW, Day NE, Nair MK, Padmakumary G. A case-control investigation of cancer of the oral tongue and the floor of the mouth in southern India. *Int J Cancer* 1989; 44:617–621.
4. Norton SA. Betel: consumption and consequences. *J Am Acad Dermatol* 1998;38:81–88.
5. Slaughter DP, Southwick HW, Smejkal W. Field cancerization in oral stratified squamous epithelium; clinical implications of multicentric origin. *Cancer* 1953;6:963–968.
6. Cooper JS, Pajak TF, Rubin P, et al. Second malignancies in patients who have head and neck cancer: incidence, effect on survival and implications based on the RTOG experience. *Int J Radiat Oncol Biol Phys* 1989;17:449–456.

7. Laccourreye O, Veivers FD, Hans S, Brasnu FD, Garcia D, Laccourreye FL. Metachronous second primary cancers after successful partial laryngectomy for invasive squamous cell carcinoma of the true vocal cord. *Ann Otol Rhinol Laryngol* 2002;111:204–209.

8. Schwartz LH, Ozsahin M, Zhang GN, et al. Synchronous and metachronous head and neck carcinomas. *Cancer* 1994;74:1933–1938.

9. Niedobitek G. Epstein-Barr virus infection in the pathogenesis of nasopharyngeal carcinoma. *Mol Pathol* 2000;53:248–254.

10. D'Souza G, Kreimer AR, Viscidi R, et al. Case-control study of human papillomavirus and oropharyngeal cancer. *N Engl J Med* 2007;356:1944–1956.

11. Mellin H, Friesland S, Lewensohn R, Dalianis T, Munck-Wikland E. Human papillomavirus (HPV) DNA in tonsillar cancer: clinical correlates, risk of relapse, and survival. *Int J Cancer* 2000;89:300–304.

12. McKaig RG, Baric RS, Olshan AF. Human papillomavirus and head and neck cancer: epidemiology and molecular biology. *Head Neck* 1998;20:250–265.

13. Van Waes C. Head and neck squamous cell carcinoma in patients with Fanconi anemia. *Arch Otolaryngol Head Neck Surg* 2005;131:640–641.

14. van Zandwijk N, Dalesio O, Pastorino U, de Vries N, van Tinteren H. EUROSCAN, a randomized trial of vitamin A and *N*-acetylcysteine in patients with head and neck cancer or lung cancer. For the European Organization for Research and Treatment of Cancer Head and Neck and Lung Cancer Cooperative Groups. *J Natl Cancer Inst* 2000;92:977–986.

15. Khuri FR, Lee JJ, Lippman SM, et al. Randomized phase III trial of low-dose isotretinoin for prevention of second primary tumors in stage I and II head and neck cancer patients. *J Natl Cancer Inst* 2006;98:441–450.

16. Khuri FR, Shin DM. Head and neck cancer chemoprevention gets a shot in the arm. *J Clin Oncol* 2008;26:345–247.

17. Omenn GS, Goodman GE, Thornquist MD, et al. Risk factors for lung cancer and for intervention effects in CARET, the Beta-Carotene and Retinol Efficacy Trial. *J Natl Cancer Inst* 1996; 88:1550–1559.

18. The effect of vitamin E and beta carotene on the incidence of lung cancer and other cancers in male smokers. The Alpha-Tocopherol, Beta Carotene Cancer Prevention Study Group. *N Engl J Med* 1994;330:1029–1035.

19. Lippman SM, Lee JJ, Karp DD, et al. Randomized phase III intergroup trial of isotretinoin to prevent second primary tumors in stage I non-small-cell lung cancer. *J Natl Cancer Inst* 2001; 93:605–618.

20. Greene FL, Page DL, Fleming ID. *AJCC Cancer Staging Manual*. 6th ed. New York: Springer-Verlag; 2002.

21. Agarwal V, Branstetter BF, Johnson JT. Indications for PET/CT in the head and neck. *Otolaryngol Clin North Am* 2008;41:23–49.

22. Chao KS, Ozyigit G, Tran BN, Cengiz M, Dempsey JF, Low DA. Patterns of failure in patients receiving definitive and postoperative IMRT for head-and-neck cancer. *Int J Radiat Oncol Biol Phys* 2003;55:312–321.

23. Lee N, Xia P, Fischbein NJ, Akazawa P, Akazawa C, Quivey JM. Intensity-modulated radiation therapy for head-and-neck cancer: the UCSF experience focusing on target volume delineation. *Int J Radiat Oncol Biol Phys* 2003;57:49–60.

24. Yao M, Dornfeld KJ, Buatti JM, et al. Intensity-modulated radiation treatment for head-and-neck squamous cell carcinoma—the University of Iowa experience. *Int J Radiat Oncol Biol Phys* 2005;63:410–421.

25. Lee NY, de Arruda FF, Puri DR, et al. A comparison of intensity-modulated radiation therapy and concomitant boost radiotherapy in the setting of concurrent chemotherapy for locally advanced oropharyngeal carcinoma. *Int J Radiat Oncol Biol Phys* 2006;66:966–974.

26. Jabbari S, Kim HM, Feng M, et al. Matched case-control study of quality of life and xerostomia after intensity-modulated radiotherapy or standard radiotherapy for head-and-neck cancer: initial report. *Int J Radiat Oncol Biol Phys* 2005;63:725–731.

27. Graff P, Lapeyre M, Desandes E, et al. Impact of intensity-modulated radiotherapy on health-related quality of life for head and neck cancer patients: matched-pair comparison with conventional radiotherapy. *Int J Radiat Oncol Biol Phys* 2007;67:1309–1317.

28. Daly ME, Lieskovsky Y, Pawlicki T, et al. Evaluation of patterns of failure and subjective salivary function in patients treated with intensity-modulated radiotherapy for head and neck squamous cell carcinoma. *Head Neck* 2007;29:211–220.

29. Mazeron JJ, Noel G, Simon JM. Head and neck brachytherapy. *Semin Radiat Oncol* 2002;12:95–108.

30. Quon H, Harrison LB. Brachytherapy in the treatment of head and neck cancer. *Oncology (Williston Park)* 2002;16:1379–1393; discussion 1393, 1395–1396.

31. Medini E, Medini A, Gapany M, Levitt SH. Radiation therapy in early carcinoma of the glottic larynx T1N0M0. *Int J Radiat Oncol Biol Phys* 1996;36:1211–1213.

32. Mendenhall WM, Amdur RJ, Morris CG, Hinerman RW. T1-T2N0 squamous cell carcinoma of the glottic larynx treated with radiation therapy. *J Clin Oncol* 2001;19:4029–4036.

33. Spayne JA, Warde P, O'Sullivan B, et al. Carcinoma-in-situ of the glottic larynx: results of treatment with radiation therapy. *Int J Radiat Oncol Biol Phys* 2001;49:1235–1238.

34. Amdur RJ, Mendenhall WM, Parsons JT, Isaacs JH Jr., Million RR, Cassisi NJ. Carcinoma of the soft palate treated with irradiation: analysis of results and complications. *Radiother Oncol* 1987;9:185–194.

35. Jackson SM, Hay JH, Flores AD, et al. Cancer of the tonsil: the results of ipsilateral radiation treatment. *Radiother Oncol* 1999;51:123–128.

36. Mendenhall WM, Morris CG, Amdur RJ, et al. Definitive radiotherapy for tonsillar squamous cell carcinoma. *Am J Clin Oncol* 2006;29:290–297.

37. Chua DT, Sham JS, Kwong DL, Au GK. Treatment outcome after radiotherapy alone for patients with stage I–II nasopharyngeal carcinoma. *Cancer* 2003;98:74–80.

38. Cooper JS, Pajak TF, Forastiere A, et al. Precisely defining high-risk operable head and neck tumors based on RTOG #85-03 and #88-24: targets for postoperative radiochemotherapy? *Head Neck* 1998;20:588–594.

39. Bonner JA, Harari PM, Giralt J, et al. Radiotherapy plus cetuximab for squamous-cell carcinoma of the head and neck. *N Engl J Med* 2006;354:567–578.

40. Frank SJ, Chao KS, Schwartz DL, Weber RS, Apisarnthanarax S, Macapinlac HA. Technology insight: PET and PET/CT in head and neck tumor staging and radiation therapy planning. *Nat Clin Pract Oncol* 2005;2:526–533.

41. Perez CA, Bradley J, Chao CK, Grigsby PW, Mutic S, Malyapa R. Functional imaging in treatment planning in radiation therapy: a review. *Rays* 2002;27:157–173.

42. Manavis J, Sivridis L, Koukourakis MI. Nasopharyngeal carcinoma: the impact of CT scan and of MRI on staging, radiotherapy treatment planning, and outcome of the disease. *Clin Imaging* 2005;29:128–133.

43. Nishioka T, Shiga T, Shirato H, et al. Image fusion between 18FDG-PET and MRI/CT for radiotherapy planning of oropharyngeal and nasopharyngeal carcinomas. *Int J Radiat Oncol Biol Phys* 2002;53:1051–1057.

44. Khoo VS, Joon DL. New developments in MRI for target volume delineation in radiotherapy. *Br J Radiol* 2006;79(Spec No 1):S2–S15.

45. Chao KS, Bhide S, Chen H, et al. Reduce in variation and improve efficiency of target volume delineation by a computer-assisted system using a deformable image registration approach. *Int J Radiat Oncol Biol Phys* 2007;68:1512–1521.

46. Gregoire V, De Neve W, Eisbruch A, Lee N, Van den Weyngaert D, Van Gestel D. Intensity-modulated radiation therapy for head and neck carcinoma. *Oncologist* 2007;12:555–564.

47. Ang KK. Altered fractionation in the management of head and neck cancer. *Int J Radiat Biol* 1998;73:395–399.

48. Allen AM, Elshaikh M, Worden FP, et al. Acceleration of hyperfractionated chemoradiation regimen for advanced head and neck cancer. *Head Neck* 2007;29:137–142.

49. Ezzat M, Shouman T, Zaza K, et al. A randomized study of accelerated fractionation radiotherapy with and without mitomycin C in the treatment of locally advanced head and neck cancer. *J Egypt Natl Canc Inst* 2005;17:85–92.

50. Langendijk JA, Bourhis J. Reirradiation in squamous cell head and neck cancer: recent developments and future directions. *Curr Opin Oncol* 2007;19:202–209.
51. Chmura SJ, Milano MT, Haraf DJ. Reirradiation of recurrent head and neck cancers with curative intent. *Semin Oncol* 2004;31:816–821.
52. Vissink A, Burlage FR, Spijkervet FK, Jansma J, Coppes RP. Prevention and treatment of the consequences of head and neck radiotherapy. *Crit Rev Oral Biol Med* 2003;14:213–225.
53. Brizel DM, Wasserman TH, Henke M, et al. Phase III randomized trial of amifostine as a radioprotector in head and neck cancer. *J Clin Oncol* 2000;18:3339–3345.
54. Li Y, Taylor JM, Ten Haken RK, Eisbruch A. The impact of dose on parotid salivary recovery in head and neck cancer patients treated with radiation therapy. *Int J Radiat Oncol Biol Phys* 2007;67:660–669.
55. Eisbruch A, Levendag PC, Feng FY, et al. Can IMRT or brachytherapy reduce dysphagia associated with chemoradiotherapy of head and neck cancer? The Michigan and Rotterdam experiences. *Int J Radiat Oncol Biol Phys* 2007;69:S40–S42.
56. Feng FY, Kim HM, Lyden TH, et al. Intensity-modulated radiotherapy of head and neck cancer aiming to reduce dysphagia: early dose-effect relationships for the swallowing structures. *Int J Radiat Oncol Biol Phys* 2007;68:1289–1298.
57. Rosenthal DI, Lewin JS, Eisbruch A. Prevention and treatment of dysphagia and aspiration after chemoradiation for head and neck cancer. *J Clin Oncol* 2006;24:2636–2643.
58. Hong WK, Schaefer S, Issell B, et al. A prospective randomized trial of methotrexate versus cisplatin in the treatment of recurrent squamous cell carcinoma of the head and neck. *Cancer* 1983;52:206–210.
59. Schornagel JH, Verweij J, de Mulder PH, et al. Randomized phase III trial of edatrexate versus methotrexate in patients with metastatic and/or recurrent squamous cell carcinoma of the head and neck: a European Organization for Research and Treatment of Cancer Head and Neck Cancer Cooperative Group study. *J Clin Oncol* 1995;13:1649–1655.
60. Grose WE, Lehane DE, Dixon DO, Fletcher WS, Stuckey WJ. Comparison of methotrexate and cisplatin for patients with advanced squamous cell carcinoma of the head and neck region: a Southwest Oncology Group Study. *Cancer Treat Rep* 1985;69:577–581.
61. Forastiere AA, Shank D, Neuberg D, Taylor SG 4th, DeConti RC, Adams G. Final report of a phase II evaluation of paclitaxel in patients with advanced squamous cell carcinoma of the head and neck: an Eastern Cooperative Oncology Group trial (PA390). *Cancer* 1998;82:2270–2274.
62. Numico G, Merlano M. Second-line treatment with docetaxel after failure of a platinum-based chemotherapy in squamous-cell head and neck cancer. *Ann Oncol* 2002;13:331–333.
63. Dreyfuss AI, Clark JR, Norris CM, et al. Docetaxel: an active drug for squamous cell carcinoma of the head and neck. *J Clin Oncol* 1996;14:1672–1678.
64. Hitt R, Amador ML, Quintela-Fandino M, et al. Weekly docetaxel in patients with recurrent and/or metastatic squamous cell carcinoma of the head and neck. *Cancer* 2006;106:106–111.
65. Catimel G, Verweij J, Mattijssen V, et al. Docetaxel (Taxotere): an active drug for the treatment of patients with advanced squamous cell carcinoma of the head and neck. EORTC Early Clinical Trials Group. *Ann Oncol* 1994;5:533–537.
66. Takimoto CH, Rowinsky EK. Dose-intense paclitaxel: deja vu all over again? *J Clin Oncol* 2003;21:2810–2814.
67. Pivot X, Raymond E, Laguerre B, et al. Pemetrexed disodium in recurrent locally advanced or metastatic squamous cell carcinoma of the head and neck. *Br J Cancer* 2001;85:649–655.
68. Murphy BA, Cmelak A, Burkey B, et al. E. The role of topoisomerases in head and neck cancer. *Oncology (Huntington)* 2001;15:47–52.
69. Catimel G, Vermorken JB, Clavel M, et al. A phase II study of Gemcitabine (LY 188011) in patients with advanced squamous cell carcinoma of the head and neck. EORTC Early Clinical Trials Group. *Ann Oncol* 1994;5:543–547.
70. Degardin M, Oliveira J, Geoffrois L, et al. An EORTC-ECSG phase II study of vinorelbine in patients with recurrent and/or metastatic squamous cell carcinoma of the head and neck. *Ann Oncol* 1998;9:1103–1107.

71. Saxman S, Mann B, Canfield V, Loehrer P, Vokes E. A phase II trial of vinorelbine in patients with recurrent or metastatic squamous cell carcinoma of the head and neck. *Am J Clin Oncol* 1998;21:398–400.

72. Cohen EE. Role of epidermal growth factor receptor pathway-targeted therapy in patients with recurrent and/or metastatic squamous cell carcinoma of the head and neck. *J Clin Oncol* 2006;24:2659–2665.

73. Jacobs C, Lyman G, Velez-Garcia E, et al. A phase III randomized study comparing cisplatin and fluorouracil as single agents and in combination for advanced squamous cell carcinoma of the head and neck. *J Clin Oncol* 1992;10:257–263.

74. Gibson MK, Li Y, Murphy B, et al. Randomized phase III evaluation of cisplatin plus fluorouracil versus cisplatin plus paclitaxel in advanced head and neck cancer (E1395): an intergroup trial of the Eastern Cooperative Oncology Group. *J Clin Oncol* 2005;23:3562–3567.

75. Browman GP, Cronin L. Standard chemotherapy in squamous cell head and neck cancer: what we have learned from randomized trials. *Semin Oncol* 1994;21:311–319.

76. Forastiere AA, Metch B, Schuller DE, et al. Randomized comparison of cisplatin plus fluorouracil and carboplatin plus fluorouracil versus methotrexate in advanced squamous-cell carcinoma of the head and neck: a Southwest Oncology Group study. *J Clin Oncol* 1992;10:1245–1251.

77. Shin DM, Khuri FR, Glisson BS, et al. Phase II study of paclitaxel, ifosfamide, and carboplatin in patients with recurrent or metastatic head and neck squamous cell carcinoma. *Cancer* 2001;91:1316–1323.

78. Shin DM, Glisson BS, Khuri FR, et al. Phase II trial of paclitaxel, ifosfamide, and cisplatin in patients with recurrent head and neck squamous cell carcinoma. *J Clin Oncol* 1998;16: 1325–1330.

79. Posner MR, Hershock DM, Blajman CR, et al. Cisplatin and fluorouracil alone or with docetaxel in head and neck cancer. *N Engl J Med* 2007;357:1705–1715.

80. Baselga J, Trigo JM, Bourhis J, et al. Phase II multicenter study of the antiepidermal growth factor receptor monoclonal antibody cetuximab in combination with platinum-based chemotherapy in patients with platinum-refractory metastatic and/or recurrent squamous cell carcinoma of the head and neck. *J Clin Oncol* 2005;23:5568–5577.

81. Bourhis J, Rivera F, Mesia R, et al. Phase I/II study of cetuximab in combination with cisplatin or carboplatin and fluorouracil in patients with recurrent or metastatic squamous cell carcinoma of the head and neck. *J Clin Oncol* 2006;24:2866–2872.

82. Induction chemotherapy plus radiation compared with surgery plus radiation in patients with advanced laryngeal cancer. The Department of Veterans Affairs Laryngeal Cancer Study Group. *N Engl J Med* 1991;324:1685–1690.

83. Lefebvre JL, Chevalier D, Luboinski B, Kirkpatrick A, Collette L, Sahmoud T. Larynx preservation in pyriform sinus cancer: preliminary results of a European Organization for Research and Treatment of Cancer phase III trial. EORTC Head and Neck Cancer Cooperative Group. *J Natl Cancer Inst* 1996;88:890–899.

84. Forastiere AA, Goepfert H, Maor M, et al. Concurrent chemotherapy and radiotherapy for organ preservation in advanced laryngeal cancer. *N Engl J Med* 2003;349:2091–2098.

85. Vermorken JB, Remenar E, van Herpen C, et al. Cisplatin, fluorouracil, and docetaxel in unresectable head and neck cancer. *N Engl J Med* 2007;357:1695–1704.

86. Hitt R, Lopez-Pousa A, Martinez-Trufero J, et al. Phase III study comparing cisplatin plus fluorouracil to paclitaxel, cisplatin, and fluorouracil induction chemotherapy followed by chemoradiotherapy in locally advanced head and neck cancer. *J Clin Oncol* 2005;23:8636–8645.

87. Dent P, Yacoub A, Contessa J, et al. Stress and radiation-induced activation of multiple intracellular signaling pathways. *Radiat Res* 2003;159:283–300.

88. Pignon JP, le Maître A, Bourhis J, MACH-NC Collaborative Group. Meta-Analyses of Chemotherapy in Head and Neck Cancer (MACH-NC): an update. *Int J Radiat Oncol Biol Phys* 2007;69(2 Suppl):S112–S114.

89. El-Sayed S, Nelson N. Adjuvant and adjunctive chemotherapy in the management of squamous cell carcinoma of the head and neck region. A meta-analysis of prospective and randomized trials. *J Clin Oncol* 1996;14:838–847.

90. Pignon JP, Bourhis J, Domenge C, Designe L. Chemotherapy added to locoregional treatment for head and neck squamous-cell carcinoma: three meta-analyses of updated individual data. MACH-NC Collaborative Group. Meta-Analysis of Chemotherapy on Head and Neck Cancer. *Lancet* 2000;355:949–955.

91. Adelstein DJ, Li Y, Adams GL, et al. An intergroup phase III comparison of standard radiation therapy and two schedules of concurrent chemoradiotherapy in patients with unresectable squamous cell head and neck cancer. *J Clin Oncol* 2003;21:92–98.

92. Taylor SG IV, Murthy AK, Vannetzel JM, et al. Randomized comparison of neoadjuvant cisplatin and fluorouracil infusion followed by radiation versus concomitant treatment in advanced head and neck cancer. *J Clin Oncol* 1994;12:385–395.

93. Vokes EE, Stenson K, Rosen FR, et al. Weekly carboplatin and paclitaxel followed by concomitant paclitaxel, fluorouracil, and hydroxyurea chemoradiotherapy: curative and organ-preserving therapy for advanced head and neck cancer. *J Clin Oncol* 2003;21:320–326.

94. Rubin Grandis J, Melhem MF, Gooding WE, et al. Levels of TGF-alpha and EGFR protein in head and neck squamous cell carcinoma and patient survival. *J Natl Cancer Inst* 1998; 90:824–832.

95. Ang KK, Berkey BA, Tu X, et al. Impact of epidermal growth factor receptor expression on survival and pattern of relapse in patients with advanced head and neck carcinoma. *Cancer Res* 2002;62:7350–7356.

96. Dassonville O, Formento JL, Francoual M, et al. Expression of epidermal growth factor receptor and survival in upper aerodigestive tract cancer. *J Clin Oncol* 1993;11:1873–1878.

97. Lee TL, Yang XP, Yan B, et al. A novel nuclear factor-kappaB gene signature is differentially expressed in head and neck squamous cell carcinomas in association with TP53 status. *Clin Cancer Res* 2007;13:5680–5691.

98. Chung CH, Parker JS, Ely K, et al. Gene expression profiles identify epithelial-to-mesenchymal transition and activation of nuclear factor-kappaB signaling as characteristics of a high-risk head and neck squamous cell carcinoma. *Cancer Res* 2006;66:8210–8218.

99. Pramana J, Van den Brekel MW, van Velthuysen ML, et al. Gene expression profiling to predict outcome after chemoradiation in head and neck cancer. *Int J Radiat Oncol Biol Phys* 2007;69: 1544–1552.

100. Van Waes C, Chang AA, Lebowitz PF, et al. Inhibition of nuclear factor-kappaB and target genes during combined therapy with proteasome inhibitor bortezomib and reirradiation in patients with recurrent head-and-neck squamous cell carcinoma. *Int J Radiat Oncol Biol Phys* 2005; 63:1400–1412.

101. Friedman J, Nottingham L, Duggal P, et al. Deficient TP53 expression, function, and cisplatin sensitivity are restored by quinacrine in head and neck cancer. *Clin Cancer Res* 2007;13:6568–6578.

102. Lui VW, Boehm AL, Koppikar P, et al. Antiproliferative mechanisms of a transcription factor decoy targeting signal transducer and activator of transcription (STAT) 3: the role of STAT1. *Mol Pharmacol* 2007;71:1435–1443.

103. Xi S, Gooding WE, Grandis JR. In vivo antitumor efficacy of STAT3 blockade using a transcription factor decoy approach: implications for cancer therapy. *Oncogene* 2005;24:970–979.

104. Brizel DM, Albers ME, Fisher SR, et al. Hyperfractionated irradiation with or without concurrent chemotherapy for locally advanced head and neck cancer. *N Engl J Med* 1998; 338:1798–1804.

105. Weber RS, Berkey BA, Forastiere A, et al. Outcome of salvage total laryngectomy following organ preservation therapy: the Radiation Therapy Oncology Group trial 91-11. *Arch Otolaryngol Head Neck Surg* 2003;129:44–49.

106. Laramore GE, Scott CB, al-Sarraf M, et al. Adjuvant chemotherapy for resectable squamous cell carcinomas of the head and neck: report on Intergroup Study 0034. *Int J Radiat Oncol Biol Phys* 1992;23:705–713.

107. Bernier J, Cooper JS, Pajak TF. Defining risk levels in locally advanced head and neck cancers: a comparative analysis of concurrent postoperative radiation plus chemotherapy trials of the EORTC (#22931) and RTOG (#9501). *HeadNeck* 2005;27:843–850.

108. Denis F, Garaud P, Bardet E. Final results of the 94-01 French Head and Neck Oncology and Radiotherapy Group randomized trial comparing radiotherapy alone with concomitant radiochemotherapy in advanced-stage oropharynx carcinoma. *J Clin Oncol.* 2004 Jan 1;22(1):19–22.

109. Al-Sarraf M, LeBlanc M, Giri PG, et al. Chemoradiotherapy versus radiotherapy in patients with advanced nasopharyngeal cancer: phase III randomized Intergroup study 0099. *J Clin Oncol* 1998;16:1310–1317.

110. Kao J, Garofalo MC, Milano MT, Chmura SJ, Citron JR, Haraf DJ. Reirradiation of recurrent and second primary head and neck malignancies: a comprehensive review. *Cancer Treat Rev* 2003;29:21–30.

111. Bourhis J, Rivera F, Mesia R et al. Phase I/II study of cetuximab in combination with cisplatin or carboplatin and fluorouracil in patients with recurrent or metastatic squamous cell carcinoma of the head and neck. *J Clin Oncol* 2006;24:2866–2872.

112. Licitra L, Grandi C, Prott FJ, Schornagel JH, Bruzzi P, Molinari R. Major and minor salivary glands tumours. *Crit Rev Oncol Hematol* 2003;45:215–225.

113. Press MF, Pike MC, Hung G, et al. Amplification and overexpression of HER-2/neu in carcinomas of the salivary gland: correlation with poor prognosis. *Cancer Res* 1994;54:5675–5682.

114. Gibbons MD, Manne U, Carroll WR, Peters GE, Weiss HL, Grizzle WE. Molecular differences in mucoepidermoid carcinoma and adenoid cystic carcinoma of the major salivary glands. *Laryngoscope* 2001;111:1373–1378.

115. Handra-Luca A, Bilal H, Bertrand JC, Fouret P. Extra-cellular signal-regulated ERK-1/ERK-2 pathway activation in human salivary gland mucoepidermoid carcinoma: association to aggressive tumor behavior and tumor cell proliferation. *Am J Pathol* 2003;163:957–967.

116. Tonon G, Modi S, Wu L, et al. Translocation in mucoepidermoid carcinoma creates a novel fusion product that disrupts a notch signaling pathway. *Nat Genet* 2003;33:208–213.

117. Okabe M, Miyabe S, Nagatsuka H, et al. MECT1–MAML2 fusion transcript defines a favorable subset of mucoepidermoid carcinoma. *Clin Cancer Res* 2006;12:3902–3907.

118. Yin HF, Okada N, Takagi M. Apoptosis and apoptotic-related factors in mucoepidermoid carcinoma of the oral minor salivary glands. *Pathol Int* 2000;50:603–609.

119. Haddad R, Colevas AD, Krane JF, et al. Herceptin in patients with advanced or metastatic salivary gland carcinomas. A phase II study. *Oral Oncol* 2003;39:724–727.

120. Glisson BS, Blumenschein G, Francisco M, et al. Phase II trial of gefitinib in patients with incurable salivary gland cancer. *J Clin Oncol* 2005;23:508S.

121. Colevas AD, Read R, Thornhill J, et al. Hypothyroidism incidence after multimodality treatment for stage III and IV squamous cell carcinomas of the head and neck. *Int J Radiat Oncol Biol Phys* 2001;51:599–604.

122. Mercado G, Adelstein DJ, Saxton JP, Secic M, Larto MA, Lavertu P. Hypothyroidism: a frequent event after radiotherapy and after radiotherapy with chemotherapy for patients with head and neck carcinoma. *Cancer* 2001;92:2892–2897.

123. Patel SG, Meyers P, Huvos AG, et al. Improved outcomes in patients with osteogenic sarcoma of the head and neck. *Cancer* 2002;95:1495–1503.

124. Pellitteri PK, Ferlito A, Bradley PJ, Shaha AR, Rinaldo A. Management of sarcomas of the head and neck in adults. *Oral Oncol* 2003;39:2–12.

125. Lengyel E, Gilde K, Remenar E, Esik O. Malignant mucosal melanoma of the head and neck. *Pathol Oncol Res* 2003;9:7–12.

126. Sok JC, Coppelli FM, Thomas SM, et al. Mutant epidermal growth factor receptor (EGFRvIII) contributes to head and neck cancer growth and resistance to EGFR targeting. *Clin Cancer Res* 2006;12:5064–5073.

SECTION 2

Thorax

2

Non–Small Cell Lung Cancer

Ronan Kelly, Martin E. Gutierrez, and Giuseppe Giaccone

EPIDEMIOLOGY

- Lung cancer, broadly divided into small cell lung cancer (SCLC) and non–small cell lung cancer (NSCLC), is the leading cause of cancer death in both men and women in the United States.
- An estimated 213,380 new cases of lung and bronchus cancer (114,760 in men and 98,620 in women) were diagnosed in 2007, resulting in 160,390 deaths (89,510 in men, 70,880 in women).
- More than 70% of patients are diagnosed with advanced disease that is not amenable to curative therapy.
- The 5-year relative survival rate for lung cancer is approximately 15%, reflecting a slow but steady improvement from 12.5% in the 1970s.
- Stage at diagnosis accounts for the most marked variation in prognosis; patient characteristics associated with poorer prognosis include older age, male gender, and African American heritage.
- In the United States, as many women now die from lung cancer as die from breast, uterine, and cervical cancers combined. The increase in lung cancer risk among women reflects changes in smoking habits during the twentieth century. By 1987, lung cancer had surpassed breast cancer as the leading cause of cancer death in women as a result of an increase in the prevalence of female smokers.
- Rates of cigarette smoking have declined in the United States in the last 10 years, but developing nations are now seeing an alarming increase in smoking rates.

ETIOLOGY AND RISK FACTORS

- The vast majority of lung cancer deaths are directly attributable to cigarette smoking.
- Tobacco smoke contains a highly complex mixture of carcinogens that have the potential to damage DNA. Polycyclic aromatic hydrocarbons, aromatic amines, and tobacco-specific nitrosamines have been implicated as the major mutagenic carcinogens responsible for DNA adduct formation. The number of DNA adducts formed is directly related to the number of cigarettes consumed; in heavy smokers they can be responsible for as many as 100 mutations per cell genome.
- Compared to those who have never smoked, smokers have an approximate 20-fold increase in lung cancer risk. The likelihood of developing lung cancer decreases among those who quit smoking compared to those who continue to smoke.
- Estimates indicate that passive smoking accounts for approximately 3,000 lung cancer deaths per year in the United States.
- Radon, a radioactive gas produced by the decay of radium 226, is the second leading cause of lung cancer in the United States, accounting for 6,000 to 36,000 cases of lung cancer each year. The decay of radium 226 produces substances that emit alpha particles, which may cause cell damage. Residential exposure has been associated with an increased risk of developing lung cancer.
- Occupational exposure to carcinogens such as asbestos, arsenic, chromates, chloromethyl ethers, nickel, polycyclic aromatic hydrocarbons, and other agents is estimated to cause approximately 9% to 15% of lung cancers. Asbestos exposure in smokers is associated with a synergistic risk of developing lung cancer. Cigarette smoking impairs bronchial clearance and thereby prolongs the presence of asbestos in the pulmonary epithelium.

- The contribution of hereditary factors to the development of lung cancer is less well understood than for any of the common forms of solid tumors in human. Proof that the familial occurrence of lung cancer has a genetic basis is complicated by the central role of cigarette smoking in the etiology of lung cancer.
- Large randomized, double-blind, placebo-controlled chemoprevention trials reported in the 1990s provided no evidence that specific dietary constituents confer protection against lung cancer.

PATHOLOGY

- NSCLC can be divided into three major subtypes (Table 2.1):
  - Adenocarcinoma
  - Squamous cell carcinoma
  - Large cell carcinoma
- Adenocarcinoma is the most frequently diagnosed form of NSCLC in both men and women in the United States and constitutes 54% of all cases of NSCLC. Tumors are classically peripheral and arise from surface epithelium or bronchial mucosal glands. Histologic examination reveals gland formation, papillary structures, or mucin production. The histologic characteristics of lung cancer in several developed countries, including the United States, have changed in the past few decades, demonstrating that the frequency of adenocarcinoma has risen while the frequency of squamous cell carcinoma has declined.
- Bronchioloalveolar carcinoma, a noninvasive subtype of adenocarcinoma, occurs more frequently in women and nonsmokers, and is associated with bilateral, multifocal pulmonary involvement, a lesser tendency for extrathoracic metastases, and a better survival rate than similar-stage NSCLC.
- Squamous cell carcinoma accounts for 35% of NSCLC and has the strongest association with cigarette smoking. This tumor arises most frequently in the central proximal bronchi and can lead to bronchial obstruction, with resultant atelectasis or pneumonia. Histologic examination reveals visible keratinization, with prominent desmosomes and intercellular bridges.
- Large cell carcinoma is the least common subtype of lung cancer, accounting for approximately 11% of all NSCLCs.

TABLE 2.1.   *Modified WHO classification of non–small cell lung cancer (1999)*

1. *Squamous cell carcinoma*
   Variants: papillary, clear cell, small cell, basaloid

2. *Adenocarcinoma*
   Acinar
   Papillary
   Bronchioloalveolar
      Nonmucinous (Clara cell/type II pneumocyte type)
      Mucinous (goblet cell type)
      Mixed mucinous and nonmucinous (Clara cell/type II) pneumocyte and goblet cell type
         or indeterminate
   Solid adenocarcinoma with mucin formation
   Mixed
   Variants: well-differentiated fetal adenocarcinoma, mucinous ("colloid"), mucinous cystadeno-
   carcinoma, signet ring, clear cell

3. *Large cell carcinoma*
   Variants: large cell neuroendocrine carcinoma, combined large cell neuroendocrine carcinoma,
   basaloid carcinoma, lymphoepithelioma-like carcinoma, clear cell carcinoma, large cell carcinoma with rhabdoid phenotype

4. *Adenosquamous carcinoma*

WHO: Word Health Organization.

TABLE 2.2. *Genetic mutations in NSCLC*

Description	Percentage
Tumor suppressor genes	
Rb mutations (13q14)	15%
p16/CDKN2 mutations (9p21)	60%
p53 mutations (17p13)	50%
3p deletions	50%
Dominant oncogene abnormalities	
K-ras mutations	30%
Her-2/neu overexpression	25%
Myc family amplification	10%
BCL-2 overexpression	25%

BIOLOGY

- Lung cancer evolves through a multistep process from normal bronchial epithelium to dysplasia to carcinoma in situ and finally to invasive cancer. These changes include activation of oncogenes, inactivation of tumor suppressor genes, and loss of genomic stability. Changes can be both genetic (via deletions or mutations) or epigenetic (methylation), leading to altered cell proliferation, differentiation, and apoptosis. Mutations in multiple tumor suppressor genes and oncogenes have been associated with the development of NSCLC (Table 2.2).
- Cytogenetic studies have revealed a large number of chromosomal abnormalities in lung cancer, such as allelic loss leading to loss of tumor suppressor genes. Two of the most studied tumor suppressor genes are p53 and retinoblastoma (RB).
  - p53 is involved in DNA repair, cell division, apoptosis, and growth regulation. In normal conditions, p53 production increases when DNA damage occurs. Increased amounts of p53 induce cell cycle arrest in the G1 phase, allowing DNA repair. If a p53 deletion or mutation exists, G1 arrest is not achieved and the abnormal cell proceeds to S phase, further dividing and propagating genetic damage. Mutations in p53 are found in 50% of NSCLC.
  - The RB gene also regulates G1 growth arrest. Hypermethylation of the CpG-rich island at the 5′ end of the RB gene is thought to lead to silencing of the RB gene and tumor progression. RB gene mutations occur in 15% of NSCLC.
- K-ras is a member of the ras family of oncogenes and codes for a 21-kDa guanine-binding protein that mediates signal transduction pathways from cell surface receptors to intracellular molecules. The ras oncogene can be activated either by a point mutation or by overexpression. To function in signal transduction, ras requires a specific posttranslational modification called farnesylation. K-ras is a critical downstream effector of the epidermal growth factor receptor (EGFR) pathway. K-ras has been found to be mutated in approximately 15% to 30% of lung adenocarcinomas and is associated with exposure to tobacco smoke.
- EGFR is highly expressed in NSCLC. Following binding of a ligand to its extracellular receptor, dimerization occurs, leading to activation of tyrosine kinases and a subsequent increase in downstream signaling pathways including Ras–Raf and Akt protein kinases. Recently, it has been shown that point mutations within the tyrosine kinase domain greatly affect tumor sensitivity to EGFR inhibitors (erlotinib, gefitinib). Sensitizing mutations in exons 19, 21, and 18 can increase the efficacy of erlotinib. Other mutations are responsible for poor disease response to tyrosine kinase inhibitors such as T790M mutation. K-ras mutations are also associated with intrinsic tyrosine kinase inhibitor resistance. EGFR and K-ras mutations are mutually exclusive in patients with lung cancer.

CLINICAL PRESENTATION

- A minority of patients present with an asymptomatic lesion discovered incidentally on chest radiograph. No set of signs or symptoms are pathognomonic of lung cancer, so diagnosis is usually delayed.
- Clinical signs and symptoms of lung cancer are outlined in Table 2.3.

TABLE 2.3. *Clinical signs and symptoms of lung cancer*

Primary disease
  Central or endobronchial tumor growth
     Cough
     Sputum production
     Hemoptysis
     Dyspnea
     Wheeze (usually unilateral)
     Stridor
     Pneumonitis with fever and productive cough (secondary to obstruction)
  Peripheral tumor growth
     Pain from pleural or chest wall involvement
     Cough
     Dyspnea
     Pneumonitis
Regional involvement (either direct or metastatic spread)
  Hoarseness (recurrent laryngeal nerve paralysis)
  Dysphagia (esophageal compression)
  Dyspnea (pleural effusion, tracheal/bronchial obstruction, pericardial effusion, phrenic nerve
    palsy, lymphatic infiltration, superior vena cava obstruction)
  Horner's syndrome (sympathetic nerve palsy)
Metastatic involvement (common sites)
  Bone (pain exacerbated by movement or weight bearing, often worse at night; fracture)
  Liver (right hypochondrial pain, icterus, altered mental status)
  Brain (altered mental status, seizures, motor and sensory deficits)
Paraneoplastic syndromes
  Hypertrophic pulmonary osteoarthropathy
  Hypercalcemia
  Dermatomyositis (Eaton-Lambert syndrome)
  Hypercoagulable state
  Gynecomastia

CLINICAL EVALUATION

Single Pulmonary Nodule (SPN)

- Definition: solitary mass, often found incidentally, surrounded by lung tissue, well circumscribed, measures <3 cm without mediastinal or hilar adenopathy.
- Benign inflammatory vascular abnormalities or infectious lesions can mimic more sinister lesions. Review of previous chest x-rays is a crucial first step. A stable lesion over a 2-year period suggests a benign condition.
- Computed tomography (CT) of the chest is required to assess for other nodules, adenopathy, or chest wall invasion.
- FDG-PET (^{18}F-fluorodeoxyglucose-positron emission tomography) is used to evaluate SPNs. False-positive PET scans may occur in conditions such as tuberculosis or histoplasmosis. False-negative results have been reported for small lesions (<1 cm) and neoplasms with low metabolic activity, such as in some cases of bronchioloalveolar carcinoma. Mean sensitivity of FDG-PET is 96%; mean specificity is 75%. The negative and positive predictive value of PET for pulmonary nodules is approximately 90%.
- A growing SPN needs a pathologic diagnosis. Tissue can be obtained by fine needle aspiration (FNA), transbronchial biopsy, or surgical resection. Flexible fiber optic bronchoscopy is appropriate for central lesions and can lead to a diagnosis in 97% of cases via biopsies, bronchial washings, and brushings.
- Observation may be reasonable in a low-risk patient (<40 years old and has never smoked) with a negative FDG-PET and a stable lesion measuring <2 cm. Reimaging with regular CT scans and follow-up clinic appointments are recommended.

Suspected Lung Cancer

- Full history and physical examination are recommended, followed by complete blood count and chemistry tests, chest x-ray, and CT of the chest and abdomen (including adrenal glands).
- Sputum analysis may be helpful in cases of central lesions.
- Bone scans and plain films of affected areas are warranted where bone pain exists, but routine imaging of the brain in asymptomatic patients is controversial.
- Peripheral lesions may require percutaneous transthoracic FNA, which can be performed under CT or fluoroscopic guidance.
- Mediastinoscopy, a more invasive method, may be needed to obtain a histologic diagnosis in difficult-to-reach primary tumors. Mediastinoscopy can reveal unsuspected tumors in mediastinal lymph nodes—a negative implication for survival. Evaluation of the mediastinum is recommended before surgery in suspected mediastinal disease and intraoperatively prior to any planned resections.
- An accurate pathologic diagnosis and staging of disease is essential in the management of lung cancer. Stage of disease determines whether surgical resection is warranted. Clinical staging often underestimates the true extent of the disease. The combination of PET evaluation and mediastinoscopy is routinely used to complete staging. In patients who undergo surgical resection, surgical/pathologic staging should be used to predict recurrence and to evaluate the need for adjuvant therapy.
- Preresection forced expiratory volume/1 second (FEV1) should be $\geq$2 L for pneumonectomy, 1 L for lobectomy, or 0.6 L for segmentectomy.
- Preresection forced vital capacity should be $\geq$1.7 L.

STAGING

- The tumor-node-metastasis (TNM) staging system bases patient prognoses on tumor size, lymph node involvement, and metastasis.
- The seventh edition of the *TNM Classification of Malignant Tumours* (UICC) has recently been published. Revisions of the TNM system (Table 2.4) raise important questions about treatment options. The most important change is the shift of node-negative patients with large tumors from stage IB, where adjuvant chemotherapy is often not recommended, to stage IIA or IIB, where chemotherapy is standard treatment after surgical resection. Under the revised system, node-negative patients with tumors >5 cm will be categorized as IIA and those with tumors >7 cm as IIB. Previously, these patients would have been categorized as IB.
- Another change involves the staging of disease in patients with malignant nodules. Currently, ipsilateral malignant nodules in the same lobe as the primary tumor are classified as stage IIIB. Under the

TABLE 2.4. *Revisions of the TNM staging in the seventh edition of the TNM classification of malignant tumors*

TX	Primary tumor cannot be assessed, or tumor proven by the presence of malignant cells in sputum or bronchial washings but not visualized by imaging or bronchoscopy
T0	No evidence of primary tumor
Tis	Carcinoma in situ
T1	Primary tumor ≤3 cm in greatest dimension, surrounded by lung or visceral pleura, without bronchoscopic evidence of invasion more proximal than the lobar bronchus (i.e., not in the main bronchus)
T1a	Tumor ≤2 cm in greatest dimension
T1b	Tumor >2 cm but ≤3 cm in greatest dimension
T2	Tumor >3 cm but ≤7 cm or tumor with any of the following features: (T2 tumors with these features are classified T2a if ≤5 cm in greatest dimension) Involves main bronchus, ≥2 cm distal to the carina Invades the visceral pleura Associated with atelectasis or obstructive pneumonitis that extends to the hilar region but does not involve the entire lung
T2a	Tumor >3 cm but ≤5 cm in greatest dimension
T2b	Tumor >5 cm but ≤7 cm in greatest dimension

(Continued)

TABLE 2.4. *(Continued)*

T3	Tumor >7 cm or that directly invades any of the following: Chest wall (including superior sulcus tumors), diaphragm, phrenic nerve, mediastinal pleura, parietal pericardium, or tumor in the main bronchus <2 cm distal to the carina but without involvement of the carina; or associated atelectasis or obstructive pneumonitis of the entire lung or separate tumor nodule(s) in the same lobe
T4	Tumor of any size that directly invades any of the following: Mediastinum, heart, great vessels, trachea, recurrent laryngeal nerve, esophagus, vertebral body, or carina; separate tumor nodule(s) in a different ipsilateral lobe, esophagus, vertebral body, heart, great vessels, malignant pleural/pericardial effusion, satellite tumor within the ipsilateral primary tumor lobe of the lung
NX	Regional lymph nodes cannot be assessed
N0	No regional lymph node metastasis
N1	Metastasis in ipsilateral peribronchial and/or ipsilateral hilar lymph nodes and intrapulmonary nodes, including involvement by direct extension of the primary
N2	Metastasis in ipsilateral, mediastinal, and/or subcarinal lymph node(s)
N3	Metastasis in contralateral, mediastinal, contralateral hilar, ipsilateral or contralateral scalene, or supraclavicular lymph node(s)
MX	Presence of distant metastasis cannot be assessed
M0	No distant metastasis
M1	Distant metastasis
M1a	Separate tumor nodule(s) in a contralateral lobe; tumor with pleural nodules or malignant pleural (or pericardial) effusion
M1b	Distant metastases

new system, same lobe nodules will be stage IIB if there is no lymph node involvement (N0) and IIIA if lymph node disease is limited (N1 or N2). This down-staging could mean that more patients with ipsilateral nodules will be considered surgical candidates.

• Staging changes will also occur in patients with an ipsilateral nodule in a different lobe. These will move from stage IV to stage IIIA (N0 or N1) or IIIB (N2 or N3). Extensive tumors with pleural or pericardial effusions will move from stage IIIB to stage IV, where they will be grouped with other nonresectable tumors. These so-called wet IIIBs have always been treated as stage IV, so this is perhaps the most obvious change required.

• A major change with no treatment implications at present is the division of metastases into two subgroups: M1a for metastases in the other lung and M1b for distant metastases. Both remain stage IV.

TREATMENT

Stages I and II

• Stage I and stage II NSCLC are considered early-stage disease. These two stages combined account for 25% to 30% of all lung cancers.

• Five-year survival rates are 60% to 80% for stage I and 40% to 50% for stage II.

• Surgical resection is the recommended treatment for patients with stage I and stage II NSCLC. In patients who are medically fit for conventional surgical resection, lobectomy or greater resection is recommended rather than sublobar resections (wedge or segmentectomy).

• Video-assisted thorascopic surgery (VATS) is an acceptable alternative to open thoracotomy.

• Intraoperative systematic mediastinal lymph node sampling or dissection is recommended for accurate pathologic staging.

• Even with complete resection, many patients with stage I and stage II NSCLC experience recurrence. Most of these relapses are distant metastases.

• For completely resected stage IA NSCLC, postoperative chemotherapy is not recommended, and most studies have found no statistically significant benefit for the subset of patients with stage IB NSCLC.

• Data on the use of adjuvant cisplatin-based chemotherapy in stage II NSCLC are convincing. The International Adjuvant Lung Trial (IALT), National Cancer Institute of Canada JBR.10, and Adjuvant

Navelbine International Trialists Association (ANITA) studies all found significant survival benefit in the use of adjuvant chemotherapy. The Lung Adjuvant Cisplatin Evaluation (LACE) meta-analysis found a 27% reduction in the risk of death (hazard ratio, 0.83; 95% CI, 0.73–0.95) in stage II patients.

- Current evidence suggests that postoperative radiotherapy is associated with decreased survival for patients with stage I (N0) and stage II (N1) NSCLC. However, most meta-analyses include several older studies that used radiotherapy methods that are inferior to current methods.
- If surgery is contraindicated in early-stage NSCLC, radiotherapy can be an effective means of local control. In clinical studies, accelerated radiotherapy (54 Gy in 12 days) was associated with better 4-year survival than conventional radiotherapy (60 Gy in 6 weeks).

Stage IIIA

- Stage IIIA (N2) NSCLC is a therapeutically challenging and controversial subset of lung cancer, with a 5-year survival rate of only 23%.
- Recent randomized trials strongly suggest a combined modality approach in stage IIIA disease. Conflicting data, however, have led to difficulties in proposing specific management guidelines.
- For patients with incidental (occult) N2 disease found at surgical resection, complete tumor resection and mediastinal lymphadenectomy is recommended, if technically possible. However, if metastatic disease is found in the N2 nodes at mediastinoscopy before thoracotomy, then further surgery at that time should be avoided based on the poor results of primary resection for stage IIIA disease.
- Postoperative radiation therapy (PORT) in completely resected stage IIIA disease is not recommended, based on the lack of evidence of improved survival.
  - The PORT meta-analysis (Meta-Analysis Trialist Group) of 2,128 patients treated in nine randomized trials of PORT concluded that this treatment was associated with a highly significant increase in risk of death (overall risk ratio 1:21; $P = 0.001$). The authors concluded that postoperative radiotherapy, as used in these studies, was detrimental and should not be used. Advocates of radiotherapy have emphasized that there are several differences between the treatment administered in several trials included in this meta-analysis and current practices in the United States.
  - Practice guidelines on postoperative radiotherapy in stage II and IIIA NSCLC were developed and published in 2004 by the Lung Cancer Disease Site Group of Cancer Care Ontario Program of Evidence-Based Care. After reviewing the literature they too concluded that no survival benefit was found with postoperative radiotherapy in completely resected stage IIIA disease and that the data for improved local control were conflicting.
- Postoperative chemotherapy in completely resected stage IIIA disease is recommended. The International Adjuvant Lung Cancer Trial of 1,867 patients with stages IB to IIIA (39% stage IIIA) randomized patients to three to four cycles of postoperative cisplatin-based chemotherapy versus surgery alone, with adjuvant 60 Gy radiotherapy given to both arms of stage IIIA patients (the use of radiotherapy was left to investigator's choice). After a median 56-month follow-up, the overall survival rate was significantly higher in the chemotherapy group (hazard ratio, 0.86), with a 5-year survival rate of 44.5% in the chemotherapy group versus 40.4% in the control arm, with the strongest benefit in patients with stage III disease.
  - The ANITA study randomized 840 completely resected patients with stages I to IIIA (35% stage IIIA) to four postoperative cycles of cisplatin and navelbine versus observation (radiotherapy as per preference of participating center). After a median follow-up of >70 months, long-term 5-year survival of stage IIIA patients in the chemotherapy arm was significantly greater at 42% versus 26% in the observation arm ($P = 0.013$). Adjuvant chemotherapy showed a benefit in stage II but not stage I patients.
- To date, evidence has yet to be established substantiating the benefit of adding adjuvant radiotherapy to adjuvant chemotherapy in fully resected stage IIIA patients.
- Poor survival rates with surgery alone in N2 disease, even with postoperative chemotherapy or radiotherapy, have led to the use of radiotherapy and/or chemotherapy in the neoadjuvant setting, with

the aim of making an unresectable tumor resectable and improving long-term survival. Theoretically, advantages include shrinking the tumor to allow for easier resection and nodal clearance, decreased surgical seeding, in vivo chemosensitivity testing of the chemotherapy regimen, and increased patient acceptance and compliance.

- Disadvantages of neoadjuvant therapy may include delayed tumor resection and increased surgical morbidity and mortality. A 2005 meta-analysis by Berghmans et al. evaluating neoadjuvant chemotherapy found only a marginal benefit in favor of induction chemotherapy.
- Two clinical trials (European Organization for Research and Treatment of Cancer 08941 and North American Intergroup 0196) showed no significant difference in overall survival between patients with stage IIIA NSCLC treated with neoadjuvant chemotherapy then surgery versus definitive chemoradiation alone (no surgery). Induction chemotherapy followed by surgery in stage IIIA disease is feasible; however, published data do not support this treatment as the standard of care.
- The use of concurrent chemotherapy/radiotherapy versus sequential treatment has been addressed in numerous trials. At present, for patients with bulky NSCLC with N2 disease, the data recommend treatment with concurrent over sequential chemotherapy/radiotherapy.
- Concurrent chemotherapy/radiotherapy followed by consolidation chemotherapy is currently not recommended as the standard of care.

Stage IIIB With No Malignant Pleural Effusion

- This stage includes patients with T4 lesions or N3 involvement. Anticipated 5-year survival for most patients with stage IIIB disease is 3% to 7%.
- Optimal treatment depends on extent of disease, age of patient, co-morbid risk factors, performance status (PS), and weight loss.
- Stage IIIB lung cancers are not amenable to curative surgical resection unless they are highly selected. Patients with clinical T4N0-1 as a result of satellite tumor nodule(s) in the same lobe, carinal involvement, or superior vena cava invasion may be considered operable based on a multidisciplinary evaluation.
- For patients with stage IIIB disease with no malignant pleural effusions, PS of 0 to 1, and minimal weight loss (<5%), platinum-based combination chemoradiotherapy is recommended.
- The most common chemotherapeutic agents used concurrently with radiotherapy have been vinorelbine, vinblastine, and etoposide in conjunction with cisplatin or weekly paclitaxel and carboplatin. No randomized phase 3 trials of concurrent chemoradiotherapy have shown the superiority of one chemotherapy regimen over another.
- Studies have shown that induction chemotherapy followed by concurrent chemoradiotherapy is not superior to initial treatment with concurrent therapy. It is uncertain how many cycles of chemotherapy are optimal in the treatment of patients with stage IIIB disease. The American Society of Clinical Oncology (ASCO) guidelines recommend two to four cycles of platinum-based chemotherapy, two of which should be administered concurrently with thoracic radiotherapy.

Stage IIIB With Malignant Pleural Effusion and Stage IV

- Prognosis for patients with advanced-stage (IIIB with malignant pleural effusions, and IV) NSCLC is extremely poor. Best supportive care produces median survival rates of 16 to 17 weeks and 1-year survival rates of 10% to 15%.
- Subsets of patients with stage IIIB disease who are treated as though they had stage IV disease include those with malignant pleural or pericardial effusions, those with advanced ipsilateral supraclavicular adenopathy, and those whose intrathoracic disease is not amenable to combined treatment modalities. For these patients, therapy options include systemic chemotherapy or supportive therapy alone if the patient's general condition is not suitable for systemic chemotherapy.
- In patients with stage IV NSCLC and good PS, chemotherapy clearly improves survival and palliates disease-related symptoms. Chemotherapeutic regimens can be divided into first-line, second-line, and third-line settings.

First-Line Therapy

- Platinum-based doublets are the standard of care for patients with stage IV NSCLC and good PS.
- There is no clearly superior regimen for first-line chemotherapy, which should not exceed four cycles, unless continuing response is seen, in which case a maximum of six cycles is recommended.
- Two chemotherapeutic agents produce superior response and survival rates compared to single agents.
- There is general agreement that either cisplatin or carboplatin combined with a taxane (paclitaxel or docetaxel), gemcitabine, vinorelbine, or irinotecan can be used as first-line treatment of patients with advanced NSCLC and good PS. Addition of a third chemotherapeutic agent to existing doublets has failed to show a superior survival benefit; response rates improved only at the cost of substantially increased toxicity.
- Clinical trials have shown evidence of survival benefit with bevacizumab in NSCLC. For example, the Eastern Cooperative Oncology Group (ECOG) E4599 trial studied patients with stage IIIB/IV disease and an ECOG performance status of 0 to 1 who were therapy naïve. Patients with squamous cell histology, hemoptysis, or brain metastases were excluded. The addition of bevacizumab to chemotherapy reduced the risk of death by 20% versus chemotherapy alone. Median survival was 12.3 months in the bevacizumab arm and 10.3 months in the control arm ($P = 0.003$). In the AVAIL (Avastin in Lung) trial bevacizumab in combination with gemcitabine/cisplatin was compared to gemcitabine/cisplatin alone. Median progression-free survival was 6.1 months in the chemotherapy-alone arm versus 6.7 months in the group receiving bevacizumab at the lower dose of 7.5 mg/kg. However, this study did not show an increase in overall survival.
- The addition of bevacizumab in eligible patients (no hemoptysis, no brain metastasis, and nonsquamous histology) may be considered in combination with carboplatin–paclitaxel.

Second-Line Therapy

- Second-line therapy has an impact on survival and quality of life in advanced NSCLC; therefore, patients with a PS of 0 to 2 should be offered further treatment following progression.
- Approved agents include docetaxel, pemetrexed, and erlotinib.
- The BR-21 trial showed an improvement in median overall survival of 6.7 versus 4.7 months in patients who received erlotinib following failure of first-line or second-line chemotherapy, compared to placebo.
- Current recommendations do not support the combination of cytotoxic chemotherapy and a tyrosine kinase inhibitor outside of a clinical trial.

Third-Line Therapy

- Erlotinib is also an approved agent in the third-line setting. If disease progression occurs after second-line or third-line chemotherapy, it is recommended that patients with a PS of 0 to 2 be enrolled in a clinical trial or treated with best supportive care.

SUGGESTED READINGS

Albain KS, Swann RS, Rusch VR, et al. Phase III study of concurrent chemotherapy and radiotherapy (CT/RT) vs CT/RT followed by surgical resection for stage IIIA (pN20) non-small cell lung cancer: outcomes update of North American Intergroup 0139 (RTOG 9309) [abstract]. *J Clin Oncol.* 2005;23(Suppl):7014.

American College of Chest Physicians (ACCP) guidelines for the diagnosis and management of lung cancer. ACCP Evidence-Based Clinical Practice Guidelines (2nd ed.). *Chest.* Sept 2007.

American Society of Clinical Oncology 43rd Annual Meeting: Abstract LBA7514. Presented June 2, 2007.

Arriagada R, Bergman B, Dunant A, et al. Cisplatin-based adjuvant chemotherapy in patients with completely resected non-small cell lung cancer. *N Engl J Med.* 2004;350:351–360.

Berghmans T, Paesmans M, Meert AP, et al. Survival improvement in resectable non-small cell lung cancer with (neo)adjuvant chemotherapy: results of a meta-analysis of the literature. *Lung Cancer.* 2005;49:13–23.

Burdett S, Stewart L. Postoperative radiotherapy in non-small cell lung cancer: update of an individual patient data meta-analysis. *Lung Cancer.* 2005;47:81–83.

Douillard J, Rosell R, Delena M, et al. ANITA: phase III adjuvant vinorelbine and cisplatin versus observation in completely resected (stage I-III) non-small cell lung cancer (NSCLC) patients: final results after 70-month median follow-up [abstract]. *J Clin Oncol.* 2005;23(Suppl):7013.

Fischer BM, Mortensen J, Hojgaard L. Positron emission tomography in the diagnosis and staging of lung cancer: a systematic, quantitative review. *Lancet Oncol.* 2001;2:659–666.

Fukuoka M, Yano S, Giaccone G, et al. Multi-institutional randomized phase II trial of gefitinib for previously treated patients with advanced non-small cell lung cancer (The IDEAL 1 Trial) [corrected]. *J Clin Oncol.* 2003;21(12):2237–2246.

Giaccone G, Herbst R, Manegold C, et al. Gefitinib in combination with gemcitabine and cisplatin in advanced non-small cell lung cancer: a phase III Trial—INTACT 1. *J Clin Oncol.* 2004;22(5): 777–784.

Gould MK, Maclean CC, Kuschner WG, Rydzak CE, Owens DK. Accuracy of positron emission tomography for diagnosis of pulmonary nodules and mass lesions: a meta-analysis. *JAMA.* 2001; 285:914–924.

Hamilton M, Wolf JL, Rusk J, et al. Effects of smoking on the pharmacokinetics of erlotinib. *Clin Cancer Res.* 2006;12:2166–2171.

Herbst R, Giaccone G, Schiller J, et al. Gefitinib in combination with paclitaxel and carboplatin in advanced non-small cell lung cancer: a phase III trial—INTACT 2. *J Clin Oncol.* 2004;22(5): 785–794.

Herbst RS, Prager D, Hermann R, et al. TRIBUTE: a phase III trial of erlotinib hydrochloride (OSI-774) combined with carboplatin and paclitaxel chemotherapy in advanced non-small cell lung cancer. *J Clin Oncol.* 2005;23(25):5892–5899.

Jemal A, Siegel R, Ward E, Murray T, Xu J, Thun MJ. Cancer statistics, 2007. *CA Cancer J Clin.* 2007;57(1):43–66.

Lubin JH, Boice JD Jr. Lung cancer risk from residential radon: meta-analysis of eight epidemiologic studies. *J Natl Cancer Inst.* 1997;89:49–57.

Mountain CF. Revisions in the International System for Staging Lung Cancer. *Chest.* 1997;111: 1710–1717.

National Comprehensive Cancer Network. Practice Guidelines in Oncology Version 2.2008.

Okawara G, Mackay JA, Evans WK, et al. Management of unresected stage III non-small cell lung cancer: a systematic review. *J Thorac Oncol.* 2006;1:377–393.

Okawara G, Ung YC, Markman BR, et al. Postoperative radiotherapy in stage II or IIIA completely resected non-small cell lung cancer: a systematic review and practice guideline. *Lung Cancer.* 2004; 44:1–11.

Pfister DG, Johnson DH, Azzoli CG, et al. American Society of Clinical Oncology treatment of unresectable non-small cell lung cancer guideline: update 2003. *J Clin Oncol.* 2004;22:330–353.

Pignon JP, Tribodet H, Scagliotti GV, et al. Lung Adjuvant Cisplatin Evaluation (LACE): a pooled analysis of five randomized clinical trials including 4,584 patients. *J Clin Oncol.* 2006;24(18S):7008.

Postoperative radiotherapy in non-small-cell lung cancer: systematic review and meta-analysis of individual patient data from nine randomized controlled trials. PORT Meta-analysis Trialist Group. *Lancet.* 1998;353:257–263.

Salgia R, Skarin AT. Molecular abnormalities in lung cancer. *J Clin Oncol.* 1998;16:1207–1217.

Sandler AB, Gray R, Brahmer J, et al. Randomized phase II/III trial of paclitaxel plus carboplatin with or without bevacizumab in patients with advanced non-squamous non-small cell lung cancer: an Eastern Cooperative Oncology Group Trial-E4599 [abstract]. *J Clin Oncol.* 2005;23(16S):4.

Saunders M, Dische S, Barrett A, Harvey A, Gibson D, Parmar M. Continuous hyperfractionated accelerated radiotherapy (CHART) versus conventional radiotherapy in non-small cell lung cancer: a randomised, multicentre trial: CHART Steering Committee. *Lancet.* 1997;350:161–165.

Shepherd FA, Pereira J, Ciuleanu TE, et al. A randomized placebo-controlled trial of erlotinib in patients with advanced non-small cell lung cancer (NSCLC) following failure of 1st line or 2nd line chemotherapy [abstract]. *J Clin Oncol*. 2004;22(Suppl 14):12.

Strauss GM, Herndon JE, Maddaus MA, et al. Adjuvant chemotherapy in stage IB non-small cell lung cancer: update of Cancer and Leukemia Group B protocol 9633 [abstract]. *J Clin Oncol*. 2006;24(18S):7007.

Thatcher N, Chang A, Parikh P, et al. Gefitinib plus best supportive care in previously treated patients with refractory advanced non–small-cell lung cancer: results from a randomised, placebo-controlled, multicentre study (Iressa Survival Evaluation in Lung Cancer). *Lancet*. 2005;366(9496):1527–1537.

Van Meerbeeck JP, Kramer G, Van Schil PE, et al. A randomized trial of radical surgery versus thoracic radiotherapy in patients with stage IIIA-N2 non-small cell lung cancer after response to induction chemotherapy (EORTC 08941) [abstract]. *J Clin Oncol*. 2005;23(Suppl):7015.

Winton T, Livingston R, Johnson D, et al. Vinorelbine plus cisplatin vs. observation in resected non–small-cell lung cancer. *N Engl J Med*. 2005;352:2589–2597.

3

Small Cell Lung Cancer

Elizabeth Smyth and Oscar S. Breathnach

Small cell lung cancer (SCLC) represents approximately 15% to 25% of lung cancers. SCLC is characterized by its high growth fraction, rapid doubling time, and its early propensity for metastases. Initial exquisite sensitivity to both chemotherapy and radiotherapy defines its treatment paradigm. Despite this, relapse frequently occurs within months and overall survival remains poor due to the aggressive clinical nature of the disease.

EPIDEMIOLOGY

In 2008, about 28,000 new cases of SCLC were estimated to occur in the United States. The incidence of SCLC decreased from 17.26% in 1986 to 12.95% in 2002. The incidence among females increased over the same period from 28% in 1973 to 50% in 2002, reflecting cigarette consumption patterns in this group. The proportion of patients presenting over the age of 70 has also increased from 31.6% in 1985 to 44.9% in 2000.

SCLC is strongly associated with cigarette smoking. It is exceptionally rare among nonsmokers. Exposure to ionizing radiation, uranium, radon, and chloromethyl ethers has also been implicated in its etiology.

PATHOLOGY

Small cell carcinoma is characterized on light microscopy by small, round, "blue" malignant cells with scant cytoplasm, finely granular chromatin, and without distinct nucleoli. The mitotic count is high and individual cell necrosis may be seen.

The 1999 WHOInternational Association for the Study of Lung Cancer (IASLC) classification characterizes SCLC in three groups:

- Classical small cell carcinoma
- Large cell neuroendocrine cancer
- Combined small cell carcinoma, composed largely of SCLC with areas of non–small cell lung cancer (NSCLC).

Up to 30% of autopsies of SCLC demonstrate areas of differentiation into non–small cell carcinoma. This differentiation is rare in untreated specimens leading to the hypothesis that pulmonary carcinogenesis may occur in a pluripotent stem cell capable of differentiation along a variety of pathways.

A majority of SCLCs are positive on immunohistochemistry for keratin, thyroid transcription factor 1 (TTF-1), and epithelial membrane antigen. Markers of neuroendocrine differentiation such as neuron-specific enolase, chromogranin A, and synaptophysin are also commonly present. However, as these may also be present on up to 10% of NSCLC they may not be used to distinguish between these two malignancies.

GENETIC ABNORMALITIES

Cumulative exposure to tobacco smoke and other mutagens lead to carcinogenesis over a period of years. The most commonly observed mutations in SCLC include:

- P53 mutations are present in 75% to 95% of SCLCs.
- Loss of heterozygosity of 10q (PTEN site) and 9p are present on most tumors.
- Tumor suppressor gene loss due to deletion of 3p may play an important role in tumorigenesis. These include FHIT (fragile histidine triad) gene, RASSF1A, and TGFBR2 (transforming growth factor 2 receptor)
- Loss of the retinoblastoma gene occurs in 60% of SCLC, the remaining 40% having abnormal gene products.
- Telomerase enzyme activity, which is responsible for stabilization of telomerase length and cellular immortality, is present in 90% of SCLCs. This is undetectable in normal somatic cells with the exception of those with the capacity to divide indefinitely, such as basal epidermal cells and hematopoietic cells.
- C-kit and phosphorylated c-kit are present in 80% to 90% of SCLCs, which may represent a growth factor loop. Imatinib has not been useful in phase 2 trials.
- Unlike NSCLC, K-ras and p16 mutations are uncommon.

CLINICAL PRESENTATION

SCLC is a disease of the central airways, typically presenting with a large hilar mass and bulky mediastinal adenopathy. Clinical symptoms of local disease include cough, dyspnoea and postobstructive pneumonia. Seventy percent of patients present with metastatic disease causing symptoms such as weight loss, debility, neurological compromise, or bone pain. SCLC commonly metastasizes to liver, adrenals, bone marrow, bone, and brain.

Presentation as a peripheral nodule in the absence of mediastinal adenopathy is uncommon. In this situation, fine-needle aspiration of the lesion may not be adequate to differentiate SCLC from typical or atypical carcinoid tumor or from large cell neuroendocrine carcinoma, and surgical resection followed by mediastinal staging is recommended.

SCLC may also present as endocrine or neurological paraneoplastic phenomena. Lambert-Eaton syndrome presents as a proximal myopathy caused by antibodies against voltage gated calcium channels. Anti-Hu antibodies which cross-react with small cell carcinoma antigen and human neuronal components may result in paraneoplastic encephalomyelitis or a sensory neuropathy. Endocrine paraneoplastic manifestations include Cushing's syndrome or hyponatremia due to ectopic ACTH and ADH hormone production respectively.

STAGING OF SCLC

The Veteran's Administration Lung Group (VALG) two-stage classification scheme is routinely used to stage SCLC.

Limited stage disease is defined as disease limited to the ipsilateral hemithorax, which may be encompassed safely within a tolerable radiation field. Contralateral mediastinal and ipsilateral supraclavicular adenopathy are included within the definition of limited stage disease. Approximately one-third of patients present with limited stage disease. The clinical relevance of this observation lies with the fact that those with limited stage disease are treated with combined modality therapy with curative intent and those with extensive stage disease are treated with palliative chemotherapy alone.

Extensive stage disease is designated as that which has spread beyond the ipsilateral hemithorax including both contralateral hilar or supraclavicular adenopathy and cytologically malignant pleural or pericardial effusions, in addition to overt distant hematogenous metastases.

Alternative Staging Systems

The IASLC advocates the use of the more complex TNM staging system for SCLC. An overlap exists between prognosis and therapy for stage groupings within this classification, limiting its clinical utility. This system defines any patient without distant metastatic disease as limited stage.

Staging Workup

All patients with SCLC should be considered for systemic chemotherapy. The significance of the staging workup lies in guiding the use of chest radiotherapy, which will be necessary for limited stage disease only. Staging will require a history and physical examination, followed by computed tomography (CT) of chest liver and adrenal glands, head CT or magnetic resonance imaging (MRI) (preferred), and a bone scan.

Bone marrow aspirate and biopsy may be recommended in the presence of neutropenia, thrombocytopenia, or nucleated red blood cells on a peripheral smear, and no other indication of metastatic disease. Bone marrow is involved in up to 30% of patients at presentation but is the solitary site of metastatic disease in less than 5% of cases. This invasive test has a low yield in the presence of a normal serum lactate dehydrogenase (LDH) level.

SCLC is a high-grade, metabolically active tumor, and positron emission tomography (PET) is likely to be useful in the future for initial staging evaluation. However, this modality has not yet been widely studied in this disease. A PET scan is therefore optional, but may be used in addition to the other recommended investigations as part of the initial evaluation.

It is recommended that thoracocentesis be attempted on all pleural effusions that are large enough to be seen by chest radiograph. If cytological analysis does not document malignant cells, thoracoscopy may be considered to document pleural involvement and thus extensive stage disease.

A nonmalignant effusion must be documented to have repeated negative cytological examinations, be nonbloody and a nonexudatative, be considered clinically to be not directly related to the cancer or be so small as not to allow image-guided sampling.

Comprehensive staging should be performed from the outset due to the high incidence of clinically occult metastatic disease. Bone scan may be positive in up to 30% of patients without bone pain or an elevated alkaline phosphatase. CT brain or MRI document disease in 10% to 15% of patients, and 5% to 8% of these are asymptomatic. Early treatment of brain metastases will lead to lower levels of subsequent neurological morbidity.

Current NCCN guidelines recommend that staging should not delay treatment by more than 1 week. Due to the rapidly progressive nature of the disease, patients may become seriously ill within that interval.

PROGNOSTIC FACTORS

The most important adverse prognostic factors are poor performance status (PS 3–4), weight loss, and markers related to high disease burden such as LDH. In limited stage disease, female gender, age <70, normal LDH and stage I disease have a favorable prognosis. In extensive stage, a single metastatic site and normal LDH are favorable prognostic markers.

SURVIVAL

Median survival for early-stage (ES) SCLC is 8 to 13 months, and 15 to 20 months for limited stage disease. Two-year survival is 20% to 40% for late-stage (LS) SCLC and <5% for ES-SCLC. Recent SEER (survival, epidemiology, and end results) program data have demonstrated a small increase in survival: for limited-stage disease the median survival has increased by 6.4 months and the 5-year survival increased by a factor of 2 (12.1% vs. 5.2%), when the period covering 1972 to 1981 is compared to that of 1982 to 1992. For patients with ES-SCLC, progress has been limited to a 2-month gain in survival (from 7 to 9 months) over the same time frame.

CHEMOTHERAPY FOR SCLC

Chemotherapy is essential in the treatment of SCLC. For LS-SCLC with good PS (<2), recommendations are for chemotherapy with concurrent radiotherapy. For ES-SCLC, chemotherapy alone is recommended. For those who have undergone surgical resection, adjuvant chemotherapy is recommended.

SCLC is exceptionally chemosensitive, and chemotherapy substantially prolongs survival versus best supportive care. This benefit to palliative chemotherapy may even be seen in patients with severe organ dysfunction.

LS-SCLC has shown response rates of 80% to 90% with concurrent chemoradiation, with 50% to 60% CR rates. ES-SCLCs show response rates of 60% to 80%, with one-quarter of these having a CR. The median duration of response is 6 to 8 months. Median survival after recurrence is 4 months.

The chemotherapeutic agents commonly used in the treatment of SCLC are as follows:

- Platinum compounds (cisplatin, carboplatin)
- Podophyllotoxins (etoposide, tenoposide)
- Camptothecins (irinotecan, topotecan)
- Alkylating agents (ifosfamide, cyclophosphamide)
- Anthracyclines (doxorubicin, epirubicin)
- Taxanes (paclitaxel, docetaxel)
- Vinca alkaloids (vincristine)

Platinum-based regimens appear to be more effective than non–platinum-based regimens. The cisplatin-plus-etoposide (PE or EP) regimen demonstrated preclinical synergism and is now the most frequently used combination in the limited stage setting, based on activity and toxicity profiles. Due to the limited risk of pneumonitis and manageable hematologic toxicity profile, this is the recommended regimen in conjunction with radiotherapy for LS-SCLC.

Clinically, carboplatin is often substituted for cisplatin due to the decreased risk of emesis, nephropathy, and neuropathy. Carboplatin use involves a higher risk of myelosuppression. Substitution of carboplatin for cisplatin in LS-SCLC has not been extensively evaluated and is recommended only if cisplatin is poorly tolerated or contraindicated. It is more acceptable in extensive stage disease as chemotherapy for these patients is not curative.

Irinotecan-Based Regimens

Multiple trials are evaluating whether the substitution of irinotecan for etoposide in ES-SCLC can improve on current outcomes. A phase 3 Japanese trial showed a higher response rate (84% vs. 66%) and longer median survival (12.8 vs. 9.4 months) and 2-year survival (19.5 vs. 5.4 months) when compared with the etoposide regimen. Hematological toxicity was less pronounced with the irinotecan regimen but diarrhea was more common.

A larger trial with a similar but not identical design conducted in the United States failed to replicate these results. An ongoing SWOG trial (SWOG 0124) is currently underway, using identical regimens to the original Japanese design. Recent initial pharmocogenomic and toxicity data were presented at the American Society of Clinical Oncology Meeting (ASCO) 2007, which showed significant differences in the toxicity between American and Japanese populations, in addition to differences in single nucleotide polymorphisms (SNPs) related to irinotecan metabolism. Whether these genetic differences account for differences in toxicities and efficacy will require further investigation.

Further evidence relating to the efficacy of irinotecan in ES-SCLC is seen in the results of a multicenter Scandinavian IRIS trial where patients were randomized to carboplatin and either irinotecan or etoposide. At a minimum 1-year follow-up presented at ASCO 2007 the irinotecan arm showed a higher response rate, longer median (8.5 vs. 7.1 months), and 1-year survival (34% vs. 24%).

Chemotherapy in the Elderly

Individuals over the age of 70 currently represent more than 40% of those diagnosed with SCLC, a figure that is likely to increase. Lower organ reserves may lead to increased toxicity due to chemotherapy. Despite this, elderly patients have similar survival rates when compared to younger patients.

Less intensive treatment is associated with decreased toxicity but inferior survival in those with a good PS (0–2) in this age group. Therefore, it is functional status rather than chronological age that must inform clinical decision making. Those who are functionally independent in their activities of daily living should undergo the recommended combination chemotherapy and radiotherapy as clinically indicated.

EXPERIMENTAL THERAPIES

Strategies to improve on standard two-drug regimens include addition of a third agent, maintenance or consolidation therapy, alternating or sequential combination therapies, and higher-dose therapies. Overall these approaches have failed to deliver significant improvements on the results yielded by standard approaches.

Additional Agents

Despite promising phase 2 data, the addition of paclitaxel to EP in ES-SCLC has shown no benefit in two phase-3 trials. In the larger trial, median survival and 1-year survival were comparable, but there was an excess of treatment-related mortality (6.5% vs. 2.4%) in the paclitaxel-containing arm. The addition of ifosfamide has been shown in one trial to be associated with a modest survival advantage, but this effect has not been uniformly observed. Multidrug regimens such as EP plus cyclophosphamide and epirubicin have shown statistically significant small increases in response rate, median survival and 1-year survival, at the expense of significantly increased hematological toxicity, including rates of febrile neutropenia and blood product transfusion.

Maintenance therapy or consolidation therapy beyond the standard 4 to 6 cycles of treatment carries a minor prolongation of response with no subsequent increase in survival and is associated with increased cumulative toxicity. Recently, maintenance therapy with bevacizumab was associated with the development of tracheoesophageal fistulae in patients with LS-SCLC receiving bevacizumab, carboplatin, and irinotecan as part of a phase 2 trial. Bevacizumab is not recommended for the treatment of SCLC.

Dose Escalation and Dose-Dense Therapy

Increased tumor cell exposure to chemotherapeutic agents can be achieved by increasing the drug dose or by decreasing the interval between cycles. This is facilitated by the use of myeloid growth factors. Numerous trials have demonstrated a higher response rate in patients receiving higher doses of chemotherapy. Most have not demonstrated a comparable increase in survival, but have documented increased toxicity. The only trial to demonstrate a survival benefit randomized 100 patients with LS-SCLC to conventional-dose cisplatin, cyclophosphamide, doxorubicin, and etoposide (CD-PCDE) or high-dose PCDE (HD-PDCE) that used 20% higher doses on the first cycle. Rates of complete response were higher with HD-PDCE (67% vs. 54%) as were survival rates at 2 and 5 years (42% vs. 20% and 26% vs. 8%, respectively).

Higher chemotherapy dose levels may be achieved using hematopoietic growth factory support (e.g., G-CSF or GM-CSF). Increasing dose intensity using these drugs has not improved survival when compared to the maximum tolerated standard chemotherapy doses without their use. Use of CSFs has been documented in two reports to be associated with increased toxicity and decreased survival. Meta-analysis of dose intensity in trials using a CAV-CAE-EP regimen and its relationship to survival showed a small and insignificant increase in median survival in patients with ES-SCLC when increased dose intensity was used.

Despite initial promising reports, the use of early or late intensification of chemotherapy with hematopoietic cell transplantation with either bone marrow or peripheral blood precursor cells has not been shown to be of benefit.

Targeted Agents

Advances in SCLC with cytotoxic chemotherapy have been small, and new approaches to treatment are required. Newer biologically targeted agents that have been investigated include bevacizumab, temosirolimus, matrix metalloproteinase inhibitors, the tyrosine kinase inhibitors imatinib and vandetanib, and the antisense oligonucleotide olibmerson. As yet, none have demonstrated significant activity in vivo, and phase 2 and 3 trials are ongoing.

THORACIC RADIOTHERAPY FOR LS-SCLC

Local recurrence or tumor progression occurs in up to 80% of those with LS-SCLC treated by chemotherapy alone. This high recurrence rate and overall survival may be improved by the addition of thoracic radiation therapy (TRT). Meta-analysis suggests that TRT is associated with an increase in local control of 23% (24% to 47%) and a 5% absolute gain in overall survival at 2 years (20.5% vs. 15%). Survival benefit is gained at an increase in toxicity.

Radiation Fields

The use of limited-field TRT is currently the gold standard. This includes all gross disease present at the time of planning (postchemotherapy volume) and all nodal regions at the time of diagnosis (prechemotherapy volume). Treatment with smaller treatment fields is associated with a reduction in toxicity from combined-modality therapy without diminishing local control rates.

Fractionation Schedule

Standard schedules consist of single daily treatments of 1.8 to 2.0 Gy 5 days per week over 6 weeks. Accelerated hyperfractionation implies treatment delivery over a shorter period of time (acceleration) with an increased number of fractions (hyperfractionation). Radiation treatment occurs two to three times daily with smaller fraction sizes. These treatment regimens are associated with more acute toxicity, increased daily treatment time, and are more complex in terms of treatment delivery. Superior survival outcomes in recent trials using hyperfractionated TRT of 45 Gy over 3 weeks of twice-daily treatment have led to the establishment of this regimen as a standard of care within the field. The CALGB 30610 trial aims to compare directly twice-daily short-course TRT (45 Gy b.i.d) to longer traditional schedules.

Integration With Chemotherapy

Concurrent, sequential, and alternating patterns of delivery have been investigated. Concurrent or alternating regimens allow uninterrupted delivery of chemotherapy—essential due to the systemic nature of SCLC. These methods have been associated with increased toxicity (esophagitis, pneumonitis, and myelosupression), but improved survival when compared to sequential treatment.

Conflicting evidence exists regarding the optimal timing of TRT relative to chemotherapy, possibly due to the heterogeneity of the chemotherapy regimens and chemotherapy dose intensity between the trials involved. Studies that showed a significant survival advantage for early TRT (given with the first cycle of chemotherapy) used cisplatin-based drug regimens and had high rates of dose delivery. Those that did not show a benefit to early TRT did not use cisplatin-based regimens and/or showed a lower rate of dose delivery in the early arms.

Despite this conflicting data regarding the optimal timing of TRT delivery, the studies using standard EP chemotherapy delivery with minimal dose reductions all showed a clear benefit to early TRT. To this end, early TRT integrated with cycle one or two of chemotherapy is the standard of care for LS-SCLC.

TREATMENT OF RELAPSED AND REFRACTORY SCLC

Despite initial chemosensitivity, most patients with SCLC will eventually relapse and require salvage chemotherapy. Disease that occurs more than 3 months after completion of first-line chemotherapy is referred to as *relapsed SCLC*. The term *refractory disease* refers to disease that has progressed through first-line chemotherapy or recurred within 3 months of treatment completion. In general, relapsed disease is more sensitive to salvage chemotherapy than refractory disease, with response rates of 25% versus 10%, respectively. Median survival of relapsed SCLC is 2 to 6 months. Prognostic indicators include disease burden (limited or extensive stage), performance status, and whether the disease is relapsed or refractory. Response rates to second-line therapy relate to time to relapse from initial treatment, response to initial treatment, first-line chemotherapy regimen used, and performance status.

Single-agent chemotherapies that have documented activity in relapsed or refractory SCLC include camptothecin derivatives toptecan and irinotecan, taxanes, oral etoposide, vinorelbine, and gemcitabine. Phase 3 trial data comparing CAV to IV topotecan in patients who had relapsed more than 2 months after completing therapy (mostly EP) showed similar response rates (18% vs. 24%) and median survival (25 vs. 24.7 weeks). The topotecan group reported better control of symptoms including dyspnea, anorexia and fatigue, and less neutropenia than the CAV group, but significantly more thrombocytopenia and anemia. This led to topotecan being recommended as the second-line agent for SCLC that has relapsed within 2 to 3 months of treatment. The efficacy and toxicity of oral topotecan is similar to the IV formulation, which is not yet commercially available in the United States.

Combination chemotherapies may have slightly higher response rates in second-line therapy, but are also more toxic. For those with relapsed disease and a long relapse-free interval, it may be feasible to reintroduce the initial induction chemotherapy.

ROLE OF SURGERY IN SCLC

SCLC is a disseminated disease at presentation, including those with apparently limited stage disease. The futility of surgery as the primary treatment modality has been documented by the historical cohort of clinical trials. Early-stage SCLC (ES-SCLC) is diagnosed in less than 5% of patients. Most data relating to resection of SCLC are uncontrolled. However, when SCLC presents as a solitary pulmonary nodule and is resected, 5-year survival ranged from 43% to 53%.

Patients with clinical stage I disease (T1-2, N0) may undergo surgical resection following standard staging and evaluation of the mediastinum by mediastinoscopy or other surgical staging to outrule occult nodal disease. Those who undergo full resection with lobectomy and mediastinal nodal dissection should be treated with postoperative chemotherapy if there is no evidence of nodal metastases and with concurrent chemotherapy and radiation to the mediastinum in the presence of positive lymph nodes. In addition, those with presumed complete remission following surgery and adjuvant chemotherapy should undergo prophylactic cranial irradiation (PCI).

PROPHYLACTIC CRANIAL IRRADIATION FOR PATIENTS WITH SCLC

The brain represents a sanctuary site for SCLC due to the relative impermeability of the blood–brain barrier to commonly used chemotherapeutic agents. This leads to a significant rate of intracerebral metastasis as a site of relapse or failure following complete response to systemic therapy. The incidence of brain metastases at 2 years is 80% leading to significant morbidity and mortality. Previously, concerns existed regarding the late neurologic toxicity of PCI—especially in LS-SCLC. This predominantly occurred in studies using high doses per fraction (>3.0 Gy), high total dose, and concurrent chemotherapy. There is less neurotoxicity when given sequentially following completion of chemotherapy and when lower doses per fraction are used.

Two meta-analyses suggest a benefit to PCI with a decrease of 25% in the cumulative 3-year incidence of brain metastases from 58% to 23% and small increase in the overall 3-year survival in the PCI group (from 15.3% to 20.1%). A recent trial of the European Organisation for Research and Treatment of Cancer (EORTC) assessed the role of PCI in the ES-SCLC population. Those who were deemed by the treating physician to have responded to 4 to 6 cycles of standard chemotherapy were randomized to PCI or observation. Radiation doses varied depending on the institution. Those who underwent PCI had a significantly decreased incidence of symptomatic brain metastases at 1 year (15% vs. 40%) and a significantly higher 1-year survival rate (27% vs. 13%). Treatment with PCI was well tolerated with most common toxicities being mild headache (42%), nausea (36%), and fatigue (10%).

PCI is currently recommended for patients with limited stage disease and ES-SCLC who achieve a complete response, who have only radiation scarring or a decrease in the tumor mass to less than 10% of the original volume on CT following induction chemoradiation. It may be considered for those with a partial response to initial treatment. It is not recommended for those with multiple co-morbidities, poor PS (3–4), or impaired cognition. It should not be given concurrently with chemotherapy due to the additive neurotoxic effects.

REGIMENS

The most important factors that predict a favorable outcome are extent of disease, good performance status, biology of the small cell tumor, and smoking cessation. Several combinations have been used successfully (Table 3.1).

TABLE 3.1. *Summary of commonly used chemotherapeutic regimens*

Regimen	Dose	Duration
EP		
Etoposide	120 mg/m^2 i.v. d 1–3	
Cisplatin	60 mg/m^2 i.v.d 1	Cycles repeated every 4 wk, for four cycles
Etoposide	100 mg/m^{2}i.v. d 1–3	
Carboplatin	AUC 6 i.v. d 1	
Etoposide	100 mg/m^2 i.v. d 1–3	
Cisplatin	25 mg/m^2 i.v. d 1–3	
Etoposide	80 mg/m^2 i.v. d 1–3	Cycles repeated every 3 wk, for four cycles
Cisplatin	80 mg/m^2 i.v. d 1	
CI		
Cisplatin	60 mg/m^2 i.v. on d 1	Every 4 wk, for four cycles
Irinotecan	60 mg/m^2 i.v. on d 1, 8, and 15	
CAV		
Cyclophosphamide	1,000 mg/m^2 i.v. d 1	Cycles repeated every 3 wk, continued for four to six cycles
Doxorubicin	45 mg/m^2 i.v. d 1	
Vincristine	1 mg/m^2 i.v. d 1	
CAE		
Cyclophosphamide	1,000 mg/m^2 i.v. d 1	Cycles repeated every 3 wk, continued for four to six cycles
Doxorubicin	45 mg/m^2 i.v. d 1	
Etoposide	50 mg/m^2 i.v. d 1–3	
CAVE		
Cyclophosphamide	1,000 mg/m^2 IV d 1	Cycles repeated every 3 wk, continued for four to six cycles
Doxorubicin	50 mg/m^2 i.v. d 1	
Vincristine	1.5 mg/m^2 i.v. d 1	
Etoposide	60 mg/m^2 i.v. d 1–5	

AUC, area under the curve; EP, etoposide/cisplatin; CI, cisplatin/irinotecan; CAV, cyclophosphamide/doxorubicin/vincristine; CAE, cyclophosphamide/doxoruicin/etoposide; CDVE, cyctophosphamide/doxorubicin/vincristine/etoposide.

SUGGESTED READINGS

Albain KS, Crowley JJ, Hutchins L, Gandara D. Predictors of survival following relapse or progression of small cell lung cancer. Southwest Oncology Group Study 8605 report and analysis of recurrent disease database. Cancer 1993;72:1184.

Auperin A, Arriagada R, Pignon JP, et al. Prophylactic cranial irradiation for patients with small-cell lung cancer in complete remission. Prophylactic Cranial Irradiation Overview Collaborative Group. N Engl J Med 1999;341:476.

Chute JP, Chen T, Feigal E, et al. Twenty years of phase III trials for patients with extensive-stage small-cell lung cancer: perceptible progress. J Clin Oncol 1999;17:1794.

Govindan R, Page N, Morgensztern D, et al. Changing epidemiology of small-cell lung cancer in the United States over the last 30 years: Analysis of the Surveillance, Epidemiologic, and End Results database. J Clin Oncol 2006;24:4539–4544.

Hanna N, Bunn PA Jr, Langer C, et al. Randomized phase III trial comparing irinotecan/cisplatin with etoposide/cisplatin in patients with previously untreated extensive-stage disease small-cell lung cancer. J Clin Oncol 2006;24:2038.

Janne PA, Freidlin B, Saxman S, et al. Twenty-five years of clinical research for patients with limited-stage small cell lung carcinoma in North America. Cancer 2002;95:1528.

Noda K, Nishiwaki Y, Kawahara M, et al. Irinotecan plus cisplatin compared with etoposide plus cisplatin for extensive small-cell lung cancer. N Engl J Med 2002;346:85.

Pijls-Johannesma M, Ruysscher D, Lambin P, et al. Early versus late chest radiotherapy for limited stage small cell lung cancer. Cochrane Database Syst Rev 2005;CD004700.

Slotman B, Faivre-Finn C, Kramer G, et al. Prophylactic cranial irradiation in extensive small-cell lung cancer. N Engl J Med 2007;357:664.

Travis WD, Colby TV, Corrin B, et al. Histological Typing of Lung and Pleural Tumours. World Health Organisation International Histological Classification of Tumours. Berlin Springer-Verlag 1999.

SECTION 3

Digestive System

4

Esophageal Cancer

Syed I. Haidar and Gregory D. Leonard

Esophageal cancer is the ninth most commonly occurring cancer worldwide and the sixth most common cause of cancer mortality (1). It is highly curable in its earliest stages; however, it usually presents with advanced disease. Despite the last two decades of progress in clinical research, the median survival time for a patient with symptoms of a primary esophageal cancer is less than 18 months. Most research and controversy in the treatment of esophageal cancer currently focuses on the role of chemoradiotherapy as either primary or adjuvant therapy for esophageal cancer.

EPIDEMIOLOGY

United States

- Esophageal cancer was estimated to account for 1% of all malignancies and 6% of all gastrointestinal malignancies in 2008 (2). The age-adjusted incidence from 2000 to 2004 is 4.6 cases per 100,000 population (http://seer.cancer.gov/csr/1975_2004).
- Approximately 16,470 new cases and 14,280 deaths were estimated for 2008.
- The median age at diagnosis is 69 years. This cancer rarely occurs in patients younger than 25 years.
- Esophageal cancer is two to four times more frequent in men than in women. Siewert type 1 tumors (adenocarcinoma [ADC]) are eight to nine times more common in men than in women.
- Rates of occurrence of esophageal cancer are approximately threefold higher among blacks than among whites.
- Squamous cell carcinoma (SCC) is more common in black men; ADC is more common in white men.
- Five-year relative survival rates were 5% from 1975 to 1977, 10% from 1984 to 1986, and 16% from 1996 to 2003 (2).

Rest of the World

- There are approximately 500,000 cases of esophageal cancer in the world, but there is marked geographic variation. Regions with clusters of high rates include China (e.g., Linxian), Iran, France, and South Africa.
- In the 1970s, approximately 90% of esophageal cancers were SCCs. The incidence of ADCs has increased dramatically and currently accounts for approximately 60% to 70% of new cases—a rate of acceleration greater than that of any other cancer in the United States.

ETIOLOGY

Adenocarcinoma

- Barrett's esophagus
- Obesity
- Gastroesophageal reflux disease (GERD), which can be caused by obesity and might result in Barrett's esophagus

57

Squamous Cell Carcinoma

- Tobacco
- Alcohol
- Predisposing conditions:
  - Tylosis (SCC)
  - Achalasia
  - Esophageal diverticula and webs (SCC)
  - Plummer-Vinson syndrome
  - Human papillomavirus (HPV)
  - Celiac disease
- Less significant causes include environmental exposure and dietary factors.

BARRETT'S ESOPHAGUS

Barrett's esophagus, perhaps as a result of GERD, is the most important risk factor (100 times risk increase over other factors) for ADC.

Screening recommendations (no randomized trial data for surveillance practices) are as follows:

- For no dysplasia, endoscopy every 2 to 3 years
- For low-grade dysplasia, endoscopy every 6 months for 12 months and then yearly
- For high-grade dysplasia, esophagectomy or three monthly endoscopies or photodynamic therapy (PDT)

CLINICAL PRESENTATION

The most common clinical presentations of esophageal cancer are listed in Table 4.1 and are usually related to local compression or infiltration symptoms or generalized malaise and anorexia.

The classic triad for presentation of esophageal cancer is as follows:

- Asthenia
- Anorexia
- Analgesia (for dysphagia)

DIAGNOSIS

- Symptoms
  - Dysphagia or odynophagia
  - Hematemesis
  - Dyspepsia

TABLE 4.1.   *Clinical presentation of esophageal cancer*

Symptoms	Patients with symptoms (%)
Dysphagia (solids usually before liquids)	80–96
Weight loss	42–46
Odynophagia	≤50
Epigastric or retrosternal pain	≤20
Cough or hoarseness	≤5
Tracheoesophageal fistula	1–13

- Hoarseness
- Dyspnea
- Anorexia
- Signs (usually late presentation)
  - Horner syndrome
  - Left supraclavicular lymphadenopathy (Virchow's node)
  - Cachexia
  - Hepatomegaly
  - Bone metastases (rare, but paraneoplastic hypercalcemia can occur)
- Upper gastrointestinal endoscopy
  - This diagnostic procedure is the gold standard. The combination of endoscopic biopsies and brush cytology has an accuracy of greater than 90% in making a tissue diagnosis of esophageal cancer.
- Barium contrast radiography
  - This diagnostic procedure can document contour and motility abnormalities and unexpected airway fistula and may be useful when the entire esophagus has not been visualized endoscopically. However, a tissue diagnosis is needed for definitive diagnosis.

PATHOLOGY

- Most newly diagnosed patients have ADC, but there are contrasting reports on their relative prognosis. Less than 1% of esophageal tumors are lymphoma, melanoma, carcinosarcoma, or small cell carcinoma.
- Fifty percent of tumors arise in the lower one-third of the esophagus, 25% arise in the upper esophagus, and 25% of tumors occur in the middle one-third of the esophagus (2).

STAGING

The American Joint Commission for Cancer (AJCC) has designated staging of cancer by TNM classification, which defines the anatomic extent of disease (3) (Table 4.2). Of note, cervical adenopathy in tumors in the lower one-third of esophagus is M1 as opposed to N1.

The Siewert classification subclassifies gastroesophageal junction tumors into three types according to their anatomic location: type I are distal esophagus tumors, type II are cardia tumors, and type III are subcardia gastric tumors (4).

Staging workup can include the following:

- Computerized tomography (CT) scan: CT scan of the chest and abdomen can demonstrate evidence of spread of tumor to lymph nodes or distant metastases to the liver (35%), lungs (20%), bone (9%), and adrenals (5%). CT scan may underestimate the depth of tumor invasion and peri-esophageal lymph node involvement in up to 50% of cases. Magnetic resonance imaging (MRI) provides similar results to CT.
- Endoscopic ultrasound (EUS): EUS may be helpful when metastases are not detected by CT or other imaging modalities. EUS is the optimal technique for locoregional staging. A meta-analysis demonstrated greater than 71% sensitivity in staging preoperative depth of invasion (T) and greater than 60% sensitivity for locoregional lymph nodes (N); specificity was greater than 67% and greater than 40%, respectively (5).
- Positron emission tomography (PET): PET is useful when CT is negative for metastatic disease, and the diagnosis can change management of cancer in 25% to 40% of patients (6,7). Bronchoscopy is required in tumors less than 25 mm from the incisors to exclude invasion of the posterior membranous trachea or tracheoesophageal fistula.

TABLE 4.2.   *Definition of TNM and stage grouping*

TNM stage

Primary tumor (T)

Primary tumor cannot be assessed
T0: No evidence of primary tumor
Tis: Carcinoma in situ
T1: Tumor invades lamina propria or submucosa
T2: Tumor invades muscularis propria
T3: Tumor invades adventitia
T4: Tumor invades adjacent structures

Regional lymph nodes (N)

N1: Regional lymph node metastasis
NX: Regional lymph nodes cannot be assessed
N0: No regional lymph node metastasis

Distant metastasis (M)

MX: Distant metastasis cannot be assessed
M0: No distant metastasis
M1: Distant metastasis
Tumors of the lower thoracic esophagus
M1a: Metastasis in celiac lymph nodes
M1b: Other distant metastasis
Tumors of the midthoracic esophagus
M1a: Not applicable
M1b: Other distant metastasis
Tumors of the upper thoracic esophagus
M1a: Metastasis in cervical nodes
M1b: Other distant metastasis

Stage grouping

Stage 0	Tis	N0	M0
Stage I	T1	N0	M0
Stage IIA	T2	N0	M0
	T3	N0	M0
Stage IIB	T1	N1	M0
	T2	N1	M0
Stage III	T3	N1	M0
	T4	Any N	M0
Stage IV	Any T	Any N	M1
Stage IVA	Any T	Any N	M1a
Stage IVB	Any T	Any N	M1b

TREATMENT

Surgery

- Surgery alone remains a standard treatment for esophageal cancer with resectable local or locoregional disease. In 1993, surgery was used as a component of treatment in 34% of patients. Surgery alone was used in 18% of patients (8).
- Recent improvements in staging techniques and patient selection have improved surgical morbidity and mortality. Operative mortality rates are now less than 5%. Surgical expertise is a major contributor to survival, with better outcomes in high-volume centers. Resection is possible in approximately 50% of patients (9). Five-year survival in patients with surgical resection is 5% to 25%.
- Surgical principles include a wide resection of the primary tumor with the goal of an R0 resection (no residual tumor), including more than 5-cm resection margins plus regional lymphadenectomy. Intraoperative frozen section can assess for residual disease, which, if present, is considered an R1 (microscopic tumor) or R2 (macroscopic tumor) resection.
- In general, patients with cervical carcinoma of the esophagus are not considered candidates for surgical resection; chemoradiation is favored in these patients.
- Surgical approaches include the following:
  - Transthoracic resection: En bloc esophagectomy requires laparotomy and thoracotomy, for example, total thoracic or transthoracic (Lewis) procedures. A three-field lymph node dissection (extended lymphadenectomy) includes superior mediastinum and cervical lymphadenectomy. It is the treatment of choice in Japan, but is associated with increased toxicity and has a questionable survival advantage.
  - Transhiatal esophagectomy: This includes laparotomy and cervical anastomosis. This technique avoids thoracotomy.

Chemoradiotherapy (Combined-Modality Approach)

Although no large prospective randomized trials have directly compared primary chemoradiation with surgery, definitive chemoradiation for locoregional carcinoma of the esophagus is considered an alternative to surgery.

Inoperable Disease

- The Radiation Therapy Oncology Group (RTOG) 85-01 trial (10) demonstrated a survival advantage (14 vs. 9 months median survival and 27% vs. 0% 5-year survival) in favor of chemoradiotherapy over radiotherapy alone (Table 4.3). A number of randomized trials of chemoradiotherapy versus radiotherapy alone have failed to duplicate the results of RTOG 85-01; however, a recent Cochrane review has confirmed the superiority of chemoradiotherapy versus radiotherapy in fit, motivated patients (11). For operable disease, chemoradiotherapy is an alternative to surgery for patients with operable esophageal cancer. Upper thoracic esophageal (above the aortic arch) tumors and T4 or N1 tumors are usually considered unresectable.

Operable Disease

Trials that used surgery after chemoradiotherapy in patients who responded and higher doses of radiation for patients who did not respond failed to show a benefit for the group receiving surgery. A better determinant of the role of surgery after chemoradiotherapy is evident from two recent trials:

- In the first trial, patients with locally advanced but resectable tumors were treated with chemoradiotherapy, and patients with at least a partial response were randomized to continued chemoradiotherapy or surgery (12). There was no difference in overall survival, but early mortality and length of hospital stay were less in the chemoradiotherapy arm (12.8% vs. 3.5% [$P = 0.03$])
- The second trial randomized patients with locally advanced tumors to either definitive chemoradiotherapy or chemoradiotherapy (lower doses of radiation) and surgery (13). There was no significant difference in survival outcomes (17.7 vs. 19.3 months, respectively) between the two groups of patients.

Radiation dose escalation has not proved to be beneficial. A recent trial examining this approach was closed after an interim analysis indicated that there would be no advantage with higher doses of radiation.

TABLE 4.3. *Radiation Therapy Oncology Group (RTOG) 85-01 trial of chemoradiotherapy versus radiotherapy alone in esophageal cancer*

Number of patients	Histology	Treatment	Median survival	5-Year survival	P-value
121	SCC = 88%	Cisplatin 75 mg/m² d 1	14.1 mo vs. 9.3 mo	27% vs. 0%	0.0001
	ADC = 12%	5-FU 1,000 mg/m²/d d 1–4 50 Gy of radiation wk 1, 5 Cisplatin/5-FU wk 8, 11 vs. 64 Gy of radiation 2 Gy/fx			

SCC, squamous cell carcinoma; ADC, adenocarcinoma; 5-FU, 5-fluorouracil; Gy, Gray of radiation; fx, fraction of radiation.
Source: From Cooper JS, Guo MD, Herskovic A, et al. Chemoradiotherapy of locally advanced esophageal cancer long-term follow-up of a prospective randomized trial (RTOG 85-01). *JAMA* 1999;281:1623–1627, with permission.

Neoadjuvant Chemoradiotherapy (Trimodality Approach)

- The rationale for preoperative chemoradiotherapy was first studied by Leichman et al. in 21 patients with SCC. Patients were treated with 3,000 cGy of radiation and with two cycles of concurrent 5-fluorouracil (5-FU) and cisplatin (14). An additional 2,000 cGy of radiation was given postoperatively when residual tumor was seen at surgery. The pathologic complete response was 37%, with a median survival of 18 months.
- A number of prospective randomized phase 3 trials have addressed the issue of whether preoperative chemoradiotherapy offers any benefit over surgery alone (15–23). Much debate exists over interpretation of these trials. Walsh et al. demonstrated a significant benefit in median survival (16 vs. 11 months, $P = 0.01$) and 3 years survival (32% vs. 6%, $P = 0.01$) for patients receiving preoperative chemoradiotherapy (15). However, limitations of this trial include poor surgical outcome, small numbers of patients studied, and the fact all patients had ADC. The Cancer and Leukemia Group B (CALGB) 9781 was designed as a prospective randomized Intergroup trial of trimodality therapy versus surgery in 56 patients with stages I–III esophageal cancer. Median survival was 4.48 years versus 1.79 years ($P = 0.002$) in favor of trimodality therapy (23).
- In a meta-analysis of 12 randomized trials, the benefit of chemotherapy and surgery was observed over surgery alone (24). Overall survival in individual patient data from nine trials showed an absolute benefit of 4% (increased from 16% to 20%). The disease-free survival over 5 years showed an absolute benefit of 4% (increased from 6% to 10%). This meta-analysis showed a small but significant benefit for neoadjuvant chemotherapy over surgery alone ($P = 0.03$).
- Neoadjuvant chemoradiation has shown a trend toward superiority versus neoadjuvant chemotherapy alone in patients with locally advanced but resectable tumors. In one randomized trial, patients received chemotherapy followed by surgery or chemotherapy followed by chemoradiation for 3 weeks, followed by surgery. A complete resection was possible in 77% versus 85% in arms A and B, respectively. Complete histologic response was 2.5% with chemotherapy and 17% after chemoradiation ($P = 0.06$). The median survival was 21.2 versus 32.8, months and 3 years survival was 27% versus 43% respectively ($P = 0.14$) (25).
- A meta-analysis in 2007 clarified the benefits of neoadjuvant chemoradiation or chemotherapy versus surgery alone. The absolute difference in survival between neoadjuvant chemoradiation versus surgery alone was 13%, while absolute difference in survival between neoadjuvant chemotherapy versus surgery alone was 7% ($P = 0.05$) (26).

Adjuvant Chemoradiotherapy

There are few data available on the use of postoperative chemoradiotherapy in esophageal cancer.

- A recent trial found a statistically significant survival advantage for postoperative chemoradiotherapy compared to surgery alone in gastroesophageal and gastric cancers (Table 4.4) (27). Based on these data, adjuvant chemoradiotherapy has been recommended for ADC tumors of the lower esophagus.

TABLE 4.4.   *Intergroup-116 trial of adjuvant chemoradiotherapy versus surgery alone in gastric or gastroesophageal adenocarcinomas*

Number of patients	Surgery	Treatment	Median survival	3-Year survival	P-value
556	D0 54%	Surgery followed by	36 mo vs. 27 mo	50% vs. 41%	0.005
	D1 36%	5-FU 425 mg/m^2/d d 1–5			
	D2 10%	LV 20 mg/m^2/d d 1–5[a]			
		4,500 cGy radiation d 28, 180 cGy/d			
		5 d/wk for 5 wk vs.			
		surgery alone			

5-FU, 5-fluorouracil; LV, leucovorin.

[a]Two further courses of chemotherapy were given 1 month apart after radiation. Additional 5-FU 400 mg/m^2 and LV 20 mg/m^2 were given on the first 4 days and the last 3 days of radiotherapy.

It is possible that the survival benefit associated with the use of chemoradiotherapy results from reductions in local recurrences and thus compensates for inadequate surgery (only 10% of patients had the recommended D2 resection).

Radiation Therapy

Radiation therapy alone is generally considered palliative and is used in patients who are unable to tolerate chemoradiotherapy. No randomized trials of preoperative single-modality radiotherapy have demonstrated a survival benefit in patients. Similarly, there is no benefit with single-modality postoperative radiotherapy in patients.

Chemotherapy

- Single-agent chemotherapy demonstrates response rates of 15% to 25%. Combination chemotherapy response rates are 25% to 45%, but this has not definitively improved survival in advanced disease states.
- Cisplatin with 5-FU is the most frequently used regimen for both combined-modality therapy in locoregional disease and systemic therapy for palliation.
- SCC may be more sensitive to chemotherapy, but there is no difference in long-term outcome between SCC and ADC.
- New chemotherapeutic agents have demonstrated encouraging response rates.

Preoperative (Neoadjuvant) Chemotherapy

- The poor survival, even for patients with clinically localized carcinoma of the esophagus, suggests that occult metastases are present at diagnosis, thereby providing the impetus to add systemic therapy early during patient management.
- In the two largest trials examining preoperative chemotherapy, the Intergroup (INT 0113) trial (28) showed no survival benefit, whereas the Medical Research Council (MRC) trial (29) demonstrated a 3-month median survival advantage for chemotherapy over surgery alone.
- The following differences in the two studies may have contributed to their different outcomes:
  - Chemotherapy was of longer duration and was with higher doses in INT 0113. This therapy may have been detrimental by delaying access to surgery and causing more toxicity.
  - Surgery was performed in only 80% of the patients in the chemotherapy arm in INT 0113 compared to 92% in the MRC trial. Outcome for surgery alone was poor in the MRC trial, thereby possibly exaggerating the benefits of chemotherapy.
  - Radiation therapy off protocol (equally distributed between treatment arms) was available in the MRC trial.
  - A larger sample size in the MRC trial may have facilitated detection of a statistically significant result.
- One Japanese study suggests neoadjuvant chemotherapy is highly superior to adjuvant chemotherapy (HR = 0.64, $P = 0.014$) (30).
- A recent trial assessed the use of perioperative epirubicin, cisplatin, and 5-FU (ECF) chemotherapy or surgery alone in esophagogastric cancer. In 503 patients, 15% had esophagogastric cancer and 11% had esophageal cancer. Adjuvant chemotherapy increased progression-free survival and resectability rates and showed a trend toward improved survival ($P = 0.06$) (31).

Palliation

- Palliative options can be split into local or systemic options.
- Local therapies include external beam and brachytherapy radiation. This approach can palliate dysphagia in approximately 80% of patients. PDT has also been approved by the U. S. Food and Drug Administration (FDA) for this indication. For rapid palliation, laser or balloon dilatation and stenting is recommended. The placement of a gastrostomy or jejunostomy tube may improve the patient's nutritional status.

- The systemic chemotherapy options in esophageal cancer are improving.
- Cisplatin combined with 5-FU is the most commonly used regimen, but this did not demonstrate a statistically significant benefit over cisplatin alone when tested in a randomized trial of patients with advanced SCC of the esophagus (32).
- Most data on chemotherapy in advanced esophageal cancer are extrapolated from trials in gastric cancer that often include gastroesophageal tumors. In Europe, ECF is frequently used because of its superior survival compared to 5-FU, doxorubicin, and methotrexate (FAMTX) in advanced esophagogastric cancer (33).
- A trial in metastatic or unresectable gastric and gastroesophageal cancer evaluated docetaxel, cisplatin, and 5-FU (DCF) and cisplatin and 5-fluorouracil (CF). Time to disease progression improved from 3.7 months to 5.2 months (hazard ratio 1.704), and median overall survival improved from 8.5 months to 10.2 months ($P = 0.0053$) in patients receiving DCF compared to those receiving CF (34).
- Another trial evaluated capecitabine and oxaliplatin as alternatives to cisplatin and flurouracil. In a two by two design, patients were randomly assigned to ECF (epirubicin/cisplatin/5-flurouracil), ECX (epirubicin/cisplatin/capecitabine), EOF (epirubicin/oxaliplatin/5-flurouracil), EOX (epirubicin/oxaliplatin/capecitabine). The median survival time was 9.9, 9.9, 9.3, and 11.2 months respectively. Overall survival was higher with EOX ($P = 0.02$) (35).
- The distribution, treatment, and survival in patients with esophageal cancer according to stage in the United States are given in Table 4.5.

TABLE 4.5. *Stage, distribution, treatment, and survival of esophageal cancers in the United States*

Stage	Distribution (%)	Treatment	5-Year relative survival rates (%)
Localized (I and II)	25	Surgery Chemoradiotherapy if surgery not possible Adjuvant chemoradiotherapy indicated for GE or lower esophageal ADC tumors	34
Regional (III)	28	Surgery if possible (e.g., T3 N0 lesions) Definitive chemoradiotherapy Neoadjuvant chemoradiotherapy followed by surgery Adjuvant chemoradiotherapy indicated for GE or lower esophageal ADC tumors	17
Distant (IV)	25	Best supportive care/palliation *Local:* Radiation therapy or brachytherapy Intraluminal intubation or dilatation Laser or endocoagulation Photodynamic therapy *Combination chemotherapy:* CF (cisplatin, 5-fluorouracil) EOX (epirubicin, oxaliplatin, capecitabine) DCF (docetaxel, cisplatin, 5-fluorouracil) ECF (epirubicin, cisplatin, 5-fluorouracil) Folfiri (5-fluorouracil, irinotecan)	3

ADC, adenocarcinoma; GE, gastroesophageal; 5-FU, 5-fluorouracil.

FOLLOW-UP FOR PATIENTS WITH LOCOREGIONAL DISEASE

There is no standard surveillance scheme.

- History and physical examination, complete blood count (CBC), urea, electrolytes, and liver function tests are recommended every 4 months for 1 year, every 6 months for 2 years, and then annually (www.nccn.org).
- Chest radiograph should be obtained as indicated.
- CT scans of the chest/abdomen should be obtained as clinically indicated.
- Upper gastrointestinal endoscopy should be performed as clinically indicated.

REFERENCES

1. Day NE, Varghese C. Oesophageal cancer. *Cancer Surv* 1994;19220:43–54.
2. Jemal A, Siegal R, Ward E, et al. Cancer statistics, 2008. *CA Cancer J Clin* 2008;58:71–96.
3. American Joint Committee on Cancer. *Cancer staging manual*, 6th ed. NewYork: Springer-Verlag, 2002:91–98.
4. Stein HJ, Feith M, Siewert JR. Cancer of the esophagogastric junction. *Surg Oncol* 2000;9:35–41.
5. Kelly S, Harris KM, Berry E, et al. A systematic review of the staging performance of endoscopic ultrasound in gastro-oesophageal carcinoma. *Gut* 2001;49:534–539.
6. Flamen P, Lerut A, Cutsem Van, et al. Utility of positron emission tomography for the staging of patients with potentially operable esophageal carcinoma. *J Clin Oncol* 2000;18:3202–3210.
7. Chatterton B.E, Ho-Shon I, Lenzo N. Multi-center prospective assessment of accuracy and impact on management of PET in oesophageal and gastro-oesophageal junction cancer. Australian PET data collection project. *Proc Am Soc Cli Onc* 2007;25 (abstract 4534).
8. Daly JM, Karnell LH, Menck HR. National cancer database report on esophageal carcinoma. *Cancer* 1996;78:1820–1828.
9. Stein HJ, Feith M, Mueller J, et al. Limited resection for early adenocarcinoma in Barrett's oesophagus. *Ann Surg* 2000;232:733.
10. Cooper JS, Guo MD, Herskovic A, et al. Chemoradiotherapy of locally advanced esophageal cancer long-term follow-up of a prospective randomized trial (RTOG 85-01). *JAMA* 1999;281:1623–1627.
11. Rebecca WO, Richard MA. Combined chemotherapy and radiotherapy (without surgery) compared with radiotherapy alone in localized carcinoma of the esophagus. *Cochrane Database Syst Rev* 2003;(1):CD002092.
12. Stahl M, Stuschke M, Lehmann N, et al. Chemoradiation with and without surgery in patients with locally advanced sqamous cell carcinoma of esophagus. *J Clin Oncol* 2005;23:2310–2317.
13. Bedenne L, Michel P, Bouche O, et al. Chemoradiation followed by surgery compared with chemoradiation alone in squamous cell cancer of esophagus. *J Clin Oncol* 2007;25:1160–1168.
14. Leichman L, Steiger Z, Seydel HG, et al. Preoperative chemotherapy and radiation therapy for patients with cancer of the esophagus: a potentially curative approach. *J Clin Oncol* 1984;2:15–79.
15. Walsh TN, Nooman N, Hollywood D, et al. A comparison of multimodal therapy and surgery for esophageal adenocarcinoma. *N Engl J Med.* 1996;335:462–467.
16. Nygaard K, Hagen S, Hansen HS, et al. Pre-operative radiotherapy prolongs survival in operable esophageal carcinoma: a randomised multicenter study of pre-operative radiotherapy and chemotherapy: the second Scandinavian trial in esophageal cancer. *World J Surg* 1992;16:1104–1110.
17. Apinop C, Puttisak P, Precha N. A prospective study of combined therapy in esophageal cancer. *Hepatogastroenterology* 1994;41:391–393.
18. Leprise E, Etienne PL, Meunier B, et al. A randomised study of chemotherapy, radiation therapy, antisurgery vs surgery for localised squamous cell carcinoma of the esophagus. *Cancer* 1994;73:1779–1784.
19. Bosset JF, Gignoux M, Triboulet JP, et al. Chemoradiotherapy followed by surgery compared with surgery alone in squamous cell cancer of the esophagus. *N Engl J Med* 1997;337:161–167.
20. Urba S, Orringer M, Turrisi JP, et al. Randomised trial of peroperative chemoradiation versus surgery alone in patients with locoregional esophageal carcinoma. *J Clin Oncol* 2001;19:305–313.

21. Burmeister BH, Smithers B, Fitzgerald L, et al. A randomized phases III trial of preoperative chemoradiation followed by surgery (CR-S) versus surgery alone(S) for localized resectable cancer of the esophagus. *Proc Am Soc Clin Oncol* 2002;21:130a (abstract 518).

22. Lee JL, Kim SB, Jung HY. A single institutional phase III trial of preoperative chemotherapy with hyperfractionation radiotherapy plus surgery (CRT-S) versus surgery(S) alone for stage II, III resectable esophageal squamous cell carcinoma (SCC): An interim analysis. *Proc Am Soc Clin Oncol* 2003;23:260 (abstract 1043).

23. Tepper JE, Krasna M, Niedzwiecki D, et al. Trial of trimodality therapywith Cisplatin, Flurouraci, Radiotherapy and surgery compared with Surgery alone for Esophageal cancer. CALGB 9781. *J Clin Oncol* 2008;26:1086–1092.

24. Thirion PG, Michiels S, Le Maitre A, et al. Individual patient data based meta-analysis assessing preoperative chemotherapy in resectable oesophageal carcinoma. *Proc Am Soc Clin Onc* 2007;25:200S (abstract 4512).

25. Stahl M, Walz MK, Stuschke M, et al. Preoperative chemotherapy (CTX) versus preoperative chemoradiotherapy (CRTX) in locally advanced esophagogastric adenocarcinomas: First results of a randomized phase III trial. *Proc Am Soc Clin Onc* 2007;25 (abstract 4511).

26. Gebski V, Burmeister B, Smithers BM, et al. Survival benefits from neoadjuvant chemoradiotherapy or chemotherapy in esophageal carcinoma. Australian gastrointestinal trial group. *Lancet Oncol* 2007;8:226–234.

27. MacDonald JS, Smalley SR, Benedetti J, et al. Chemoradiotherapy after surgery compared with surgery alone for adenocarcinoma of the stomach or gastroesophageal junction. *N Engl J Med* 2001;345:725–730.

28. Kelsen D, Ginsberg R, Pajak TF, et al. Chemotherapy followed by surgery compared with surgery alone for localized esophageal cancer. *N Engl J Med* 1998;339:1979–1984.

29. Medical Research Council Oesophageal Cancer Working Party. Surgical resection with or without preoperative chemotherapy in oesophageal cancer: a randomised controlled trial. *Lancet* 2002;359:1727–1733.

30. Ando N, Kato H, Shinoda M, et al. A randomized trial of postoperative adjuvant chemotherapy with cisplatin and 5-fluorouracil versus neoadjuvant chemotherapy for localized squamous cell carcinoma of the thoracic esophagus (JCOG 9907). *Proc Gastrointestinal Cancers Symposium.* 2008;74 (abstract 10).

31. Cunningham D, Allum WH, Stenning SP, et al. Perioperative chemotherapy versus surgery alone for resectable gastroesophageal cancer. *N Engl J Med* 2006;355:11–20.

32. Bleiberg H, Conroy T, Paillot B, et al. Randomised phase two study of Cisplatin and 5-Flurouracil versus cisplatin alone in advanced squamous cell oesophageal cancer. *Eur J Cancer* 1997;33: 1216–1220.

33. Webb A, Cunningham D, Scarffe JH, et al. A randomised trial comparing ECF with FAMTX in advanced esophagogastric cancer. *J Clin Oncol* 1997;15:261–267.

34. Ajani JA, Van Cutsem E, Moiseyenko S, et al. Phase 111 study of docetaxel and cisplatin plus flurouracil compared with cisplatin and 5 flurouracil as first-line therapy for advanced gastric cancer. *J Clin Oncol* 2006;31:4991–4997.

35. Cunningham D, Starling N, Rao S, et al. Capecitabine and oxaliplatin for advanced esophagogastric cancer. *N Engl J Med* 2008;358:36–46.

5

Gastric Cancers

Thomas J. George, Jr.

EPIDEMIOLOGY

Worldwide, gastric carcinoma represents the third or fourth most common malignancy. The frequency of occurrence of gastric carcinoma at different sites within the stomach has changed in the United States over recent decades. Cancer of the distal half of the stomach has been decreasing in the United States since the 1930s. However, over the last two decades, the incidence of cancer of the cardia and gastroesophageal junction has been rapidly rising, particularly in patients younger than 40 years. There were nearly 22,000 new cases and 10,800 deaths from gastric carcinoma in the United States in 2008.

RISK FACTORS

- Age at onset is fifth decade
- Male-to-female ratio is 1.7:1
- African American-to-white ratio is 1.8:1
- Precursor conditions include chronic atrophic gastritis and intestinal metaplasia, pernicious anemia (10–20% incidence), partial gastrectomy for benign disease, *Helicobacter pylori* infection (especially childhood exposure—three- to fivefold increase), Ménétrier's disease, and gastric adenomatous polyps. These precursor lesions are largely linked to distal (intestinal type) gastric carcinoma.
- Family history: first degree (two- to threefold); the family of Napoléon Bonaparte is an example; familial clustering; patients with hereditary nonpolyposis colorectal cancer (Lynch syndrome II) are at increased risk; recently, germline mutations of E-cadherin (*CDH1* gene) have been linked to the rare entity of familial diffuse gastric cancer and lobular breast cancer.
- Tobacco use results in a 1.5- to threefold increased risk for cancer.
- High salt and nitrosamine food content from fermenting and smoking process
- Deficiencies of vitamins A, C, and E; β-carotene; selenium; and fiber
- Blood type A
- Alcohol
- The marked rise in the incidence of gastroesophageal and proximal gastric adenocarcinoma appears to be strongly correlated to the rising incidence of Barrett's esophagus.

SCREENING

In most countries, screening of the general populations is not practical because of a low incidence of gastric cancer. However, screening is justified in Japan where the incidence of gastric cancer is high. Japanese screening guidelines include initial upper endoscopy at age 50, with follow-up endoscopy for abnormalities. No screening guidelines are available in the United States.

PATHOPHYSIOLOGY

Most gastric cancers are adenocarcinomas (more than 90%) of two distinct histologic types: intestinal and diffuse. In general, the term "gastric cancer" is commonly used to refer to adenocarcinoma of the stomach. Other cancers of the stomach include non-Hodgkin's lymphomas (NHL), leiomyosarcomas, and gastrointestinal stromal tumors (GIST). Differentiating between adenocarcinoma and lymphoma is critical because the prognosis and treatment for these two entities differ considerably. Although less common, metastases to the stomach include melanoma, breast, and ovarian cancers.

Intestinal Type

The *epidemic* form of cancer is further differentiated by gland formation and is associated with precancerous lesions, gastric atrophy, and intestinal metaplasia. The intestinal form accounts for most distal cancers with a stable or declining incidence. These cancers in particular are associated with *H. pylori* infection. In this carcinogenesis model, the interplay of environmental factors leads to glandular atrophy, relative achlorhydria, and increased gastric pH. The resulting bacterial overgrowth leads to production of nitrites and nitroso compounds causing further gastric atrophy and intestinal metaplasia, thereby increasing the risk of cancer.

This form is more common in areas of the world where gastric carcinoma is endemic. The recent decline in gastric carcinoma in the United States is likely the result of a decline in the incidence of intestinal type lesions. Intestinal type lesions are associated with an increased frequency of overexpression of epidermal growth factor receptor *erbB-2* and *erbB-3*.

Diffuse Type

The *endemic* form of carcinoma is more common in younger patients and exhibits undifferentiated signet-ring histology. There is a predilection for diffuse submucosal spread because of lack of cell cohesion, leading to linitis plastica. Contiguous spread of the carcinoma to the peritoneum is common. Precancerous lesions have not been identified. Although a carcinogenesis model has not been proposed, it is associated with *H. pylori* infection. Genetic predispositions to endemic forms of carcinoma have been reported, as have associations between carcinoma and individuals with type A blood. These cancers occur in the proximal stomach where increased incidence has been observed worldwide. Stage for stage, these cancers have a worse prognosis than do distal cancers.

Diffuse lesions have been linked to abnormalities of fibroblast growth factor systems, including the *K-sam* oncogene as well as E-cadherin mutations. The latter results in loss of cell-cell adhesions.

Molecular Analysis

- Loss of heterozygosity of chromosome 5q or APC gene (deleted in 34% of gastric cancers), 17p, and 18q (DCC gene)
- Microsatellite instability, particularly of transforming growth factor-β type II receptor, with subsequent growth-inhibition deregulation
- p53 is mutated in approximately 40% to 60% caused by allelic loss and base transition mutations.
- Mutations of E-cadherin expression (*CDH1* gene on 16q), a cell adhesion mediator, is observed in diffuse-type undifferentiated cancers and is associated with an increased incidence of lobular breast cancer.
- Epidermal growth factor receptor overexpression, specifically *Her2/neu* and *erbB-2/erbB-3* especially in intestinal forms
- Epstein-Barr viral genomes are detected.
- *Ras* mutations are rarely reported (less than 10%) in contrast to other gastrointestinal cancers.

DIAGNOSIS

Gastric carcinoma, when superficial and surgically curable, typically produces no symptoms. Among 18,365 patients analyzed by the American College of Surgeons, patients presented with the following symptoms: weight loss (62%), abdominal pain (52%), nausea (34%), anorexia (32%), dysphagia (26%), melena (20%), early satiety (18%), ulcer-type pain (17%), and lower-extremity edema (6%).

Clinical findings at presentation may include: anemia (42%), hypoproteinemia (26%), abnormal liver functions (26%), and fecal occult blood (40%). Medically refractory or persistent peptic ulcer should prompt endoscopic evaluation.

Gastric carcinomas primarily spread by direct extension, invading adjacent structures with resultant peritoneal carcinomatosis and malignant ascites. The liver, followed by lung, are the most common sites of hematogenous dissemination. The disease may also spread as follows:

- To intra-abdominal nodes and left supraclavicular nodes (Virchow's node)
- Along peritoneal surfaces, resulting in a periumbilical nodule (Sister Mary Joseph node, named after the operating room nurse at the Mayo Clinic, or periumbilical lymph nodes, which form as tumor spreads along the falciform ligament to subcutaneous sites)
- To a left anterior axillary lymph node resulting from the spread of proximal primary cancer to lower esophageal and intrathoracic lymphatics (Irish node)
- To enlarged ovary (Krukenberg tumor; ovarian metastases)
- To a mass in the cul-de-sac (Blumer shelf), which is palpable on rectal examination

Paraneoplastic Syndromes

- Skin syndromes: acanthosis nigricans, dermatomyositis, circinate erythemas, pemphigoid, and acute onset of seborrheic keratoses (Leser–Trélat sign)
- Central nervous system syndromes: dementia and cerebellar ataxia
- Miscellaneous: thrombophlebitis, microangiopathic hemolytic anemia, membranous nephropathy

Tumor Markers

Carcinoembryonic antigen (CEA) is elevated in 40% to 50% of cases. It is useful in follow-up and monitoring response to therapy, but not for screening. α-Fetoprotein and CA 19-9 are elevated in 30% of patients with gastric cancer.

STAGING

The American Joint Committee on Cancer (AJCC) has designated staging by TNM classification (Table 5.1). Of note, alternative staging systems are used by Japanese cancer centers.

TABLE 5.1. *TNM classification of gastric cancer staging designated by the American Joint Committee on Cancer 2002*

Primary tumor	
Tis	Carcinoma in situ
T1	Invasion of lamina propria or submucosa
T2	Invasion of muscularis propria or subserosa
T3	Penetration of serosa (visceral peritoneum) without invasion of adjacent structures
T4	Invasion of adjacent structures
Lymph node status (N)	
N0	No regional lymph node involvement
N1	Metastases in 1 to 6 regional lymph nodes
N2	Metastases in 7 to 15 regional lymph nodes
N3	Metastases in more than 15 regional lymph nodes
Metastatic disease (M)	
M0	No distant metastases
M1	Distant metastases present

(Continued)

TABLE 5.1.   *(Continued)*

Stage grouping

Stage	T	N	M
0	Tis	N0	M0
IA	T1	N0	M0
IB	T1	N1	M0
	T2	N0	M0
II	T1	N2	M0
	T2	N1	M0
	T3	N0	M0
IIIA	T2	N2	M0
	T3	N1	M0
	T4	N0	M0
IIIB	T3	N2	M0
IV	T4	N1–3	M0
	T1–3	N3	M0
	T1–4	N0–2	M1

Lymphadenectomy should contain at least 15 lymph nodes for proper staging.
Source: American Joint Committee on Cancer. *TNM classification of gastric cancer staging.* 6th ed. 2002.

- Initial upper gastrointestinal endoscopy and double-contrast barium swallow identify suggestive lesions and have diagnostic accuracy of 95% and 75%, respectively, but add little to preoperative staging otherwise.
- Endoscopic ultrasonography assesses the depth of tumor invasion (T staging) and nodal involvement (N staging) with accuracies up to 90% and 75%, respectively.
- Computerized tomographic scanning is useful for assessing local extension, lymph node involvement, and presence of metastasis, although understaging occurs in most cases.
- Whole-body 2-[18F]fluoro-2-deoxyglucose (FDG)–positron emission tomography (PET) is currently under investigation in gastric cancer, but appears to be less reliable than in esophageal cancer.

PROGNOSIS

Pathologic staging remains the most important determinant of prognosis (Table 5.2). Other prognostic variables that have been proposed to be associated with an unfavorable outcome include the following:

- Older age
- Male gender
- Location of tumor
- Weight loss greater than 10%
- Diffuse versus intestinal histology (5-year survival after resection, 16% vs. 26%, respectively)

TABLE 5.2.   *Disease-specific survival (DSS) after complete resection by American Joint Committee on Cancer stage grouping*

Stage	2-Year DSS (%)	5-Year DSS (%)
IA	100	90
IB	95	83
II	80	55
IIIA	60	30
IIIB	30	10
IV[a]	30	<10

[a]Majority of stage IV cases cannot undergo complete resection; therefore these survival data are far higher than would be expected in clinical practice.
Source: Modified from Kattan MW, et al. *J Clin Oncol.* 2003 Oct 1;21(19):3647–3650.

- High-grade or undifferentiated tumors
- Four or more lymph nodes involved
- Aneuploid tumors
- Elevations in epidermal growth factor or P-glycoprotein level
- Overexpression of thymidylate synthase
- Overexpression of ERCC1, p53, and Her-2
- Loss of p21 and p27

MANAGEMENT OF GASTRIC CANCER

Standard of Care

Although surgical resection remains the cornerstone of gastric cancer treatment, the optimal extent of nodal resection remains controversial, with randomized studies failing to show that more extensive procedures improve survival when compared with less extensive. The high rate of recurrence and poor survival of patients following surgery provides a rationale for the use of adjuvant or perioperative treatment. Adjuvant radiotherapy alone does not improve survival following resection. After complete surgical resection, either adjuvant chemoradiotherapy (chemoRT) or perioperative chemotherapy alone appear to confer survival advantages. The results of the Intergroup 0116 study show that the combination of 5-fluorouracil (5-FU)–based chemoRT significantly prolongs disease-free and overall survival when compared to no adjuvant treatment. Similarly, the use of polychemotherapy pre- and postoperatively can increase disease-free and overall survival compared to observation.

In advanced gastric cancer, chemotherapy enhances quality of life and prolongs survival when compared with the best supportive care. There are numerous therapeutic options in this setting without a clear standard of care. Of the commonly used regimens, triple combination chemotherapy with either docetaxel, cisplatin, and 5-FU (DCF) or epirubicin, oxaliplatin, and capecitabine (EOX) probably have the strongest claims to this role. However, there is a pressing need for assessing new agents, both cytotoxic and molecularly targeted, in both the advanced and adjuvant settings.

Resectable Disease

Surgery

Complete surgical resection of the tumor and adjacent lymph nodes remains the only chance for cure. Unfortunately, only 20% of U.S. patients with gastric cancer have disease at presentation amenable to such therapy. Resection of gastric cancer is indicated in patients with stages I, II, and III disease, with minimal lymph node involvement. Tumor size and location dictate the type of surgical procedure to be used. Current surgical issues include subtotal versus total gastrectomy, extent of lymph node dissection, and palliative surgery.

SUBTOTAL VERSUS TOTAL GASTRECTOMY

Subtotal gastrectomy (SG) may be performed for proximal cardia or distal lesions, provided that the fundus or cardioesophageal junction is not involved (Fig. 5.1). Total gastrectomy (TG) is more appropriate if tumor involvement is diffuse and arises in the body of the stomach, with extension to within 6 cm of the cardia. TG is associated with increased postoperative complications, mortality, and quality-of-life decrement, necessitating thorough consideration of complete gastric resection (Fig. 5.2).

EXTENT OF LYMPH NODE DISSECTION

Regional lymph node dissection is important for accurate staging and may have therapeutic benefit as well. The extent of lymphadenectomy is categorized by the regional nodal groups removed (Table 5.3). At least 15 lymph nodes must be reported for accurate AJCC staging. D2 lymphadenectomy is reported to improve survival in patients with T1, T2, and some serosa-involved T3 lesions as compared to D1. However, factors such as operative time, hospitalization length, and transfusion requirements,

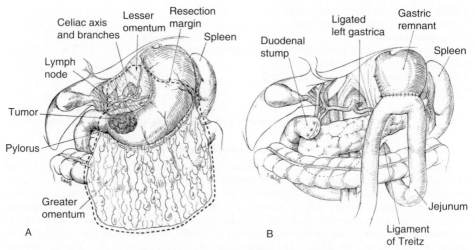

Fig. 5.1. A and B: Subtotal gastrectomy.

and thus morbidity, are all increased. The routine inclusion of splenectomy in D2 resections is no longer advocated given higher postoperative complications. The greatest benefit of more extensive lymph node dissection may occur in early gastric cancer lesions with small tumors and superficial mucosal involvement as up to 20% of such lesions have occult lymph node involvement.

Radiation Therapy

- For patients with locally advanced or metastatic disease, moderate doses of external-beam radiation can be used to palliate symptoms of pain, obstruction, and bleeding, but do not routinely improve survival.

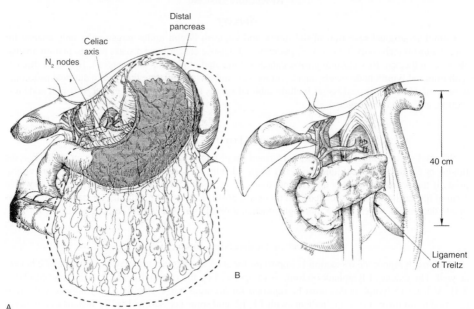

Fig. 5.2. A and B: Total gastrectomy.

TABLE 5.3. *Classification of regional lymph node dissection*

Dissection (D)	Regional lymph node groups removed
D0	None
D1	Perigastric
D2	D1 plus nodes along hepatic, left gastric, celiac, and splenic arteries; splenic hilar nodes; +/− splenectomy
D3[a]	D2 plus periaortic and portahepatis

[a]Periaortic and portahepatis nodes are typically considered distant metastatic disease.

- Local or regional recurrence in the gastric or tumor bed, the anastomosis, or regional lymph nodes occurs in 40% to 65% of patients after gastric resection with curative intent (Table 5.4). The high frequency of such relapses has generated interest in perioperative therapy. Radiotherapy (RT) in this setting is limited by the technical challenges inherent in abdominal irradiation, optimal definition of fields, diminished performance status, and nutritional state of many patients with gastric cancer.
- A prospective randomized trial from the British Stomach Cancer Group failed to demonstrate a survival benefit for postoperative adjuvant radiation alone, although locoregional failures had decreased from 27% to 10.6%.
- Attempts to improve the efficacy and minimize toxicity with newer RT techniques have been investigated. Sixty patients who underwent curative resection at the National Cancer Institute were randomized to either receive adjuvant intraoperative radiotherapy (IORT) or conventional RT. IORT failed to afford a benefit over conventional therapy in overall survival and remains unavailable to many outside of a clinical trial.
- In patients with locally unresectable pancreatic and gastric adenocarcinoma, the Gastrointestinal Tumor Study Group (GITSG) has shown that combined-modality therapy is superior to either RT or chemotherapy alone. On the basis of this concept, combined chemoRT (typically in combination with 5-FU) has been evaluated both in the neoadjuvant (preoperative) and the adjuvant (postoperative) settings.

Perioperative Chemoradiotherapy

Aside from gastroesophageal junction tumors, the available data on the role of neoadjuvant chemoRT for gastric cancer are not conclusive. Although neoadjuvant therapy may reduce the tumor mass in many patients, several randomized, controlled trials have shown that, compared with primary resection, a multimodal approach does not result in a survival benefit in patients with potentially resectable tumors. In contrast, for some patients with locally advanced tumors (i.e., patients in whom complete tumor removal with upfront surgery seems unlikely), neoadjuvant chemoRT may increase the likelihood of complete tumor resection on subsequent surgery. However, predicting those likely to benefit from this approach remains an ongoing research question.

Adjuvant chemoRT has been evaluated in the United States. In a phase 3 Intergroup trial (INT-0116), 556 patients with completely resected stage IB to stage IV M0 adenocarcinoma of the stomach and gastroesophageal junction were randomized to receive best supportive care or adjuvant chemotherapy (5-FU and leucovorin) and concurrent radiation therapy (45 Gy). With >6-year median follow-up, median survival was 35 months for the adjuvant chemoRT group as compared to 27 months for the

TABLE 5.4. *Failure areas following curative surgery*

	MGH clinical	MINN reoperation	MCNEER autopsy
Failure area	130 no. (%)	105 no. (%)	92 no. (%)
Gastric bed	27 (21%)	58 (55%)	48 (52%)
Anastomosis or stump	33 (25%)	28 (27%)	55 (60%)
Lymph nodes	11 (8%)	45 (43%)	48 (52%)

no., total number of patients; MGH, Massachusetts General Hospital; MINN, Minnesota; MCNEER, Massey Cancer Center.

surgery-alone arm ($P = 0.006$). Both 3-year overall survival (50% vs. 41%; $P = 0.006$) and relapse-free survival (48% vs. 31%; $P < 0.0001$) favored adjuvant chemoRT. Although treatment-related mortality was 1% in this study, only 65% of patients completed all therapy as planned and many had inadequate lymph node resections (54% D0). Regardless, adjuvant chemoRT is considered a standard of care in the United States.

Perioperative Chemotherapy

In Japan, patients who underwent complete surgical resection for stage II and III gastric cancer with D2 lymphadenectomy appeared to benefit from adjuvant S-1, a novel oral fluoropyrimidine. In a randomized controlled trial, patients were randomized to 1 year of monotherapy or surveillance only. The study was closed early after interim analysis confirmed a 3-year overall survival (80% vs. 70%; $P = 0.002$) and relapse-free survival (72% vs. 60%; $P = 0.002$) advantage in favor of adjuvant chemotherapy.

In Europe, focus has recently been on the role of more potent polychemotherapy regimens in the perioperative setting without RT. The UK Medical Research Council recently reported the results of a randomized controlled trial of three cycles of pre- and postoperative epirubicin, cisplatin, and 5-FU (ECF) to surgery alone in patients with resectable stage II–IV nonmetastatic gastric cancer; 503 patients were stratified according to surgeon, tumor site, and performance status. Perioperative chemotherapy improved 5-year overall survival (36% vs. 23%; $P = 0.009$) and reduced local and distant recurrence. There appeared to be significant downstaging by chemotherapy treatment, with more patients deemed by the operating surgeon to have had a "curative" resection (79% vs. 70%; $P = 0.03$), had smaller tumors (median 3 vs. 5 cm; $P < 0.001$), had T1/T2 stage tumors (52% vs. 37%; $P = 0.002$), and had N1/N2 stage disease (84% vs. 71%; $P = 0.01$). Toxicity was feasible with postoperative complications comparable; however nearly one-third of patients who began with preoperative chemotherapy did not receive postoperative chemotherapy due to progressive disease, complications, or patient request. In Europe, perioperative polychemotherapy is now considered a standard of care.

Unresectable or Metastatic Disease

Primary goals of therapy should focus on improvement in symptoms, delay of disease progression, pain control, nutritional support, and quality of life. Although a role for palliative surgery and radiotherapy exist (see previous sections), chemotherapy remains the primary means of palliative treatment in this setting. The most commonly administered chemotherapeutic agents with objective response rates in advanced gastric cancer include mitomycin, antifolates, anthracyclines, fluoropyrimidines, platinums, taxanes, and topoisomerase inhibitors.

Palliative Surgery

This should be considered in patients with obstruction, bleeding, or pain, despite operative mortalities of 25% to 50%. Gastrojejunostomy bypass surgery alone may provide a twofold increase in mean survival. The selection of patients most likely to benefit from this palliative effort requires further evaluation.

Use of Stents

Plastic and expansile metal stents are associated with successful palliation of obstructive symptoms in more than 85% of patients with tumors in the gastroesophagus and in the cardia.

Chemotherapy Versus Best Supportive Care

Four randomized studies in patients with metastatic gastric cancer have demonstrated a survival advantage to combination chemotherapy over best supportive care (BSC) (Table 5.5). Two studies used

TABLE 5.5. *Chemotherapy versus best supportive care (BSC)*

Regimen	n patients	Survival BSC (mo)	Survival chemo (mo)
FAMTX	36	3	12
FAMTX	40	3	10
ELF	37	3	7.5+
ELF	18	4	10

BSC, best supportive care; FAMTX, 5-FU, doxorubicin, and methotrexate; ELF, etoposide, 5-FU, and leucovorin.

fluorouracil, doxorubicin, and methotrexate (FAMTX) and two studies used etoposide, fluorouracil, and leucovorin (ELF) as the primary regimens.

SINGLE-AGENT CHEMOTHERAPY

Monotherapy with single agents (Table 5.6) results in a 10% to 30% response rate with mild toxicities. 5-FU is the most extensively studied, producing a 20% response rate. Complete responses with single agents are rare and disease control is relatively brief.

COMBINATION CHEMOTHERAPY

Various combinations of active agents have been reported to improve the response rate (20–50%) among patients with advanced gastric carcinoma (Table 5.7). While utilizing 5-FU as a backbone, FAMTX (5-FU, doxorubicin, methotrexate) became an international standard after direct comparison to FAM (5-FU, doxorubicin, mitomycin) supporting a superiority with a survival advantage for FAMTX. The addition of cisplatin into combination regimens was supported by subsequent studies in both Europe and the United States.

Historically, the most commonly used combination regimens include FAMTX, FAM, FAP, ECF, ELF, FLAP (5-FU, leucovorin, doxorubicin, cisplatin), PELF (cisplatin, epidoxorubicin, leucovorin, 5-FU with glutathione and filgrastim), and FUP or CF (5-FU, cisplatin).

NEWER CHEMOTHERAPY AGENTS

Newer chemotherapeutic agents, including irinotecan, docetaxel, paclitaxel, and alternative platinums and fluoropyrimidines, have shown promising activity as single agents and are being actively incorporated into combination therapy (see Tables 5.6 and 5.7). A complete review of all agents is beyond the scope of this chapter.

Docetaxel has recently become FDA approved in combination with cisplatin and 5-FU (DCF) in patients with advanced or metastatic gastric cancer based on the results of a large phase 3 international trial; 445 patients were randomized to receive cisplatin and 5-FU with or without docetaxel. The addition of docetaxel resulted in an improvement in tumor response (37% vs. 25%; $P = 0.01$), time to progression (5.6 vs. 3.7 months; $P < 0.001$), and median survival (9.2 vs. 8.6 months; $P = 0.02$) with a doubling of 2-year survival (18% vs. 9%). These findings were at the cost of anticipated increased

TABLE 5.6. *Single-agent chemotherapy with activity in advanced gastric cancer*

Class	Examples
Antifolates	Methotrexate
Anthracyclines	Doxorubicin, epirubicin
Fluoropyrimidines	5-FU, capecitabine, S-1, UFT
Platinums	Cisplatin, carboplatin, oxaliplatin
Taxanes	Docetaxel, paclitaxel
Topoisomerase inhibitors	Etoposide, irinotecan

TABLE 5.7. *Randomized studies of combination chemotherapy in advanced gastric cancer*

	n patients	RR (%)	Median survival
FAMTX vs. FAM	213	41 vs. 9[a]	42 vs. 29 wk[a]
PELF vs. FAM	147	43 vs. 15[a]	35 vs. 23 wk
FAMTX vs. EAP	60	33 vs. 20	7.3 vs. 6.1 mo
ECF vs. FAMTX	274	45 vs. 21[a]	8.9 vs. 5.7 mo[a]
DCF vs. CF	445	37 vs. 25[a]	9.2 vs. 8.6 mo[a]
EOX vs. ECF	488	48 vs. 40	11.2 vs. 9.9 mo[a]

RR, response rate; FAMTX, 5-FU, doxorubicin, and methotrexate; FAM, 5-FU, doxorubicin, mitomycin-C; PELF, cisplatin, epidoxorubicin, leucovorin, 5-FU with glutathione and filgrastim; EAP, etoposide, doxorubicin, cisplatin; ECF, epirubicin plus cisplatin and 5-FU; EOX, epirubicin, oxaliplatin, capecitabine; DCF, docetaxel, cisplatin, 5-FU; CF, cisplatin, 5-FU.
[a]Difference is statistically significant.

toxicity, however, maintenance of quality of life and performance status indices were longer for DCF. In a Japanese study, 20% of patients who showed no response to previous chemotherapy had a partial response to monotherapy with docetaxel. Predictable neutropenia can be managed by dose modification or by using prophylactic granulocyte colony stimulating factor.

S-1 is a novel oral fluoropyrimidine derivative composed of tegafur (5-FU prodrug), 5-chloro-2, 4-dihydroxypyridine (inhibitor of 5-FU degradation), and potassium oxonate (inhibitor of gastrointestinal toxicities). In Japanese patients with advanced gastric cancer, a phase 2 trial has revealed a response rate of 53.6%, whereas a retrospective study showed an overall response rate of 32% (44% of patients were chemo-naïve).

Capecitabine is an oral fluoropyrimidine that has been substituted for infusional 5-FU in a variety of settings. It was formally evaluated with encouraging results in combination with a platinum alternative (see oxaliplatin).

Oxaliplatin is a third-generation platinum with much less nephrotoxicity, nausea, and bone marrow suppression than cisplatin. In a recently reported two-by-two designed study in patients with advanced gastric cancer, standard ECF chemotherapy was modified with oxaliplatin substituted for cisplatin and capecitabine substituted for 5-FU; 1,002 patients were randomly allocated between the four arms (ECF, EOF, ECX, and EOX). Capecitabine and oxaliplatin appeared as effective as 5-FU and cisplatin, respectively. Response rates and progression-free survival were nearly identical between the groups, with the EOX regimen showing superiority in overall survival over ECF (11.2 vs. 9.9 months; $P = 0.02$).

Biologic/Targeted Agents

New biologic therapies aimed to inhibit or modulate targets of aberrant signal transduction in gastric cancer are actively being investigated. Inhibition of angiogenesis, vascular endothelial growth factor (VEGF), and epidermal growth factor (EGFR) pathways are an early focus (Table 5.8) based on the

TABLE 5.8. *Efficacy data on selected targeted therapy use in advanced gastric cancer*

Target	Treatment	n patients	Response rate (%)	Median survival
EGFR	Cetuximab + 5-FU/irinotecan	34	44	16 mo
	Cetuximab + 5-FU/oxaliplatin	46	65	9.5 mo
	Erlotinib	68	9	
HER2	Trastuzumab + cisplatin	17	35	
VEGF	Bevacizumab + cisplatin/irinotecan	35	65	12.3 mo
	Bevacizumab + docetaxel	17	17	

availability of effective agents and success in advanced colorectal cancer. Until the results of ongoing large randomized studies are known, use of these agents should be restricted to clinical trials.

TREATMENT OF GASTRIC CANCER ACCORDING TO STAGE

Stage 0 Gastric Cancer

Stage 0 indicates gastric cancer confined to the mucosa. Based on the experience in Japan, where stage 0 is diagnosed more frequently, it has been found that more than 90% of patients treated by gastrectomy with lymphadenectomy will survive beyond 5 years. An American series has confirmed these findings. No additional perioperative therapy is necessary.

Stage I Gastric Cancer

1. One of the following surgical procedures is recommended for stage I gastric cancer:
   - Distal SG (if the lesion is not in the fundus or at the cardioesophageal junction)
   - Proximal SG or TG, with distal esophagectomy (if the lesion involves the cardia)
   - TG (if the tumor involves the stomach diffusely or arises in the body of the stomach and extends to within 6 cm of the cardia or distal antrum)
   - Regional lymphadenectomy is recommended with all of the previously noted procedures
   - Splenectomy is not routinely performed
2. Postoperative chemoRT is recommended for patients with stage IB disease.

Stage II Gastric Cancer

1. One of the following surgical procedures is recommended for stage II gastric cancer:
   - Distal SG (if the lesion is not in the fundus or at the cardioesophageal junction)
   - Proximal SG or TG, with distal esophagectomy (if the lesion involves the cardia)
   - TG (if the tumor involves the stomach diffusely or arises in the body of the stomach and extends to within 6 cm of the cardia)
   - Regional lymphadenectomy is recommended with all of the previously noted procedures
   - Splenectomy is not routinely performed
2. Postoperative chemoRT or perioperative chemotherapy is recommended.

Stage III Gastric Cancer

1. Radical surgery: Curative resection procedures are confined to patients who do not have extensive nodal involvement at the time of surgical exploration.
2. Postoperative chemoRT or perioperative chemotherapy is recommended.

Stage IV Gastric Cancer

Patients Without Distant Metastases (M0)

Neoadjuvant polychemotherapy can be considered to improve resectability. Radical surgery is performed if possible, either followed by postoperative chemoRT or perioperative chemotherapy.

Patients With Distant Metastases (M1)

All newly diagnosed patients with hematogenous or peritoneal metastases should be considered as candidates for clinical trials. For many patients, chemotherapy may provide substantial palliative benefit and occasional durable remission, although the disease remains incurable. Balancing the risks to benefits of therapy in any individual patient is recommended.

Peritoneal Carcinomatosis

In approximately 50% of patients with advanced gastric cancer, the disease recurs locally or at an intra-peritoneal site, and this recurrence has a negative effect on quality of life and survival. Intraperitoneal (IP) 5-FU, cisplatin, and/or mitomycin have been used at select centers. IP chemotherapy administration does not routinely alter survival and should be reserved for clinical trial or practice at an experienced center.

POSTSURGICAL FOLLOW-UP

- Follow-up in patients following complete surgical resection should include routine history and physi-cal, with liver function tests and CEA measurements being performed.
- Evaluation intervals of every 3 to 6 months for the first 3 years, then annually thereafter have been suggested.
- Symptom-directed imaging and laboratory workup is indicated, without routine recommendations otherwise.
- If TG is not performed, annual upper endoscopy is recommended due to a 1% to 2% incidence of second primary gastric tumors.
- Vitamin B_{12} deficiency develops in most TG patients and 20% of SG patients, typically within 4 to 10 years. Replacement must be administered at 1,000 mcg subcutaneously or intramuscularly every month indefinitely.

PRIMARY GASTRIC LYMPHOMA

Gastric lymphomas are uncommon malignancies representing 3% of gastric neoplasms and 10% of lymphomas.

Classification and Histopathology

Gastric lymphomas can be generally classified as primary or secondary:

- Primary gastric lymphoma (PGL) is defined as a lymphoma arising in the stomach, typically origi-nating from mucosa-associated lymphoid tissue (MALT). PGL can spread to regional lymph nodes and can become disseminated. Most are of B-cell NHL origin, with occasional cases of T-cell and Hodgkin's lymphoma seen. Examples of PGLs include extranodal marginal zone B-cell lymphoma of MALT type previously called low-grade MALT lymphoma, diffuse large B-cell lymphoma (DLBCL) previously called high-grade MALT lymphoma, and Burkitt's and Burkitt's-like lymphoma. This sec-tion will primarily address PGLs.
- Secondary gastric lymphoma indicates involvement of the stomach associated with lymphoma aris-ing elsewhere. The stomach is the most common extranodal site of lymphoma. In an autopsy series, patients who died from disseminated NHL showed involvement of the gastrointestinal tract in 50% to 60% of cases. Examples of secondary gastric lymphoma include several common advanced-stage systemic NHLs, particularly mantle cell lymphoma.

Epidemiology

- The prevalence of PGL has been increasing over the last 20 years without a clear explanation.
- PGL incidence rises with age, with a peak in the sixth to seventh decades with a slight male predomi-nance.
- Risk factors include *H. pylori*-associated chronic gastritis (particularly low-grade MALT lymphoma), autoimmune diseases, and immunodeficiency syndromes including AIDS and chronic immunosup-pression.

Diagnosis

Clinical symptoms that are most common at presentation include abdominal pain, weight loss, nausea, vomiting, and early satiety. Frank bleeding is uncommon and patients rarely present with perforation.

Findings on upper endoscopy are diverse and may be identical to typical adenocarcinoma.

Since PGL can infiltrate the submucosa without overlying mucosal changes, conventional pinch biopsies may miss the diagnosis. Deeper biopsy techniques should be employed. If an ulcer is present, the biopsy should be at multiple sites along the edge of the ulcer crater. Specimens should be pathologically evaluated by both standard techniques to determine histology and *H. pylori* positivity as well as flow cytometry to determine clonality and characteristics of any infiltrating lymphocytes. The latter requires fresh tissue placed in saline, not preservative.

Staging

Staging of gastric lymphoma is identical to systemic lymphoma staging using the Ann Arbor system. For example, stage IE indicates disease limited to the stomach, without nodal spread. Stage IIE_1 is a tumor in the stomach that spreads to adjacent contiguous lymph nodes. Stage IIE_2 is a tumor in the stomach that spreads to lymph nodes that are noncontiguous with the primary tumor.

Patients present with stage IE and stage IIE PGL with an equal prevalence ranging between 28% and 72%.

Presentation with high-grade and low-grade disease is also equal, with 34% to 65% of disease presenting as high-grade lymphoma and 35% to 65% presenting as low-grade lymphoma.

CT scanning of the chest and abdomen is important to determine the extent of lymphoma nodal involvement. FDG-PET scanning and bone marrow biopsy may be useful in high-grade PGL staging.

Treatment

Treatment of PGL is dependent primarily by stage and histologic grade of the lymphoma. However, given the rarity of the disease and lack of clinical trial data, treatment recommendations are based primarily on retrospective studies.

Extranodal marginal zone B-cell lymphoma of MALT type is usually of low-grade histology (40–50%) and confined to the stomach (70–80% stage IE). Very good epidemiologic data support *H. pylori*-induced chronic gastritis as a major etiology for this tumor. Eradication of *H. pylori* infection with antibiotics should be the initial standard treatment. Complete histologic regression of the lymphoma has been demonstrated in 50% to 80% of patients treated in this manner with good long-term disease free survival. Radiation therapy can provide durable remission for cases that relapse or are *H. pylori*-negative. More advanced stage or aggressive histologies at presentation should be treated like DLBCL.

Previously called high-grade MALT lymphoma, DLBCL is a more aggressive PGL. Eradication of *H. pylori* provides less reliable and durable disease control. Gastrectomy was the traditional treatment of choice; however, this appears to be no longer necessary. Five hundred eighty-nine patients with stage IE and IIE_1 DLBCL PGL were randomized to receive surgery, surgery plus radiotherapy, surgery plus chemotherapy, or chemotherapy alone. Chemotherapy was 6 cycles of cyclophosphamide, doxorubicin, vincristine, and prednisone (CHOP). Overall survivals at 10 years were 54%, 53%, 91%, and 96% respectively. Late toxicity and complications were more frequent and severe in those receiving surgery. Gastric perforation or bleeding as a result of initial chemotherapy was not evident. Organ preservation has been a major advance for this disease with the use of chemotherapy.

Highly aggressive PGLs including Burkitt's and Burkitt's-like lymphoma have seen dramatic improvement in survival over the past decade as a result of potent chemotherapy combinations for systemic disease as well as better treatment of underlying immunodeficiency states (i.e., highly effective antiretroviral therapy for AIDS).

SUGGESTED READINGS

Adachi Y, Yasuda K, Inomata M, et al. Pathology and prognosis of gastric carcinoma: well versus poorly differentiated type. *Cancer* 2000;89(7):1418–1424.

Aviles A, Nambo MJ, Neri N, et al. The role of surgery in primary gastric lymphoma: results of a controlled clinical trial. *Ann Surg* 2004;240:44–50.

Bonenkamp JJ, Hermans J, Sasako M, et al. Extended lymph-node dissection for gastric cancer: Dutch Gastric Cancer Group. *N Engl J Med* 1999;340:908–914.

Chang HM, Jung KH, Kim TY, et al. A phase III randomized trial of 5-fluorouracil, doxorubicin, and mitomycin C versus 5-fluorouracil and mitomycin C versus 5-fluorouracil alone in curatively resected gastric cancer. *Ann Oncol* 2002;13(11):1779–1785.

Cullinan SA, Moertel CG, Wieard HS, et al. Controlled evaluation of three drug combination regimens versus fluorouracil alone for the therapy of advanced gastric cancer: North Central Cancer Treatment Group. *J Clin Oncol* 1994;12:412–416.

Cunningham D, Allum WH, Stenning SP, et al. Perioperative chemotherapy versus surgery alone for resectable gastroesophageal cancer. *N Engl J Med* 2006;355:11–20.

Cunningham D, Starling N, Rao S, et al. Capecitabine and oxaliplatin for advanced esophagogastric cancer. *N Engl J Med* 2008;358:36–46.

Earle CC, Maroun JA, Adjuvant chemotherapy after curative resection for gastric cancer non-Asian patients: revisiting a meta-analysis of randomised trials. *Eur J Cancer* 1999;35(7):1059–1064.

Gastrointestinal Tumor Study Group. A comparison of combination chemotherapy and combined modality therapy for locally advanced gastric carcinoma. *Cancer* 1982;49:1771–1777.

Gunderson LL, Sosin H. Adenocarcinoma of the stomach: areas of failure in a re-operation series (second or symptomatic look) clinicopathologic correlation and implications for adjuvant therapy. *Int J Radiat Oncol Biol Phys* 1982;8(1):1–11.

Hermans J, Bonenkamp JJ, Boon MC, et al. Adjuvant therapy after curative resection for gastric cancer: meta-analysis of randomized trials. *J Clin Oncol* 1993;11:1441–1447.

Kattan MW, Karpeh MS, Mazumdar M, et al. Postoperative nomogram for disease-specific survival after an R0 resection for gastric carcinoma. *J Clin Oncol* 2003;21:3647–3650.

Macdonald JS, Smalley SR, Benedetti J, et al. Chemoradiotherapy after surgery compared with surgery alone for adenocarcinoma of the stomach or gastroesophageal junction. *N Engl J Med* 2001;345(10): 725–730.

Sakuramoto S, Sasako M, Yamaguchi T, et al. Adjuvant chemotherapy for gastric cancer with S-1, and oral fluoropyrimidine. *N Engl J Med* 2007;357:1810–1820.

Stephens J, Smith J. Treatment of primary gastric lymphoma and gastric mucosa-associated lymphoid tissue lymphoma. *J Am Coll Surg* 1998;187(3):312–320.

Van Cutsem E, Moiseyenko VM, Tjulandin S, et al. Phase III study of docetaxel and cisplatin plus fluorouracil compared with cisplatin and fluorouracil as first-line therapy for advanced gastric cancer: a report of the V325 study group. *J Clin Oncol* 2006:24:4991–4997.

6

Biliary Tract Cancer

Linda E. Coate and Gregory D. Leonard

Carcinomas of the biliary tract include those cancers arising in either the gallbladder or the bile duct. There were estimated to be 9,250 new cases of gallbladder and biliary tract cancers (excluding intra-hepatic biliary tract cancer) and 3,340 deaths from these cancers in 2006 (1). Gallbladder cancer is twice as common as cholangiocarcinoma. The term cholangiocarcinoma was initially used to designate tumors of the intrahepatic bile ducts; it is now taken to refer to the entire spectrum of tumors arising in the intrahepatic, perihilar, and distal bile ducts. The epidemiology, clinical features, staging, and surgical treatment are distinct for carcinomas arising in the gallbladder and bile duct, and these are described separately. The palliative treatment options are similar and are discussed together at the end of the chapter.

CARCINOMA OF THE GALLBLADDER

Epidemiology

- The age-adjusted incidence of carcinoma of the gallbladder is 1.2 per 100,000 population in the United States from 2000 to 2004 (http://seer.cancer.gov/csr/1975_2004/).
- Carcinoma of the gallbladder is the fifth most common GI malignancy.
- It affects women two to six times more commonly than men and has a 50% greater incidence in whites as compared to black individuals (2). There is a prominent geographic variation in the incidence of gallbladder cancer, and the highest is among Native Americans and in South America (particularly Chile), Japan, and Eastern Europe, and the lowest incidence is in Singapore, Nigeria, and the United States.
- The mean age at diagnosis of the carcinoma is 65 years.

Etiology

- Cholelithiasis (gallstones): Of patients with gallbladder carcinoma, 70% to 90% have gallstones, whereas only 1% to 3% of patients with gallstones develop gallbladder cancer. The risk increases with increase in size of the stones (2).
- Infection: Chronic infection with *Salmonella typhi*, *Escherichia coli*, and *Helicobacter pylori* may also cause gallbladder carcinomas.
- Gallbladder polyps or porcelain gallbladder: Polyps >1 cm diameter have the greatest malignancy potential. Porcelain gallbladder due to extensive calcium deposition in the wall is a pathologic finding and is associated with cholelithiasis in nearly all cases. The reported incidence of gallbladder cancer in patients with this condition ranges from 12.5% to 60%.
- Miscellaneous: Anomalous pancreaticobiliary duct junction resulting in backflow of pancreatic juice and biliary stasis may cause gallbladder cancer. Obesity, estrogens, and chemicals from the rubber industry have also been associated with this disease.

Clinical Features

Early disease may be asymptomatic or present with very nonspecific symptoms, including the following:

- Pain (82%)
- Weight loss (72%)
- Anorexia (74%)
- Nausea or vomiting (68%)
- Mass in the right upper quadrant (65%)
- Jaundice (44%)
- Abdominal distension (30%)
- Pruritus (20%)
- Incidental (15–20%)
- Courvoisier's law states that if the gallbladder is enlarged and if the patient has painless jaundice, the cause is unlikely to be gallstones.
- In elderly patients, gallbladder cancer may present as cholecystitis.

Diagnosis

- The majority of gallbladder cancers are diagnosed as an incidental finding during exploration of presumed benign disease. Approximately 1% to 2% of patients undergoing exploration of presumed benign disease will have gallbladder cancer.
- Ultrasound is usually abnormal (thickened wall, mass, and loss of gallbladder or liver interface) but may not be specific for gallbladder cancer.
- Plain radiograph of the abdomen may detect calcifications from porcelain gallbladder.
- Endoscopic ultrasound (EUS) is more accurate than transabdominal ultrasound; it is useful in differentiating polyps from cancer and also in preoperative staging as it provides information on depth of tumor invasion and on regional lymph node appearance. It is however highly operator dependent and not available in all centers (3).
- Laboratory studies are generally not diagnostic but abnormal serology can occur with elevations in levels of alkaline phosphatase, γ-glutamyl transpeptidase, bilirubin, carcinoembryonic antigen (CEA), or CA 19-9, but these factors are more commonly elevated in cholangiocarcinoma.
- Computerized tomography (CT) scan allows visualization of the extent of tumor growth and nodal status and is useful in radiological staging of gallbladder cancer where distant metastases are common.
- Magnetic resonance cholangiopancreatography (MRCP) and cholangiography by endoscopic retrograde cholangiopancreatography (ERCP) are the optimal imaging modalities to outline local anatomy for preoperative planning (2).
- Biopsies prior to surgery may result in tumor seeding; therefore, the diagnosis is usually made at the time of surgery.

Pathology

- Adenocarcinoma accounts for more than 85% of cases. It is subcharacterized into papillary, tubular, mucinous, or signet cell type. Other histologies include anaplastic, squamous cell, small cell, carcinoid, and lymphoma.

Staging

- Gallbladder cancers are classified by Nevin et al. (4) or by using the TNM staging system (5) (Table 6.1).
- A staging laparoscopy is a useful adjunct to imaging modalities because it may detect intra-abdominal metastases, thereby sparing radical and potentially morbid surgery in patients.

TABLE 6.1. *TNM Staging systems for gallbladder cancer*

Stage IA	T1 N0 M0	T1a: invades lamina propria
		T1b: invades the muscle layer
Stage IB	T2 N0 M0	T2: invades perimuscular connective tissue
Stage IIA	T3 N0 M0	T3: perforates the serosa and/or directly invades the liver or one other adjacent organ
Stage IIB	T1–3 N1 M0	N1: metastases in cystic duct, choledochal, and/or hilar lymph nodes
Stage III	T4 N0–1 M0	T4: tumor invades portal vein or hepatic artery or multiple extrahepatic organs or structures
Stage IV	Any T any N M1	M1: distant metastases

Nevin stage

Stage I	Intramucosal only
Stage II	Extends to muscularis
Stage III	Extends through serosa
Stage IV	Transmural involvement and cystic lymph nodes are involved
Stage V	Direct extension to liver or distant metastases

Source: *AJCC Cancer Staging Manual*, 6th ed., 2002.

Treatment

Surgery

- Surgery is the only potentially curative therapy.
- Only 10% to 30% of patients can be considered for potentially curative surgery (2).
- Contraindications to surgery include liver or peritoneal metastases, ascites, extensive involvement of the hepatoduodenal ligament, and encasement or occlusion of major vessels. Direct involvemt of adjacent organs is not an absolute contraindication.
- Surgery can be a simple cholecystectomy or a radical (extended) cholecystectomy.
- A radical procedure involves wedge resection of the gallbladder bed, excision of the supraduodenal extrahepatic bile duct, en bloc dissection of regional lymph nodes, and resection of segments V and IVB of the liver (some physicians advocate pancreaticoduodenectomy) (6).
- Stage I disease can be treated successfully with a simple cholecystectomy, with survival rate being greater than 85%, but some physicians advocate radical surgery (Table 6.2).
- Up to 40% of stage IIA (formerly stage II) cancers are found to have lymph node involvement at surgery, upstaging them to pathological stage IIB (formerly stage III). Because of this upstaging, most surgeons advocate radical surgery for stage II and above. Many studies have demonstrated

TABLE 6.2. *Treatment and 5-year survival of gallbladder cancers according to stage*

TNM stage	Treatment	Median survival	5-year survival (%)
I	Simple cholecystectomy	19 mo	60–100
	Radical cholecystectomy		
II	Radical cholecystectomy	7 mo	10–20
	+/− Radiation therapy (not standard)		
III	Radical cholecystectomy	4 mo	5
	+/− Radiation therapy (not standard)		
IV	Palliation with stent placement	2 mo	0
	Surgery or radiation or chemotherapy or combination of these		

improvements in survival in patients reoperated with a radical procedure compared to those receiving only a simple cholecystectomy (7).
* Some authors have reported extended survivals with radical surgery even in stage IV patients studied by Nevin et al. (8).

Radiation
* In patients with unresectable tumors, radiation alone is rarely a successful palliative procedure (9).
* A number of reports have documented improvements in survival rates in cases of intraoperative or postoperative adjuvant radiotherapy. No prospective randomized controlled trials have been performed to address this issue.

Chemotherapy and Palliation
The benefits and options available for chemotherapy and palliation of carcinoma of the gallbladder are the same as those for cholangiocarcinoma.

Survival
The various aspects of survival following treatment of gallbladder cancers according to stage are given in Table 6.2.

CARCINOMA OF THE BILE DUCTS (CHOLANGIOCARCINOMA)

Epidemiology
* Cholangiocarcinomas arise from the epithelial cells of the intrahepatic and extrahepatic bile ducts.
* Cholangiocarcinoma accounts for 3% of all GI malignancies (9).
* Cholangiocarcinoma is subdivided into proximal extrahepatic (perihilar or Klatskin tumor; 50–60%), distal extrahepatic (20–25%), intrahepatic (peripheral tumor; 20–25%), and multifocal (5%) tumors (10).
* The incidence of intrahepatic bile duct tumors was 0.9 cases per 100,000 population between 1996 and 2000, and for other biliary tumors was 1.5 cases per 100,000 population. For unclear reasons the incidence of intrahepatic cholangiocarcinoma has increased, but this may be because of increased recognition.
* The incidence increases with age and is more common in men (11).

Etiology
* Inflammatory conditions: Primary sclerosing cholangitis is associated with a 10% to 15% lifetime risk. Ulcerative colitis and chronic intraductal gallstone disease also increase risk. Nearly 30% of cholangiocarcinomas are diagnosed in patients with coexistent ulcerative colitis and primary sclerosing cholangitis.
* Bile duct abnormalities: Caroli disease (cystic dilatation of intrahepatic ducts), bile duct adenoma, biliary papillomatosis, and choledochal cysts increase risk.
* Infection: In Southeast Asia, risk can be increased 25- to 50-fold by parasitic infestation from *Opisthorchis viverrini* and *Clonorchis sinensis*. Hepatitis C cirrhosis is also a risk factor.
* Genetic: Lynch syndrome II and multiple biliary papillomatosis are associated with an increased risk of developing cholangiocarcinoma.
* Miscellaneous: Smoking, thorotrast (a radiologic contrast agent), asbestos, radon, and nitrosamines are also known to increase risk (6).

Clinical Features
Cholangiocarcinomas usually become symptomatic when the biliary system becomes blocked.

* Intrahepatic cholangiocarcinoma may present as a mass, be asymptomatic, or produce vague symptoms such as pain, anorexia, weight loss, night sweats, and malaise.

- Extrahepatic cholangiocarcinoma usually presents with symptoms and signs of cholestasis (icterus, pale stools, dark urine, and pruritus or cholangitis, which includes pain, icterus, and fever).

Diagnosis

The diagnosis of cholangiocarcinoma can be challenging.

- Ultrasonography is the first-line investigation for suspected cholangiocarcinoma. Biliary dilatation is usually seen. This technique can often overlook masses and is poor at delineating anatomy.
- ERCP provides anatomical information (cholangiography) that is useful for planning surgery, but, more importantly, it may provide a tissue diagnosis. However, because these tumors are desmoplastic, cytology brushings have a low yield (30%) in making the diagnosis. When brushings and biopsy are combined, the yield improves to 40% to 70%. Endoscopic ultrasound and positron emission tomography (PET) may provide further information on local and distant disease, respectively.
- Endoscopic ultrasound may be useful in visualizing the extent of tumor and lymph node involvement of distal bile duct lesions. Its role in proximal bile duct lesions is less clear
- A cholestatic serologic picture (as discussed in gallbladder cancer) may be seen. A value of CA 19-9 >100 U per mL is highly suggestive of malignancy and is elevated in up to 85% of patients with cholangiocarcinoma (9).
- CT scan defines anatomy and can be used to direct CT scan–guided biopsies.
- MRCP is the optimal imaging modality.
- The diagnosis of cholangiocarcinoma is frequently based on the clinical scenario, serology, and radiology but without histologic confirmation, but such a diagnosis in the absence of tissue should be made only after efforts are taken to prove the diagnosis by use of cytologic or pathologic evaluation preoperatively.

Pathology

- Adenocarcinomas account for 95% of tumors. They are graded as well, moderately, and poorly differentiated and are further divided into sclerosing, nodular, and papillary subtypes.

Staging

- Up to 50% of patients have lymph node involvement at presentation and 10% to 20% have peritoneal involvement. In one series, laparoscopy prevented unnecessary surgery in one-third of patients (12).
- Staging is based on the TNM classification (5). Other classifications such as the classification by Bismuth et al. (13) define the extent of ductal involvement (Table 6.3).

TABLE 6.3. *Staging systems for extrahepatic bile duct cancers*

Stage IA	T1 N0 M0	T1: tumor confined to the bile duct
Stage IB	T2 N0 M0	T2: tumor invades beyond the bile duct wall
Stage IIA	T3 N0 M0	T3: tumor invades liver, gallbladder, pancreas, unilateral branches of portal vein, or hepatic artery
Stage IIB	T1–T3 N1 M0	N1: regional lymph node
Stage III	T4 any N M0	T4: tumor invades main portal vein or bilateral branches, common hepatic artery, or other adjacent structures
Stage IV	Any T any N M1	M1: distant metastases

(Continued)

TABLE 6.3.   *(Continued)*

Bismuth classification	
Type I	Tumors below the confluence of left and right hepatic ducts
Type II	Tumors reaching the confluence but not involving the left or right hepatic ducts
Type III	Tumors occluding the common hepatic duct and either the right or left hepatic duct
Type IV	Tumors that are multicentric or that involve the confluence of the right and left hepatic ducts

Source: AJCC Cancer Staging Manual, 6th ed., 2002.

Treatment

Surgery

- Surgery is the only curative option and may be possible in 30% to 60% of patients (14). The goals of surgery are (a) tumor removal and (b) establishing or restoring biliary drainage.
- Surgery for extrahepatic hilar cholangiocarcinomas is based on the stage of disease, and the goal of surgical intervention is to obtain a tumor-free margin >5 cm (Table 6.4).
- Long-term survival has been reported after liver transplantation in three studies, but transplantation is not a standard approach (6).
- Trimodality therapy is also advocated by some groups.

Radiation/Chemoradiation

- In patients with unresectable locally advanced disease or resected disease with positive margins there have been reports of long-term survival with combined-modality chemoradiotherapy. One report documented a median survival of 21 months in patients with unresectable cancer or those with residual disease after surgery (15,16).
- Definitive evidence from phase 3 studies to support this practice, however, remains lacking.

TABLE 6.4.   *Treatment and survival of cholangiocarcinomas according to location*

Location	Treatment	Median survival	5-year survival (%)
Extrahepatic (hilar)	Type I + II: en bloc resection of extrahepatic bile ducts, gallbladder, regional lymphadenectomy, and Roux-en-Y hepaticojejunostomy Type III: as above plus right/left hepatectomy Type IV: as above plus extended right/left hepatectomy	12–24 mo	9–18
Extrahepatic (distal)	Pancreaticoduodenectomy	12–24 mo	20–30
Intrahepatic	Resect involved segments or lobe of liver	18–30 mo	10–45

- In locally advanced disease radiation with or without chemotherapy may ameliorate painful symptoms and contribute towards biliary decompression.
- Adjuvant radiation is not a standard recommendation because there is limited and conflicting data on this subject.

Chemotherapy

- Chemotherapy appears to provide palliative benefit to patients with biliary tract cancer, although definitive proof of a survival benefit is lacking (17). Similarly, its role in the adjuvant setting is uncertain.
- Many trials supporting the use of chemotherapy in biliary cancer contain small numbers of patients and include a heterogeneous mix of bile duct tumors, gallbladder cancer, pancreatic cancer, and hepatic cancer.
- There are now many chemotherapy options for cholangiocarcinoma and gallbladder cancer (6,18). Many of these trials are reported in abstract form or sample sizes are small, so the treatment of choice has not been established. Usual response rates are between 10% and 20%, and high response rates found in single-institution studies have not been reproducible in larger multi-institution trials.
- Historically, fluoropyrimidines have been the cytotoxic therapy of choice, but the likelihood of response is less than 10%. Increasingly, gemcitabine is considered a standard of care.
- Gemcitabine combinations, for example, cisplatin and gemcitabine, have demonstrated high response rates of 20% to 60% and median survival up to 20 months. Gemcitabine combined with capecitabine is a frequently used regimen (19,20) but as yet, there have been no randomized comparisons showing clear-cut superiority over single-agent therapy.
- Other gemcitabine combinations that have demonstrated efficacy in the treatment of advanced biliary tumors are oxaliplatin and irinotecan.
- Mitomycin, as a single agent or in combination therapy, has demonstrated response rates of up to 47% and median survivals of 9.5 months.
- Other single agents with activity include docetaxel, irinotecan, raltitrexed, anthracyclines, carboplatin, and oxaliplatin.

Targeted Therapy

- A phase 2 study has shown erlotinib, a tyrosine kinase inhibitor of the epidermal growth factor receptor to have efficacy in a small study of previously treated and chemo-naive patients with biliary cancer (21).
- Antitumor activity was also noted in a small phase 2 trial combining erlotinib with bevacizumab the monoclonal antibody directed against the vascular endothelial growth factor (22). Similarly small trials have also combined targeted therapy with chemotherapy (23). Clinical trials are ongoing to investigate this area.

Palliation

- Patients with unresectable or metastatic disease may benefit from palliative surgery, radiation, chemotherapy, or a combination of these.
- Biliary drainage can be achieved by Roux-en-Y choledochojejunostomy, bypass of the site of obstruction to left or right hepatic duct, or endoscopic or percutaneously placed stents (metal-wall stents have a larger diameter and are less prone to occlusion or migration and are preferably used in patients with a life expectancy of greater than 6 months and/or in those who have unresectable disease).
- Photodynamic therapy is another option for patients with locally advanced inoperable disease (24). This involves injecting a porphyrin photosensitizer and then endoscopically applying light to the tumor. Although the data are derived from small studies to support this practice, the survival benefit derived from photodynamic therapy appears impressive with one report showing an improvement in median survival of 14 months (25).
- Celiac plexus blockade may also ameliorate symptoms of pain in the patient with inoperable disease.

REFERENCES

1. Jemal A, Murray T, Samuels A, et al. Cancer statistics, 2008. *CA Cancer J Clin* 2008;58:1–96.
2. Misra S, Chaturvedi A, Misra NC, et al. Carcinoma of the gallbladder. *Lancet Oncol* 2003; 4:167–176.
3. Sadamoto Y, Kubo H, Harada N, Tanaka M, Eguchi T, Nawata H. Preoperative diagnosis and staging of gallbladder carcinoma by EUS. *Gastrointest Endosc* 2003;58:536–541.
4. Nevin JE, Moran TJ, Kay S, et al. Carcinoma of the gallbladder, staging, treatment and prognosis. *Cancer* 1976;37:141–148.
5. American Joint Committee on Cancer. *Cancer staging manual*, 6th ed. New York: Springer-Verlag, 2002:139–156.
6. Yee K, Sheppard BC, Domreis J, et al. Cancers of the gallbladder and biliary ducts. *Oncology* 2002;16:939–957.
7. Todoroki T, Kawamoto T, Takahashi H, et al. Treatment of gallbladder cancer by radical resection. *Br J Surg* 1999;86:622–627.
8. Fong Y, Jarnagin W, Blumgart LH. Gallbladder cancer: comparison of patients presenting initially for definitive operation with those presenting after prior noncurative intervention. *Ann Surg* 2000;232:557–569.
9. Vauthey JN, Blumgart LH, Recent advances in the management of cholangiocarcinomas. *Semin Liver Dis* 1994;14:109–114.
10. Houry S, Haccart V, Huguier M, et al. Gallbladder cancer: role of radiation therapy. *Hepatogastro-enterology* 1999;46:1578–1584.
11. Khan SA, Davidson BR, Goldin R, et al. Guidelines for the diagnosis and treatment of cholangi-ocarcinoma: consensus document. *Gut* 2002;51(Suppl. VI):vi1–vi9.
12. Corvera CU, Weber SM, Jarnagin WR. Role of laparoscopy in the evaluation of biliary tract cancer. *Surg Oncol Clin North Am* 2002;11:877–891.
13. Bismuth H, Castaing D, Traynor O, et al. Resection or palliation: priority of surgery in the treatment of hilar cancer. *World J Surg* 1988;12:39–47.
14. de Groen PC, Gores GJ, LaRusso NF, et al. Biliary tract cancers. *N Engl J Med* 1999;341:1368–1378.
15. Morganti AG, Trodella L, Valentini V, et al. Combined modality treatment in unresectable extrahe-patic biliary carcinoma. *Int J Radiat Biol Phys* 2000;46:913–999.
16. Shinohara E.T, Mitra N, Guo M, et al. Effect of radiation therapy on survival in the adjuvant and definitive treatment of cholangiocarcinoma *Proc GI Cancers Symposium* 2008:140; (abstr 143)
17. Glimelius B, Hoffman K, Sjoden PO, et al. Chemotherapy improves survival and quality of life in advanced biliary and pancreatic cancer. *Ann Oncol* 1996;7(6):793–600.
18. Henja M, Pruckmayer M, Raderer M. The role of chemotherapy and radiation in the management of biliary cancer: a review of the literature. *Eur J Cancer* 1998;34:977–986.
19. Knox JJ, Hedley D, Oza A, et al. Combining gemcitabine and capecitabine in patients with advanced biliary cancer: a phase II trial. *J Clin Oncol* 2005;23:2332–2334.
20. Cho JY, Paik YH, Chang YS, et al. Capecitabine combined with gemcitabine (CapGem) as first-line treatment in patients with advanced/metastatic biliary tract carcinoma. *Cancer* 2005;104: 2753–2756.
21. Philip P. Mahoney M, ALlmer C, et al. Phase II Study of Erlotinib in patients with advanced biliary cancer. *J Clin Oncol* 2006;24:3069–3074.
22. LoConte NK, Holen KD, Mahoney MR, et al. Interim report of a multicenter phase II clinical trial testing a combination of biweekly bevacizumab and daily erlotinib in patients with metastatic bile tract carcinoma: a phase II consortium (P2C). *Proc GI Cancers Symposium* 2008:196; (abstr 255).
23. Clark JW, Meyerhardt JA, Sahani DV, et al. Phase II study of gemcitabine, oxaliplatin in combina-tion with bevacizumab (GEMOX-B) in patients with unresectable or metastatic biliary tract and gallbladder cancers. *Proc Am Soc Clin Oncol* 2007;25:18S (abstr 4625).
24. Berr F, Wiedmann M, Tannapfel A, et al. Photodynamic therapy for advanced bile duct cancer: evidence for improved palliation and extended survival. *Hepatology* 2000;31:291–298.
25. Zoepf T, Jakobs R, Arnold JC, et al. Palliation of nonresectable bile duct cancer improved survival after photodynamic therapy. *Am J Gastroenerol* 2005;100:2426–2430.

7

Primary Cancers of the Liver

Syed J. Asghar, Carmen J. Allegra, and Gregory D. Leonard

Primary liver cancers arise predominantly from the parenchymal liver cells or hepatocytes (90%) and are called hepatocellular carcinoma (HCC). The incidence of HCC continues to increase rapidly in the United States, with rates increasing the fastest in men (1). Research on vaccinations for hepatitis B and their use have impacted the development of HCC in many regions of the world.

EPIDEMIOLOGY

- In the United States, the incidence of clinically significant metastatic carcinoma to the liver is 20 times more common than primary liver cancer.
- Based on November 2006 SEER data submission, the incidence for all races was 9.9 per 100,000 men and 3.5 per 100,000 women (http://seer.cancer.gov/statfacts/html/livibd.html).
- There are fewer than 10,000 new patients annually, accounting for less than 2% of all malignancies.
- There is marked geographic variation in the incidence of HCC, with the highest incidences occurring in sub-Saharan Africa and Asia. Over 40% of all cases of HCC occur in the People's Republic of China, which has an annual incidence of 137,000 cases (2).
- Men are affected twice as often as women (mean 3.7:1). The mean age at diagnosis is between 50 and 60 years.

ETIOLOGY

- Cirrhosis is present in 80% of patients with HCC. Therefore, risk factors for cirrhosis are also risk factors for HCC.
- Hepatitis B virus (HBV) infection increases the risk of developing HCC by 100-fold. HBV causes 80% of HCC in the world. HCC develops from chronic hepatitis due to HBV at a rate of 0.5% per year; 15% to 80% have HBs antigenemia.
- Hepatitis C virus (HCV) infection accounts for 30% to 50% of HCC in the United States. In contrast to HBV infection, HCC in patients with hepatitis C occurs almost exclusively in those with cirrhosis.
- Alcoholic cirrhosis accounts for 15% of HCC.
- Hemochromatosis (HH), hereditary tyrosinemia, and autoimmune chronic active hepatitis are other causes of cirrhosis and are associated with a significant risk for developing HCC. In all, 3% to 27% of patients with long-standing HH develop HCC.
- There is less convincing evidence for the risk of developing HCC from Aflatoxin B_1 (chemical product of *Aspergillus*), androgenic steroids, thorotrast (radiology contrast agent), oral contraceptives, and non-alcoholic fatty liver disease. In diabetes mellitus, the risk was increased by approximately 2.5 times.

CLINICAL FEATURES

The most common symptoms or signs of HCC are:

- Pain (91%)
- Weight loss (35%)

89

- Vomiting (8%)
- Hepatomegaly (89%)
- Abdominal swelling (43%)
- Jaundice (7–41%).

Paraneoplastic manifestations can also occur. They include hypoglycemia, hypercalcemia, carcinoid, erythrocytosis, hypercholesterolemia, hyperthyroidism, and osteoporosis. The physical findings in most patients with HCC (splenomegaly, ascites, jaundice, or other manifestations of decompensated cirrhosis) reflect the underlying liver disease. Hepatomegaly or a bruit heard over the liver are occasionally present.

DIAGNOSIS

The diagnosis of HCC is often suspected in a patient with underlying liver disease (i.e., cirrhosis, chronic viral hepatitis), who develops a rising serum alfa-fetoprotein (AFP) level (3).

Recommendations for diagnosis of HCC have been issued in a guideline from the American Association for the Study of Liver Diseases (3).

- Nodules found on ultrasound surveillance that are smaller than 1 cm should be followed with ultrasound at intervals of 3 to 6 months. If there has been no growth over a period of up to 2 years, one can revert to routine surveillance.
- Nodules between 1 and 2 cm found on ultrasound screening of a cirrhotic liver should be investigated further with two dynamic studies, whether computed tomography (CT) scan, contrast ultrasound, or magnetic resonance imaging (MRI) with contrast. If the appearances are typical of HCC (i.e., hypervascular with washout in the portal/venous phase) in two techniques the lesion should be treated as HCC. If the findings are not characteristic or the vascular profile is not coincidental among techniques, the lesion should be biopsied.
- If the nodule is larger than 2 cm at initial diagnosis and has the typical features of HCC on a dynamic imaging technique, biopsy is not necessary for the diagnosis of HCC. Alternatively, if the AFP is >200 ng/mL biopsy is also not required. However, if the vascular profile on imaging is not characteristic or if the nodule is detected in a noncirrhotic liver, biopsy should be performed.
- Biopsies of small lesions should be evaluated by expert pathologists. If the biopsy is negative for HCC, patients should be followed by ultrasound or CT scanning at 3 to 6 month intervals until the nodule disappears, enlarges, or displays diagnostic characteristics of HCC. If the lesion enlarges but remains atypical for HCC, a repeat biopsy is recommended.

Serum Markers

The most commonly used marker for HCC is the serum AFP concentration. Several other serologic markers (such as des-gamma-carboxy prothrombin—these other markers are not used in routine clinical practice) may indicate the presence of HCC, and used alone or in combination with the serum AFP may improve the diagnostic accuracy.

It is generally accepted that serum levels greater than 500 mcg/L (normal in most laboratories is between 10 and 20 mcg/L) in a high-risk patient is diagnostic of HCC. However, HCC is often diagnosed at a lower AFP level in patients undergoing screening (4), as not all tumors secrete AFP, and serum concentrations are normal in up to 40% of small HCCs, eppsecially where alcohol is the etiological factor (5). AFP levels are normal in the majority of patients with fibrolamellar carcinoma, a variant of HCC.

Imaging Studies

The imaging tests most commonly used for the diagnosis of HCC are ultrasound, CT, MRI, and angiography. A classic appearance on one of these imaging modalities combined with an elevated serum AFP concentration in the appropriate clinical setting is usually sufficient for establishing the diagnosis of HCC.

PET Scanning

The ability of a PET scan to distinguish benign lesions from malignant lesions is unclear. A new tracer, ^{11}C-acetate, appears to improve sensitivity and specificity when used in conjunction with F-FDG PET. Until further data are available, the role of PET scanning in the evaluation of patients with HCC remains uncertain (6,7).

- Laparoscopy is recommended to improve staging and to prevent unnecessary laparotomy (8).

PATHOLOGY

- Ninety percent of primary cancers of the liver are HCC, the remaining include cholangiocarcinoma, hepatoblastoma, angiosarcoma, and other sarcomas. There are many histologic types of HCC including trabecular, pseudoglandular or acinar, compact, scirrhous, clear cell, and fibrolamellar.
- Fibrolamellar carcinoma is a histologic variant accounting for 1% of HCC. It occurs more commonly in women, is not associated with cirrhosis, and has a better prognosis than HCC.

STAGING

- The TNM staging system (Table 7.1) has been criticized because it does not evaluate the underlying liver disease, which is clearly a major prognostic factor in patients regardless of tumor stage.
- The Child-Pugh grading system has been incorporated into the management of HCC because it evaluates the status of the underlying liver function and influences treatment (Table 7.2).

TREATMENT

Surgery

- Surgery remains the only possibility for cure in HCC. Surgery is applicable to only about 5% of the U.S. population.
- The treatment of HCC is determined by two factors: tumor extent and the severity of the underlying hepatic parenchymal disease.

TABLE 7.1. *The American Joint Committee on Cancer (AJCC) sixth edition TNM stage groupings*

Stage I	T1 N0 M0	T1: solitary tumor with no vascular invasion	5-year survival rates—55%
Stage II	T2 N0 M0	T2: solitary tumor with vascular invasion or multiple tumors none >5 cm	5-year survival rates—37%
Stage IIIA	T3 N0 M0	T3: multiple tumors 5 cm or involving a major branch of the portal or hepatic vein(s)	
Stage IIIB	T4 N0 M0	T4: tumor directly invading adjacent organs other than gallbladder or perforating visceral peritoneum	5-year survival rates—15%
Stage IIIC	Any T N1 M0	N1: regional lymph node metastases	
Stage IV	Any T any N M1	M1: distant metastases	

TABLE 7.2. *Child-Pugh scoring system*

Chemical and biochemical parameters	Score attributed to each parameter		
	1	2	3
Encephalopathy	None	1–2	3–4
Ascites	None	Slight	Moderate
Albumin (g/dL)	>3.5	2.8–3.5	<2.8
Prothrombin time prolonged (s)	1–4	4–6	>6
INR	<1.7	1.7–2.3	>2.3
Bilirubin (mg/dL)	1–2	2–3	>3

Class A = 5–6 points, Class B = 7–9 points, Class C = 10–15 points. These grades correlate with 1- and 2-year patient survival—grade A: 100% and 85%; grade B: 80% and 60%; and grade C: 45% and 35%.

- Partial hepatectomy: Only 13% to 35% are surgical candidates. Small tumors have the best outcomes. Recurrence is most commonly seen in the remnant liver. Repeat hepatectomy is possible in 10% to 29% of patients. Operative mortality is <5%, but is higher in the presence of cirrhosis. Long-term relapse-free survival rates average 40% or better, and 5-year survival rates as high as 90% are reported in carefully selected patients.
- Total hepatectomy and liver transplantation: Transplantation is indicated in patients with severe cirrhosis or where extensive resection leaving minimal liver reserve is required.
- Orthotopic liver transplantation (OLT) is a suitable option for unresectable patients who have a solitary HCC ≤5 cm in diameter or up to three separate lesions none of which is larger than 3 cm, no evidence of gross vascular invasion, and no regional nodal or distant metastases (The Milano/Mazzaferro criteria). Based on these criteria, 4-year survival was reported as 75% to 85% (9).
- Survival outcomes may be further improved by living donor transplantation, although this remains controversial.
- Disadvantages of transplantation are the expense, the lack of specialty centers performing operations, and the lack of donor livers.

Ablative Techniques

- Although there is no absolute tumor size beyond which radiofrequency ablation (RFA) should not be considered, the best outcomes are in patients with a single tumor <4 cm in diameter. For cirrhotic patients, some clinicians restrict RFA to those with Child-Pugh class A or B severity only.
- Ablation of large tumors (>5 cm) has been shown to be associated with very high local recurrence rates.
- Percutaneous ethanol or acetic acid into tumors is frequently used for up to three localized tumors of <5 cm that are not surgical candidates usually due to cirrhosis. It is relatively inexpensive and well tolerated.
- RFA is performed percutaneously using ultrasound guidance and causes focal coagulative necrosis of tumors via thermal energy. It is most efficacious for tumors <3 cm where complete necrosis can occur in up to 90% of tumors.
- Cryotherapy is also safe and more effective than RFA for larger tumors, but is less suited to a percutaneous approach.
- Hepatic artery chemoembolization (transarterial chemoembolization [TACE]) is based on the principal that 80% of the blood supply to tumors is from the hepatic artery, which supplies only 20% to 30% of normal liver parenchyma. Ligation or embolization of the hepatic artery can induce temporary tumor responses, but when combined with chemotherapy can be more efficacious.
- TACE is used most often for the treatment of large unresectable HCCs that are not amenable to other treatments such as resection or RFA; its use as a "bridging therapy" prior to transplant is less well defined. Bland particle embolization alone (i.e., without chemotherapy) has also been used for both unresectable and locally recurrent HCC.

- This approach is currently progressing, resulting in an improved median survival rate and quality of life. In a study of 16 patients with stage II–IV unresectable or recurrent HCC, hepatic arterial infusion (HAI) of oxaliplatin was administered. HAI-oxaliplatin was shown to be feasible, well-tolerated, and to demonstrate activity in patients with advanced HCC (10).
- Absolute contraindications to this technique include the absence of hepatopetal blood flow (portal vein thrombosis), encephalopathy, and biliary obstruction.

Radiation

- Liver can only tolerate about 20 Gy. However, safe and effective doses can be given to palliate the pain.
- Radioactive isotopes have demonstrated efficacy in the adjuvant treatment of HCC.
- Stereotactic radiotherapy: Stereotactic body radiation therapy (SBRT) is a technique in which a single (sometimes called sterotactic radiosurgery) or limited number of high-dose radiation fractions are delivered to a small, precisely defined target by using multiple, nonparallel radiation beams. The beams converge precisely on the target lesion, minimizing radiation exposure to adjacent normal tissue. This targeting allows treatment of small- or moderate-sized tumors in extracranial sites in either a single or limited number of dose fractions.
- Stereotactic approaches to RT are increasingly being used for treatment of metastatic liver tumors.
- Selective internal irradiation: For example, iodine-131 (^{131}I)-labeled lipiodol or yttrium-90 (^{90}Y)-tagged glass microspheres are delivered selectively to the tumor via the hepatic artery. Early reports suggest that radioembolization using intrahepatic artery administration of (^{90}Y)-tagged glass microspheres is safe, and induces objective responses in patients with unresectable HCC. However, long-term follow-up of these studies and additional experience are needed with this technique.

Chemotherapy

- Hepatocellular cancer has been considered to be a relatively chemotherapy-refractory tumor.
- Systemic therapy is appropriate for patients with advanced unresectable disease who are unsuitable for locoregional therapy.
- Single-agent chemotherapy has demonstrated response rates of approximately 15% to 30%, which increases to 20% to 35% with combination therapy. Cisplatin and anthracycline combinations have been studied most extensively, but there is no reference regimen for this disease (11). Despite objective responses that are occasionally complete, median survival in all of these studies has been short (4–11 months), with the exception of those in which resection/transplantation is attempted after chemotherapy.
- Interferon-alfa (IFNa) and chemoimmunotherapy: Combinations of chemotherapy with IFNa appear active.
- The PIAF regimen (intravenous cisplatin, recombinant interferon-alfa 2b, doxorubicin, and 5-fluorouracil) demonstrated a 50% objective response rate in 50 patients with unresectable disease from Hong Kong (12), but failed to show superiority versus Doxorubicin (13).

Molecularly Targeted Therapy

- Sorafenib (a multikinase inhibitor with antiangiogenic, proapoptotic, and Raf kinase–inhibitory activity) was well tolerated and is the first agent to demonstrate a statistically significant improvement in overall survival (OS) for patients with advanced HCC. The OS was significantly longer in the sorafenib-treated patients (10.7 vs. 7.9 months; HR = 0.69, $P = 0.0006$), as was the time to progression (5.5 vs. 2.8 months; HR = 0.58, $P = 0.000007$). This effect is clinically meaningful and establishes sorafenib as first-line treatment for patients with advanced HCC (14). It has also demonstrated encouraging results with doxorubicin (15).

VEGF Receptor Targeting

- Bevacizumab: Bevacizumab (an anti-VEGFR monoclonal antibody [MoAb]) alone is active in HCC. A preliminary report of a trial documented a partial response in 2 of 27, and disease stabilization in 18 patients (16).
- The combination of bevacizumab with gemcitabine and oxaliplatin (GEMOX) was safe and moderately effective in a small phase 2 trial.
- Sunitinib: Sunitinib is an orally active TKI that targets a variety of TKs in addition to VEGFR, including platelet-derived growth factor receptors (PDGFRs), KIT, RET, and FLT3. Some antitumor activity is suggested with early studies (17).

Anti-EGFR Strategies

- Small-molecule TK inhibitors: Limited activity for erlotinib (Tarceva), a small-molecule TKI with specificity for EGFR, was suggested in a phase 2 study of 38 patients with unresectable or metastatic HCC, one-half of whom had previously received cytotoxic chemotherapy (18).
- Cetuximab: Cetuximab (Erbitux) is a MoAb that binds to the EGFR. Early results suggest activity for cetuximab in combination with GEMOX (19).

PREVENTION AND NOVEL THERAPIES

- Hormone therapy: Tamoxifen, megestrol, antiandrogen therapy, and octreotide have been extensively investigated but do not have a beneficial effect on patients with HCC. HMG-CoA reductase inhibitors such as pravastatin have shown conflicting results (20).
- IFNa reduces the onset of liver damage and its progression to cirrhosis in 10% to 30% of patients with chronic hepatitis B.
- Refrigerated storage of food grains and transportation of grains in refrigerated vehicles should help reduce the risk of ingesting aflatoxin.
- Acyclic retinoid polyprenoic acid, reduces the incidence of second primary of HCC after initial resection and requires further investigation.
- Screening of high-risk populations with AFP at 4-month intervals and with ultrasound at yearly intervals has been shown to identify patients with earlier stages of HCC and may improve survival in high-risk groups (21).

REFERENCES

1. Jemal A, Siegel R, Ward E, et al. Cancer statistics, 2008. *CA Cancer J Clin.* 2008;58:71–96.
2. Skolnick, AA. Armed with epidemiologic research, China launches programs to prevent liver cancer (news). *JAMA.* 1996;13;276:1458–1459.
3. Bruix J, Sherman M. Management of hepatocellular carcinoma. *Hepatology.* 2005;42:1208–1236.
4. Wu JT. Serum alpha-fetoprotein and its lectin reactivity in liver disease: a review. *Ann Clin Lab Sci.* 1990;20:98–105.
5. Fasani P, Sangiovanni A, De Fazio C, et al. High prevalence of multinodular hepatocellular carcinoma in patients with cirrhosis attributable to multiple risk factors. *Hepatology.* 1999;29:1704–1747.
6. Ho YJ, Jeng LB, Yang MD, et al. A trial of single photon emission computed tomography of the liver with technetium-99m tetrofosmin to detect hepatocellular carcinoma. *Anticancer Res.* 2003; 23:1743–1746.
7. Iwata Y, Shiomi S, Sasaki N, et al. Clinical usefulness of positron emission tomography with fluorine-18-fluorodeoxyglucose in the diagnosis of liver tumors. *Ann Nucl Med.* 2000;14:121–126.
8. Llovet JM, Fuster J, Bruix J. Intention-to-treat analysis of surgical treatment of early hepatocellular carcinoma: resection versus transplantation. *Hepatology.* 1999;30:1434–1440.
9. Mazzaferro V, Regalia E, Doci R, et al. Liver transplantation for the treatment of small hepatocellular carcinomas in patients with cirrhosis. *N Engl J Med.* 1996;334:693–699.

10. Rathore R, Soares G, Bass J, et al. Hepatic arterial infusion (HAI) of oxaliplatin in advanced hepatocellular cancer (HCC): a phase I Brown University Oncology Group study. *Proc Gastrointestinal Cancers Symposium* 2008;183 (abstr 230).

11. Johnson PJ. Are there indications for chemotherapy in hepatocellular carcinoma. *Surg Oncol Clin North Am.* 2003;12:127–134.

12. Leung TW, Patt YZ, Lau WY, et al. Complete pathological remission is possible with systemic combination chemotherapy for inoperable hepatocellular carcinoma. *Clin Cancer Res.* 1999;5: 1676–1681.

13. Yeo W, Mok TS, Zee B, et al. A phase III study of doxorubicin (A) versus cisplatin (P)/interferona-2b (I)/doxorubicin (A)/fluorouracil (F) combination chemotherapy (PIAF) for inoperable hepatocellular carcinoma (HCC). *J Natl Cancer Inst.* 2005;19;97:1532–1538.

14. Llovet J, Ricci S, Mazzaferro V, Hilgard P, et al. Sorafenib improves survival in advanced Hepatocellular Carcinoma (HCC): results of a Phase III randomized placebo-controlled trial (SHARP trial). *Proc Am Soc Clin Oncol.* 2007;25:18s (abstr LBA1).

15. Abou-Alfa G. Preliminary results from a Phase II, randomized, double-blind study of sorafenib plus doxorubicin versus placebo plus doxorubicin in patients with advanced hepatocellular carcinoma. *Proc Gastrointestinal Cancers Symposium* 2008;132 (abstr 128).

16. Schwartz JD, Schwartz M, Lehrer D, et al. Bevacizumab in unresectable hepatoceullar carcinoma (HCC) for patients without metastasis and without invasion of the portal vein. *Proc Am Soc Clin Oncol.* 2006; 24:18s (abstr 4144).

17. Zhu AX, Sahani DV, di Tomaso E, et al. A phase II study of sunitinib in patients with advanced hepatocellular carcinoma. *Proc Am Soc Clin Oncol.* 2007;25:18s (abstr 4637).

18. Philip PA, Mahoney MR, Allmer C, et al. Phase II study of Erlotinib (OSI-774) in patients with advanced hepatocellular cancer. *J Clin Oncol.* 2005;23:6657–6663.

19. Asnacios A, Fartoux L, Romano O, et al. Gemcitabine plus oxaliplatin (GEMOX) combined with cetuximab in patients with progressive advanced stage hepatocellular carcinoma: results of a multicenter phase 2 study. *Cancer.* 2008 Apr 15 (Epub ahead of print).

20. Kawata S, Yamasaki E, Nagase T, et al. Effect of pravastatin on survival in patients with advanced hepatocellular carcinoma. A randomized controlled trial. *Br J Cancer.* 2001;84:886–891.

21. Yang B, Zhang B, Xu Y, et al. Prospective study of early detection for primary liver cancer. *J Cancer Res Clin Oncol.* 1997;123:357–360.

8

Colorectal Cancer

Thomas J. George, Jr.

EPIDEMIOLOGY

- Colorectal cancer (CRC) is the second leading cause of cancer death among men and women combined in the United States and is the third most common cause of cancer, separately, in men and in women.
- Nearly 149,030 new cases of CRC were diagnosed in 2008 in the United States, and one-third of patients would have died as a result of the disease (1).
- The lifetime risk of developing CRC is 1:18.
- Surgery will cure almost 50% of all diagnosed patients, although almost 80,000 people develop metastatic CRC each year.
- The incidence of colon cancer is higher in the more economically developed regions, such as the United States or Western Europe, than in Asia, Africa, or South America.
- U.S. mortality rates from CRC continue to decline (2.3% decrease from 1998 to 2004) as a result of effective screening programs, diagnosing early disease, and effective therapies.

RISK FACTORS

Although certain conditions predispose patients to develop colon cancer, up to 70% of patients have no identifiable risk factors:

- Age: More than 90% of colon cancers occur in patients older than 50 years.
- Gender: The incidence of colon cancer is higher in women, whereas rectal cancer is more common in men.
- Ethnicity: The occurrence of cancer is more common in African Americans than in whites, and mortality is 10% higher in African Americans.
- Personal history of colorectal cancer or adenomas:
  - tubular adenomas (lowest risk)
  - tubulovillous adenomas (intermediate risk)
  - villous adenomas (highest risk)
- Tobacco use: About 2.5-fold increased risk of adenomas is observed in smokers.

Obesity

- Dietary factors: High-fiber, low caloric intake, and low animal fat diets may reduce the risk of cancer.
- Calcium deficiency: Daily intake of 1.25 to 2.0 g of calcium was associated with a reduced risk of recurrent adenomas in a randomized placebo-controlled trial.
- Micronutrient deficiency: Folate, selenium, and vitamins E and D deficiency may increase the risk of cancer.
- Inflammatory bowel disease: Ulcerative colitis increases risk by 7-fold to 11-fold, especially with the duration of colitis (8–12 years) and with the detection of dysplasia. Crohn's disease is associated with a twofold increased risk of CRC.

- Nonsteroidal anti-inflammatory drugs: An American Cancer Society study reported 40% lower mortality in regular aspirin users, and similar reductions in mortality were seen in prolonged nonsteroidal anti-inflammatory drug use in patients with rheumatologic disorders. The cyclooxygenase-2 (COX-2) inhibitor celecoxib is approved by the U.S. Food and Drug Administration (FDA) for adjunctive treatment of patients with familial adenomatous polyposis (FAP). Chemoprevention with selective COX-2 inhibitors must be balanced against increased cardiovascular risks (2).
- Family history: In the general population, if one first-degree relative develops cancer, it increases the relative risk for other family members to 1.72, and if two relatives are affected, the relative risk increases to 2.75. Increased risk is also observed when a first-degree relative develops an adenomatous polyp before age 60. True hereditary forms of cancer account for only 6% of CRCs.

FAMILIAL CANCER SYNDROMES

Familial Adenomatous Polyposis

Familial adenomatous polyposis (FAP) is an autosomal-dominant inherited syndrome with more than 90% penetrance, manifested by hundreds of polyps developing by late adolescence. The risk of developing invasive cancer over time is virtually 100%. Germline mutations in the adenomatous polyposis coli (APC) gene on chromosome 5q21 have been identified. The loss of the APC gene results in altered signal transduction with increased transcriptional activity of β-catenin. Several FAP variants with extraintestinal manifestations also exist:

- Attenuated FAP: This variant generates flat adenomas that arise at an older age. Mutations tend to occur in the proximal and distal portions of the APC gene.
- Gardner's syndrome: Associated with desmoid tumors, osteomas, lipomas, and fibromas of the mesentery or abdominal wall.
- Turcot's syndrome: Involves tumors (esp. medulloblastoma) of the central nervous system.
- Peutz–Jeghers syndrome: Includes non-neoplastic hamartomatous polyps throughout the gastrointestinal tract and perioral melanin pigmentation.
- Juvenile polyposis: Associated with hamartomas in colon, small bowel, and stomach.

Hereditary Nonpolyposis Colorectal Cancer (HNPCC)

The Lynch syndromes, named after Henry T. Lynch, include Lynch I or the colonic syndrome, which is an autosomal-dominant trait characterized by distinct clinical features including proximal colon involvement, mucinous or poorly differentiated histology, pseudodiploidy, and the presence of synchronous or metachronous tumors. Increased survival has been observed in patients despite colon cancer developing before 50 years, with a lifetime risk of cancer approximating 75%. In Lynch II or the extracolonic syndrome, individuals are susceptible to malignancies in the endometrium, ovary, stomach, hepatobiliary tract, small intestine, and genitourinary tract.

The Amsterdam criteria (3-2-1 rule) were established to identify potential kindreds and include:

- Histologically verified CRC in at least three family members, one being a first-degree relative of the other two members
- CRC involving at least two successive generations
- At least one family member being diagnosed by 50 years

Inclusion of extracolonic tumors and clinicopathological and age modifications were introduced by the Bethesda criteria in 1997. Germline defects in DNA mismatch-repair genes (*hMSH2, hMLH1, hPMS1,* and *hPMS2*) have been detected, and resultant microsatellite instability (MSI) can be identified in virtually all HNPCC kindred and in 15% to 20% of sporadic colon cancers.

SCREENING

Several professional societies have developed screening guidelines for the early detection of colon cancer. There are a number of early detection tests for colon cancer in average-risk asymptomatic

TABLE 8.1. *American Cancer Society Recommended Colorectal Cancer Screening Guidelines for asymptomatic average-risk individuals*

Beginning at age 50, all patients should have one of the five screening options listed.

Test	Frequency
Fecal Occult Blood Test (FOBT)	Every year
Flexible sigmoidoscopy	Every 5 years
FOBT plus flexible sigmoidoscopy (preferred option of the first three options)	Every year
	Every 5 years
Double-contrast barium enema	Every 5 years
Colonoscopy*	Every 10 years

*Colonoscopy should be done if the FOBT shows blood in the stool, if sigmoidoscopy results show a polyp, or if double-contrast barium enema studies show anything abnormal. If possible, all polyps should be completely removed during the colonoscopy.

patients. The American Cancer Society screening guidelines (Table 8.1) are the most widely cited. Starting at age 50, both men and women should discuss the full range of testing options with their physician. Any positive or abnormal screening test should be followed up with colonoscopy. Individuals with a family or personal history of colon cancer or polyps, or a history of chronic inflammatory bowel disease, should be tested earlier and possibly more often.

Virtual Colonoscopy

A virtual colonoscopy, or computerized tomographic colonography, is an emerging technology in which a spiral computerized tomography (CT) scan of the colon is obtained and three-dimensional images are created and reviewed by a radiologist. Specificity for detection of polyps and cancer appear reasonable, but there is a wide range of sensitivities reported despite improved experience by providers and consistent technology (3). Patients still require bowel preparation and colonic distension as well as ingestion of oral contrast. Detected abnormalities require investigation with endoscopy. Additional studies are required before this technique can be recommended routinely.

Carcinoembryonic Antigen

Carcinoembryonic antigen (CEA) is not useful for general CRC screening purposes. CEA has a low positive predictive value whereby approximately 60% of cancers are missed. It is routinely recommended in surveillance programs.

K-*ras* Detection

The K-*ras* gene is mutated in 30% to 50% of CRCs, and the detection in stool represents a potentially powerful screening strategy. This is currently an active area of clinical investigation.

PATHOPHYSIOLOGY

More than 90% of CRC is adenocarcinoma, the focus of this chapter. Other primary cancers of the colon and rectum include Kaposi's sarcoma, non-Hodgkin's lymphomas, small cell carcinoma, and carcinoid tumors. Although uncommon, metastases to the large bowel include melanoma, ovarian, and gastric cancer. Anatomic location and symptoms at presentation are the primary differences between right colon, left colon, and rectal adenocarcinomas.

Colon carcinogenesis involves progression from hyperproliferative mucosa to polyp formation, with dysplasia, and transformation to noninvasive lesions and subsequent tumor cells, with invasive and metastatic capabilities. CRC is a unique model of multistep carcinogenesis resulting from the accumulation of multiple genetic alterations. Stage-by-stage molecular analysis has revealed that this progression involves several types of genetic instability, including loss of heterozygosity, with chromosomes 8p, 17p, and 18q representing the most common chromosomal losses. The 17p deletion accounts for loss of p53 function, and 18q contains the tumor-suppressor genes deleted in colon cancer (i.e., DCC) and the gene deleted in pancreatic 4 (i.e., DPC4).

Colon carcinogenesis also occurs as a consequence of defects in the DNA mismatch-repair system. The loss of *hMLH1* and *hMSH2*, predominantly, in sporadic cancers leads to accelerated accumulation of additions or deletions in DNA. This MSI contributes to the loss of growth inhibition mediated by transforming growth factor-β due to a mutation in the type II receptor. Mutations in the APC gene on chromosome 5q21 are responsible for FAP and are involved in cell signaling and in cellular adhesion, with binding of β-catenin. Alterations in the APC gene occur early in tumor progression. Mutations in the proto-oncogene *ras* family, including K-*ras* and N-*ras*, are important for transformation and also are common in early tumor development.

DIAGNOSIS

Signs and Symptoms

- Abdominal pain, typically intermittent and vague
- Weight loss
- Bowel changes for left-sided colon and rectal cancers, including constipation, decreased stool caliber (pencil stools), and tenesmus
- Early satiety
- Fatigue
- Obstruction, perforation, acute or chronic bleeding, or liver metastasis, all of which contribute to symptom development
- Unusual presentations include deep venous thrombosis, *Streptococcus bovis* bacteremia or endocarditis, and nephrotic-range proteinuria
- Clinical findings include iron-deficiency anemia, weight loss, electrolyte abnormalities, and liver enzyme elevations

Diagnostic Evaluation

- A double-contrast barium enema may be more cost effective as an initial evaluation, but endoscopic studies provide histologic information, potential therapeutic intervention, and overall greater sensitivity and specificity.
- CEA elevations occur in non–cancer-related conditions, reducing the specificity of CEA measurements alone in the initial detection of colon cancer.
- Basic laboratory studies including complete blood count, electrolytes, liver and renal function tests, and CT scan of the abdomen and pelvis (with or without chest evaluation) are useful in initial cancer diagnosis and staging.
- In colon cancers, CT scan sensitivity for detecting distant metastasis is higher (75–87%) than for detecting nodal involvement (45–73%) or the extent of local invasion (~50%). CT scanning is very sensitive for detection of malignant pelvic lymph nodes in rectal cancer as any perirectal adenopathy is presumed to be malignant, since benign adenopathy is not typically seen in this area.
- Contrast-enhanced magnetic resonance imaging (MRI) can help determine the status of suspicious lesions in the liver as well as the characteristics (not just size) of perirectal adenopathy.
- PET scanning adds little over conventional imaging in the initial staging and diagnosis of CRC.

Endoscopic rectal ultrasound is a valuable tool in the preoperative evaluation of rectal cancer, with high accuracy of determining the extent of the primary tumor (63–95%) and perirectal nodal status (63–82%).

STAGING

The American Joint Committee on Cancer staging of CRC using the TNM classification was updated in 2002 (Fig. 8.1 and Table 8.2). Patients with stage II and III disease have been further stratified, and vascular or lymphatic invasion has been included. The tumor designation, or T stage, defines the extent of bowel wall penetration, as opposed to tumor size. The Dukes or MAC staging system is no longer used.

PROGNOSIS

Pathologic staging remains the most important determinant of prognosis (Table 8.3). Stage for stage, rectal cancer confers a worse prognosis than colon cancer (4). Other prognostic variables that have been proposed to be associated with an unfavorable outcome include:

- Advanced age of patient
- High tumor grade
- High CEA level

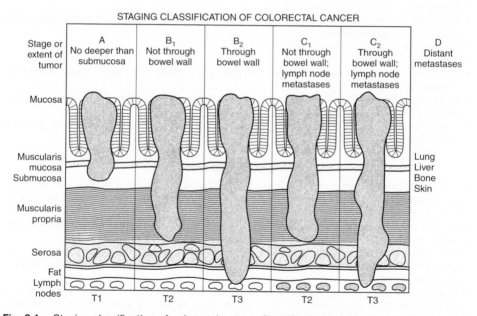

Fig. 8.1. Staging classification of colorectal cancer. Classification is based on modifications of Dukes' system. Stages B3 and C3 (not shown) signify invasion of contiguous organs or structures (TF). Prognosis is also determined by the number of positive lymph nodes: more than four (N2) lymph nodes predicts a worse outcome than one to three (N1) lymph nodes, and a poor histopathologic differentiation, vascular or lymphatic invasion, and a positive preoperative CEA value of >5 ng/mL implies a worse outcome. According to the revised TNM classification system, stage I equals T1 or T2 N0 (Dukes' stage A and B_1); stage II equals T2 or T4 N0 (Dukes' stage B_2 and B_3); stage III equals any T plus N1, N2, or N3 (Dukes' stage C_1, C_2, and C_3); and stage IV equals any T any N plus M1 (Dukes' stage D).

TABLE 8.2. *TNM classification of colorectal cancer staging designated by the American Joint Committee on Cancer (AJCC), sixth edition (2002).*

Primary tumor (T)[a]

T0	No evidence of primary tumor
Tis	Carcinoma in situ—intraepithelial or invasion of the lamina propria
T1	Invasion of submucosa
T2	Invasion of muscularis propria
T3	Invasion through the muscularis propria into the subserosa or into nonperitonealized pericolic or perirectal tissues
T4	Tumor directly invades other organs or structures, and/or perforates visceral peritoneum

Lymph node status (N)[b]

N0	No regional lymph node involvement
N1	Metastases in one to three regional lymph nodes
N2	Metastases in four or more regional lymph nodes

Metastatic disease (M)

M0	No distant metastases
M1	Distant metastases present

Stage grouping

Stage	T	N	M
0	Tis	N0	M0
I	T1–T2	N0	M0
IIA	T3	N0	M0
IIB	T4	N0	M0
IIIA	T1–T2	N1	M0
IIIB	T3–T4	N1	M0
IIIC	T1–T4	N2	M0
IV	T1–T4	N0–2	M1

Lymphadenectomy should contain at least 12 lymph nodes for adequate staging.
[a]The V and L substaging should be used to identify the presence or absence of vascular or lymphatic invasion.
[b]Smooth metastatic nodules in the pericolic or perirectal fat are considered lymph node metastases and will be counted in the N status. In contrast, irregularly contoured metastatic nodules in the peritumoral fat are considered as a vascular invasion and will be coded as an extension of the T category as either V1 (microscopic vascular invasion) if it is only microscopically visible or as V2 (macroscopic vascular invasion) if it is grossly visible.

- Bowel obstruction or perforation at presentation
- Biochemical and molecular markers such as elevated thymidylate synthase, p53 mutations, or loss of heterozygosity of chromosome 18q (DCC gene) are associated with a poor prognosis (5,6). MSI caused by a defective DNA mismatch-repair system (altered *MLH1*, *MSH2*; associated with HNPCC) is associated with an improved outcome.

MANAGEMENT ALGORITHM

Surgery

- For colon cancers, the primary curative intervention requires en bloc extirpation of the involved bowel segment and mesentery, with pericolic and intermediate lymphadenectomy for both staging and therapeutic intent. Negative proximal, distal, and lateral surgical margins are of paramount importance.
- For rectal cancers, en bloc resection of the primary tumor with negative proximal, distal, and radial margins is critical as well as a sharp dissection of the mesorectum (total mesorectal excision) to optimally reduce local recurrence. The location of the tumor in relation to the anal sphincter is the

TABLE 8.3. *Prognosis by stage for colon and rectal cancers*

Stage	5-Year overall survival (%)	
	Colon	*Rectal*
0–I	93	90
IIA	85	75
IIB	72	65
IIIA	83	55
IIIB	64	35
IIIC	44	24
IV	8	6

primary determinant in a low anterior resection (LAR) versus an abdominoperineal resection (APR). The latter generates a permanent colostomy. For highly selected very early stage rectal cancer cases, transanal endoscopic microsurgery may be a reasonable option.
• Surgical intervention is indicated if polypectomy pathology reveals muscularis mucosal involvement or penetration.
• Surgical palliation may include colostomy or even resection of metastatic disease for symptoms of acute obstruction or persistent bleeding.
• The number of lymph nodes resected and pathologically examined is critical to accurate staging. The probability of determining true node negativity increases with the number of nodes sampled. At least 12 lymph nodes should be examined and reported.

Radiation Therapy

• Routine administration of abdominal radiotherapy (RT) is limited by bowel-segment mobility, adjacent small bowel toxicity, previous surgery with adhesion formation, and other medical comorbidities.
• Local control and improved disease-free survival (DFS) have been reported in retrospective series of patients with T4 lesions or perforations, nodal disease, and subtotal resections, who have been treated with 5,000 to 5,400 cGy directed at the primary tumor bed and draining lymph nodes. However, there are no randomized data to support the routine use of RT in the management of colon cancer.
• In contrast, RT is utilized in rectal cancers to reduce local recurrence and improve resectability.

Adjuvant Chemotherapy Studies for Colon Cancer

Intergroup 0035

This large Intergroup trial of 5-fluorouracil (5-FU) and levamisole (Lev) is of historic importance because it reported a 41% reduction in the relapse rate and a 33% decrease in overall cancer mortality (7). This study resulted in the National Institutes of Health consensus panel recommending that 5-FU–based adjuvant therapy be administered to all patients with resected stage III colon cancer.

Intergroup 0089

Intergroup 0089 randomized 3,759 patients with stage II or III disease to one of four therapeutic arms (8, 9). The results demonstrated that the 5-FU and leucovorin (LV) containing schedules (Mayo Clinic and Roswell Park) were equivalent without the need for Lev. A 6-month schedule of the 5-FU and LV was similar to a protracted 12 months of therapy.

The 5-year DFS and overall survival (OS) for each of the four arms in the study were as follows:

- 5-FU + Lev for 12 months; DFS = 56%, OS = 63%
- 5-FU + high-dose LV (Roswell Park) for 8 months; DFS = 60%, OS = 66%
- 5-FU + low-dose LV (Mayo) for 6 months; DFS = 60%, OS = 66%
- 5-FU + LV + Lev; DFS = 60%, OS = 67%

X-ACT

Utilization of an oral fluoropyrimidine (capecitabine) was evaluated in patients with stage III disease. Capecitabine (1,250 mg/m^2 b.i.d. for 14 days, every 3 weeks) was compared with the Mayo Clinic bolus of 5-FU and LV (10). The study was designed to demonstrate equivalency, with a primary endpoint of 3-year DFS. The capecitabine arm was noninferior and demonstrated a trend toward superiority in DFS (64% vs. 60%, HR 0.87; 95% CI, 0.75–1.00; P = 0.0526). Toxicity was improved in all categories except hand–foot syndrome. A 3-year DFS endpoint was chosen because a retrospective analysis of more than 20,000 patients demonstrated equivalency to the conventional 5-year OS benchmark (11).

MOSAIC

In Europe, 2,219 patients with stage II (40%) and III (60%) disease treated with infusional 5-FU with LV modulation versus the same combination with oxaliplatin (FOLFOX4) every 2 weeks for 6 months (12), which demonstrated a 3-year DFS benefit favoring the FOLFOX4 combination over standard 5-FU with LV (78.2% vs. 72.9%, HR 0.77; 95% CI, 0.65–0.92; P = 0.002). With a median 6-year follow-up, the DFS advantage was confirmed with a trend toward improved OS (13). Treatment with FOLFOX4 was well tolerated, with 41% patients having grade 3 and 4 neutropenia, with only 0.7% being associated with fever. Anticipated grade 3 peripheral neuropathy or paresthesias were observed (12%) which almost entirely resolved 1 year later (1%).

NSABP C-07

The addition of oxaliplatin to three cycles of adjuvant Roswell Park 5-FU with LV (FLOX) was evaluated in 2,407 stage II (30%) and III (70%) patients (14). The combination improved 3-year DFS (76.1% vs. 71.8%; HR 0.80; 95% CI, 0.69–0.93; P =0.003). Grade 3 diarrhea (38%) and peripheral neuropathy (8%) were significantly worse with FLOX without any difference in treatment-related mortality.

CALGB 89803, PETACC-3, and ACCORD

Unlike oxaliplatin, at least three studies failed to confirm a benefit for the use of adjuvant irinotecan. CALGB 89803 was a study of irinotecan with bolus 5-FU and LV (IFL) versus weekly 5-FU in patients with stage III disease (15). Increased grade 3 and 4 neutropenia and early deaths were observed in the experimental arm, and a higher number of patients withdrew from the study. Overall, IFL was not better than the 5-FU and LV arm. The two European studies (PETACC-3 and ACCORD) together randomized over 3,500 patients to infusional 5-FU with or without irinotecan. Both studies failed to reach their primary endpoint of 3-year DFS, although toxicities were less than in the IFL study. The use of irinotecan cannot be recommended in the adjuvant setting.

Adjuvant Chemotherapy Regimens for Colon Cancer

Based on these studies, adjuvant chemotherapy is recommended for patients with stage III colon cancer. Several acceptable options exist (Table 8.4), with combination regimens offering increased efficacy and toxicity. The incorporation of biologic targeted therapy into the adjuvant setting is the topic of numerous, ongoing, large clinical trials.

TABLE 8.4. *Acceptable adjuvant chemotherapy regimens for stage III colon cancer*

Name	Regimen and dose	Repeated (days)	Total cycles
Mayo Clinic	LV 20 mg/m^2/day IV followed by 5-FU 425 mg/m^2/day IV days 1–5	28	6
Roswell Park	LV 500 mg/m^2 IV followed by 5-FU 500 mg/m^2 IV weekly × 6	8 wk	3–4
Capecitabine	1,250 mg/m^2 PO twice daily × 14 days	21	8
FOLFOX4	Oxaliplatin 85 mg/m^2 IV on day 1 followed by LV 200 mg/m^2/day IV on days 1 and 2 followed by 5-FU 400 mg/m^2/day IV on days 1 and 2 followed by 5-FU 600 mg/m^2/day CIVI for 22 hours on days 1 and 2	14	12
FOLFOX6	Oxaliplatin 85–100 mg/m^2 IV on day 1 followed by LV 400 mg/m^2/day IV on day 1 followed by 5-FU 400 mg/m^2/day IV on day 1 followed by 5-FU 2,400 mg/m^2 CIVI for 46 hours	14	12
FLOX	LV 500 mg/m^2 IV followed by 5-FU 500 mg/m^2 IV on days 1, 8, 15, 22, 29, 36 and Oxaliplatin 85 mg/m^2 IV on days 1, 15 and 29	8 wk	3

There is no role for biologic targeted therapy or irinotecan-containing regimens in the adjuvant setting at this time.

LV, leucovorin; IV, intravenous; 5-FU, 5-fluorouracil; CIVI, continuous intravenous infusion.

Fluoropyrimidines

Reasonable options include 5-FU with LV via the Mayo Clinic or Roswell Park regimen or capecitabine. The toxicity profile of the regimens differs. Myelosuppression and oral mucositis are more common with the daily Mayo Clinic regimen, whereas diarrhea may be more severe with the weekly Roswell Park schedule. Cryotherapy with ice held in the mouth during the 5-FU infusion may help lessen the mucositis associated with the therapy. Hand–foot syndrome (HFS) and diarrhea are primary toxicities of capecitabine.

Oxaliplatin Combinations

Increased efficacy as well as toxicity is seen with the addition of oxaliplatin to either bolus or infusional 5-FU and LV. FOLFOX6 represents a modification to FOLFOX4, which omits the day 2 bolus 5-FU and LV and gives more continuously infused 5-FU over 46 hours, and appears to have activity equivalent to that of FOLFOX4 in the advanced disease setting. It has been incorporated into numerous adjuvant clinical trials given the improved ease of administration.

Adjuvant Chemotherapy for Stage II Colon Cancer

Despite the 75% 5-year survival with surgery alone, some patients with stage II disease have a higher risk of relapse, with outcomes being similar to those of node-positive patients. Adjuvant chemotherapy provides up to 33% relative risk reduction in mortality, resulting in an absolute treatment benefit of approximately 5%.

Several analyses have reported varying outcomes in patients with stage II disease who received adjuvant treatment:

- The National Surgical Adjuvant Breast and Bowel Project (NSABP) summary of protocols (C-01 to C-04) of 1,565 patients with stage II disease reported a 32% relative reduction in mortality (cumulative odds, 0.68; 95% CI, 0.50–0.92; $P = 0.01$). This reduction in mortality translated into an absolute survival advantage of 5% (16).
- A meta-analysis by Erlichman et al. (17) detected a nonsignificant 2% benefit (82% vs. 80%; $P = 0.217$) in 1,020 patients with high-risk T3 and T4 cancer treated with 5-FU and LV for 5 consecutive days.
- Schrag et al. reviewed Medicare claims for chemotherapy within the Surveillance, Epidemiology, and End Results (SEER) database and identified 3,700 patients with resected stage II disease among whom 31% received adjuvant treatment (18). No survival benefit was detected with 5-FU compared to surgery alone (74% vs. 72%) even with patients considered to be at high risk because of obstruction, perforation, or T4 lesions.
- The Quasar Collaborative Group study reported an OS benefit of 3.6% in 3,239 patients (91% Dukes B colon cancer) prospectively randomized to chemotherapy versus surgery alone (19). With a median follow-up of 5.5 years, the risk of recurrence (HR 0.78; 95% CI, 0.67–0.91; $P = 0.001$) and death (HR 0.82; 95% CI, 0.70–0.95; $P = 0.008$) favored 5-FU and LV chemotherapy.
- In the MOSAIC study, FOLFOX4 chemotherapy showed nonsignificant benefits in DFS over 5-FU and LV in patients with stage II disease (86.6% vs. 83.9%, HR 0.82, 95% CI, 0.57–1.17).
- The American Society of Clinical Oncology Panel concluded in 2004 that the routine use of adjuvant chemotherapy for patients with stage II disease could not be recommended (20). A review of 37 randomized controlled trials and 11 meta-analyses found no evidence of a statistically significant survival benefit with postoperative treatment of stage II patients. However, treatment should be considered for specific subsets of patients (e.g., T4 lesions, perforation, poorly differentiated histology, or inadequately sampled nodes), and patient input is critical.
- Utilization of molecular prognostic markers in stage II disease is being incorporated into active clinical trial protocols to help determine which patients may maximally benefit from adjuvant therapy.

Perioperative Treatment for Rectal Cancer

In contrast to colon cancer, local treatment failures after potentially curative resections represent a major clinical problem. Combined-modality chemotherapy with radiation therapy (chemoRT) is now the standard therapy for patients with stages II and III rectal cancer (T3, T4, and nodal involvement).

Intergroup 0114

A four-arm study of 1,695 patients compared 5-FU alone, 5-FU and LV combination, 5-FU and Lev combination, and 5-FU and LV and Lev combination (21). Two cycles of chemotherapy were administered before and after chemotherapy in combination with 5,040 cGy of external beam radiation (4,500 cGy with 540 cGy boost). The chemotherapy during the radiation was given as a bolus with or without LV. The DFS and OS was similar in all treatment arms, leading to the conclusion that 5-FU alone was as effective as other combinations.

NCCTG

Both DFS and OS advantages were observed in patients receiving continuous infusion of 5-FU during radiation when compared with those receiving bolus 5-FU (22). This survival benefit has led to continuous infusion of 5-FU during radiation being considered as a standard.

German Rectal Cancer Study Group

The benefit of delivering chemoRT in a preoperative (neoadjuvant) fashion was evaluated in 421 patients compared to 401 similar patients randomized to receive postoperative chemoRT (23). In both groups, 5-FU was administered in a continuous fashion during the first and fifth weeks of radiation. All patients received an additional four cycles of adjuvant 5-FU after chemoRT and surgery. Results of neoadjuvant treatment provided improvement in local recurrence (6% vs. 13%; $P = 0.006$), but no difference in 5-year OS. Both acute toxic effects (27% vs. 40%; $P = 0.001$) and long-term toxicities (14% vs. 24%; $P = 0.01$) were less common with neoadjuvant treatment. Preoperative chemoRT followed by surgical resection with postoperative 5-FU–based chemotherapy represents a standard approach to patients with rectal cancer.

Combined-Modality Options for Rectal Cancer

1. Following initial treatment with surgery:
   - Intravenous 5-FU bolus (500 mg/m^2/day) on days 1 to 5 and on days 36 to 40.
   - Followed by radiation therapy given in 180 cGy fractions over 5 weeks, starting day 64, to a total dose of 4,500 to 5,400 cGy along with 5-FU (225 mg/m^2/day) by ambulatory infusion pump during the entire 5-week period of radiation therapy.
   - Followed by intravenous 5-FU bolus (450 mg/m^2/day) given daily for 5 days on days 134 to 138 and on days 169 to 173 for a total treatment period of 6 months.
2. Neoadjuvant therapy:
   - Intravenous 5-FU continuous infusion (1,000 mg/m^2/day) given daily for 5 days during the first and fifth week of radiation therapy, which is given in 180 cGy fractions to a total dose of 5,040 cGy.
3. Followed by surgery:
   - Upon recovery from surgery, intravenous 5-FU bolus (500 mg/m^2/day) on days 1 to 5 repeated every 28 days for 4 cycles.

The oral fluoropyrimidine capecitabine mimics infusional 5-FU and has been investigated in conjunction with radiation. Additionally, oxaliplatin is being evaluated as a radiation sensitizer for patients with rectal disease. Given the previously discussed data for adjuvant chemotherapy regimens in colon cancer, several different regimens (see Table 8.4) may be considered in select cases as components of the systemic adjuvant chemotherapy phase of therapy in rectal cancer.

FOLLOW-UP AFTER ADJUVANT TREATMENT

Eighty percent of recurrences are seen within 2 years of initial therapy. The American Cancer Society recommends total colonic evaluation with either colonoscopy or double-contrast barium enema within 1 year of resection, followed every 3 to 5 years if findings remain normal. Synchronous cancers must be excluded during initial surgical extirpation, and metachronous malignancies in the form of polyps must be detected and excised before more malignant behavior develops.

History and physical evaluations with serum CEA measurements should be performed every 3 to 6 months for the first few years after therapy. These evaluations can be further reduced during subsequent years. Surveillance imaging should be reserved for those individuals who would be considered operable candidates if localized metastases were to be identified. Elevations of CEA postoperatively may suggest residual tumor or early metastasis. Patients with initially negative levels of CEA can subsequently exhibit positive levels; therefore, serial CEA measurements after completion of treatment may identify patients who are eligible for a curative reresection, in particular, patients with a solitary liver or lung metastasis.

TREATMENT FOR ADVANCED COLORECTAL CANCER

Unprecedented improvements in survival have been recognized during the past decade with systemic chemotherapy in advanced or metastatic disease. Median survival has improved from 6 months with best supportive care to over 2 years with incorporation of all active agents (24).

5-Fluorouracil–Based Chemotherapy

5-FU and LV chemotherapy regimens in advanced CRC have objective response rates of 15% to 20%, with median survival of 8 to 12 months. Toxicity is predictable and manageable.

Continuous Infusion of 5-Fluorouracil

The efficiency of continuous infusion of 5-FU may be equivalent to or slightly better than that of bolus 5-FU and LV and is generally well tolerated despite the inconvenience of a prolonged intravenous infusion apparatus (25, 26). Toxicities include mucositis and palmar–plantar erythrodysesthesia (hand–foot syndrome); however, myelosuppression is less common. Continuous infusions of 5-FU may have activity in patients who have progressed on a bolus 5-FU regimen.

Capecitabine

Capecitabine, an oral fluoropyrimidine prodrug, undergoes a series of three enzymatic steps in its conversion to 5-FU. The final enzymatic step is catalyzed by thymidine phosphorylase, which is expressed in tumor tissues. Two phase 3 studies have compared single-agent capecitabine to the Mayo Clinic 5-FU and LV regimen and demonstrated higher response rates for the former but equivalent time to progression and median survival (27). The toxicity profile favored the capecitabine arm with decreased gastrointestinal and hematologic toxicities and fewer hospitalizations. An increased frequency of hand–foot syndrome and hyperbilirubinemia were noted with capecitabine.

Oxaliplatin

Oxaliplatin is an agent that differs structurally from other platinums in its 1,2-diaminocyclohexane (DACH) moiety, but acts similary by generating DNA adducts. Oxaliplatin exhibits synergy with 5-FU with response rates as high as 66% even in patients who are refractory to 5-FU. Despite its unique toxicities (i.e., reversible peripheral neuropathy, laryngopharyngeal dysesthesias, and cold hypersensitivities), oxaliplatin lacks the emetogenic and nephrogenic toxicities of cisplatin.

Oxaliplatin was initially approved for second-line therapy in metastatic CRC based on a study comparing FOLFOX4 with oxaliplatin alone and with infusional or bolus 5-FU and LV. In this study, response rate, time to progression, and relief of tumor-related symptoms were improved with FOLFOX4, when compared to the other treatment arms. Despite the improved time to progression, the OS difference was not statistically significant (9.8 vs. 8.7 and 8.1 months, respectively).

The North Central Cancer Treatment Group (NCCTG-9741) conducted a trial (28) comparing first-line FOLFOX4 versus IFL versus IROX (irinotecan in combination with oxaliplatin). Of the original six arms in the study, three were eliminated based on changes in the standard of care or toxicity. In addition, higher 60-day mortality was detected in the IFL arm, resulting in a dose reduction in the protocol. The response rate, time to progression, and OS were significantly better in the FOLFOX4 arm than in the modified IFL arm. However, imbalances in the second-line chemotherapy administered to patients in this study may confound the survival differences. Approximately 60% of the oxaliplatin failures were treated with irinotecan, whereas only 24% of patients who are refractory to irinotecan received oxaliplatin. In addition, the study was not designed to address the effect of infusional 5-FU. The observed toxicities in the study were reflective of the specific drug combinations and included grade 3 or higher paresthesias (18%) in the FOLFOX arm and a 28% incidence of diarrhea in the IFL arm. Despite a higher degree of neutropenia (60% in FOLFOX vs. 40% in IFL) with FOLFOX, febrile neutropenia was significantly greater in the IFL arm. IROX also exhibited significant toxicities. Oxaliplatin was approved by the FDA for use in the first-line treatment of patients with metastatic CRC largely based on this study.

Although FOLFOX is clearly a superior regimen compared to IFL, the use of infusional 5-FU with irinotecan (FOLFIRI) may produce results similar to those seen using FOLFOX. Tournigand et al. reported an equivalent median survival of 21.5 months with FOLFIRI followed by FOLFOX and a median survival of 20.6 months with the opposite sequence ($P = 0.99$) (29). The conclusion is that similar survival is observed in patients receiving either sequence.

Irinotecan/CPT-11

Irinotecan is a topoisomerase I inhibitor, with activity in patients with advanced CRC and in patients deemed refractory to 5-FU. As a single agent, response rates as high as 20% are observed, and an additional 45% of patients achieve disease stabilization. Significant survival advantages have been shown for irinotecan as second-line therapy after 5-FU compared with supportive care or with continuous-infusion 5-FU regimens. Several schedules are typically administered with and without 5-FU, however, the cumulative data suggest that irinotecan should not be utilized with bolus 5-FU (i.e., IFL) due to excessive treatment-related mortality.

Irinotecan obtained FDA approval based on a study (30) comparing IFL to the 5-FU bolus Mayo Clinic regimen. A higher response rate (39% vs. 21%; $P = 0.0001$) and OS (14.8 vs. 12.6 months; $P = 0.042$) were observed favoring IFL.

Delayed-onset diarrhea is common and requires close monitoring and aggressive management (high-dose loperamide, 4 mg initially and then 2 mg every 2 hours until diarrhea stops for at least 12 hours). Neutropenia, mild nausea, and vomiting are common. This combination of toxicities can be severe and life-threatening, which was evident in NCCTG 9741 (see previous oxaliplatin section). A higher 60-day mortality was observed (4.5% vs. 1.8%), and the dose of the irinotecan required reduction.

Infusional 5-FU with biweekly irinotecan offered improvements in response (35% vs. 22%; $P < 0.005$), median survival (17.4 vs. 14.1 months; $P = 0.031$), and quality of life over 5-FU (31). Neutropenia was equivalent to that found in the weekly irinotecan regimen, although febrile neutropenia and diarrhea were markedly reduced.

As monotherapy, irinotecan every 3 weeks produced responses in 13.7% of patients and stable disease in another 44% of cases (32). In patients who are refractory to 5-FU, a median survival of 10.5 months was reported. Administration of weekly irinotecan alone has also been reported by Pitot et al (33). In patients receiving 5-FU earlier, a 13% response rate and an 7.7 median response duration were observed.

Bevacizumab

Bevacizumab (BEV) is a recombinant humanized antivascular endothelial cell growth factor (VEGF) monoclonal antibody with amino acid sequence similarity of 97% to that of human IgG1. BEV blocks VEGF-induced angiogenesis with an exceptionally high affinity for VEGF. One of the initial trials with BEV in untreated CRC patients combined BEV with weekly bolus 5-FU and LV. Interestingly, a 40% response rate and 21.5-month median survival was observed. The major toxicities included arterial thrombosis (13 patients with three treatment discontinuations and one patient death), proteinuria, and hypertension. Updated toxicity data reveals that full-dose anticoagulation can be administered with BEV and that there is no increased risk of deep venous thrombus formation. When added to IFL, BEV increased the response rate (45% vs. 35%; $P = 0.004$) and had a longer median survival (20.3 vs. 15.6 months; $P < 0.001$) (34). When added to FOLFOX in the second-line setting, response rates are again increased (23% vs. 9%; $P < 0.001$) along with OS (12.9 vs. 10.8 months; $P = 0.0011$) (35). BEV has been approved by the FDA for the treatment of patients with advanced CRC in combination with any intravenous 5-FU–based regimen. The optimal duration of treatment remains controversial and under intense investigation.

Cetuximab and Panitumumab

The epidermal growth factor receptor (EGFR) and pathway represent a targeted approach to CRC therapy. Two monoclonal antibodies are FDA approved for use in patients with metastatic CRCs. Importantly, tumor EGFR positivity by immunohistochemistry staining does not correlate with treatment response; however, K-*ras* mutational status does. K-*ras* is an intracellular tyrosine kinase involved in the EGFR signal transduction pathway. There appears to be no clinical benefit to the use of EGFR inhibition if K-*ras* is mutated (i.e., not wild-type), which is the case in approximately 40% of patients (36). Commercial testing for K-*ras* mutational status is available.

Cetuximab is a chimerized IgG1 antibody that prevents ligand binding to the EGFR and its heterodimers. Cetuximab exhibits higher affinity (subnanomolar) or approximately 1-log greater binding than the natural ligands for EGFR. Panitumumab is a fully humanized IgG2 antibody also targeting EGFR. These agents block receptor dimerization, tyrosine kinase phosphorylation, and subsequent downstream signal transduction. Both agents can cause a skin rash and diarrhea, but are without myelosuppression. A correlation between the intensity of the skin rash and survival has been consistently noted.

Cetuximab is FDA approved based on a study in patients refractory to irinotecan. They were randomized to the combination of cetuximab and irinotecan versus cetuximab alone with improvements in the response rate (22.9% vs. 10.8%; $P = 0.0074$) and time to progression (4.1 vs. 1.5 months; $P < 0.0001$) favoring the combination (37). Despite manageable toxicity, no improvements in survival outcomes were observed.

Panitumumab is FDA approved as monotherapy given improvement in progression-free survival over best supportive care in heavily pretreated patients (HR, 0.54; 95% CI, 0.44–0.66; $P < 0.0001$), although no overall survival advantage was noted (38). Attempts to combine this agent with FOL-FOX or FOLFIRI plus BEV in first-line management of advanced disease did not provide benefit over placebo for unclear reasons.

CHEMOTHERAPY REGIMENS FOR METASTATIC COLORECTAL CANCER

See Tables 8.4 and 8.5. Investigations into the optimal timing and sequence of treatment combinations both with and without EGFR and VEGF inhibition continue.

CONTROVERSIES

Hepatic-only Metastasis

The liver is the most common site for metastasis, with one-third of cases involving only the liver. Approximately 25% of liver metastases are resectable, with certain patient subsets showing 30% to 40% 5-year survival after resection and 3% to 5% operative morbidity and mortality. Nonoperative ablative techniques (i.e., cryoablation, radiofrequency ablation, and hepatic artery embolization with or without chemotherapy) have not shown consistent durable survival benefits. Intraoperative ultrasound is the most sensitive test for initial detection, followed by CT scan or MRI. PET scanning can help identify occult extrahepatic disease in select patients being considered for resection. Optimal therapy to improve survival after surgical resection is controversial.

Patients with unresectable disease limited to the liver can be treated with locoregional hepatic artery infusion (HAI) or systemic chemotherapy. Kemeny et al. (39) reported a 4-year DFS and hepatic

TABLE 8.5. *Select chemotherapy regimens for advanced colorectal cancer[a]*

Name	Regimen and dose	Repeated (days)
XELOX	Oxaliplatin 100–130 mg/m² IV on day 1 Capecitabine 850 mg/m² PO twice daily on days 1–14	21
Irinotecan	300–350 mg/m² IV	21
Irinotecan	125 mg/m² IV on days 1, 8, 15, and 22	6 wk
FOLFIRI	Irinotecan 180 mg/m² IV on day 1 followed by LV 400 mg/m²/day IV on day 1 followed by 5-FU 400 mg/m²/day IV on day 1 followed by 5-FU 2,400 mg/m² CIVI for 46 hours	14
Bevacizumab[b]	5 mg/kg IV on day 1	14
Cetuximab[c]	400 mg/m² IV on day 1 followed by 250 mg/m² IV weekly thereafter	weekly
Panitumumab	6 mg/kg IV	14

LV, leucovorin; IV, intravenous; 5-FU, 5-fluorouracil; CIVI, continuous intravenous infusion.

[a]These are in addition to those presented in Table 8.4.

[b]In combination with any 5-FU–containing regimen.

[c]Alone or in combination with irinotecan.

disease-free benefit in patients with resected liver metastases who had received intra-arterial floxuridine with systemic 5-FU compared to those who did not receive any postoperative therapy, although there was no statistically significant difference in OS (62% vs. 53%; $P = 0.06$). Such an approach has typically been reserved for select centers and its utility has been challenged by the advent of more effective systemic chemotherapy.

The feasibility of converting initially unresectable disease to a potentially curative disease has been investigated by Bismuth and colleagues (40). Resection was possible in 99 patients with either down-staged or stable disease, and the 3-year survival was encouraging (58% for responders, 45% for patients with stable disease). Similar observations have been reported by Alberts using preoperative FOLFOX4 on 41% of patients undergoing resection with an observed median survival of 31.4 months (95% CI, 20.4–34.8) for the entire cohort (41). Indeed, current management of resectable liver disease typically includes perioperative systemic chemotherapy. This is based, in part, on the results of a European study showing a progression-free survival advantage to the use of 3 months of FOLFOX4 chemotherapy pre- and post-resection compared to surgery alone (42). However, attention must be paid to the potential hepatotoxicity and surgical complications from perioperative chemotherapy. The role of targeted therapies in the perioperative setting is an area of active investigation.

REFERENCES

1. American Cancer Society. Cancer facts and figures 2008. <http://www.cancer.org> Accessed March 1, 2009.
2. Pasty BM, Potter JD. Risks and benefits of celecoxib to prevent recurrent adenomas. *N Engl J Med* 2006;355:950–952.
3. Mulhall BP, Veerappan GR, Jackson JL. Meta-analysis: computed tomographic colonography. *Ann Intern Med* 2005;142(8):635–650.
4. Gunderson LL, Sargent DJ, Tepper JE, et al. Impact of T and N stage and treatment on survival and relapse in adjuvant rectal cancer: a pooled analysis. *J Clin Oncol* 2004;22(10):1785–1796.
5. Johnston PG, Fisher ER, et al. The role of thymidylate synthase expression in prognosis and outcome of adjuvant chemotherapy in patients with rectal cancer. *J Clin Oncol* 1994;12:2640–2647.
6. Popat S, Matakidou A, Houlston RS. Thymidylate synthase expression and prognosis in colorectal cancer: a systematic review and meta-analysis. *J Clin Oncol* 2004;22:529–536.
7. Moertel CG, Fleming TR, Macdonald JS, et al. Levamisole and fluorouracil for adjuvant therapy of resected colon carcinoma. *N Engl J Med* 1990;322:352–358.
8. Haller DG, Catalano PJ, MacDonald JS, et al. Fluorouracil (FU), leucovorin (LV) and levamisole (LEV) adjuvant therapy for colon cancer: five-year final report of INT-0089. *Proc Am Soc Clin Oncol* 1998;16:256a.
9. Haller DG, Catalano PJ, Macdonald JS, et al. Phase III study of fluorouracil, leucovorin, and levamisole in high-risk stage II and III colon cancer: final report of Intergroup 0089. *J Clin Oncol* 2005;23(34):8671–8678.
10. Twelves C, Wong A, Nowacki MP, et al. Capecitabine as adjuvant treatment for stage III colon cancer. *N Engl J Med* 2005;352(26):2696–2704.
11. Sargent DJ, Wieand HS, Haller DG, et al. Disease-free survival versus overall survival as a primary end point for adjuvant colon cancer studies: individual patient data from 20,898 patients on 18 randomized trials. *J Clin Oncol* 2005;23(34):8664–8670.
12. Andre T, Boni C, Mounedji-Boudiaf L, et al. Multicenter international study of oxaliplatin/ 5-fluorouracil/leucovorin in the adjuvant treatment of colon cancer (MOSAIC) investigators. Oxaliplatin, fluorouracil, and leucovorin as adjuvant treatment for colon cancer. *N Engl J Med* 2004;350:2343–2351.
13. de Gramont A, Boni C, Navarro M, et al. Oxaliplatin/5FU/LV in adjuvant colon cancer: updated efficacy results of the MOSAIC trial, including survival, with a median follow-up of six years. *J Clin Oncol* 2007 ASCO Annual Meeting Proceedings (Post-Meeting Edition). 25(18S):4007.
14. Kuebler JP, Wieand HS, O'Connell MJ, et al. Oxaliplatin combined with weekly bolus fluorouracil and leucovorin as surgical adjuvant chemotherapy for stage II and III colon cancer: results from NSABP C-07. *J Clin Oncol* 2007;25(16):2198–2204.

15. Saltz LB, Niedzwiecki D, Hollis D, et al. Irinotecan plus fluorouracil/leucovorin (IFL) versus fluorouracil/leucovorin alone (FL) in stage III colon cancer (CALGB C89803). *J Clin Oncol* 2007;25(23):3456–3461.

16. Mamounas E, Wieand S, Wolmark N, et al. Comparative efficacy of adjuvant chemotherapy in patients with Dukes' B versus Dukes' C colon cancer: results from four National Surgical Adjuvant Breast and Bowel Project adjuvant studies (C01, C02, C03, and C04). *J Clin Oncol* 1999;17:1349–1355.

17. Erlichman. Efficacy of adjuvant fluorouracil and folinic acid in B2 colon cancer. International multicenter pooled analysis of B2 colon cancer trials (IMPACT B2) investigators. *J Clin Oncol* 1999;17(5):1356–1363.

18. Schrag D, Rifas-Shiman S, Saltz L, et al. Adjuvant chemotherapy use for Medicare beneficiaries with stage II colon cancer. *J Clin Oncol* 2002;20:3999–4005.

19. Quasar Collaborative Group, Gray R, Barnwell J, McConkey C, et al. Adjuvant chemotherapy versus observation in patients with colorectal cancer: a randomised study. *Lancet* 2007;370(9604): 2020–2029.

20. Benson AB, Schrag D, Somerfield MR, et al. American Society of Clinical Oncology recommendations on adjuvant chemotherapy for stage II colon cancer. *J Clin Oncol* 2004;22:3408–3419.

21. Krook JE, Moertel CG, Gunderson LL, et al. Effective surgical adjuvant therapy for high-risk rectal carcinoma. *N Engl J Med* 1991;324:709–715.

22. O'Connell MJ, Martenson JA, Wieand HS, et al. Improving adjuvant therapy for rectal cancer by combining protracted infusion fluorouracil with radiation therapy after curative surgery. *N Engl J Med* 1994;331:502–507.

23. Sauer R, Becker H, Hohenberger W, et al. Preoperative versus postoperative chemoradiotherapy for rectal cancer. *N Engl J Med* 2004;351(17):1731–1740.

24. Grothey A, Sargent D, Goldberg RM, et al. Survival of patients with advanced colorectal cancer improves with the availability of fluorouracil-leucovorin, irinotecan, and oxaliplatin in the course of treatment. *J Clin Oncol* 2004;22(7):1209–1214.

25. Leichman CG, Fleming TR, Muggia FM, et al. Phase II study of fluorouracil and its modulation in advanced colorectal cancer: a Southwest Oncology Group study. *J Clin Oncol* 1995;13:1303–1311.

26. Falcone A, Allegrini G, Lenconi M, et al. Protracted continuous infusion of 5-fluorouracil and low-dose leucovorin in patients with metastatic colorectal cancer resistant to 5-fluorouracil bolus-based chemotherapy: a Phase II study. *Cancer Chemother Pharmacol* 1999;44:159–163.

27. Van Cutsem E, Hoff PM, Harper P, et al. Oral capecitabine vs intravenous 5-fluorouracil and leucovorin: integrated efficacy data and novel analyses from two large, randomised, phase III trials. *Br J Cancer* 2004;90:1190–1197.

28. Goldberg RM, Sargent DJ, Morton RF, et al. A randomized controlled trial of fluorouracil plus leucovorin, irinotecan, and oxaliplatin combinations in patients with previously untreated metastatic colorectal cancer. *J Clin Oncol* 2004;22:23–30.

29. Tournigand C, Andre T, Achille E, et al. FOLFIRI followed by FOLFOX6 or the reverse sequence in advanced colorectal cancer: a randomized GERCOR study. *J Clin Oncol* 2004;22(2):229–237.

30. Saltz LB, Cox JV, Blanke C, et al. Irinotecan Study Group. Irinotecan plus fluorouracil and leucovorin for metastatic colorectal cancer. *N Engl J Med* 2000;343:905–914.

31. Douillard JY, Cunningham D, Roth AD, et al. Irinotecan combined with fluorouracil compared with fluorouracil alone as first-line treatment for metastatic colorectal cancer: a multicentre randomised trial. *Lancet* 2000;355:1041–1047.

32. Cunningham D, Pyrhonen S, James RD, et al. Randomised trial of irinotecan plus supportive care versus supportive care alone after fluorouracil failure for patients with metastatic colorectal cancer. *Lancet* 1998;352:1413–1418.

33. Pitot HC, Wender DB, O'Connell MJ, et al. Phase II trial of irinotecan in patients with metastatic colorectal carcinoma. *J Clin Oncol* 1997;15(8):2910–2919.

34. Hurwitz H, Fehrenbacher L, Novotny W, et al. Bevacizumab plus irinotecan, fluorouracil, and leucovorin for metastatic colorectal cancer. *N Engl J Med* 2004;350:2335–2342.

35. Giantonio BJ, Catalano PJ, Meropol NJ, et al. Bevacizumab in combination with oxaliplatin, fluorouracil, and leucovorin (FOLFOX4) for previously treated metastatic colorectal cancer:

results from the Eastern Cooperative Oncology Group Study E3200. *J Clin Oncol* 2007;25(12): 1539–1544.

36. Van Cutsem E, Köhne CH, Hitre E, et al. Cetumaxib and chemotherapy as initial treatment for metastatic colorectal cancer. *NEJM* 2009;360(14):1408–1417.
37. Cunningham D, Humblet Y, Siena S, et al. Cetuximab monotherapy and cetuximab plus irinotecan in irinotecan-refractory metastatic colorectal cancer. *N Engl J Med* 2004;351:337–345.
38. Van Cutsem E, Peeters M, Siena S, et al. Open-label phase III trial of panitumumab plus best supportive care compared with best supportive care alone in patients with chemotherapy-refractory metastatic colorectal cancer. *J Clin Oncol* 2007;25(13):1658–1664.
39. Kemeny MM, Adak S, Gray B, et al. Combined-modality treatment for resectable metastatic colorectal carcinoma to the liver: surgical resection of hepatic metastases in combination with continuous infusion of chemotherapy—an Intergroup study. *J Clin Oncol* 2002;20:1499–1505.
40. Bismuth H, Adam R, Levi F, et al. Resection of nonresectable liver metastases from colorectal cancer after neoadjuvant chemotherapy. *Ann Surg* 1996;224:509–520.
41. Alberts SR, Donohue JH, Mahoney MR, et al. Liver resection after 5-fluorouracil, leucovorin and oxaliplatin for patients with metastatic colorectal cancer (MCRC) limited to the liver. *A North Central Cancer Treatment Group (NCCTG) Phase II Study Meeting:2003 ASCO Annual Meeting* (abstr 1053).
42. Nordlinger B, Sorbye H, Glimelius B, et al. Perioperative chemotherapy with FOLFOX4 and surgery versus surgery alone for resectable liver metastases from colorectal cancer. *Lancet* 2008;371(9617):1007–1016.

9

Pancreatic Cancer

George P. Kim

EPIDEMIOLOGY

- In 2008, approximately 37,680 new cases of pancreatic cancer were diagnosed and 34,290 patients died from this disease (1).
- Pancreatic cancer remains the fourth leading cause of cancer death in the United States.
- The 5-year survival of patients with pancreatic cancer is less than 5%.
- Men and African Americans are at a higher risk for developing pancreatic cancer and have higher mortality rates.
- Incidence of pancreatic cancer increases at the age of 50 and peaks in the seventh decade (Table 9.1).

Pathophysiology

The pancreas performs both endocrine and exocrine functions; however, approximately 80% of the cells in the pancreas are acinar cells and 10% to 15% are ductal cells. Approximately 95% of malignant pancreatic cancer arises in the exocrine pancreas, with two-thirds arising in the head of the pancreas. The sites where the cancer arises determine the symptoms: lesions arising in the head of the pancreas cause duct obstruction, jaundice, and pain, whereas tumors arising in the body or tail of the pancreas are less likely to cause symptoms until metastatic disease develops.

- Pain caused by localized disease is usually described as mid to upper back pain resulting from tumor invasion of the celiac and mesenteric plexi.

TABLE 9.1. *Risk factors*

Environmental	
Cigarette smoking	N-nitrosoamines may increase risk by twofold to threefold. Accounts for roughly 30% of pancreatic cancers.
Dietary factors	Decreased risk with fruits and vegetables, increased risk with fat and meat. No caffeine association, and alcohol link is controversial.
Disease states	
Diabetes mellitus	Maximal risk at time of diagnosis of diabetes and for the subsequent 5 years.
Chronic pancreatitis	Relative risk as high as 16-fold.
Genetic	
FAMM	p16 mutation, 13- to 22-fold increased risk
Hereditary pancreatitis	PRSS1 or cationic trypsinogen gene, 20-fold increased risk
HNPCC	Lynch syndrome II
BRCA2	10-fold risk
Peutz-Jeghers syndrome	Manifested by hamartomatous gastrointestinal polyps and perioral pigmented spots, mutation of serine–threonine kinase (STK) (11)
Occupational	
Chemicals	Petrochemical products, benzidine, and β-naphthylamine

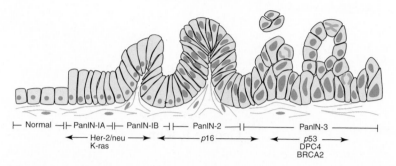

Fig. 9.1. Neoplastic progression model—pancreatic intraepithelial neoplasia (PanIN-1 through PanIN-3). (Used with permission from Hruban RH, Goggins M, Parsons J, et al. Progression model for pancreatic cancer. *Clin Can Res* 2000;6:2969–2972.)

- Most patients develop glucose intolerance and some degree of pancreatic insufficiency. An analysis of 512 pancreatic cancer patients and 933 age-matched controls revealed diabetes mellitus to be more prevalent (47% vs. 7%; $P < 0.001$) and of recent, $<$2-year onset (74% vs. 53%; $P = 0.002$) in the cancer cases (2).
- K-*ras* mutations are common in pancreatic cancer (Fig. 9.1).
- Intraductal papillary mucinous neoplasm and mucinous cystic neoplasm are relatively benign lesions, but the presence of severe dysplasia or invasion warrant further investigation and probable resection (3). Lesions that are 2 cm or less can be followed as there is low risk for development of invasive cancer over 5 to 10 years. Incidental cysts that enlarge over time to greater than 3 cm and/or a change in morphology (presence of solid component) should be considered for resection. Despite the evolution of malignant clones within these lesions, the overall survival is better than with ductal adenocarcinoma.

STAGING

The American Joint Committee for Cancer/International Union Against Cancer (AJCC/UICC) staging classification of pancreatic cancer is done using the TNM classification, as shown in Table 9.2 (4).

PROGNOSIS

Tumor size, presence of lymph node metastasis, and histologic differentiation each have independent prognostic values, with larger tumors, lymph node metastasis, and poor differentiation having worse prognoses. The 36-month survival for node-negative patients is between 25% and 30%, whereas survival can be significantly shortened for node-positive patients. Long-term survival is seen in about 20% of patients who successfully undergo a potentially curative surgical resection (Fig. 9.2).

DIAGNOSIS

- Screening tests: There are no approved screening tests for pancreatic cancer. CA 19-9, a sialated Lewis antigen, is elevated in 70% to 90% of patients with pancreatic cancer; however, it is not useful as a screening test because of low specificity. A recent analysis of resected patients revealed that 34% of patients were Lewis-antigen–negative (5). The CA 19-9 may have greater utility for surveillance in detecting recurrent or advanced disease. Changes or trends during treatment should not be used to alter therapy.
- Imaging techniques: Imaging techniques include chest radiographs, abdominal computerized tomography (CT), ultrasound, endoscopic retrograde cholepancreatography (ERCP), and endoscopic ultrasound (EUS)

TABLE 9.2. *American Joint Committee for Cancer/International Union Against Cancer staging classification (2002)*

Primary tumor

TX	Primary tumor cannot be assessed
T0	No evidence of primary tumor
Tis	Carcinoma in situ
T1	Tumor limited to the pancreas ≤2 cm
T2	Tumor limited to the pancreas 2 cm
T3	Tumor extends beyond the pancreas but without involvement of the celiac axis or the superior mesenteric artery (SMA)
T4	Tumor involves the celiac axis or the SMA (unresectable primary tumor)

Regional lymph nodes

NX	Regional lymph nodes cannot be assessed
N0	No regional lymph node metastasis
N1	Regional lymph node metastasis

Distant metastasis

MX	Distant metastasis cannot be assessed
M0	No distant metastasis
M1	Distant metastasis

Stage grouping

Stage 0	Tis	N0	M0
Stage IA	T1	N0	M0
Stage IB	T2	N0	M0
Stage IIA	T3	N0	M0
Stage IIB	T1–3	N1	M0
Stage III	T4	Any N	M0
Stage IV	Any T	Any N	M1

Source: From Exocrine Pancreas. In: American Joint Committee on Cancer. *AJCC Cancer Staging Manual,* sixth edition. New York, NY: Springer, 2002, 157–164.

- Dual-phase contrast, helical CT: Its sensitivity is 67% for lesions <1.5 cm and almost 100% for tumors >1.5 cm; it has a 95% positive predictive value in defining resectability if major vessel tumor encasement is present.
- Endoscopic ultrasound is excellent for tumor and nodal staging, and also for detecting the presence of portal vein invasion; fine-needle aspiration (FNA) provides tissue for pathologic diagnosis with minimal risk of tumor seeding; hepatic lesions can be visualized and sampled; limitations include assessment of blood vessel encasement or superior mesenteric artery (SMA) invasion.
- Pathologic diagnosis may be achieved with ERCP, laparoscopy, peritoneal cytology, or CT-guided biopsy.

MANAGEMENT

For management considerations, pancreatic cancer can be divided into resectable disease (potentially curable), locally advanced disease, and metastatic disease (Fig. 9.3).

Resectable Disease

Unfortunately, less than 10% of patients with pancreatic cancer have resectable disease at diagnosis. Resectable disease is defined as tumor confined to the pancreas that is not encasing the celiac axis or SMA and, at many institutions, not involving the superior mesenteric vein–portal vein confluence. However, patients may have isolated involvement of the superior mesenteric vein, portal vein, or hepatic artery. A Whipple or modified, pylorus-sparing procedure is the surgical procedure of choice. The stomach (distal third), gallbladder, cystic and common bile ducts, duodenum, and proximal jejunum are

Resectable disease

5-year Survival
17.5%

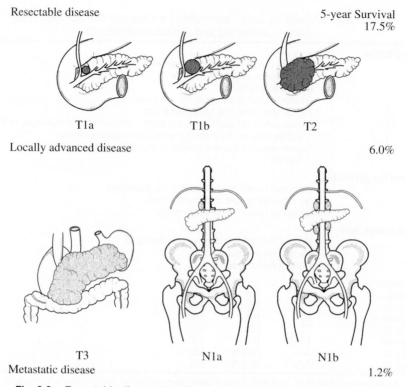

T1a   T1b   T2

Locally advanced disease   6.0%

T3   N1a   N1b

Metastatic disease   1.2%

Fig. 9.2. Resectable disease, locally advanced disease, metastatic disease.

resected, with resultant pancreatico-, choledocho-, and gastrojejunostomy. The peripancreatic, superior mesenteric, and hepatoduodenal lymph nodes are also staged. Pathologic review of the surgical margins must include assessment of the retroperitoneal margin (space directly adjacent to the proximal 3–4 cm of the SMA) by inking the margin and sectioning the tumor perpendicular to the margin.

Even after complete resection, the risk of locoregional recurrence is as high as 70%. This risk provides strong rationale for the use of adjuvant therapy. The historic Gastrointestinal Study Group (GITSG) trial (6) randomized patients to chemoradiation ($n = 21$) versus surgery alone ($n = 22$). The chemoradiation arm consisted of split-course 4,000 cGy radiation in combination with bolus 5-fluorouracil (5-FU; 500 mg/m^2/day for the first 3 days of each 2,000-cGy segment of radiotherapy). Unmodulated 5-FU (500 mg/m^2/week) was administered thereafter for up to two additional years. A significantly prolonged median survival of 20 months for the patients treated with chemoradiation versus 11 months for controls was observed. In addition, 43% 2-year actuarial survival (versus 18% for the control arm) and 25% 5-year overall survival were observed.

This small trial established the benefit from postoperative combined-modality therapy. More contemporary approaches include: (a) administration of up to 5,040 cGy radiation as a continuous-course schedule instead of the split-course schedule; (b) combination with 5-FU (bolus, continuous infusion, capecitabine) or gemcitabine; and (c) the postradiation treatment of weekly 5-FU has also been shortened from 2 years to 4–6 months, and maintenance therapy with weekly gemcitabine (1,000 mg/m^2 for 3 of every 4 weeks) is preferred.

Several randomized trials have provided additional information about the effectiveness of conventional adjuvant therapy.

Management algorithm

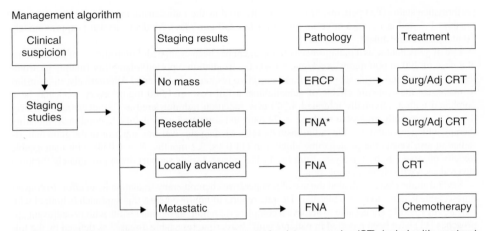

Fig. 9.3. Staging studies should include computerized tomography (CT) (spiral with contrast preferred) or magnetic resonance imaging (MRI), endoscopic ultrasound (EUS), as well as laparoscopy for potentially respectable cancers. (*) indicates that for CT-guided FNA there is a controversy about tumor seeding in potentially curable (i.e., resectable) disease, and in some centers patients undergo a planned Whipple procedure to obtain tissue at the time of surgery. Adj CRT, adjuvant chemoradiation; FNA, fine needle aspiration; ERCP, endoscopic retrograde cholangiopancreatography.

In a follow-up trial using the same GITSG regimen but without maintenance 5-FU chemotherapy, the European Organization for Research and Treatment of Cancer trial (7) treated, 114 patients but found no survival benefits with combined-modality therapy—median survival 17.1 months versus 12.6 months in surgery-alone patients ($P = 0.099$), and 2-year survival—37% versus 23%.

A trial from the European Study Group for Pancreatic Cancer (ESPAC-1) (8) used a 2×2 factorial randomization design and suggested that chemotherapy alone in the adjuvant setting was more effective than chemotherapy–radiation—CRT. The 5-year survival rate was 21% for patients receiving chemotherapy alone ($n = 147$, chemotherapy arm and CRT-then-chemotherapy arm) and 8% among patients who did not receive chemotherapy ($n = 142$, CRT arm and observation arm; $P = 0.009$). Despite these intriguing results, conclusions from the study are limited by significant selection bias and considerable treatment variability.

The Radiation Therapy Oncology Group trial 9704 compared gemcitabine to 5-FU alone 1 month prior to and for three additional months after combined-modality therapy (5,040 cGy external beam radiation and continuous infusion 5-FU at a dose of 225 mg/m²) (5). In the primary analysis of patients with cancers in the head of the pancreas ($n = 388$), the gemcitabine-treated patients experienced an improved median survival (20.5 vs. 16.9 months) and 3-year survival (31% vs. 22%; HR, 0.82 [95% CI, 0.65–1.03]; $P = 0.09$). Subset analyses revealed that patients (13%) with a CA19-9 greater than 180 U/mL after surgery and prior to initiation of adjuvant therapy had a worse survival (median 9 months).

The Charité Onkologie (CONKO-001) (9) compared postoperative therapy consisting of gemcitabine alone (6 cycles on days 1, 8, and 15 every 4 weeks) versus observation in completely resected R0 patients (>81%). In the primary analysis, disease free survival was more favorable in the gemcitabine arm (13.4 vs. 6.9 months, $P < 0.001$). In a subsequent report, overall survival also was improved in the gemcitabine-treated patients (22.8 vs. 20.2 months, $P = 0.005$).

Locally Advanced Disease

Approximately 25% to 35% of patients have regional involvement at diagnosis, and treatment with combined chemotherapy and radiation has been shown to improve survival. In locally advanced, good performance status (PS) patients, 5FU is typically used as the radiosensitizing agent (500 mg/m^2/day for days 1–3 and last 3 days or continuous infusion 250 g/m^2/day). Median survival is approximately 10 months with treatment.

Use of gemcitabine as a radiation-sensitizing agent has been evaluated. Initial studies of gemcitabine at a dose of 400 to 600 mg/m^2/week and 5,040 cGy irradiation reported tolerability (mainly gastrointestinal toxicity and myelosuppresion) and objective responses in patients. Alternatively, in an effort to maximize the systemic effects of gemcitabine, a full dose of 1,000 mg/m^2 every week has been combined with a maximally tolerated 4,200 cGy radiation (administered as 280-cGy fractions over 3 weeks). A recently presented study ($n = 74$ patients) compared gemcitabine to combined- modality therapy with gemcitabine as the radiosensitizer (10). Median survival was superior in the gemcitabine-radiation arm versus the gemcitabine alone arm (11.0 vs. 9.2 months, $P = 0.034$) with manageable toxicity observed. Subset analyses from recent U.S. phase 3 trials support the approximately 9-month survival seen with chemotherapy alone

Several studies have evaluated the use of preoperative chemotherapy–radiation in an effort to convert unresectable patients to resectable state. Despite reports of improvements, this approach is limited with only 8% to 13% of patients able to achieve a complete resection. Intriguing results with neoadjuvant approaches (11) have been reported in patients with "borderline resectable disease" as defined by the following tumor-vessel relationships: SMV–PV confluence that can be reconstructed (i.e., a suitable portal vein above, and SMV below the area of occlusion); tumor abutment of the SMA of <180 degrees; or short segment encasement of the hepatic artery amenable to resection and reconstruction (usually at the origin of the gastroduodenal artery).

Metastatic Disease

Approximately 50% of newly diagnosed pancreatic cancer patients have metastasis, and palliative treatment with systemic chemotherapy should be offered to patients with a good PS (Eastern Cooperative Oncology Group [ECOG] 0–1). Gemcitabine is the first-line standard treatment in patients with metastatic pancreatic cancer (12). This is based on a study in which 126 untreated patients were randomized to receive gemcitabine, 1,000 mg/m^2 intravenously weekly for 3 of 4 weeks, or single-agent 5-FU, 600 mg/m^2 intravenous bolus weekly. Despite an objective response rate of less than 10%, a benefit in quality-of-life scores (clinical benefit response 23.8% vs. 4.8%, [$P = 0.0022$]) and median survival (5.7 vs. 4.4 months, $P = 0.0025$) was observed with the gemcitabine therapy. The 1-year survival also favored the gemcitabine arm (18% vs. 2%).

Several clinical trials attempting to surpass survival outcomes with gemcitabine alone have been reported. In the National Cancer Institute-Canada phase 3 trial PA.3, 569 patients were randomly assigned to receive standard gemcitabine and erlotinib (100 or 150 mg/d orally) or gemcitabine plus placebo (13). The primary end point, overall survival, was significantly longer with erlotinib/gemcitabine (median 6.24 vs. 5.91 months, HR 0.82 (95% CI, 0.69–0.99); $P = 0.038$). One-year survival (23% vs. 17%; $P = 0.023$) and progression-free survival (HR of 0.77; $P = 0.004$) were also improved with the combination. Exploratory analyses revealed that patients who developed ≥ grade 2 skin rash had better survival (10.5 months) while trends for improved outcome were seen with wild-type k-ras status and EGFR negativity as measured by FISH.

The combination of gemcitabine and capecitabine (GEM-CAP) was evaluated by the National Cancer Research Institute of the United Kingdom (14). Although only presented as an interim analysis (70% of the expected events), survival (median—GEM-CAP 7.4 vs. Gem 6.0 months; 1-year—GEM-CAP 26% vs. Gem 19%) was improved with the combination. Capecitabine was given as 1,660 mg/m^2/day for 21 consecutive days of a 4-week cycle while gemcitabine 1000 mg/m^2 was administered weekly 3 times every 4 weeks. Responses were also higher with GEM-CAP (14.2% vs. 7.1%, $P = 0.008$). Presentation of the final results is awaited prior to declaring this the new chemotherapy standard although the regimen may be considered for patients with good PS.

The role of combination chemotherapy in the treatment of metastatic patients has been explored using two- and three-drug regimens. Unfortunately despite signs of early promise in small, single institution studies with selected patient populations, the regimens proved inferior to gemcitabine alone upon formal phase 3 testing. Noteworthy combinations include gemcitabine and platinums or gemcitabine with fluoropyrimidines. Several meta-analyses have been performed that support these combinations in patients with good PS. For example, with the gemcitabine-platinum combination, a HR of 0.85 ($P = 0.010$) is detected and with gemcitabine-fluoropyrimidine the HR is 0.90 ($P = 0.030$). In the subgroup with a Karnofsky PS of 90% to 100% or ECOG 0–1, survival benefits are more pronounced (HR = 0.76, $P < 0.001$) with combination chemotherapy (15). Another meta-analysis reported a consistent survival benefit (HR = 0.83, 95% CI, 0.72–0.96) with the combination of gemcitabine and capecitabine (16). Unfortunately, more detailed analysis derived from pooled individual patient data has not been presented.

Targeted agents such as bevacizumab (Avastin) and cetuximab (Erbitux) have been evaluated in combination with gemcitabine in pancreatic cancer.

- Gemcitabine in combination with cetuximab (loading dose 400 mg/m^2 followed by 250 mg/m^2 weekly) was evaluated in a phase 3 trial (17) by SWOG with a nonstatistically significant, yet similar to erlotinib, 2-week benefit being detected (6.4 vs. 5.9 months gemcitabine, HR 1.09 [0.93–1.27], $P = 0.14$).
- Despite significant activity in a phase 2 trial, the CALGB study with gemcitabine with and without Avastin (10 mg/kg every 2 weeks) failed to demonstrate any survival advantage with the combination (5.8 vs. 6.1 months gemcitabine, HR = 1.03, $P = 0.78$). Trials with EGFR inhibitors (erlotinib or cetuximab) and bevacizumab have also failed to demonstrate any significant activity with the combined biologic approach.

Palliation

Pain remains a significant problem with pancreatic cancer and can be palliated with narcotics, external beam radiation, and, if indicated, a nerve block to an involved plexus. Biliary and intestinal obstruction is also a common local issue and can be relieved with stents or surgical bypass.

TREATMENT OPTIONS

Localized Disease

Whipple procedure followed by adjuvant chemoradiation with a continuous course of 45- to 50.4-Gy external beam radiation in 1.8-Gy fractions combined with:

- 5-FU, 225 to 250 mg/m^2/day continuous infusion concomitantly with radiation or 5-FU, 500 mg/m^2/day by intravenous bolus for the first 3 days and last 3 days of radiotherapy (total dose per 3-day course of fluorouracil, 1,500 mg/m^2), or capecitabine 825 mg/m^2 BID Monday through Friday, followed by
- gemcitabine, 1,000 mg/m^2/week intravenously weekly for 3 weeks (days 1, 8, and 15) followed by 1 week without gemcitabine for 4 to 6 months.

Locally Advanced Disease

The goal of treatment for locally advanced and metastatic disease is to decrease symptoms and ultimately prolong survival. For those patients with poor PS, supportive care can be considered.

For those patients with good performance status (PS 0–1), clinical trials are the preferred mode of treatment; otherwise, chemoradiation or gemcitabine-based chemotherapy are considered standard treatments. The chemoradiation is given as described earlier, and chemotherapy after chemoradiation consists of gemcitabine, 1,000 mg/m^2/week intravenously weekly for 3 weeks (days 1, 8, and 15) followed by 1 week rest. Treatment cycles are repeated every 28 days.

Metastatic Disease

For patients with good PS, clinical trials are the preferred mode of treatment. Gemcitabine or gemcitabine in combination with erlotinib, a fluoropyrimidine or a platinum are each considered standard treatments.

- Gemcitabine, 1,000 mg/m²/week intravenous weekly for 3 weeks (days 1, 8, and 15), followed by 1 week rest. Treatment cycles are repeated every 28 days.
- Gemcitabine-erlotinib 100 mg/day continuous
- Gemcitabine-capecitabine 1,660 mg/m²/day days 1 to 21, 1-week rest of a 4-week cycle
- Gemcitabine (either standard or prolonged infusion 10 mg/m²/min) given every 2 weeks with oxaliplatin 100 mg/m² every 2 weeks of a 4-week cycle
- Gemcitabine and cisplatin 50 mg/m² given every 2 weeks of a 4-week cycle

REFERENCES

1. Jemal A, Siegel R, Ward E, et al. Cancer statistics, 2008. *CA Cancer J Clin.* Mar-Apr 2008;58(2): 71–96.
2. Pannala R, Leirness JB, Bamlet WR, Basu A, Petersen GM, Chari ST. Prevalence and clinical profile of pancreatic cancer-associated diabetes mellitus. *Gastroenterology.* Apr 2008;134(4):981–987.
3. DiMagno EP. The pancreatic cyst incidentaloma: Management consensus. *Clin Gastroenterol Hepatol.* 2007;5(7):797–798.
4. Greene FL, Fleming ID, et al. *Exocrine Pancreas. In American Joint Committee on Cancer Cancer Staging Manual.* 6th ed. New York, NY: Springer-Verlag; 2002.
5. Regine WF, Winter KA, Abrams RA, et al. Fluorouracil vs gemcitabine chemotherapy before and after fluorouracil-based chemoradiation following resection of pancreatic adenocarcinoma: a randomized controlled trial. *JAMA.* Mar 5 2008;299(9):1019–1026.
6. Kaiser MH, Ellenberg SS. Pancreatic cancer: Adjuvant combined radiation and chemotherapy following curative resection. *Arch Surg* 1985;120:899–903.
7. Klinkenbijl JH, Jeekel J, Sahmoud T, et al. Adjuvant radiotherapy and 5-fluorouracil after curative resection of cancer of the pancreas and periampullary region: phase III trial of the EORTC gastrointestinal tract cancer cooperative group. *Ann Surg.* Dec 1999;230(6):776–782; discussion 782–774.
8. Neoptolemos JP, Stocken DD, Friess H, et al. A randomized trial of chemoradiotherapy and chemotherapy after resection of pancreatic cancer. *N Engl J Med.* Mar 18 2004;350(12):1200–1210.
9. Oettle H, Post S, Neuhaus P, et al. Adjuvant chemotherapy with gemcitabine vs observation in patients undergoing curative-intent resection of pancreatic cancer: a randomized controlled trial. *JAMA.* Jan 17 2007;297(3):267–277.
10. Loehrer PJ, Powell ME, Cardenes HR, et al. A randomized phase III study of gemcitabine in combination with radiation therapy versus gemcitabine alone in patients with localized, unresectable pancreatic cancer: E4201. *J Clin Oncol.* 2008;26(May 20 suppl; abstr 4506).
11. Varadhachary G, Tamm E, Abbruzzese J, et al. Borderline resectable pancreatic cancer: definitions, management, and role of preoperative therapy. *Ann Surg Oncol.* 2006;13(8):1035–1046.
12. Burris HA, Moore MJ, Andersen J, et al. Improvements in survival and clinical benefit with gemcitabine as first-line therapy for patients with advanced pancreas cancer: a randomized trial. *J Clin Oncol.* 1997;15(6):2403–2413.
13. Moore MJ, Goldstein D, Hamm J, et al. Erlotinib plus gemcitabine compared with gemcitabine alone in patients with advanced pancreatic cancer. A phase III trial of the National Cancer Institute of Canada Clinical Trials Group. *J Clin Oncol.* 2007;25(15):1960–1966.
14. Cunningham D, Chau I, Stocken D, et al. Phase III randomised comparison of gemcitabine (GEM) versus gemcitabine plus capecitabine (GEM-CAP) in patients with advanced pancreatic cancer. *Eur J Cancer.* 2005;3(4).
15. Heinemann V, Boeck S, Hinke A, Labianca R, Louvet C. Meta-analysis of randomized trials: evaluation of benefit from gemcitabine-based combination chemotherapy applied in advanced pancreatic cancer. *BMC Cancer.* 2008;8(1):82.
16. Sultana A, Smith CT, Cunningham D, Starling N, Neoptolemos JP, Ghaneh P. Meta-analyses of chemotherapy for locally advanced and metastatic pancreatic cancer. *J Clin Oncol.* June 20;2007: 25(18):2607–2615.
17. Philip PA, Benedetti J, Fenoglio-Preiser C, et al. Phase III study of gemcitabine [G] plus cetuximab [C] versus gemcitabine in patients [pts] with locally advanced or metastatic pancreatic adenocarcinoma [PC]: SWOG S0205 study. *J Clin Oncol.* 2007;25(18S).

10

Anal Cancer

M. Wasif Saif and Bryan W. Chang

Anal cancer is an uncommon malignancy, accounting for only a small percentage (4%) of all cancers of the lower alimentary tract. There are approximately 4,000 cases per year in the United States. Individuals with human papillomavirus (HPV) and homosexual men, in particular, are at increased risk of anal cancer. Most studies have included small numbers of patients accrued over several years, and in some situations, there is a lack of data from randomized trials on which to base treatment decisions. Small, early-stage carcinomas of the anal margin can be managed with local excision. Concurrent chemoradiation with 5-fluorouracil (5-FU) and mitomycin C (MMC) is the standard of care for more advanced anal canal and anal margin cancers, although 30% of patients will fail after this organ-sparing approach. Patients who recur locally after definitive chemoradiation can undergo salvage with an abdominoperineal resection (APR) with a reasonable expectation of long-term survival.

EPIDEMIOLOGY

Anal cancer has an annual incidence of 0.6 per 100,000 in whites in the United States and is more frequent in women than in men by a ratio of 2:1. However, cancer of the anal margin is more frequent in men. More than 80% of anal cancers develop between the ages of 50 and 60 years. Epidemiologic studies during the last decade suggest that the incidence of anal cancer in men younger than 35 years has increased, and the gender ratio is reversed in this age group. The San Francisco study revealed an incidence of anal carcinoma in homosexual men of between 25 and 87 cases per 100,000. The incidence appears to be rising in this population, likely due to increased overall survival from the use of highly active antiretroviral medications.

ETIOLOGY AND RISK FACTORS

Environmental factors are predominantly implicated in the carcinogenesis of anal cancer. The most common risk factors can be classified as those with strong evidence and those with moderately strong evidence.

Risk factors with strong evidence include:

1. HPV, particularly serotypes 16 and 18. HPV is associated with anal intraepithelial neoplasia (AIN), which is a precursor lesion. The same subtypes of HPV that cause malignant transformation in cervical cancer are also implicated in anal cancer. Patients may present with anogenital warts.
2. History of receptive anal intercourse
3. History of sexually transmitted disease
4. More than 10 sexual partners
5. History of cervical, vulvar, or vaginal cancer
6. Immunosuppression after solid-organ transplantation

Risk factors with moderately strong evidence include:

1. Human immunodeficiency virus (HIV) infection. HIV-infected patients with severe immunosuppression, as evidenced by CD4 counts less than 50/mm³, may present with more aggressive and advanced disease.

2. Long-term use of corticosteroids
3. Cigarette smoking

PATHOLOGY

Anatomy

1. The anal canal extends from the anorectal ring (where the rectum enters the puborectalis sling at the apex of the sphincter complex) to the anal verge (where the anal squamous mucosa merges with the epidermis of the perianal skin). The length of the canal is approximately 3 to 4 cm.
2. The anal margin consists of the anal area distal to the anal canal, including perianal skin. Some authors have suggested a radius of 5 cm from the anal verge as the distal boundary of the anal margin (Fig. 10.1).

HISTOLOGY

The histology and features of the different types of anal carcinoma are described in Table 10.1.

Frequency

Table 10.2 shows the frequency of occurrence of each histologic type of anal cancer. Squamous cell carcinoma is the most common form of anal cancer.

Presentation

Symptoms

The incidence of presenting symptoms for three types of anal carcinoma is shown in Table 10.3.

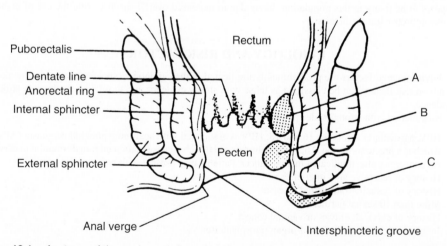

Fig. 10.1. Anatomy of the anal canal. A tumor in location A is always considered anal canal cancer; in location C, it is anal margin cancer. A tumor in location B has been called canal or margin cancer, depending on institutional preference, but now should be called anal canal cancer by the AJCC/UICC definition.

TABLE 10.1. *Characteristics of different types of anal cancer*

Histologic types	Features
Squamous cell (epidermoid) carcinoma	Occurs in the lower anus, often ulcerating
Cloacogenic (also known as basaloid, cuboidal, or transitional) carcinoma	Develops high in the anal canal in the transitional zone between glandular mucosa of the rectum and the squamous epithelium of the distal anus
Intraepithelial squamous cell carcinoma (Bowen's disease)	Premalignant lesion of the perirectal skin
Intraepithelial mucous adenocarcinoma (Paget's disease)	Develops in apocrine or mucous glands

TABLE 10.2. *Frequency of occurrence of different types of anal cancer*

Squamous cell carcinoma	113 (55%)
Cloacogenic (basaloid) carcinoma	64 (31%)
Intraepithelial adenocarcinoma (Paget's disease)	8 (4%)
Melanoma	7 (3%)
Basal cell carcinoma	6 (3%)
Adenocarcinoma	6 (3%)
Total	**204**

Signs

- Rectal bleeding or discharge
- Perianal mass
- Change in bowel habits or stool caliber

BIOPSY

An incisional biopsy is preferred to confirm diagnosis. Clinically suspicious inguinal lymph nodes should be examined to rule out metastatic disease.

STAGING AND PROGNOSTIC FACTORS

Workup should include history, physical examination with special attention to digital rectal examination and palpation of the inguinal nodes, chest radiograph, pelvic CT or MRI, PET scan, liver function

TABLE 10.3. *Frequency of occurrence of symptoms in different types of anal cancer*

Presenting symptoms	Squamous cell carcinoma	Perianal	Basaloid squamous carcinoma
Bleeding	50	9	32
Pain	41	5	17
Mass	27	5	16
Constipation	11	1	10
Diarrhea	5	0	7
Pruritus[a]	22	17	1
Other	16	6	12
Asymptomatic	25	6	14

[a]$P = <0.001$; differences not significant for other lesions.

Source: From Beahrs OH, Wilson SM. Carcinoma of the anus. *Ann Surg* 1976;184(4):422–8, with permission.

tests, and biopsy. Women should also undergo pelvic examination to rule out vaginal invasion by tumor and cervical cancer screening with a Pap smear. An endoscopic ultrasound of the anal canal may be helpful in assessing the perirectal lymph nodes. An HIV test and CD4 count should be considered.

The UICC (Union Internationale Contre le Cancer) and AJCC (American Joint Committee on Cancer) have proposed a practical staging system for anal cancers. The staging systems for both types of tumors are outlined in Tables 10.4 and 10.5.

MAJOR PROGNOSTIC FACTORS

There are four major prognostic factors:

- Site: Cancers of the anal margin have a more favorable prognosis than those of the anal canal.
- Size: Patients with primary tumors <5 cm have a more favorable prognosis than those with tumors >5 cm.
- Differentiation: Well-differentiated tumors are more favorable than poorly differentiated tumors.
- Lymph node involvement: Absence of nodal involvement or local extension indicates a better prognosis.

TABLE 10.4.   *AJCC classification of anal canal tumors*

Primary tumor (T)
TX	Primary tumor cannot be assessed
T0	No evidence of primary tumor
Tis	Carcinoma in situ
T1	Tumor ≤2 cm in greatest dimension
T2	Tumor >2 cm but <5 cm in greatest dimension
T3	Tumor >5 cm in greatest dimension
T4	Tumor of any size that invades adjacent organs (e.g., vagina, bladder, urethra; involvement of sphincter muscle(s) alone is not classified as T4)

Regional lymph nodes (N)
NX	Regional lymph nodes cannot be assessed
N0	No regional lymph node metastasis
N1	Metastasis in perirectal lymph node(s)
N2	Metastasis in unilateral internal iliac and/or inguinal lymph node(s)
N3	Metastasis in perirectal and inguinal lymph node(s) and/or bilateral internal iliac and/or inguinal lymph nodes

Distant metastasis (M)
MX	Distant metastasis cannot be assessed
M0	No distant metastasis
M1	Distant metastasis

Grade (G)
GX	Grade of differentiation cannot be assessed
G1	Well differentiated
G2	Moderately differentiated
G3	Poorly differentiated
G4	Undifferentiated

Stage groupings
Stage 0	Tis	N0	M0
Stage I	T1	N0	M0
Stage II	T2	N0	M0
	T3	N0	M0
Stage IIIA	T1-3	N1	M0
	T4	N0	M0
Stage IIIB	T4	N1	M0
	Any T	N2-3	M0
Stage IV	Any T	Any N	MI

TABLE 10.5. *TNM classification of anal margin tumors*

Primary tumor (T)[a]			
T4	Tumor invades deep extradermal structures		
Regional lymph nodes (N)			
N1	Ipsilateral inguinal nodes		
Metastases (M)			
M1	Distant metastases		
Stage groupings[b]			
Stage III	T4	N0	M0
	Any T	N1	M0

[a]Designation as for anal canal tumors, except T4.

[b]Stage groupings as for anal canal tumors, except stage III (no stage IIA or IIIB).

Source: Adapted from Sobin LH, Wittekind C (eds). *UICC International Union Against Cancer: TNM classification of malignant tumors.* 5th ed. New York: John Wiley & Sons, 1997, with permission.

When balanced for other factors, the prognosis for patients with squamous cell carcinoma of the anus and cloacogenic carcinoma is similar.

TREATMENT

Surgery

Anal Canal Lesions

Historically, the standard (and sole) form of therapy of the anal canal was surgical resection, often involving an APR with bilateral inguinal node dissection and formation of a colostomy. Despite such radical procedures, the most frequent site of failure is the pelvis, with local recurrences occurring in 30% of patients (Table 10.6).

Although postoperative radiation therapy has been utilized in an effort to reduce the local recurrence rate, the benefit of this practice has not been documented through a controlled trial.

Local excision may be sufficient to cure patients with small T1 N0 cancers of the anal canal, although patients treated in this manner need to be followed very closely. Local excision is not appropriate in cases where surgery would result in incontinence, or where the risk of involved lymph nodes exceeds 5%. Therefore, tumors that (a) involve the dentate line, or (b) are >2 cm (T2), or (c) involve greater than half the anal circumference, or (d) are moderately or poorly differentiated, are probably best managed with combined-modality treatment with chemotherapy and radiation. This integrated approach improves overall survival and may allow radical surgery to be avoided, preserving anal sphincter function. APR is used as salvage therapy in patients with chemoradiation-resistant disease, with a 50% 5-year survival rate.

Anal Margin Lesions

- For well-differentiated T1 N0 anal margin lesions, a wide local excision without the need for a colostomy seems to be adequate (Table 10.7).
- Larger (T2-4N0) or node-positive anal margin cancers should be treated with chemoradiation with 5-FU and MMC, similar to anal canal carcinomas.

TABLE 10.6. *Surgical results for anal canal lesions*

Nodal status	5-year survival (%)
Nodes negative	54–70
Metachronous nodal spread	51
Synchronous nodal spread	16

TABLE 10.7.   *Five-year survival after local excision in anal margin cancer in 31 patients*

	Tumor size (cm)				
	0–2	2–5	>5	NC	Total
Alive without recurrence	7	9	3	1	20
Alive with recurrence	0	1	0	0	1
Lost to follow-up	0	1	0	0	1
Died from recurrence	2	0	0	1	3
Died from unrelated causes	2	4	0	0	6
Total	11	15	3	2	31

Source: From Greenall MJ, Quan SH, Stearns MW, et al. Epidermoid cancer of the anal margin. Pathologic features, treatment, and clinical results. *Am J Surg* 1985;149(1):95–101, with permission.

Radiation Therapy

Radiation therapy has been given by external beam treatment, interstitial treatment. and combined external beam and interstitial treatment.

The overall 45% to 50% rate of cure reported in the series of selected patients who were treated with primary radiation therapy is quite similar to that seen in patients treated with radical surgery. Definitive radiation and surgery cannot be prospectively compared since the issue of a permanent colostomy is an unacceptable variable in a clinical trial. While the APR has remained a standard procedure during the last 25 years, radiotherapy techniques and equipment have advanced markedly, permitting the delivery of a higher, more precisely defined dose (approaching 60 Gy) with less toxicity. Recent series utilizing external beam and interstitial treatment or high-dose external beam irradiation are encouraging, suggesting local control rates of 70% to 80%, but will require further confirmation before receiving full acceptance. Advantages of primary radiation-based treatment over surgery include avoidance of perioperative morbidity and mortality, avoidance of a colostomy, and a lower risk of impotence in men. Disadvantages include the inability to determine the pathological nodal stage.

Combined Radiation Therapy and Chemotherapy

In 1972, Nigro and colleagues at Wayne State University began treating patients with preoperative concomitant radiation (30 Gy external beam) and chemotherapy (continuous infusion 5-FU and MMC) in an attempt to enhance the efficacy of radical surgery in patients with anal canal cancer. When this experience was last updated, 45 patients had been followed for a median of 50 months; 38 of 45 (84%) achieved a complete biopsy-proven response after only radiation and chemotherapy including all patients whose initial lesion was <5 cm in size. None of the 38 patients developed local or distant tumor recurrence, but all seven of the patients who had recurrent disease after preoperative treatment developed distant spread and subsequently died despite salvage APR.

While the original treatment plan called for an APR following the radiation and chemotherapy, this program was altered after it was found that five of the first six patients who had undergone the radical operation had no tumor in the operative specimen; subsequently, surgery has been performed only for those patients with residual tumor in the anal canal at the time of the posttreatment biopsy. The vast majority of patients have experienced cures of their anal cancers without the need for a colostomy and with manageable toxicity. These highly encouraging results from the Wayne State group have now been confirmed and extended by others in randomized trials. Tables 10.8 and 10.9 show results of some trials of chemoradiation for anal canal carcinoma.

Radiation Therapy Alone Versus Combined-Modality Therapy

The European Organization for Research and Treatment of Cancer (EORTC) randomized 110 patients with bulky tumors to receive 45 to 65 Gy of pelvic RT alone or in combination with 5-FU/MMC. Statistically significant benefits for complete response rate, local regional control, and colostomy-free survival all favored the combined-modality approach. The United Kingdom Coordinating Committee on Cancer Research (UKCCCR) randomized 585 patients to receive 45 Gy of pelvic RT alone or in combination with 5-FU/MMC (1). The local failure rate was reduced by 46% in patients

(text continues on page 129)

TABLE 10.8. *Selected results of concurrent radiation, 5-fluorouracil, and mitomycin C*

Chemotherapy regimens	Radiation (dose/ fractions/time)	Primary tumor control	Regional nodal control	5-year survival	Reference
5-FU 1,000mg/m² /d CIVI for 8 d, d 1–4, d 29–32 (total dose/course 8,000 mg/m²) MMC, 15 mg/m² IV bolus d 1	30 Gy/15/d –21	31/34 (91%) (≤5 cm)	NS	80% crude	15
5-FU 1,000 mg/m² /d CIVI d 2–5, d 28–31 (total dose/course, 8,000 mg/m²) MMC, 10 mg/m² IV bolus d 1	40.8 Gy/24/d 1–35	22/26 (85%) (≤3 cm)	NA	73%, 3 yr actual	16
5-FU 1,000 mg/m² /d, CIVI d 1–4, d 43–46 (total dose/course 8,000 mg/m²) MMC 10 mg/m² IV bolus, d 1 and 43 (total dose/course 20 mg/m²)	48–50 Gy/20–24/ d 1–58 (split course)	25/27 (93%) (≤5 cm)	4/5	65%, actuarial	17
5-FU 1,000 mg/m² /d, CIVI d 1–4, d 29–32 (total dose/course 8,000 mg/m²) MMC 10 mg/m² IV bolus, d 1 and 29 (total dose/course 20 mg/m²)	50 Gy/25–28/d 1–35 ± boost	21/22 (95%) (≤5 cm)	3/4	77%, actuarial	18
5-FU 600 mg/m² /d, CIVI d 1–5 MMC 12 mg/m² IV bolus d 1	42 Gy/10/d 1–19 plus interstitial iridium-192 boost	No data in origi- nal publication	NS	NS	8
5-FU 1,000 mg/m² /d CIVI d 1–4 (total dose/course 4,000 mg/m²)	50–54 Gy/25–27/ d 1–35	28/30 (93%) (≤5 cm)	NS	72%, actuarial	19

(Continued)

TABLE 10.8. (Continued)

Chemotherapy regimens	Radiation (dose/fractions/time)	Primary tumor control	Regional nodal control	5-year survival	Reference
MMC 10–15 mg/m² IV bolus d 1 5-FU 1,000 mg/m²/d CIVI d 1–4 (total dose/course, 4,000 mg/m²)	50 Gy/20/d 1–28	3/3 (100%) (≤5 cm) 11/13 (85%) (>5 cm or T4)	3/3	75%, actuarial	20
MMC 10 mg/m² IV bolus d 1 5-FU 750 mg/m²/d CIVI d 1–5, d 43–7 (total dose/course, 4,000 mg/m²)	54–60 Gy/30–33/d 1–53 (split course)	28/38 (74%) (≤5 cm) 9/17 (53%) (>5 cm)	8/8	81%, actuarial	21
MMC 15 mg/m² IV bolus d 1, 43, 85 (total dose/course, 45 mg/m²) 5-FU 1,000 mg/m²/d, d 1–4, d 29–32 (total dose/course, 8,000 mg/m²)	40 Gy/20–24/d 1–24 then 10–13 Gy boost (split course)	13/17 (77%) (≤5 cm) 18/33 (55%) (>5 cm or T4)	NS	74%	22
MMC 10 mg/m² IV bolus d 2 5-FU 600–800 mg/m²/d d 1–5 (total dose/course 3,000–4,000 mg/m²)	38 Gy/19/d 1–21 then 18 Gy interstitial iridium-192 boost (split course)	23/33 (70%) (≤5 cm) 22/35 (63%) (>5 cm or T4)	NS	65.5%	23
MMC 0.4 mg/kg IV bolus d 1 (maximum 20 mg)					

5-FU, 5-fluorouracil; MMC, mitomycin C; CIVI, continuous intravenous infusion; NS, not stated; NA, not applicable; T, tumor invading adjacent organs; T4, tumor invading deep extradermal structures.

TABLE 10.9. *Randomized trials comparing radiation alone and chemoradiation*

Group	Arm	N	Complete responses[a] (%)	3-year local control[b] (%)	Crude metastasis rate (%)	3-year survival (%)
EORTC	RT	52	54	55	21	64
	RT/5-FU/ MMC	51	80	69[c]	18	69
UKCCCR	RT	285	30	39	17	58
	RT/5-FU/ MMC	292	39	61[c]	10	65

EORTC, European Organization for Research and Treatment of Cancer; UKCCCR, United Kingdom Coordinating Committee on Cancer Research; RT, radiation therapy; 5-FU, 5-fluorouracil; MMC, mitomycin C.

[a]Local control was assessed 6 weeks after completion of 45 Gy in EORTC trial (before boost) and 6 weeks after completion of 60 to 65 Gy radiation in the UKCCCR trial.

[b]Patients requiring surgery to achieve local control after radiation were considered locally controlled in the EORTC trial. Patients who had surgery after completion of radiation or for treatment-related morbidity were counted as local failures in the UKCCCR trial.

[c]Difference statistically significant at $P < 0.05$.

given the combined-modality approach (Table 10.9). A planned subset analysis revealed a significant local control benefit even in T1-2N0 patients.

Value of MMC in the Combined-Modality Regimen

The RTOG/Intergroup study randomized 310 patients to receive 45 to 50.4 Gy of pelvic RT with 5-FU or the same radiation and 5-FU/MMC (2). A statistically significant increase in 4-year disease-free survival was observed in the patient cohort that received MMC, although toxicity was significantly greater. Substitution of cisplatin for MMC in combination with 5-FU and radiation therapy has been explored in phase 2 trials (3) with promising initial results. Induction therapy with 5-FU/cisplatin followed by RT/5-FU/cisplatin was compared with "standard" RT/5-FU/MMC in RTOG 98-11 (Table 10.10). The results showed equal overall survival of 69% at 5 years and equivalent 5-year disease-free survival (48% in the experimental arm and 56% in the standard arm). Hematologic toxicity was worse in the MMC-containing arm, although nonhematologic toxicities were similar. However, the colostomy rate was higher in the experimental arm (19% vs. 10%). The authors concluded that the experimental regimen was not superior to standard chemoradiation with 5-FU/MMC (4).

Toxicity of Combined-Modality Therapy

The acute toxicities of chemoradiation for anal cancer can be severe and include anemia, thrombocytopenia, desquamation and skin breakdown, diarrhea, infection, fluid and electrolyte derangements, pain, and fatigue. The RTOG/ECOG trial (2) reported a 3% rate of treatment-related death in the 5-FU/MMC arm. Aggressive use of barrier creams and emollients on the inguinal and perianal regions and antidiarrheal medications such as loperamide and diphenoxylate/atropine can be helpful in reducing the risk of infection and trauma to the perianal region. Opioid analgesics are often necessary for pain control and help decrease the frequency of stools. Blood counts should be monitored closely, particularly if MMC is used. Fecal contamination of areas of compromised perianal skin in the setting of neutropenia can pose a high-risk of sepsis. Overall, however, treatment breaks should be avoided if possible. A protocol of split-course chemoradiation with a planned 2-week treatment break produced a significantly higher local failure and colostomy rate (5). Late complications of chemoradiation for anal cancer can include painful fibrosis, lymphedema, anal stenosis and sphincter dysfunction, fistula formation, rectal bleeding, impotence, infertility, femoral neck fractures, and small-bowel injury.

TABLE 10.10. *Randomized trials comparing radiation with 5-fluorouracil and mitomycin C to other chemoradiation regimens*

Trial	Arm	N	Disease-free survival (%)	Colostomy rate (%)	Toxicity	Overall survival (%)
RTOG/ ECOG	RT/5-FU	145	51	22	8% Grade 4–5	67
	RT/5-FU/ MMC	146	73*	9*	26%* Grade 4–5	76
RTOG 98-11	Induction 5- FU/CDDP then RT/5-FU/ CDDP	598 ana- lyzable 324	56	19	75% non- heme 47% heme Grade 3–4	69
	RT/5-FU/ MMC	320	48	10*	76% non- heme 67% heme* Grade 3–4	69

RTOG, Radiation Therapy Oncology Group; ECOG, Eastern Cooperative Oncology Group; RT, radiation therapy; 5-FU, 5-fluorouracil; MMC, mitomycin C; CDDP, cisplatin; heme, hematologic toxicity; nonheme, nonhematologic toxicity.

*Statistically significant at $P < 0.05$.

Chemoradiation in HIV-Positive Patients

HIV-positive patients are more likely to require treatment breaks and hospitalization during treatment. Dose reduction of chemotherapy and radiation or alterations of the treatment plan (such as omission of MMC) may be necessary for HIV-positive patients with a history of HIV/AIDS-related complications. However, sequential chemoradiation in anal cancer is markedly inferior to concurrent treatment and should not be used.

Combined External Beam and Interstitial Radiation Therapy

Lower-dose external beam radiation has been combined with chemotherapy and an interstitial iridium-192 implant in an effort to improve the therapeutic radio. Several European investigators have reported series showing average local control rates of 81% (range 73–89%), with 5-year survival of 70% (range 60–84%) (6–11). The rate of anal necrosis ranged from 2% to 76%, and many of these patients required salvage with APR, even if they were free of disease. Interstitial implantation after external beam radiotherapy may help some patients with residual disease to have a complete response.

Dose of Radiation

Although series have been published suggesting that highly selected early-stage patients can be cured with only 30 Gy with concurrent 5-FU/MMC after a local excision, several reports have suggested that radiation doses above 54 Gy are associated with improved local control and survival (12). Recently, attempts have been made to escalate the radiation dose used in combined-modality therapy, including the recent RTOG 98-11 randomized protocol. However, local control and survival for the best arm of this trial, which used doses up to 59.4 Gy with 5-FU/MMC, were not substantially better than the results obtained in the RTOG/ECOG study with 45 to 50.4 Gy and 5-FU/MMC. Increases in dose have also been associated with greater toxicity. Daily fraction sizes should not exceed 2 Gy with concurrent chemotherapy due to enhanced acute and late toxicity. In select cases, radiation alone in doses of 60 to 70 Gy has been used to safely and successfully treat small, early-stage tumors.

Intensity-Modulated Radiation Therapy (IMRT)

IMRT can achieve tight conformality of the prescribed radiation dose to the target volume while increasing sparing normal tissues, and is particularly useful in situations where the target is complex or concave in shape. In anal cancer, IMRT has been investigated as a means of decreasing dose to the skin, bone marrow, and bowel while maintaining or escalating the tumor dose. Salama et al. reported preliminary results from a series of 53 anal cancer patients treated with IMRT and concurrent chemotherapy (13). The median dose to the pelvic and inguinal lymph nodes was 45 Gy; the primary site and involved nodes were boosted to a median dose of 51.5 Gy; 48 of the patients received 5-FU/MMC and 15% of patients developed acute grade 3 gastrointestinal toxicity and 34% had grade 3 dermatologic toxicity, significantly better than the results from RTOG 98-11 (34% and 48%, respectively). There were no nonhematologic toxicities of grade 4 or higher. Local control was excellent with a 93% complete response rate and 84% colostomy-free survival at 18 months. These encouraging results are being confirmed in RTOG 0529, a phase 2 protocol.

Tumor Regression After Chemoradiation

The median time to complete tumor regression after combined-modality treatment is 12 weeks, and most local recurrences manifest within 2 years. Regression after treatment with radiation alone may be even more prolonged, and up to a year may need to elapse before a complete response is evident. Biopsy should only be performed if tumor persists on serial exams. Results from a phase 3 study suggested benefit to adding a radiation boost with cisplatin for patients with persistent disease after chemoradiation (2), but this was more likely due to continued prolonged tumor regression from the initial therapy

TREATMENT OPTIONS ACCORDING TO STAGE

Treatment options according to stage for anal cancer are contained in Table 10.11.

Stage 0

• Surgical resection is the treatment of choice for the lesions of the perianal area that do not involve the anal sphincter.

TABLE 10.11. *Treatment options for anal cancer*

Stage	Treatment options
0	Surgery
I	Radiation
	Chemoradiation
	Surgery
II	Chemoradiation
	Surgery
III	Chemoradiation
	Surgery
IV	Palliative surgery
	Palliative irradiation
	Palliative chemoradiation
	Clinical trial

Stage I

- Small, well-differentiated tumors of the anal margin not involving the anal sphincter can be treated with wide local excision.
- All other stage I tumors of the anal margin and anal canal are treated with chemoradiation with 5-FU/MMC.
- Patients who cannot tolerate chemotherapy may be treated with radiation alone.
- Surgical salvage with APR is reserved for residual cancer in the anal canal after chemoradiation.

Stage II

- Chemoradiation with 5-FU/MMC is the recommended initial approach.
- Patients who cannot tolerate chemotherapy may be treated with radiation alone.
- Surgical salvage with APR is reserved for residual disease in the anal canal after chemoradiation.

Stage IIIA

Stage IIIA anal cancer presents clinically as stage II anal cancer in most patients but is upstaged to IIIA by presence of perirectal nodal disease or adjacent organ involvement. Endoscopic ultrasound (endoanal or endorectal) may aid in assessing perirectal lymph nodes.

- Chemoradiation with 5-FU/MMC is the recommended initial approach.
- Surgical salvage with APR is reserved for residual disease in the anal canal after chemoradiation.

Stage IIIB

Though the cure of this stage is possible, the involvement of inguinal lymph nodes (unilateral or bilateral) constitutes a poor prognostic sign.

- Chemoradiation with 5-FU/MMC is the recommended initial approach.
- Surgical salvage with APR is reserved for residual disease in the anal canal after chemoradiation.
- Because of the poor prognosis of these patients, they should be recruited for clinical trials whenever possible.

Stage IV

There is no standard chemotherapy regimen for stage IV disease. Chemotherapy with 5-FU/MMC or cisplatin has been reported to give a 50% response rate, with a median survival of 12 months (14). Palliation of symptoms constitutes the backbone of management. Patients with stage IV anal cancer should be enrolled in clinical trials.

- Palliative chemotherapy
- Palliative radiation therapy to localized symptomatic metastases
- Palliative surgery
- Palliative combined chemotherapy and radiation therapy
- Clinical trials

PERSISTENT OR RECURRENT ANAL CANCER

Persistent anal cancer can be managed according to Fig. 10.2.

Local recurrences after initial treatment with either chemoradiation or surgical resection can be effectively controlled by alternate treatment options, including:

- Surgical resection after chemoradiation (salvage APR)
- Salvage radiation with or without chemotherapy if normal tissue tolerances permit
- Isolated recurrence in the inguinal area may be managed with inguinal node dissection or, if possible, with local radiation with or without chemotherapy

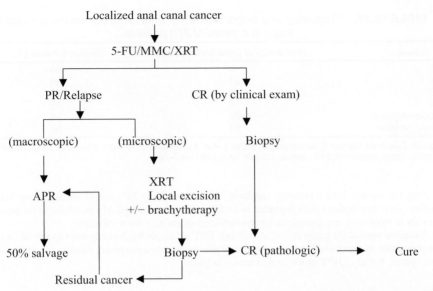

Fig. 10.2. Management of anal cancer after definitive chemoradiation. (PR, partial response; CR, complete response; APR, abdominoperineal resection; XRT, radiation therapy.)

Follow-up

Patients with anal cancer should be monitored as follows:

- Every 3 months for the first 3 years
- Every 6 months for an additional 2 years
- Annually thereafter

The following specific recommendations should be undertaken:

- Medical history
- Physical examination, including digital rectal exam and palpation of inguinal nodes
- Complete blood counts
- Liver function tests
- Chest radiograph yearly
- CT scan of the pelvis every 6 to 12 months for the first 3 years

Prognosis

Frequency and 5-year survival of anal canal carcinoma patients by stage is shown in Table 10.12.

Prevention

Awareness of the disease by the physician and the recognition of a high-risk group (homosexual men, women with cervical or vulvar cancer) may aid patients by early detection. There are currently no standard recommendations for screening for anal cancer in high-risk populations. Anoscopy with anal cytology should be undertaken in patients with abnormal discharge, bleeding, pruritis, bowel irregularity, rectal or pelvic pain, and those with a history of previous preinvasive lesions or abnormal Pap smears. Other patients who should be screened include HIV-negative men with a history of anal-receptive intercourse, HIV-positive men and women with CD4 cell counts less than 500/mm^3, and HIV-positive and -negative women with a history of high-grade cervical intraepithelial neoplasia (CIN).

TABLE 10.12. *Frequency and 5-year survival of anal canal carcinoma patients by stage in a series of 270 patients*

Stage	Frequency at presentation (%)	5-year survival (%)
T1	9	86
T2	51	86
T3	30	60
T4	10	45
Node-negative	87	76
Node-positive	13	54

Source: Data from Touboul E, Schlienger M, Buffat L et al. Epidermoid carcinoma of the anal canal. Results of curative-intent radiation in 270 patients. *Cancer* 1994;73(6):1569–79.

Anal Pap smears have a reported sensitivity of approximately 70% (equal to that associated with uterine cervix Pap testing). AIN is graded like CIN and the treatment of AIN is similar to the treatment for CIN in women. It may include electrocautery, cryoablation, or laser ablation.

A vaccine against the transmission of high-risk HPV serotypes has recently been approved for use in the prevention of cervical cancer in women, and this represents a promising strategy for prevention of anal cancer. A trial of HPV prevention in men is ongoing.

REFERENCES

1. UKCCCR Anal Cancer Trial Working Party. Epidermoid anal cancer: results from the UKCCCR randomized trial of radiotherapy alone versus radiotherapy, 5-fluorouracil, and mitomycin. *Lancet* 1996;348:1049–1054.
2. Flam M, John M, Pajak TF, et al. Role of mitomycin in combination with fluorouracil and radiotherapy, and of salvage chemoradiation in the definitive nonsurgical treatment of epidermoid carcinoma of the anal canal: results of a phase III randomized Intergroup study. *J Clin Oncol* 1996;14:2527–2539.
3. Doci R, Zucali R, LaMonica G, et al. Primary chemoradiation therapy with fluorouracil and cisplatin for cancer of the anus: results in 35 consecutive patients. *J Clin Oncol* 1996;14:3121–3125.
4. Ajani JA, Winter KA, Gunderson LA, et al. Fluorouracil, mitomycin, and radiotherapy vs fluorouracil, cisplatin, and radiotherapy for carcinoma of the anal canal. A randomized controlled trial. *JAMA* 2008;299(16):1914–1921.
5. John M, Pajak TJ, Flam MS, et al. Dose escalation in chemoradiation for anal cancer. Preliminary results of RTOG 92-08. *Cancer J Sci Am* 1996;2:205–211.
6. Gerard JP, Ayzac L, Hun D, et al. Treatment of anal carcinoma with high dose radiation therapy and concurrent fluoruracil-cisplatin. Long-term results of 95 patients. *Radiother Oncol* 1998;46(3):249–256.
7. Allal AS, Mermillod B, Roth AD, et al. Impact of clinical and therapeutic factors on major late complications after radiotherapy with or without concomitant chemotherapy for anal carcinoma. *Int J Radiat Oncol Biol Phys* 1997;39(5):1099–1105.
8. Papillon J, Montbaron F. Epidermoid carcinoma of the anal canal. A series of 276 cases. *Dis Colon Rectum* 1987;30(5):224–233.
9. Sandhu AP, Symonds RP, Robertson AG, et al. Interstitial iridium-192 implantation combined with external radiotherapy in anal cancer: ten years experience. *Int J Radiat Oncol Biol Phys* 1998;40(3):575–578.
10. Roed H, Engelholm SA, Svendsen LB, et al. Pulsed dose rate (PDR) brachytherapy of anal carcinoma. *Radiother Oncol* 1996;44(3):296–297.
11. Loenhert M, Doniec JM, Kovacs G, et al. New method of radiotherapy for anal cancer with three-dimensional tumor reconstruction based on endoanal ultrasound and ultrasound-guided afterloading therapy. *Dis Colon Rectum* 1998;41(2):169–176.

12. Constantinou EC, Daly W, Fung CY, et al. Time-dose considerations in the treatment of anal cancer. *Int J Radiat Oncol Biol Phys* 1997;39 (3):651–657.
13. Salama JK, Mell LK, Schomas DA, et al. Concurrent chemotherapy and intensity-modulated radiation therapy for anal canal cancer patients: a multicenter experience. *J Clin Oncol* 2007;25(29): 4581–4586.
14. Tanum G. Treatment of relapsing anal carcinoma. *Acta Oncol* 1993;32:33–35.
15. Leichman L, Nigro N, Vaitkericus VK, et al. Cancer of the anal canal. Model for preoperative adjuvant combined modality therapy. *Am J Med* 1985;78(2):211–215.
16. Sischy B, Doggett RL, Krall JM, et al. Definitive irradiation and chemotherapy for radiosensitization in management of anal carcinoma: Interim report on radiation therapy oncology group study no. 8314. *J Nat Cancer Inst* 1989;81:850–856.
17. Cummings B, Keane T, Thomas G, et al. Results and toxicity of treatment of anal canal carcinoma by radiation therapy or radiation therapy and chemotherapy. *Cancer* 1984;54(10):2062–2068.
18. Schneider IH, Grabenbauer GG, Reck T, et al. Combined radiation and chemotherapy for epidermoid carcinoma of the anal canal. *Int J Colorectal Dis* 1992;7(4):192–196.
19. Tanum G, Tveit K, Karlsen KO, et al. Chemotherapy and radiation therapy for anal cacrcinoma: Survival and late morbidity. *Cancer* 1991;67(10):2462–2466.
20. Cummings BJ, Rider WA, Harwood AR, et al. Combined radical radiation therapy and chemotherapy for primary squamous cell carcinoma of the anal canal. *Cancer Treat Rep* 1982;66(3): 489–492.
21. Doci R, Zucali R, Bombelli L, et al. Combined chemoradiation therapy for anal cancer: A report of 56 cases. *Ann Surg* 1992;215(2):150–156.
22. Martenson JA, Lipsitz SR, Lefkopoulou M, et al. Results of combined modality therapy for patients with anal cancer (E7283). An Eastern Cooperative Oncology Group study. *Cancer* 1995;76(10):1731–1736.
23. Allal A, Kurtz JM, Pipard G, et al. Chemoradiotherapy versus radiotherapy alone for anal cancer: A retrospective comparison. *Int J Radiat Oncol Biol Phys* 1993;27(1):59–66.

SUGGESTED READINGS

Bartelink H, Roelofson F, Eschwege F, et al. Concomitant radiotherapy and chemotherapy is superior to radiotherapy alone in the treatment of locally advanced anal cancer: results of a phase III randomized trial of the European Organization for Research and Treatment of Cancer radiotherapy and gastrointestinal cooperative groups. *J Clin Oncol* 1997;15:2040–2049.

Martenson JA Jr, Gunderson LL. External radiation therapy without chemotherapy in the management of anal cancer. *Cancer* 1993;71:1736–1740.

Melbye M, Cote TR, Kessler L, et al. High incidence of anal cancer among AIDS patients. *Lancet* 1994;343:636–639.

Palefsky JM, Holly EA, Hogoboom CJ, et al. Anal cytology as a screening tool for anal squamous intraepithelial lesion. *J Acquir Immun Defic Syndr Hum Retrovirol* 1997;14:415–422.

Peddada AV, Smith DE, Rao AR, et al. Chemotherapy and low-dose radiotherapy in the treatment of HIV-infected patients with carcinoma of the anal canal. *Int J Radiat Oncol Biol Phys* 1997;37: 1101–1105. *Radiother Oncol* 1996;41(2):131–134.

Ryan DP, Compton CC, Mayer RJ. Carcinoma of the anal canal. *N Engl J Med* 2000;342:792–800.

Schraut WH, Wang CH, Dawson PI, Block GE. Depth of invasion, location, and size of cancer of the anus dictate operative treatment. *Cancer* 1983;51:1291–1296.

Toubol E, Schlienger M, Buffat L, et al. Epidermoid carcinoma of the anal canal. Results of curative-intent radiation therapy in a series of 270 patients. *Cancer* 1994;73(6):1569–1579.

11

Other Gastrointestinal Tumors

M. Wasif Saif

GASTROINTESTINAL STROMAL TUMOR

Gastrointestinal stromal tumors (GISTs), a type of sarcoma, are the most common nonepithelial tumors of the digestive tract that arise from precursors of connective tissue cells located in the gastrointestinal (GI) tract. Most GI soft tissue neoplasms, previously classified as leiomyomas, schwannomas, leiomyoblastomas, or leiomyosarcomas, are presently classified as GIST on the basis of molecular and immunohistologic features. Such tumors usually have activating mutations in either KIT (75%–80%) or platelet-derived growth factor receptor alpha (PDGFRa) (5%–10%) which lead to ligand-independent signal transduction. Targeting these activated proteins with imatinib mesylate, a small-molecule kinase inhibitor, has proven useful in the treatment of recurrent or metastatic GISTs.

Epidemiology

The incidence of GIST is estimated to be approximately 10 to 20 cases per 1,000,000 population; the median age at diagnosis has been reported to be 55 to 65 years. GISTs most commonly occur in the stomach (60%) or duodenum, followed by the small intestine (25%), rectum (5%), and esophagus (2%); 5% are found in the colon, mesentery, and retroperitoneum. Early-stage GIST typically manifests as a localized tumor (i.e., in the stomach). Approximately 50% of patients present with metastatic disease at first diagnosis, predominantly in the liver or peritoneum.

Pathology

GISTs are believed to originate from interstitial cells of Cajal. The majority of cases can be classified into two categories: spindle cell type (70%) and epithelioid type (20%). The spindle cell type has uniform eosinophilic spindle cells organized in short fascicles or in a short storiform growth pattern (Fig. 11.1). The epithelioid cell type has round-shaped cells exhibiting eosinophilic or clear cytoplasm that tend to exhibit a nested growth pattern (Fig. 11.2).

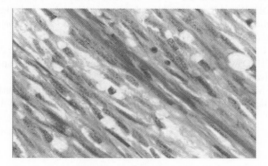

Fig. 11.1.   Spindle cell.

136

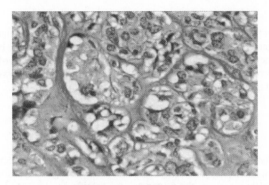

Fig. 11.2. Epitheloid.

Diagnosis

Approximately 85% of GISTs express KIT, a type 3 transmembrane receptor tyrosine kinase. It is the single most common tumor marker for GIST and is identified with anti-CD117 antibodies. PDGFR alpha (PDGFRA) mutations are homologous to those responsible for KIT– and Flt-3L–independent kinase activation in other malignancies, including acute myeloid leukemia, mast cell disorders, and seminomas. KIT and PDGFRA mutations and overexpression are usually mutually exclusive in GIST. Similarly, GISTs have high levels of either phospho-KIT or phospho-PDGFRA, but not both. Thirty-five percent of KIT wild-type GISTs have PDGFRA mutations. Downstream activation of many targets of KIT are also activated by PDGFRA mutations in GIST and include: AKT, MAPK, and STATs (STAT1 and STAT3) (Fig. 11.3).

Positron emission tomography (PET) and computerized tomography (CT) scans are sensitive and reliable indicators of tumor response to therapy, particularly with imatinib 2-fluoro-2-deoxy-D-glucose (FDG). PET improves staging, accurately separates responders from nonresponders in an early phase, and is helpful during follow-up of patients.

Clinical Presentation

The clinical presentation of GIST depends on the location of the tumor and may include the following:

- Abdominal discomfort or pain
- Sense of abdominal fullness
- Nausea
- Vomiting
- GI bleeding
- Fatigue related to anemia

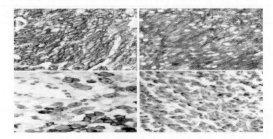

Fig. 11.3. Different KIT-staining patterns in GIST.

Prognostic Factors

Current clinical practice guidelines now recognize that all GISTs have malignant potential. Because GISTs are widely diverse in terms of clinical presentation, morphology, and biologic behavior, the prediction of malignancy in these tumors on the basis of pathologic features is often difficult. To date, proposed prognostic features indicative of malignancy or high risk for aggressive clinical behavior include tumor size and mitotic index (Table 11.1).

Treatment

Surgery

Surgery is the primary treatment of choice for localized or potentially resectable GIST. However, surgery alone is inadequate for the treatment of GIST due to the high rate of local and distant recurrence. Following complete resection, the 5-year disease-specific survival rate is about 50%. Median time to recurrence after resection of primary high-risk GIST is about 2 years. Metastases can develop 10 to 15 or more years after primary surgery, necessitating long-term clinical follow-up. Metastasis into the abdominal cavity or liver are more common than in lymph nodes and extremely rare in the lungs and other extra-abdominal locations.

Chemotherapy

Recurrent or malignant GIST does not respond to conventional cytotoxic agents; the response rate of this fatal disease to doxorubicin has been reported to be lower than 5%. Other commonly used chemotherapeutic agents yield similarly poor responses in GIST.

Radiotherapy

The effectiveness of radiation therapy in treating GIST also has not been proven.

Targeted Therapy

The development of a tyrosine kinase inhibitor has changed the management of unresectable GIST. Imatinib mesylate (STI571, Glivec), a tyrosine kinase inhibitor that inhibits the c-kit receptor, has been proven to be highly effective against GIST and has improved survival in metastatic GIST. Early results from clinical trials confirm the high activity of this novel treatment, with response rates of approximately 60% and arrest of tumor progression seen in more than 80% of patients, which results in fast relief of symptoms (see Table 11.2).

Imatinib is approved at a dose of 400 to 600 mg daily for GIST. Some investigators have attempted to determine the most effective dose of imatinib in GIST patients. A large international randomized

TABLE 11.1. *The prognostic factors that define different risk groups for GISTs*

Risk	Size (cm)	Mitotic count (per 50 HPF)	5-Year survival[a] (%)
Very low	<2	<5	~70
Low	2–5	<5	
Intermediate	<5	6–10	~56
	5–10	<5	
High	>5	>5	~22
	>10	>Any mitotic rate	
	Any tumor	>10	

HPF, high-power field.

Note: Size represents the single largest dimension.

[a]Retrospective analysis of disease-specific survival by tumor size in patients with primary disease who underwent complete resection (*n* = 80).

TABLE 11.2. *Responses to imatinib mesylate in a phase 2 trial of patients with advanced GISTs*

Confirmed overall responses[a]	400-mg dose of imatinib (n = 73) (%)	600-mg dose of imatinib (n = 74) (%)	Either dose (n = 147) (%)
Partial response	62	65	63
Stable disease	15	20	20
Progressive disease	16	18	12
Clinical benefit	77	85	83

[a]15-month follow-up.

phase 3 trial compared the efficacy of two different doses of imatinib in GIST patients. The study randomized 946 patients to receive either 400 mg of imatinib once daily (with crossover to 800 mg/day with disease progression) or 400 mg twice daily (for a daily dose of 800 mg). The interim analysis presented at the 2002 American Society of Clinical Oncology (ASCO) meeting showed that patients responded well to both doses of imatinib, with an objective response of 43% observed in each arm of the trial. Complete response was similar between the two arms—5.6% and 3.9%, respectively, for the 400-mg and 800-mg groups. Most patients, however, showed either partial response (44.7% and 47.2%, respectively) or stable disease (32.7% and 33.3%, respectively). Data also showed that progression-free survival (PFS), the primary endpoint of the study, was significantly higher in patients who received the 800-mg dose of imatinib ($P = 0.0216$).

Treatment with imatinib is generally well tolerated, although most common toxicities include grade 1 or 2 adverse events—most commonly nausea, diarrhea, periorbital edema, muscle cramps, fatigue, headache, and dermatitis.

Post-surgery (Adjuvant) Imatinib

The FDA has not yet approved the use of imatinib (Glivec) after complete resection of a primary GIST. Trials are underway to determine whether administering imatinib for some period of time after complete resection (1, 2, or 3 years) of a primary tumor will reduce the percentage of patients who develop recurrences or metastases of GIST. In the United States, the American College of Surgeons Oncology Group (ACOSOG) Intergroup Adjuvant GIST Study Team performed a phase 3 trial (ACOSOG Z9001) in which 708 patients were randomized in a double-blind fashion to 1 year of imatinib 400 mg daily or placebo following complete gross resection of a primary GIST measuring at least 3 centimeters and expressing KIT. Upon recurrence, treatment assignment was unblinded and patients were allowed to cross over to imatinib if they had been on placebo or increase the daily dose of imatinib to 800 mg if they were already receiving the drug. The primary endpoint of the trial was recurrence-free survival (RFS). An interim analysis, RFS at 1 year, is shown in Table 11.3.

A single-arm, open-label, phase 2 multicenter study was performed in patients who underwent complete gross resection of a KIT-expressing primary GIST that was at high risk of recurrence (tumor size ≥10 cm, tumor rupture, or <5 peritoneal metastases). Patients received imatinib at a daily dose of 400 mg for 1 year. The primary endpoint was overall survival. Among 107 evaluable patients, 1-, 2-, and 3-year overall survival rates were 99%, 97%, and 97%, respectively at a median follow-up of 4 years. The 1-, 2-, and 3-year RFS rates were 94%, 73%, and 61%, respectively. This study suggested that imatinib given at a daily oral dose of 400 mg for 1 year following the resection of a high-risk primary GIST prolongs RFS and is associated with improved overall survival compared with historical controls.

TABLE 11.3. *Interim analysis of post-surgery imatinib*

Recurrence-free survival at the 1-year mark	Tumor size 3–6 cm	6–10 cm	>10 cm
Imatinib group	100%	96%	96%
Placebo group	95%	80%	67%
Significant difference	No	$P < 0.01$	$P < 0.001$

The mechanisms of acquired resistance to imatinib are heterogeneous, with most involving the emergence of secondary mutations in KIT exons 13, 14, or 17 and is of interest to investigators.

Neoadjuvant Therapy

RTOG 0132/ACRIN 6665, a prospective phase 2 study, evaluated safety and efficacy of neoadjuvant imatinib mesylate (600 mg/day) for patients with primary GIST or the preoperative use of imatinib mesylate in patients with operable metastatic GIST. The trial continued post-op imatinib mesylate for 2 years. Early results among 63 patients, of whom 52 were analyzable, 30 patients with primary GIST (group A) and 22 with recurrent metastatic GIST (group B) showed response (RECIST) as follows: group A, 7% partial, 83% stable, 10% unknown; group B, 4.5% partial, 91% stable, 4.5% progression. Two-year PFS was 83% for group A and 77% for group B. Estimated overall survival was 93% for group A and 91% for group B. Complications of surgery and imatinib mesylate toxicity were minimal. This trial represents the first prospective report of pre-op imatinib mesylate in GIST. This approach is feasible, requires multidisciplinary consultations, and is not associated with notable postoperative complications.

SU11248 (sunitinib; sutent)

Sunitinib malate is a novel oral multitargeted tyrosine kinase inhibitor with antitumor and antiangiogenic activities. Sunitinib is approved for the treatment of patients with GIST after disease progression or intolerance to imatinib mesylate therapy. A double-blind placebo-controlled, multicenter, randomized phase 3 trial confirmed the efficacy and safety of sunitinib as second-line therapy in 312 patients with GIST showing disease progression or intolerance under imatinib mesylate therapy. Patients were randomized in a 2:1 ratio to receive sunitinib 50 mg daily for 4 weeks, with 2 weeks off ($n = 207$) or placebo ($n = 105$). Objective response rate in the sunitinib arm and in the placebo arm were 8% and 0%, respectively. Median time to progression was significantly longer in the sunitinib arm (6.3 vs. 1.5 months). Fifty-nine patients in the placebo group crossed over to sunitinib therapy due to disease progression. Ten percent had subsequent partial responses, suggesting that the optimal therapeutic effect of sunitinib may be observed when it is administered in the early disease phase. Hypertension and asthenia are the most common side effects with sunitinib. The further role of sunitinib is under investigation in clinical trials.

Other Treatments

Experimental treatment options beyond those currently available consist of other KIT-targeting tyrosine kinase inhibitors, such as nilotinib, or agents targeting alternative pathways, such as antiangiogenic agents, mammalian target of rapamycin, RAF kinase, and chaperone inhibitors.

SMALL BOWEL ADENOCARCINOMA

Introduction

Malignant neoplasms of the small bowel are among the rarest types of cancer, accounting for only 2% of all GI cancers. Research into the natural history and prognosis of patients with small bowel cancer has been limited by the number of cases and the heterogeneity of tumor types, including adenocarcinomas, carcinoids, sarcomas, and lymphomas. Each of these tumor subtypes has its own distinct clinical behavior and, therefore, dictates a different treatment approach. Unfortunately, malignant lesions are often discovered when they have metastasized to distant sites or at surgery when indicated for other diagnosis or intestinal obstruction.

Epidemiology

Cancer of the small bowel is a relatively rare malignancy, accounting for approximately 2% of GI tumors. Approximately 5,300 new cases of small bowel adenocarcinoma and 1,100 deaths from the disease are reported annually in the United States. Approximately 64% of all small bowel tumors are malignant, and approximately 40% of these tumors are adenocarcinomas, 40% are carcinoids, 15% are sarcomas (GIST), and fewer than 5% are lymphomas.

Etiology

Genetic Risk Factors

- Familial adenomatous polyposis: Patients with this condition develop multiple adenomas throughout the small bowel and colon, which may lead to adenocarcinomas. After the colon, the duodenum is the most common site of adenocarcinoma. A 1993 study from Johns Hopkins by Offerhaus et al. found that patients with familial adenomatous polyposis have a relative risk of more than 300 for duodenal adenocarcinoma but no elevated risk for gastric or nonduodenal small bowel cancer. Molecular genetic studies of duodenal polyps in patients with familial adenomatous polyposis performed by Kashiwagi et al. in 1997 found a high frequency of p53 overexpression in dysplastic adenomas, although the frequency of TP53 and k-ras gene mutations was much lower.
- Hereditary nonpolyposis colorectal cancer: Aside from colorectal carcinoma, patients with this genetic syndrome also develop endometrial, gastric, small bowel, upper urinary tract, and ovarian carcinomas. The lifetime risk of small bowel adenocarcinoma in patients with hereditary nonpolyposis colorectal cancer is 1% to 4%, which is more than 100 times the risk in the general population. Small bowel adenocarcinomas in persons with hereditary nonpolyposis colorectal cancer are distributed evenly throughout the small bowel. They occur at younger age and appear to have a better prognosis than sporadic small bowel cancers. The most commonly mutated genes in the germline of patients with hereditary nonpolyposis colorectal cancer are HMLH1 *and* HMSH2, which are involved in DNA mismatch repair.

Environmental Risk Factors

- Diet: A 1977 study by Lowenfels and Sonni found animal fat intake to be correlated with small bowel cancer. A 1993 study by Chow et al. reported that consumption of red meat and salt-cured or smoked foods raised the risk of small bowel cancer 2 to 3 times.
- Tobacco and alcohol: Studies from 1994 by Chen et al. found an association between smoking and small bowel adenocarcinoma and between alcohol consumption and small bowel adenocarcinoma, but this has not been confirmed in other studies.

Predisposing Medical Conditions

- Crohn's disease: The relative risk of small bowel adenocarcinoma is estimated to be between 15 and more than 100 in patients with Crohn's disease. Unlike most small bowel adenocarcinomas, Crohn-related tumors generally occur in the ileum, reflecting the distribution of Crohn's disease. The risk of adenocarcinoma does not begin until at least 10 years after the onset of Crohn's disease, and the adenocarcinoma typically occurs more than 20 years afterward.
- Celiac disease (nontropical sprue): Patients with celiac disease appear to be at increased risk of small bowel lymphoma and adenocarcinoma. A 2001 survey of adult celiac disease patients in the United States performed by Green et al. found a relative risk of 300 for the development of lymphoma and 67 for the development of adenocarcinoma. Small bowel adenocarcinomas associated with celiac disease appear to have an increased incidence of defective DNA mismatch repair compared with those not associated with celiac disease, and are associated with an earlier stage at diagnosis and a better prognosis.
- Peutz-Jeghers syndrome: Hemminki has reported an approximately 18-fold increase in the incidence compared to that in the general population.

Pathology

Small bowel adenocarcinoma includes adenocarcinomas arising in the duodenum, jejunum, and ileum. Whereas adenocarcinomas arising from the ampulla of Vater and the periampullary region are typically included in the category of small bowel adenocarcinomas, those arising from the ileocecal valve, appendix, and Meckel diverticulum are excluded.

Epidemiologically, small bowel adenocarcinomas have a striking resemblance to large bowel adenocarcinomas. For example, although small bowel adenocarcinomas are only one-fiftieth as common as large bowel adenocarcinomas, they share a similar geographic distribution, with predominance in Western countries. In addition, they tend to co-occur in the same individuals, with an increased risk of small bowel adenocarcinoma in survivors of colorectal cancer and vice versa.

Furthermore, similar to adenocarcinomas in the colon, those in the small bowel arise from premalignant adenomas. This occurs both sporadically and in the context of familial adenomatous polyposis. Through a stepwise accumulation of genetic mutations, these adenomas become dysplastic and progress to carcinomas in situ and then to invasive adenocarcinomas. They metastasize via the lymphatics or portal circulation to the liver, lung, bone, brain, and other distant sites. Despite these similarities with colon cancer, small bowel adenocarcinomas tend to cluster away from the colon, toward the gastric end of the small intestine. Approximately 50% arise in the duodenum, 30% in the jejunum, and 20% in the ileum. The duodenum is the first portion of the small bowel to be exposed to ingested chemicals and pancreaticobiliary secretions. This fact, combined with the higher prevalence of cancer in the duodenum, may indicate that the substances (i.e., ingested chemicals, pancreaticobiliary secretions) may have carcinogenic properties. Animal studies have demonstrated that diverting bile decreases the prevalence of experimentally induced small bowel cancers, which suggests that bile may be carcinogenic.

In addition, genetic analyses of sporadic small bowel adenocarcinomas suggest similarities and differences from the pathogenesis from colorectal carcinomas. Although K-ras mutation and p53 overexpression appear to be as common in small bowel adenocarcinoma as in colorectal carcinoma, mutation of the APC tumor suppressor gene, which is characteristic of colorectal carcinoma, does not commonly occur in small bowel adenocarcinoma. The SMAD4/DPC4 gene, which is often mutated in pancreatic and colorectal carcinomas, also appears to be inactivated in small bowel adenocarcinomas.

Most small bowel adenocarcinomas are solitary, sessile lesions, often appearing in association with adenomas. They are usually moderately well-differentiated and are almost always positive for acid mucin.

Small bowel adenocarcinomas can be positive for carcinoembryonic antigen (CEA), carbohydrate antigen 19-9 (CA 19-9), and p53. Expression of c-erbB-2, Ki-67, and tenascin has also been described. Small bowel adenocarcinomas arising from the ileum may show staining with neuroendocrine markers.

Clinical Presentation

The clinical presentation of small-bowel adenocarcinoma depends on the location of the primary tumor, its growth pattern, and the extent of metastatic spread. In general, symptoms are initially nonspecific and include anemia, bleeding, abdominal pain, nausea and vomiting, or obstruction and/or perforation in cases of locally advanced tumor. Because of a vague presentation of small bowel adenocarcinoma, the time between initial development of symptoms and diagnosis is often relatively long, approximately 6 to 8 months, and contributes to the higher percentage of advanced cases at the time of diagnosis (in contrast to colorectal cancer). Common sites of metastases include locoregional lymph nodes, liver, lung, and the peritoneum.

Diagnosis

Lab Studies

- Complete blood count (CBC) may show mild anemia related to chronic blood loss.
- Liver function tests may reveal hyperbilirubinemia, which may be related to biliary obstruction from periampullary tumors. Elevated transaminase levels also may be found in the presence of liver metastases.
- CEA levels may be elevated. Although cases with elevation of CA 19-9, or CA 125 levels have been reported, no clear role for such tumor markers has been established for diagnosis.

Imaging Studies

- Plain abdominal x-ray films may reveal partial or complete small bowel obstruction.
- Upper GI series with small bowel follow through show abnormalities in 53% to 83% of patients with small bowel cancer.
- Small bowel enteroclysis studies are done with double-contrast barium enema, which has a sensitivity of 95%. However, it is difficult to perform as it requires a long tube to be inserted in the small bowel to instill air and contrast.
- Abdominal CT scan may elucidate the site and extent of local disease and the presence of liver metastases.

Other Tests

In those rare cases of bleeding due to a small bowel tumor, the diagnostic approach is the same for all cases of lower GI bleeding. In case of negative upper and lower endoscopy, tagged red blood cell scan and angiography can be helpful in localizing the disease process. A newer test, called capsule endoscopy, has a better sensitivity and specificity and is being performed for occult GI bleeding.

Procedures

- Upper GI endoscopy with small bowel enteroscopy (push enteroscopy) may identify and allow biopsy of lesions in the duodenum and jejunum. Push enteroscopy is difficult to perform. The endoscopes are long and difficult to manipulate. The procedure is lengthy.
- Colonoscopy with retrograde ileoscopy may be useful in identifying ileal tumors.
- Capsule endoscopy: This test is done with a capsule with dimensions of 11×26 mm that weighs 4 g. The capsule contains a small video camera, batteries, and a radiofrequency transmitter. The batteries last 8 hours. The capsule takes about 50,000 pictures as it passes through the GI system. The pictures are captured in a device that is strapped to the waist. The test was FDA approved for small bowel use in 2001. Cobrin et al. reported that 9% of cases of occult GI bleeding were caused by small bowel tumors.

Staging

Small bowel adenocarcinomas are staged according to the tumor–node–metastasis (TNM) criteria, as used for colon cancer. Staging is based on the extent to which the tumor is present in the bowel wall, the regional nodal status, and the presence or absence of distant metastasis.

The American Joint Committee on Cancer staging system is shown in Table 11.4.

The staging for the duodenal polyps found in familial adenomatous polyposis is that of Spigelman.

Prognosis

Resectability is the key prognostic factor. Other factors include age older than 75 years, performance status, well-differentiated and moderately differentiated versus undifferentiated small bowel adenocarcinomas, tumor location (arising in the duodenum), and presence of distant metastasis. The prognostic significance of lymph node status for survival is controversial.

Survival

The median survival of patients with localized, locally advanced, and metastatic disease is 50.1, 22.2, and 8.6 months, respectively.

TABLE 11.4. *American Joint Committee on Cancer Staging System*

Primary Tumor (T)

TX	Primary tumor cannot be assessed.
T0	No evidence of primary tumor is present.
Tis	Carcinoma in situ is present.
T1	Tumor invades the lamina propria or submucosa.
T2	Tumor invades the muscularis propria.
T3	Tumor invades through the muscularis propria into subserosa or into nonperitonealized perimuscular tissue (mesentery or retroperitoneum), with extension of less than 2 cm.
T4	Tumor penetrates the visceral peritoneum or directly invades other organs or structures.

Regional Lymph Nodes (N)

NX	Regional lymph nodes cannot be assessed.
N0	No regional lymph node metastasis is present.
N1	Regional lymph node metastasis has occurred.

Distant Metastases (M)

MX	Presence of distant metastasis cannot be assessed.
M0	No distant metastasis is present.
M1	Distant metastasis has occurred.

Stage Grouping

Stage 0	Tis	N0	M0
Stage I	TI-2	N0	M0
Stage II	T3-4	N0	M0
Stage III	Any T	N1	M0
Stage IV	Any T	any N	M1

Treatment of Localized Disease

Surgery

Surgical resection provides the only hope of cure for patients with small bowel adenocarcinomas. This is possible in approximately two-thirds of patients.

A review of the Department of Defense tumor registry database from 1970 to 1996 found that 47% of 144 small bowel malignancies were small bowel adenocarcinomas; 91% of these patients underwent surgical resection, 45% with curative surgery. During a median follow-up of 38.9 months (range 1–405. months), the median survival was 182 versus 33 months and the 5-year survival rate was 81% versus 42% after curative surgery and incomplete resection, respectively. In patients not amenable to surgery, the median survival was 10 months with a 5-year survival of 39%. Rose et al. found that among 79 patients with primary duodenal small bowel adenocarcinomas, the patients with completely resected disease (node-negative) had a median survival of 86 months and a 5-year survival of 60%, whereas patients with completely resected disease (node-positive) had a median survival of 41 months and a 5-year survival of 43% (5). Patients who had palliative surgery or who did not undergo surgery had a median survival of 9 months, and no patient was alive at 5 years. This study, although small, suggested that resection of the primary tumor, even with known locoregional involvement, may provide survival benefit.

The remaining have unresectable disease as a result of extensive local disease or metastases to regional lymph nodes, the liver, or the peritoneum. Wide local excision is recommended on lesions in the distal duodenum, jejunum, or ileum. Patients with lesions in the proximal duodenum, including those in the periampullary region, should undergo pancreaticoduodenectomy, which now has an operative mortality rate of less than 5%. Ileal tumors are more likely to develop intestinal obstruction than jejunal tumors. Emergency surgery for these patients relieves the obstruction but precludes a complete and negative margin resection.

Adjuvant Therapy

ADJUVANT CHEMOTHERAPY

Data for adjuvant therapy involving agents such as 5-fluorouracil (5-FU), obtained from the experience gained in the treatment of colorectal cancer and the information obtained from patients with metastatic small bowel disease are scarce. No prospective phase 2 or randomized phase 3 data are currently available. A review of the National Cancer Center Database from 1985 to 1995 revealed an increasing use of adjuvant chemotherapy for regionally advanced disease—from 28% for the period 1985 to 1990 to more than 40% from 1990 to 1995—a practice based on the current treatment standards for colorectal cancer. It is estimated that 14% of patients in the United States with only localized small bowel adenocarcinoma receive some form of adjuvant chemotherapy. An intensified adjuvant therapy (protracted intravenous infusion of 5-FU modulated with leucovorin with an intense-dose external-beam radiotherapy to liver, regional lymph nodes, and tumor bed) was evaluated in patients with pancreatic or periampullary adenocarcinoma. The regimen was found to be very toxic, with no survival benefit when compared to the historical data from patients who were receiving more conventional doses of chemotherapy or radiation. Median disease-free survival was approximately 8 months, with earlier recurrences suggesting that the disease may promptly develop resistance to chemotherapy and radiation.

In 2003, Bettini and colleagues found that the FOLFOX 4 regimen (i.e., combination infusional 5-FU, oxaliplatin, and leucovorin) was safely administered as adjuvant chemotherapy in three patients with resected small bowel adenocarcinoma associated with celiac disease.

CHEMORADIATION

Coia et al. treated four patients with resectable duodenal cancer at Fox Chase Cancer Center as part of a clinical study for pancreatic cancer with neoadjuvant or preoperative chemoradiation (6). The regimen consisted of two cycles of 5-FU at a dosage of 1 g/m^2/day for 4 days on days 2 to 5 and days 29 to 32 and mitomycin C at a dosage of 10 mg/m^2 on day 2 given with concurrent radiation administered at a dose of 1.8 Gy/day to a total dose of 50.4 Gy. Surgical resection was performed 4 to 6 weeks after completion of chemoradiation. All four patients underwent surgical resection and achieved complete pathologic response. At a median follow-up of 4.5 years, all patients were alive without recurrence, with actual survival durations of 12, 23, 35, and 90 months, respectively.

Treatment of Metastatic Disease

Surgery

The role of surgical resection is limited to either palliative measures or prevention of bowel obstruction or bleeding in patients with metastatic small bowel adenocarcinoma.

Chemotherapy

The choice of chemotherapeutic agents and the actual efficacy of such treatment in metastatic disease are less well-defined. This is partly because of the lack of well-controlled clinical trials and partly because the disease is uncommon. The National Cancer Database indicates that 37% of all patients with advanced disease received some form of chemotherapy, 12% received external-beam radiation with or without surgery, and 25% received no cancer-related therapy. Historically, the most commonly used chemotherapy includes 5-FU alone or 5-FU–based regimens. Other chemotherapy regimens include tegafur, thiotepa, mitomycin C, and cisplatin, anthracyclines, or alkylating agents. Regimens such as ECF (epirubicin, cisplatin, and 5-FU) have been tested in a small group of patients with advanced small bowel cancer at the Royal Marsden Hospital (7). Patients received epirubicin at 50 mg/m^2, cisplatin at 60 mg/m^2, each given every 3 weeks, and protracted venous infusion (PVI) of 5-FU at a dose of 200 mg/m^2. The overall response rate was 37%. The median PFS was 7.8 months, with a median overall survival of 13 months. The authors concluded that small bowel adenocarcinoma is sensitive to infusional

5-FU and that chemotherapy appears to have clinical benefit over palliative surgery alone. As reported by Polyzos and colleagues in 2003, three subjects with 5-FU–refractory small bowel adenocarcinoma were treated with salvage irinotecan therapy. Two patients achieved a minor response and had improvement of their symptoms. In summary, lack of prospective, randomized trials; the minimal benefit, if any, reported in clinical series; and the associated toxicity should be taken into account. The decision to treat should be individualized, and the risks and benefits should be carefully explained to the patient.

Follow-up

Patients who have undergone surgical resection for localized disease should have a follow-up visit in the outpatient setting every 3 months to assess for symptoms or signs suggestive of recurrent disease.

- CBC and liver function test results may be checked periodically to identify anemia related to blood loss or abnormal liver enzymes related to hepatic metastases or biliary obstruction, respectively.
- Abdominal CT scan images should be obtained every 6 months to identify subclinical recurrent disease early, which may be amenable to repeat surgical resection.
- Patients with small bowel adenocarcinoma should also undergo colorectal cancer screening (i.e., colonoscopy) because of the high risk of secondary malignancies.
- Patients with advanced metastatic disease may be treated with chemotherapy in an outpatient setting. They should also be observed for hematologic and other toxicity related to chemotherapy.

Complications

- Partial or complete small bowel obstruction may occur because of an obstructing intraluminal tumor. This may be treated either conservatively (i.e., nasogastric tube decompression and parenteral nutrition) or with surgery (i.e., small bowel resection or bypass).
- Intestinal bleeding is common with small bowel sarcomas and may require transfusion support and surgical intervention.
- Biliary obstruction may result from compression of the extrahepatic common bile duct by a periampullary or proximal duodenal tumor. Biliary stenting via endoscopic retrograde cholangiopancreatography or transhepatic biliary drainage may be performed if feasible.

SUGGESTED READINGS

Gastrointestinal Stromal Tumor

Abrams RA, Grochow LB, Chakravarthy A, et al. Intensified adjuvant therapy for pancreatic and periampullary adenocarcinoma: survival results and observations regarding patterns of failure, radiotherapy dose and CA 19-9 levels. *Int J Radiat Oncol Biol Phys.* 1999;44:1039–1046.

Buemming P, Meis-Kindblom JM, Kindblom LG, et al. Is there an indication for adjuvant treatment with imatinib mesylate in patients with aggressive gastrointestinal stromal tumors (GISTs)?. Presented at: 39th Annual Meeting of the American Society of Clinical Oncology, Chicago, IL, May 31, June 3, 2003, Abstract 3289.

Casali G, Verweij J, Zalcberg J, et al. Imatinib (Gleevec) 400 and 800 mg daily in patients with gastrointestinal stromal tumors (GIST): a randomized phase III trial from EORTC Soft Tissue and Bone Sarcomas Group, the Italian Sarcoma Group (ISG), and the Australasian Gastrointestinal Trials Group (AGITG). A toxicity report. Presented at: 38th Annual Meeting of the American Society of Clinical Oncology, Orlando, FL, May 1824, 2002, Abstract 1650.

Choi H, Charnsangavej C, Macapinlac HA, et al. Correlation of computerized tomography (CT) and proton emission tomography (PET) in patients with metastatic GIST treated at a single institution with imatinib mesylate. Presented at: 39th Annual Meeting of the American Society of Clinical Oncology, Chicago, IL, May 31, June 3, 2003, Abstract 3290.

Crawley C, Ross P, Norman A, et al. The Royal Marsden Experience of small bowel adenocarcinoma treated with protracted venous infusion 5-fluorouracil. *Br J Cancer.* 1998;78:508–510.

DeMatteo R, Owzar K, Maki R, et al. Ballman and the American College of Surgeons Oncology Group (ACOSOG) Intergroup Adjuvant GIST Study Team. Adjuvant imatinib mesylate increases recurrence free survival (RFS) in patients with completely resected localized primary gastrointestinal stromal tumor (GIST): North American Intergroup Phase III trial ACOSOG Z9001. 2007 ASCO Annual Meeting; Abstract # 10079.

DeMatteo RP, Owzar K, Antonescu CR, et al. Efficacy of adjuvant imatinib mesylate following complete resection of localized, primary gastrointestinal stromal tumor (GIST) at high risk of recurrence: The U.S. Intergroup phase II trial ACOSOG Z9000. 2008 Gastrointestinal Cancers Symposium; Abstract # 8.

Demetri GD, van Oosterom AT, Garrett CR, et al. Efficacy and safety of sunitinib in patients with advanced gastrointestinal stromal tumour after failure of imatinib: a randomised controlled trial. *Lancet.* 2006 Oct 14;368(9544):1329–1338.

Demetri GD, von Mehren M, Blanke CD, et al. Efficacy and safety of imatinib mesylate in advanced gastrointestinal stromal tumors. *N Engl J Med.* 2002;347:472–480.

Eisenberg BL, Harris J, Blanke CD, et al. Phase II trial of neoadjuvant/adjuvant imatinib mesylate (IM) for advanced primary and metastatic/recurrent operable gastrointestinal stromal tumor (GIST): early results of RTOG 0132/ACRIN 6665. *J Surg Oncol.* 2009;99(1):42–47.

Howe JR, Karnell LH, Menck HR, et al. Adenocarcinoma of the small bowel, review of the National Cancer Data Base, 1985–1995. *Cancer* 1999;86:2693–2696.

Joensuu H, Roberts PJ, Sarlomo-Rikala M, et al. Effect of the tyrosine kinase inhibitor STI571 in a patient with a metastatic gastrointestinal stromal tumor. *N Engl J Med* 2001;344:1052–1056.

Small Bowel Adenocarcinoma

Arai M, Shimizu S, Imai Y, et al. Mutations of the Ki-ras, p53 and APC genes in adenocarcinomas of the human small intestine. *Int J Cancer.* Feb 7 1997;70(4):390–395.

Bakaeen FG, Murr MM, Sarr MG, et al. What prognostic factors are important in duodenal adenocarcinoma?. *Arch Surg.* Jun 2000;135(6):635–641; discussion 641–642.

Bauer RL, Palmer ML, Bauer AM, et al. Adenocarcinoma of the small intestine: 21-year review of diagnosis, treatment, and prognosis. *Ann Surg Oncol.* May 1994;1(3):183–188.

Beebe-Dimmer JL, Schottenfeld D. Cancers of the small intestine. In: Schottenfeld D, Fraumeni J, eds. *Cancer: Epidemiology and Prevention.* 3rd ed. Oxford University Press; 2006:801–808.

Bettini AC, Beretta GD, Sironi P, et al. Chemotherapy in small bowel adenocarcinoma associated with celiac disease: a report of three cases. *Tumori.* Mar-Apr 2003;89(2):193–195.

Blanchard DK, Budde JM, Hatch GF III, et al. Tumors of the small intestine. *World J Surg.* Apr 2000; 24(4):421–429.

Chen CC, Neugut AI, Rotterdam H. Risk factors for adenocarcinomas and malignant carcinoids of the small intestine: preliminary findings. *Cancer Epidemiol Biomarkers Prev.* Apr-May 1994;3(3):205-207.

Chow WH, Linet MS, McLaughlin JK, et al. Risk factors for small intestine cancer. *Cancer Causes Control.* Mar 1993;4(2):163–169.

Cobrin GM, Pittman RH, Lewis BS. Increased diagnostic yield of small bowel tumors with capsule endoscopy. *Cancer.* Jul 1 2006;107(1):22–27.

Crawley C, Ross P, Norman A, et al. The Royal Marsden experience of a small bowel adenocarcinoma treated with protracted venous infusion 5-fluorouracil. *Br J Cancer.* Aug 1998;78(4):508–510.

Dabaja BS, Suki D, Pro B, Bonnen M, Ajani J. Adenocarcinoma of the small bowel: presentation, prognostic factors, and outcome of 217 patients. *Cancer.* Aug 1 2004;101(3):518–526.

Haselkorn T, Whittemore AS, Lilienfeld DE. Incidence of small bowel cancer in the United States and worldwide: geographic, temporal, and racial differences. *Cancer Causes Control.* Sep 2005;16(7): 781–787.

Hemminki A. Inherited predisposition to gastrointestinal cancer: The molecular backgrounds of Peutz-Jeghers syndrome and hereditary nonpolyposis colorectal cancer. Dissertation/master's thesis. University of Helsinki; 1998.

Hemminki A. The molecular basis and clinical aspects of Peutz-Jeghers syndrome. *Cell Mol Life Sci.* May 1999;55(5):735–750.

Howe JR, Karnell LH, Menck HR, Scott-Conner C. The American College of Surgeons Commission on Cancer and the American Cancer Society. Adenocarcinoma of the small bowel: review of the National Cancer Data Base, 1985–1995. *Cancer.* Dec 15 1999;86(12):2693–706.

Jemal A, Murray T, Ward E, et al. Cancer statistics, 2005. *CA Cancer J Clin.* Jan-Feb 2005;55(1): 10–30.

Jigyasu D, Bedikian AY, Stroehlein JR. Chemotherapy for primary adenocarcinoma of the small bowel. *Cancer.* Jan 1 1984;53(1):23–25.

Kashiwagi H, Spigelman AD, Talbot IC, et al. p53 and K-ras status in duodenal adenomas in familial adenomatous polyposis. *Br J Surg.* Jun 1997;84(6):826–829.

Lowenfels AB, Sonni A. Distribution of small bowel tumors. *Cancer Lett.* Jul 1977;3(1-2):83–86.

Neugut AI, Marvin MR, Rella VA, Chabot JA. An overview of adenocarcinoma of the small intestine. *Oncology (Huntingt).* Apr 1997;11(4):529–536; discussion 545, 549–550.

Offerhaus GJ, Giardiello FM, Krush AJ, et al. The risk of upper gastrointestinal cancer in familial adenomatous polyposis. *Gastroenterology* Jun 1992;102(6):1980–1982.

Ouriel K, Adams JT. Adenocarcinoma of the small intestine. *Am J Surg.* Jan 1984;147(1):66–71.

Polyzos A, Kouraklis G, Giannopoulos A, et al. Irinotecan as salvage chemotherapy for advanced small bowel adenocarcinoma: a series of three patients. *J Chemother.* Oct 2003;15(5):503–506.

Potter DD, Murray JA, Donohue JH, et al. The role of defective mismatch repair in small bowel adenocarcinoma in celiac disease. *Cancer Res.* Oct 1 2004;64(19):7073-7077.

Rodriguez-Bigas MA, Vasen HF, Lynch HT, et al. Characteristics of small bowel carcinoma in hereditary nonpolyposis colorectal carcinoma. International Collaborative Group on HNPCC. *Cancer.* Jul 15 1998;83(2):240–244.

Ryder NM, Ko CY, Hines OJ, et al. Primary duodenal adenocarcinoma: a 40-year experience. *Arch Surg.* Sep 2000;135(9):1070–1074; discussion 1074–1075.

Sturgeon C, Chejfec G, Espat NJ. Gastrointestinal stromal tumors: a spectrum of disease. *Surg Oncol.* Jul 2003;12(1):21–26.

Suster S. Gastrointestinal stromal tumors. *Semin Diagn Pathol.* Nov 1996;13(4):297–313.

Talamonti MS, Goetz LH, Rao S, Joehl RJ. Primary cancers of the small bowel: analysis of prognostic factors and results of surgical management. *Arch Surg.* May 2002;137(5):564–570; discussion 570–571.

Wheeler JM, Warren BF, Mortensen NJ, et al. An insight into the genetic pathway of adenocarcinoma of the small intestine. *Gut.* Feb 2002;50(2):218–223.

Zeh H III. Cancer of the small intestine. In: DeVita VT Jr, Hellman S, Rosenberg SA, eds. *Cancer: Principles and Practice of Oncology.* 7th ed. Philadelphia, PA: Lippincott Williams & Wilkins; 2005:1035–1048.

SECTION 4

Breast

12

Breast Cancer

Manish Sharma and Jame Abraham

Breast cancer is the most common cancer diagnosed in women in North America, and it is second only to lung cancer as a cause of death from cancer in women. When diagnosed early, breast cancer can be treated primarily using surgery, radiation, and systemic therapy (chemotherapy or hormonal therapy or both). In Western countries, at the time of diagnosis, more than 90% of patients will have only localized disease.

EPIDEMIOLOGY

- In the United States, in 2008, about 182,460 women were diagnosed with an invasive breast cancer and 67,770 were diagnosed with ductal carcinoma in situ (DCIS).
- In 2008, about 40,480 women died from breast cancer in the United States.
- Approximately 1,990 men will get a diagnosis of breast cancer in 2008.
- Lifetime risk of developing breast cancer in North American women (who live up to the age of 85) is one in eight.
- The incidence of breast cancer decreased from mid-2002 to 2003 by 6.7%. This decrease in incidence was observed mainly in postmenopausal women, who were more likely to have ER(+) breast cancer. This unprecedented drop could be due to dramatic decrease in hormone replacement therapy (HRT) use after the publication of the Women's Health Initiative study in 2001.

RISK FACTORS

The risk factors for developing breast cancer in women are listed in Table 12.1.

Most breast cancers are sporadic and due to multiple factors, including hormonal and environmental. About 5% to 10% of breast cancers are familial or hereditary.

TABLE 12.1. *Risk factors for breast cancer in women*

History of breast cancer
BRCA1 or *BRCA2* mutations
Increasing age
Early menarche
Late menopause
Nulliparity
First birth after the age of 30
Atypical lobular hyperplasia or atypical ductal hyperplasia
Prior breast biopsies
Long-term postmenopausal estrogen replacement
Early exposure to ionizing radiation

151

Genetics

- Approximately 5% to 10% of all women with breast cancer may have a germ-line mutation of the genes *BRCA1* or *BRCA2*.
- Mutations of *BRCA1* (chromosome 17q21) and *BRCA2* (chromosome 13q12–13q13) are responsible for 85% of hereditary breast cancer.
- Specific mutations of *BRCA1* and *BRCA2* are more common in women of Ashkenazi Jewish ancestry.
- The estimated lifetime risk for developing breast cancer in women with a *BRCA1* or *BRCA2* mutation is 56% to 87%, and the risk for developing bilateral/contralateral breast cancer is about 20% to 40%.
- Mutations in either gene also confer about 20% to 40% increased lifetime risk for developing ovarian cancer.

Indications for Genetic Testing

Genetic testing is available commercially (Myriad Genetics). All patients should undergo genetic counseling before doing the test. There are three possible outcomes of genetic testing for the *BRCA* mutations: positive, undetermined, or negative. A negative result indicates no increased risk of breast cancer due to a germ-line mutation of the *BRCA 1/2* genes. An indeterminate test result indicates that no conclusive evidence exists to indicate that the mutation does or does not carry an increased risk for the development of breast cancer due to an inherited genetic mutation. A positive result indicates that there exists a mutation in the *BRCA 1* or *2* genes that has been associated with an inherited risk of developing breast cancer (Table 12.2).

Management of Patients with Positive BRCA Test

Management recommendations for patients with a known genetic mutation are highly individualized and should be made by an expert. Recommendations include the following:

- Early screening using mammogram and/or magnetic resonance imaging (MRI)
- Chemoprevention using tamoxifen may be considered. The role of raloxifene and aromatase inhibitors (AIs) is not clear.
- Bilateral prophylactic mastectomy could prevent breast cancer in 90% to 100%.
- Prophylactic salpingo-oophorectomy alone reduces breast cancer incidence by 50% and prevents ovarian cancer by 95%.

PATHOLOGY

Infiltrating or invasive ductal cancer is the most common breast cancer histologic type and comprises 70% to 80% of all cases (Table 12.3).

TABLE 12.2. *Indications for genetic testing*

Age less than 40 years at the time of diagnosis of breast cancer
Ashkenazi Jewish ancestry
History of ovarian cancer or first- or second-degree relative with a history of ovarian cancer
A first-degree relative with breast cancer diagnosed at an age less than 50 years
History of bilateral breast cancer or a first- or second-degree relative with bilateral breast cancer
A male relative with a history of breast cancer

Source: Adapted from U.S. Task Force for Prevention and NCCN guidelines.

TABLE 12.3. *Pathologic classification of breast cancer*

Ductal	Lobular
Intraductal (in situ)	In situ
Invasive with predominant intraductal component	Invasive with predominant in situ component
	Invasive
Invasive, NOS	**Nipple**
Comedo	Paget's disease, NOS
Inflammatory	Paget's disease with intraductal carcinoma
Medullary with lymphocytic infiltrate	Paget's disease with invasive ductal carcinoma
Mucinous (colloid)	**Other types (not typical breast cancer)**
Papillary	Phyllodes tumor
Scirrhous	Angiosarcoma
Tubular	Primary lymphoma
Other	
Other	
Undifferentiated	

NOS, not otherwise specified.

CHEMOPREVENTION

Risk Assessment

- The Gail model (http://www.nci.nih.gov) is a statistical model that calculates a woman's absolute risk of developing breast cancer by using the following criteria: age, age at menarche, age at first live birth, number of previous biopsies, history of atypical ductal hyperplasia (ADH), and number of first-degree relatives with breast cancer. This model is not intended to be used in patients with an existing history of invasive cancer, DCIS or lobular carcinoma in situ (LCIS).

Prevention Studies

The National Surgical Adjuvant Breast and Bowel Project (NSABP)

- The NSABP P-1 study showed a 49% reduction in the incidence of invasive breast cancer in high-risk subjects who took tamoxifen at a dose of 20 mg daily for 5 years.
- Women eligible for this trial were at least 35 years old and were assessed to have an absolute risk of at least 1.67% over the period of 5 years using Gail model or a pathologic diagnosis of LCIS.
- Use of tamoxifen for breast cancer should be individualized, and must be considered after weighing the risk:benefit ratio for each patient.

Study of Tamoxifen and Raloxifene (STAR)

In the NSABP P-2 study, tamoxifen 20 mg daily was compared with raloxifene 60 mg daily in post-menopausal high-risk (Gail risk model 1.66%) women for prevention of breast cancer. The results of the study revealed that raloxifene was equivalent to tamoxifen in preventing invasive breast cancer (about 50% reduction). Raloxifene did not reduce the risk of DCIS or LCIS unlike tamoxifen.

Raloxifene had a better side effect profile, which resulted in a lower incidence of uterine hyperplasia, hysterectomy, cataracts, and a lower rate of thromboembolic events. In postmenopausal patients, due to equal efficacy and better side effect profile, raloxifene 60 mg daily could be used instead of tamoxifen for breast cancer prevention.

Aromatase Inhibitors

The role of AIs is being investigated for breast cancer prevention. There are ongoing trials with exemestane and letrozole in patients with high risk for breast cancer.

Screening Mammograms and MRI

- Regular mammographic screening results in early diagnosis of breast cancer and a 25% to 30% decrease in mortality in women older than 50 years.
- A 17% reduction in mortality is seen in women between 40 and 49 years.
- The National Cancer Institute and American Cancer Society recommend annual mammography for women aged 40 years and older.

Digital Mammogram

The diagnostic superiority of digital mammography was demonstrated in the Digital Mammographic Imaging Screening Trial (DMIST). This study concluded that pre- or perimenopausal women under the age of 50, or women at any age with dense breasts, had a more accurate detection of breast cancer with the digital mammogram. The amount of radiation exposure in digital mammograms is less than film mammograms.

Magnetic Resonance Imaging

According to the American Cancer Society, any patient who has more than 20% lifetime risk of developing breast cancer can be screened with an MRI.

Breast Cancer Screening for High-Risk Family

Women with families at high risk for breast cancer, especially with *BRCA1* and *BRCA2* mutations, are often advised to undergo screening with mammogram and MRI from the age of 25, or 5 years earlier than the earliest age at which another family member was diagnosed with breast cancer.

CLINICAL FEATURES OF BREAST CANCER

Clinical features could include a breast lump, skin thickening or alteration, peau d'orange, dimpling of the skin, nipple inversion or crusting (Paget's disease), unilateral nipple discharge, and so on. Patients could instead present with signs and symptoms of metastatic disease.

DIAGNOSIS

1. History and physical examination
2. Bilateral mammogram (80% to 90% accuracy)
3. Biopsy: Any distinct mass should be considered for a biopsy, even if the mammograms are negative. The standard methods of diagnosis for palpable lesions are:
   - Core-needle biopsy
   - Incisional or excisional biopsy

   The options in nonpalpable breast lesions are:
   - Ultrasound-guided core-needle biopsy
   - Stereotactic core-needle biopsy under mammographic localization
   - Needle localization under mammography, followed by surgical excision
   - MRI-guided biopsy
4. Laboratory studies
   - Complete blood count, liver function tests, and alkaline phosphatase level
   - Routine use of breast cancer markers such as CA 27:29 and 15:3 is not recommended
5. Pathology and special studies
   - Histology and diagnosis (invasive versus in situ)
   - Pathologic grade of the tumor
   - Tumor involvement of the margin

- Tumor size
- Lymphovascular invasion
- Special studies: estrogen receptor/progesterone receptor (ER/PR) status, HER2/neu status, and indices of proliferation (e.g., mitotic index, Ki-67, or S phase)
- HER2/neu status can be assessed by immunohistochemistry (IHC) or fluorescent in situ hybridization 3^+ is considered as positive. If the IHC result is 2^+ (indeterminate), fluorescent in situ hybridization (FISH) should be performed for gene amplification.
6. Radiology: Radiographic studies are performed on the basis of the findings of the history and physical examination and screening blood tests: computerized tomography (CT) scan of the chest and abdomen, brain and bone scan.
7. Breast MRI is indicated in the following:
   - Evaluating the extent of disease in known cancer patients
     - Multifocal and multicentric disease
     - Pectoralis and chest wall involvement
     - Contralateral breast cancer
   - Evaluating response to neoadjuvant chemotherapy
   - Axillary adenopathy, primary unknown
   - Post lumpectomy for residual disease (close or positive margins)
   - Suspected recurrence of breast cancer
     - Inconclusive mammographic/clinical findings
     - Reconstruction with tissue flaps or implants
   - Lesion characterization
     - Inconclusive findings on mammogram, ultrasound, physical examination
8. Positron emission tomography (PET) scan. PET scans are of low yield in patients with early (stage I and II) breast cancer. The PET scan may be useful in patients with locally advanced or metastatic breast cancer.

STAGING OF BREAST CANCER

The American Joint Committee on Cancer (AJCC) staging of breast cancer and the pathologic classification are listed in Tables 12.4, 12.5, and 12.6.

TABLE 12.4. *Staging of breast cancer (American Joint Committee on Cancer)*

Primary Tumor (T)

TX	Primary tumor cannot be assessed
T0	No evidence of primary tumor
Tis	Carcinoma in situ; intraductal carcinoma, lobular carcinoma in situ, or Paget's disease of the nipple with no associated tumor. Note: Paget's disease associated with a tumor is classified according to the size of the tumor.
T1	Tumor ≤2.0 cm in greatest dimension
T1mic	Microinvasion ≤0.1 cm in greatest dimension
T1a	Tumor >0.1 but ≤0.5 cm in greatest dimension
T1b	Tumor >0.5 cm but ≤1.0 cm in greatest dimension
T1c	Tumor >1.0 cm but ≤2.0 cm in greatest dimension
T2	Tumor >2.0 cm but ≤5.0 cm in greatest dimension
T3	Tumor >5.0 cm in greatest dimension
T4	Tumor of any size with direct extension to (a) chest wall or (b) skin
T4a	Extension to chest wall
T4b	Edema (including peau d'orange) or ulceration of the skin of the breast or satellite skin nodules confined to the same breast
T4c	Both of the above (T4a and T4b)
T4d	Inflammatory carcinoma

(Continued)

TABLE 12.4. *(Continued)*

Regional Lymph Nodes (N)

NX	Regional lymph nodes cannot be assessed (e.g., previously removed)
N0	No regional lymph node metastasis
N1	Metastasis to movable ipsilateral axillary lymph node(s)
N2a	Metastasis to ipsilateral axillary lymph node(s) fixed or matted
N2b	Metastasis in clinically apparent[a] ipsilateral internal mammary nodes in the absence of clinically evident axillary lymph node metastasis
N3a	Metastasis in ipsilateral infraclavicular lymph node(s)
N3b	Metastasis to ipsilateral internal mammary lymph node(s) and axillary node(s)
N3c	Metastasis in ipsilateral supraclavicular lymph node(s)

[a]Clinically apparent is defined as being detected by imaging studies (excluding lymphoscintigraphy) or by clinical examination or being grossly visible on histopathologic evaluation.

TABLE 12.5. *Pathologic classification (pN)*

pNX	Regional lymph nodes cannot be assessed (not removed for pathologic study or previously removed)
pN0	No regional lymph node metastasis histologically, no additional examination for isolated tumor cells (ITC)
pN0(i−)	No regional lymph node metastasis histologically, negative IHC
pN0(i+)	No regional lymph node metastasis histologically, positive IHC, no IHC cluster >0.2 mm
pN0(mol−)	No regional lymph node metastasis histologically, negative molecular finding (RT-PCR)
pN0(mol+)	No regional lymph node metastasis histologically, positive molecular finding (RT-PCR)
pN1	Metastasis in 1–3 axillary lymph node(s) and/or in internal mammary node(s), with microscopic disease detected by sentinel lymph node dissection but not clinically apparent[a]
pN1mi	Only micrometastasis (>0.2 mm, <2.0 mm)
pN1a	Metastasis in 1–3 axillary lymph node(s)
pN1b	Metastasis in internal mammary node(s), with microscopic disease detected by sentinel lymph node dissection but not clinically apparent[a]
pN1c	Metastasis in 1–3 axillary lymph node(s) and in internal mammary node(s), with microscopic disease detected by sentinel lymph node dissection but not clinically apparent[a]
pN2	Metastasis in 4–9 axillary lymph nodes or in clinically apparent[b] internal mammary lymph nodes in the absence of axillary lymph node metastasis
pN2a	Metastasis in 4–9 axillary lymph nodes (at least one tumor deposit >2.0 mm)
pN2b	Metastasis in clinically apparent[b] internal mammary lymph nodes in the absence of axillary lymph node metastasis
pN3	Metastasis in 10 or more axillary lymph nodes, or in infraclavicular lymph nodes, or clinically apparent[b] ipsilateral internal mammary lymph nodes in the presence of one or more positive axillary lymph nodes; or in more than three axillary lymph nodes, with clinically microscopic metastasis in internal mammary lymph nodes or in ipsilateral supraclavicular lymph nodes
pN3a	Metastasis in 10 or more axillary lymph nodes (at least one tumor deposit >2.0 mm), or metastasis to the infraclavicular lymph nodes
pN3b	Metastasis in clinically apparent[b] ipsilateral internal mammary lymph nodes in the presence of one or more positive axillary lymph nodes; or in more than three axillary lymph nodes and in internal mammary lymph nodes, with microscopic disease detected by sentinel lymph node dissection but not clinically apparent[a]
pN3c	Metastasis in ipsilateral supraclavicular lymph nodes

(Continued)

TABLE 12.5. *(Continued)*

Distant Metastasis (M)

MX	Presence of distant metastasis cannot be assessed
M0	No distant metastasis
M1	Distant metastasis present

[a]Not clinically apparent is defined as not being detected by imaging studies (excluding lymphoscintigraphy) or clinical examination, or by not being grossly visible on histopathologic evaluation.

[b]Clinically apparent is defined as being detected by imaging studies (excluding lymphoscintigraphy) or clinical examination, or by being grossly visible pathologically.

IHC, immunohistochemistry; RT-PCR, reverse-transcription polymerase chain reaction.

Source: From AJCC Cancer Staging Manual. Sixth edition 2002. Springer Publications, with permission.

Prognostic Factors

Anatomic features such as tumor size and lymph node status are important prognostic features. But biologic features of the tumor are equally important or possibly even more important than anatomic features.

1. Number of positive axillary lymph nodes
   - This is an important prognostic indicator. Prognosis is worse with increasing number of lymph nodes.
2. Tumor size
   - In general, tumors smaller than 1 cm have a good prognosis in patients without lymph node involvement.
3. Histologic or nuclear grade
   - Patients with poorly differentiated histology and high nuclear grade have a worse prognosis than others.
   - Scarff–Bloom–Richardson grading system and Fisher nuclear grade are commonly used systems. The Modified Scarff-Bloom-Richardson grading system assigns a score (1–3 points) for features such as size, mitosis, and tubule formation. These scores are added and tumors are labeled low grade (3–5 points), intermediate grade (6–7 points), or high grade (8–9 points).
4. ER/PR status
   - ER- and/or PR-positive tumors have better prognosis and these patients are eligible to receive endocrine therapy.

TABLE 12.6. *American Joint Committee on Cancer stage groupings*

Stage	T	N	M
Stage 0	Tis	N0	M0
Stage I	T1	N0	M0
Stage IIA	T0	N1	M0
	T1	N1	M0
	T2	N0	M0
Stage IIB	T2	N1	M0
	T3	N0	M0
Stage IIIA	T0	N2	M0
	T1	N2	M0
	T2	N2	M0
	T3	N1	M0
	T3	N2	M0
Stage IIIB	T4	N0–N2	M0
Stage IIIC	Any T	N3	M0
Stage IV	Any T	Any N	M1

Source: From AJCC Cancer Staging Manual, sixth edition 2002, Springer Publications, with permission.

5. Histologic tumor type
   - Prognoses of infiltrating ductal and lobular carcinoma are similar.
   - Mucinous (colloid) and tubular histologies have good prognosis
   - Inflammatory breast cancer is one of the most aggressive forms of breast cancer.
6. HER2/neu expression
   - HER2/neu overexpression is a poor prognostic marker and patients with HER2/neu overexpression are candidates for HER2-targeted therapies. Her2/neu testing can be done with IHC or FISH. A positive result means that greater than 30% (3+) of tumor cells stain for HER2/neu, a FISH result of more than six *HER2* gene copies per nucleus or a FISH ratio (*HER2* gene signals to chromosome 17 signals) of more than 2.2. A negative result means less than 10% (1+) stain positive, FISH result of less than four gene copies per nucleus, or FISH ratio of less than 1.8. An IHC score of 2+, or a FISH result of 4 to 6 copies per nucleus of the HER2 gene amplified, or a FISH ratio of 1.8–2.2 is inconclusive. (But in all the published clinical trials patients received trastuzumab for FISH ratio more than 2).
7. Gene expression profiles
   - Oncotype DX is a diagnostic genomic assay based on *RT-PCR* on paraffin-embedded tissue. This assay was initially developed to quantify the likelihood of cancer recurrence in women with newly diagnosed, stage I or II, node-negative, ER-positive breast cancer. Patients are divided into low-risk, intermediate-risk, and high-risk groups on the basis of the expression of a panel of 21 genes. The recurrence score determined by this assay is found to be a better predictor of outcome than standard measures such as age, tumor size, and tumor grade. A recent study validated the role of Oncotype DX patients with node-positive and ER-positive tumors.
   - MammaPrint is a DNA microarray assay of 70 genes designed to predict the risk of recurrence of early-stage breast cancer. In February 2007, the FDA approved the use of MammaPrint in patients less than the age of 61, with a tumor size less than 5 cm and lymph node negative. This requires fresh tumor samples. It is currently being studied in the MINDACT trial in Europe.

MANAGEMENT

High-Risk Lesions

Patients with high-risk lesions may be eligible for breast cancer prevention studies.

Atypical Ductal Hyperplasia

- There is a fourfold to fivefold increase in the risk of developing breast cancer in patients with ADH.
- There is wide variation in the criteria used in the diagnosis of ADH.
- ADH is managed by close follow-up of patients.
- Clinical breast examination and mammogram are the preferred screening methods.
- Tamoxifen 20 mg PO for 5 years: NSABP P-1 study showed 86% reduction in the risk for developing invasive breast cancer in patients who received tamoxifen.
- The NSABP P-2 study showed similar efficacy for raloxifene 60 mg daily for 5 years, but with fewer adverse effects. Hence, in postmenopausal patients, raloxifene could be considered as the preferred treatment option.

Lobular Carcinoma In Situ

- LCIS is not considered a form of cancer, but a marker of increased risk for developing invasive breast cancer.
- It is usually multicentric and bilateral.
- There is a 21% chance of developing breast cancer in patients within 15 years of developing LCIS.

- It is managed by close follow-up of patients.
- Patients can be followed by clinical breast examination every 4 to 12 months, annual mammogram, and/or MRI.
- Tamoxifen or raloxifene (postmenopausal) may be used for prevention of breast cancer (56% reduction in risk as per the NSABP P-1 and P-2 studies).

Noninvasive Breast Cancer

Ductal Carcinoma In Situ

- With the extensive use of mammograms, the diagnosis of DCIS has increased over the last several years.
- Microcalcification or soft tissue abnormality is seen in the mammogram of DCIS.

Different Histologic Types of Ductal Carcinoma In Situ

- Comedocarcinoma has a poor prognosis.
- Noncomedocarcinoma includes micropapillary, papillary, solid, and cribriform carcinoma.

Treatment

- Lumpectomy followed by radiation treatment plus tamoxifen is the standard treatment option. Other treatment options are:
  - Total mastectomy with or without tamoxifen
  - Breast-conserving surgery (BCS) without radiation therapy, which could be considered in select patients with low Van Nuys Prognostic Index (VNPI), which combines four predictors of local recurrence (tumor size, margin width, pathologic classification, and age).
  - In patients who previously had lumpectomy and radiation, tamoxifen reduced the risk of breast cancer recurrence (ipsilateral and contralateral; NSABP B-24). The benefit is limited only for patients with ER/PR-positive DCIS.
  - The role of AIs in receptor-positive DCIS is being investigated in many clinical trials, some of which have closed for accrual (NSABP B-35). Another phase 3 clinical trial, the CRUK-IBIS-II-DCIS, is still accruing patients.

Invasive Breast Cancer

The following are treatment options for for invasive, early-stage breast cancer.

Surgery

No survival difference is seen in patients who are treated with modified radical mastectomy versus lumpectomy plus radiation. Lumpectomy plus radiation therapy is the preferred treatment for early breast cancer.

Contraindications for lumpectomy are:

- Two or more tumors in separate quadrants of the breast
- Diffuse, indeterminate, or malignant-appearing microcalcifications
- Central location of the tumor mass

Contraindications for radiation are:

- A history of therapeutic irradiation to the breast
- Connective tissue disorders (scleroderma)
- Pregnancy

Axillary Lymph Node Dissection (ALND)

- ALND primarily provides prognostic information. It has minimal therapeutic benefit, especially in clinically negative axilla.
- Among patients with clinically negative axillary lymph nodes, 30% will have positive histology after dissection.
- It is associated with approximately 10% to 25% risk of lymphedema, which can be mild to severe. This varies with the level and type of axillary node dissection.

Sentinel Node Biopsy

- This is a minimally invasive procedure for axillary staging.
- A radioactive substance or blue dye is injected into the area around the tumor.
- The ipsilateral axilla is explored and the node that has taken up the dye or radioactive material is excised and examined pathologically.
- In expert hands, this procedure identifies a node in more than 92% to 98% of patients.

Reconstruction

Reconstructive surgery may be used for patients who opt for a mastectomy. It may be done at the time of the mastectomy (immediate reconstruction) or at a later time. In stage I and IIA patients, after mastectomy, immediate reconstruction should be offered. In stage IIB or III patients, it may be reasonable to offer delayed reconstruction.

Reconstruction may include either an implant or an autologous tissue graft. An example of an autologous tissue graft includes: TRAM (transverse rectus abdominus myocutaneous) flaps and the latissimus dorsi flap. The DIEP (deep inferior epigastric perforator) flap is analogous to the TRAM flap, however the rectus muscle is not raised to the breast site. This allows quicker recovery of abdominal strength. The latissimus dorsi flap may be safer in patients who are obese or have compromised vasculature due to diabetes mellitus or smoking.

Radiotherapy

- Radiotherapy (RT) is an integral part of breast-conserving treatment (lumpectomy).
- Radiation boost of up to 4,500 to 5,000 cGy $\pm$ 1,000 to 1,500 cGy to the tumor bed of the breast is effective.
- In patients who need chemotherapy, RT is usually done after chemotherapy.
- Postmastectomy radiation treatment to the chest wall and supraclavicular lymph nodes decreases the risk of locoregional recurrence in patients with four or more positive lymph nodes and in patients with tumor size >5 cm.
- Two randomized trials showed improvement in overall survival (OS) for postmastectomy radiation in patients with one to three positive lymph nodes, and it is being evaluated in more clinical trials. In selected patients, this should be discussed with them.

Accelerated Partial Breast Irradiation (APBI)

The primary goal of APBI is to shorten the duration of radiation therapy while maintaining adequate local control. There are several APBI techniques currently under study; however, brachytherapy is the most widely used. Brachytherapy attempts to give irradiation to the tumor bed or cavity while sparing normal breast tissue. Of the various brachytherapy approaches, Mammosite is FDA approved.

The Mammosite Breast Brachytherapy System delivers 34 Gy of radiation in 10 fractions within 5 days through a balloon inserted at the lumpectomy site during surgery.

- Indications for Mammosite include: age $\geq$45, tumor $\leq$3 cm, negative lymph node status, negative margins (up to 2 mm), skin distance $\geq$5–7 mm, and no evidence of extensive intraductal carcinoma.
- Partial breast brachytherapy (PBB) or interstitial brachytherapy is also undergoing clinical trials in stage I and II patients with free resected margins and zero to three positive lymph nodes. In the PBB method, patients receive 10 fractions of radiations of 3.4 Gy within 5 days.

Adjuvant Systemic Therapy

Adjuvant therapy decisions are made based upon the stage, nodal status, and tumor biology. Important tumor biological factors are ER/PR, HER2-neu, tumor grade and gene expression profiles (e.g., Oncotype DX) (Fig. 12.1).

- In general, chemotherapy is recommended for patients with lymph node–positive disease. Chemotherapy can be considered for patients with lymph node–negative invasive cancer (ductal, lobular, mixed, and metaplastic) if they have one of the following high-risk features (Fig. 12.2):
    - ER/PR-negative tumor
    - Patients who are younger than 35
    - If the tumor is more than 2 cm in size
    - Intermediate to high nuclear or histologic grade
- For tubular and colloid histology, adjuvant chemotherapy is usually recommended when the tumor size is more than 3 cm.
- Patients with locally advanced breast cancer should be considered for neoadjuvant chemotherapy.
- Endocrine therapy is recommended for patients with hormone receptor–positive disease.
- Gene expression profiles (Fig. 12.3) such as oncotype DX (RT-PCR-based 21-gene assay) or Mammaprint (DNA microarray-based technology) can be used in selected patients to stratify the risk and treatment selection.
- Trastuzumab is recommended for node-positive patients with HER2-neu over expression and hormone receptor–negative patients with HER2-neu overexpression, irrespective of the node status.
- Trastuzumab could be considered for node-negative patients with HER2-neu overexpression if they have one of the following high risk features:
    - ER/PR-negative tumors
    - Histologic and/or nuclear grade 2 or 3 diseases
    - Pathologic tumor size greater than 2 cm
    - Age ≤35 years

ADJUVANT THERAPY IN HER2-NEU–NEGATIVE PATIENTS

- Node-negative patients: Many regimens are available including AC, FEC, TC, CMF, FAC, etc. In North America, the most commonly used regimen is four cycles of AC. But a recent study has shown that four cycles of TC (docetaxel and cyclophosphamide) has improved disease-free survival (DFS) and OS compared to 4 cycles of AC. The TC regimen is being tested in many clinical trials now. NSABP B-36 comparing AC versus FEC has completed accrual.
- Node-positive patients: A taxane-based chemotherapy is commonly used in node-positive patients based upon NSABP B-28, CALGB 9344, CALGB 9741 and BCIRG 001. Some of the commonly used regimens in the United States are AC followed by paclitaxel given every 2 (dose dense) or 3 weeks, docetaxel/adriamycin/Cyclophosphamide (TAC) every 3 weeks for 6 cycles, AC followed by docetaxel given every 3 weeks and FAC for six cycles.

Clinical trials are evaluating the role of many biologic agents including bevacizumab in adjuvant setting (Fig. 12.1 and Table 12.7).

ADJUVANT THERAPY HER2-NEU–POSITIVE PATIENTS

Incorporation of trastuzumab in the adjuvant therapy is the most important development in the treatment of breast cancer in the past 10 years. Many trastuzumab-containing regimens have been tested and all are equally effective. Clinical trials have shown more than 50% improvement in DFS and more than 30% improvement in OS for patients who received trastuzumab in an adjuvant setting. The major difference is in the cardiac toxicity. Non–anthracycline-containing regimen (TCH-BCIRG 006) and HERA trial (sequential herceptin) had less cardiac toxicity compared to other anthracycline-containing regimens.

Patients can be treated with AC followed by paclitaxel and herceptin for 1 year as per the NSABP B-31 and N9831. The non–anthracycline-containing regimen TCH (docetaxel/carboplatin/trastuzumab) given every 3 weeks for six cycles, followed by trastuzumab for 1 year as per the BCIRG 006 study

(text continues on page 165)

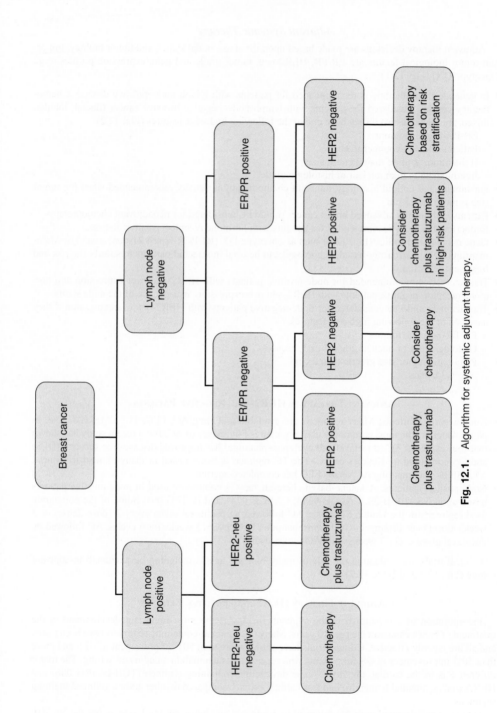

Fig. 12.1. Algorithm for systemic adjuvant therapy.

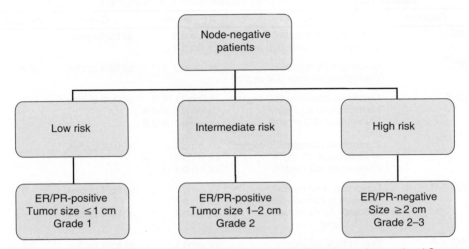

Fig. 12.2. Risk stratification of lymph node–negative patients. (Based upon International Consensus Panel Recommendation.)

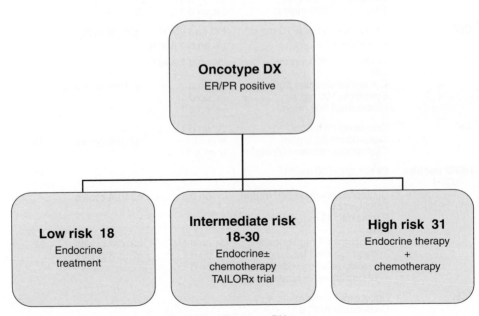

Fig. 12.3. Oncotype DX assay.

TABLE 12.7. *Commonly used combination chemotherapy regimens*

Regimen	Drugs	Route	Cycles	Reference
AC	Doxorubicin 60 mg/m^2 Cyclophosphamide 600 mg/m^2	i.v. on d 1 i.v. on d 1	q21d/4 cycles	1
TC	Docetaxel 75 mg/m^2 Cyclophosphamide 600 mg/m^2	i.v. on d 1	q21d/4 cycles	2–4
CMF	Cyclophosphamide 100 mg/m^2 Methotrexate 40 mg/m^2 Fluorouracil 600 mg/m^2 *OR* Cyclophosphamide 600 mg/m^2 Methotrexate 40 mg/m^2 Fluorouracil 600 mg/m^2	PO on 1–14 d i.v. on d 1 and 8 i.v. on d 1 and 8 i.v. on d 1 i.v. on d 1 i.v. on d 1	q28d/6 cycles q21d/4 cycles	
AC + P	Doxorubicin 60 mg/m^2 Cyclophosphamide 600 mg/m^2 *Followed by* Paclitaxel 175 mg/m^2	i.v. on d 1 i.v. on d 1 i.v. on d 1	q21d/4 cycles q21d/4 cycles	5

AC + P
  (dose dense)
	Doxorubicin 60 mg/m^2
	
	Cyclophosphamide 600 mg/m^2
	Followed by paclitaxel
	  175 mg/m
	Filgrastim with each cycle
		i.v. on d 1
		
		i.v. on d 1
		i.v. on d 1
			q14d/4 cycles
			
			q14d/4 cycles
			q14d/4 cycles
				6
				
				7

CAF	Cyclophosphamide 500 mg/m^2 Doxorubicin 50 mg/m^2 Fluorouracil 500 mg/m^2	i.v. on d 1 i.v. on d 1 i.v. on d 1	q21d/4 cycles 8,9	
CEF	Cyclophosphamide 75 mg/m^2 Epirubicin 60 mg/m^2 Fluorouracil 500 mg/m^2 *OR* Cyclophosphamide 500 mg/m^2 Epirubicin 100 mg/m^2 Fluorouracil 500 mg/m^2	PO on 1–14 d i.v. on d 1 and 8 i.v. on d 1 and 8 i.v. on d 1 i.v. on d 1 i.v. on d 1	q28d/6 cycles q21d/4–6 cycles	
TAC	Docetaxel 75 mg/m^2 Doxorubicin 50 mg/m^2 Cyclophosphamide 500 mg/m^2	i.v. on d 1 iv on d 1 iv on d 1	q21d/6 cycles	10

HER2 positive
  ACTH
	Doxorubicin 60 mg/m^2
	
	Cyclophosphamide 600 mg/m^2
	Followed by
	Paclitaxel 175 mg/m^2
	Plus
	Trastuzumab 4 mg/kg loading
	  dose followed by 2 mg/kg
	  weekly (starting with first cycle
	  of paclitaxel for total of 1 yr)
		
		i.v. on d 1
		
		i.v. on d 1
		i.v. on d 1
		i.v. on d 1
			
			q21d/4 cycles
			
			q21d/4 cycles
			q21d/6 cycles
				11
				
				12

TCH	Docetaxel 75 mg/m^2
	Carboplatin AUC 6
	Plus
	Trastuzumab (weekly during
	  chemotherapy and then
	  trastuzumab 6 mg/kg q21
	  days for 1 yr)			

is equally effective and has less cardiac toxicity. As per the HERA study, patients can be treated with any of the commonly used adjuvant chemotherapy regimens, followed by trastuzumab for 1 year.

NEOADJUVANT OR PREOPERATIVE CHEMOTHERAPY

Neoadjuvant or preoperative chemotherapy can be considered for any patients with IIA, IIB, IIIA, IIIB, IIIC, and inflammatory breast cancer. But in locally advanced breast cancer, especially IIIA, IIIB and IIIC, and inflammatory breast cancer it is the treatment of choice.

- Initial surgery is limited to biopsy to confirm the diagnosis and to identify the receptor and HER2/neu status.
- Preoperative evaluation of the breast mass by mammogram, ultrasound, or MRI is recommended.
- Potentially, the neoadjuvant chemotherapy can reduce the size of the primary tumor so BCS can be performed.
- Usually, a preoperative regimen contains an anthracycline and a taxane. One of the largest neoadjuvant clinical trials is NSABP B-27 trial (four cycles of AC followed by docetaxel for four cycles given every 3 weeks).
- In HER2-neu–positive patients, an M.D. Anderson study has shown that trastuzumab with paclitaxel for four cycles followed by FEC with trastuzumab for four cycles is highly active.
- Several clinical trials are ongoing in both HER2-neu–positive and HER2-neu–negative patients to define the role of combination of chemotherapy and biological agents, such as trastuzumab (NSABP B-41) and bevacizumab (B-40), respectively.
- The majority of the neoadjuvant trials did not show an improvement in OS (NSABP B-18 and B-27).
- But some of the trials (B18) showed an increase in breast conservation in the neoadjuvant group, but not in NSABP B27.
- Response to neoadjuvant chemotherapy is a predictor of survival.

ADJUVANT ENDOCRINE THERAPY

Unless there is any contraindication, endocrine therapy should be considered for all patients with for ER-positive and/or PR-positive patients. As per the Oxford overview, tamoxifen can decrease mortality by about 30% in hormone receptor patients (Fig. 12.4 and Table 12.8).

POSTMENOPAUSAL WOMEN

Several large randomized studies have shown superiority of AIs over tamoxifen in adjuvant setting. If the patient has no contraindication, AIs are the preferred agents in postmenopausal patients. Anastrozole, letrozole, and exemestane are three third-generation AIs approved by the FDA for adjuvant use. The major side effects include arthralgia, ostopenia, osteoporosis, and fracture.

Anastrozole: One of the largest adjuvant breast cancer trial, of comparing tamoxifen with anastrazole and combination of both anastrozole and tamoxifen (ATAC) has shown that anastrozole is superior than tamoxifen in improving DFS, reduction in contralateral breast cancer, and has favorable side-effect profile. For postmenopausal patients, the recommended dose is anastrozole 1 mg PO daily for 5 years.

Letrozole: The Breast International Group (BIG) 1-98 showed a similar magnitude of improvement (like the ATAC trial) in DFS and a reduction of distant metastasis with letrozole. For postmenopausal patients, the recommended dose is letrozole 2.5 mg PO daily for 5 years.

Switching from tamoxifen to an aromatase inhibitor: In the IES study, exemestane therapy after 2 to 3 years of tamoxifen therapy significantly improved DFS and reduced the incidence of contralateral breast cancer as compared with the standard 5 years of tamoxifen therapy. FDA has approved exemestane 25 mg daily after 2 to 3 years of tamoxifen in postmenopausal patients (total of 5 years of endocrine therapy).

The Italian Tamoxifen Anastrozole (ITA) trial, and Austrian Breast Colorectal Study Group (ABCSG 8) and Arimidex, Noveldex (ARNO) study have shown an improvement in DFS and OS in patients

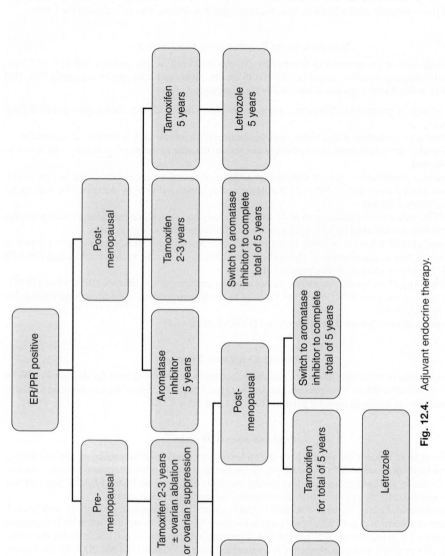

Fig. 12.4. Adjuvant endocrine therapy.

TABLE 12.8. *Endocrine agents used in treatment of breast cancer*

Selective estrogen-receptor modifier (SERM) with combined estrogen agonist and estrogen antagonist activity
Tamoxifen (Nolvadex, others), 20 mg/d PO
Toremifene (Fareston), 60 mg/d PO
Estrogen receptor-down regulator
Faslodex, 250 mg/mo i.m.
Aromatase inhibitors
Anastrozole (Arimidex), 1 mg/d PO
Letrozole (Femara), 2.5 mg/d PO
Exemestane (Aromasin), 25 mg/d PO
LHRH agonist analog in premenopausal women
Leuprolide (Lupron Depot), 7.5 mg/dose i.m. monthly, or
Leuprolide (Lupron Depot), 22.5 mg/dose i.m. every 3 mo, or
Leuprolide (Lupron Depot), 30 mg/dose i.m. every 4 mo
GnRH agonist analog
Goserelin (Zoladex), 3.6 mg/dose s.c. implant into the abdominal wall every 28 d or
Goserelin (Zoladex), 10.8 mg/dose s.c. implant into the abdominal wall every 12 wk
Used in patients who have tumors that express either ER or PR receptors or both receptors.

LHRH, leuteinizing hormone-releasing hormone; GnRH, gonadotropin-releasing hormone; ER, estrogen receptor; PR, progesterone receptor.

who were initially treated with 2 to 3 years of tamoxifen and subsequently randomized to 2 to 3 years of anastrozole.

Extended adjuvant: The MA-17 study showed approximately 43% reduction in recurrence in post-menopausal patients receiving 2.5 mg of letrozole after completing 5 years of tamoxifen (extended adjuvant therapy).

The role of extended use of AIs beyond 5 years of adjuvant AIs is being studied in the NSABP B-42 clinical trial.

ENDOCRINE THERAPY: PREMENOPAUSAL PATIENTS

Hormone receptor–positive, premenopausal patients are in general treated with tamoxifen with or without ovarian suppression or ablation. Combination of ovarian ablation or suppression with endocrine therapy (tamoxifen or aromatize inhibitors) is being investigated in many clinical trials.

Tamoxifen: Tamoxifen is a selective estrogen-receptor modulator (SERM), with both estrogen agonist and antagonist potential. In premenopausal patients, tamoxifen 20 mg daily for 5 years is the treatment of choice, unless the patient has any contraindications such as history of thromboembolic disease, stroke, endometrial cancer etc. Major adverse effects include a higher incidence of cerebrovascular accidents, thrombosis, endometrial cancer, hot flashes, mood changes, and weight gain.

The duration of tamoxifen was studied in many clinical trials. The current guidelines still recommends 5 years of tamoxifen based on NSABP B-14 clinical trial. Recent presentations of ATLAS and ATTOM trials are revisiting this question. Both trials showed continued benefit of tamoxifen beyond 5 years. Therefore, it is reasonable to consider tamoxifen beyond 5 years in premenopausal patients.

Ovarian Ablation or Ovarian Suppression

The Oxford overview and several studies have found that premenopausal patients who stopped having periods after completion of chemotherapy have better survival than those who continued to have periods. Ovarian ablation can be achieved by surgery, radiation, or with LHRH agonists (goserelin, triptorelin). The definite roles of ovarian suppression or ablation in patients who are receiving tamoxifen or AIs are not clear yet. Several ongoing phase 3 clinical trials using LHRH agonists (SOFT, TEXT, PERCHE) will answer this question. Ovarian ablation may be considered in a subset of premenopausal patients after carefully considering the risk and benefit of this procedure versus cancer recurrence.

BREAST CANCER IN PREGNANCY

- Breast cancer during pregnancy was thought to be more aggressive, but the overall poor outcome is likely related to advanced stage at the time of diagnosis.
- Breast biopsy is safe in all stages of pregnancy and should be done for any suggestive mass.

Treatment

- Lumpectomy and axillary dissection can be performed in the third trimester, and RT can be safely delayed until after delivery.
- Modified radical mastectomy is the treatment of choice in the first and second trimesters because radiation treatment is contraindicated during pregnancy.

Chemotherapy

- Chemotherapy should not be administered during the first trimester.
- No chemotherapeutic agent has been found to be completely safe during pregnancy.
- An anthracycline combined with cyclophosphamide (e.g., AC given every 3 weeks for four cycles) has been used safely in the adjuvant setting during the second or third trimesters.
- Chemotherapy should be scheduled to avoid neutropenia and thrombocytopenia at the time of delivery.
- Paclitaxel is teratogenic and should not be used during pregnancy.
- Tamoxifen is teratogenic and should not be used in pregnant women.
- Therapeutic abortion does not change the survival rate.

MALE BREAST CANCER

- Male breast cancer is uncommon.
- Risk factors are family history, *BRCA2* germ-line mutation, Klinefelter syndrome, and radiation to the chest wall.
- Presence of gynecomastia is not a risk factor for breast cancer.
- It is first seen as a mass beneath the nipple or ulceration.
- The mean age of occurrence is 60 to 70 years.
- Eighty percent of male breast cancer is hormone-receptor positive.

Treatment

- Modified radical mastectomy
- Lumpectomy is rarely done because it does not offer any cosmetic benefit.
- Systemic treatment with chemotherapy and endocrine therapy should follow the general guidelines for female patients.
- None of the adjuvant treatment modalities has been tested in a randomized clinical trial setting in men.

Phylloides Tumor

Phylloides tumor is clinically suspected when the tumor is growing rapidly and clinical and radiological features suggestive of fibroadenoma. It is treated with wide excision without an axillary node dissection. In patients who has recurrent phylloides tumor, radiation therapy can be considered after wide excision.

Paget's Disease of the Nipple

Patients should be evaluated for any evidence of invasive or noninvasive breast cancer by appropriate imaging and biopsy. If the patient has only Paget's disease of the nipple areolar complex (NAC), the patient can be treated with mastectomy with axillary lymph node dissection or wide excision of the NAC and axillary node surgery with whole breast radiation. Patients with invasive or noninvasive breast cancer should be managed appropriately.

Metastatic Breast Cancer

Principles of Treatment

- In newly diagnosed metastatic breast cancer, it is recommended to confirm the diagnosis, hormone receptor, and HER2/neu status by repeat biopsy.
- All patients should be considered for clinical trials.
- Quality of life should be taken into consideration prior to starting any treatment.
- In majority of the patients the goal of the treatment is palliation.
- But in a subset of patients long-term remission is possible.
- ER/PR–positive patients with slow-growing bone or soft-tissue disease can be treated with endocrine therapy. Premenopausal patients should be considered for oophorectomy.
- HER2-neu–positive patients could be treated with a trastuzumab-containing regimen or if they progressed on trastuzumab, consider lapatinib-containing regimen or continue on trastuzumab with a different chemotherapy.
- Since there is no significant survival advantage, but increased toxicity for combination chemotherapy, single-agent chemotherapy is the preferred treatment.
- Many combination chemotherapy regimens have shown an increased response rate and some of them showed an increase in DFS. But the majority of the combination therapy regimens have increased toxicity.
- Combination of paclitaxel and bevacizumab has shown doubling of DFS compared to single-agent paclitaxel without significant increase in side effects in the first-line treatment.
- All patients with bone metastatic disease should be considered for treatment with bisphosphanates (Fig. 12.5).

Targeted Therapy

Trastuzumab (Herceptin): About 25% of patients overexpress HER2/neu. Trastuzumab is a monoclonal antibody, which is found to be highly effective in metastatic and adjuvant breast cancer therapy. The dose is usually 4 mg/kg as a loading dose and 2 mg/kg weekly. It can be given every 3 weeks, with a loading dose of 8 mg/kg followed by 6 mg/kg.

It is well tolerated; rarely it can cause infusion reaction and pulmonary toxicity. The major side effect from trastuzumab is cardiac toxicity when it is used with or after anthracyclines. In anthracycline-containing regimen, the congestive heart failure rate is about 2% to 4%. Nonanthracycline regimens such as TCH did not show increased cardiac toxicity. It is important to monitor cardiac function with an ECHO cardiogram or MUGA scan carefully for patients who are receiving trastuzumab.

Lapatinib (Tykerb): A potent, small molecule inhibitor of the HER1 and HER2 tyrosine kinases. The inhibitory effects, though reversible, result in blockade of receptor-mediated activation and propagation of downstream signaling involved in regulation of cell proliferation and cell survival. This is the first drug to demonstrate significant clinical benefits in patients with HER2-positive, advanced breast cancer progressing on previous therapy which included trastuzumab, an anthracycline, and a taxane. It is a dual tyrosine kinase inhibitor, which blocks both EGFR (HER1) and HER2 pathway intracellularly. The FDA-approved dose of lapatinib is 1,250 mg daily PO. The side effects include diarrhea and rash. Some of the preliminary data supports its efficacy in patients with brain metastatic disease. It is being tested in combination with many different combinations in early and metastatic breast cancer.

Bevacizumab (Avastin): It is a monoclonal antibody against vascular endothelial growth factor (VEGF), which is a mediator of angiogenesis. It is approved by FDA for breast cancer in the first-line metastatic setting, in combination with paclitaxel. In the phase 3 randomized study, it is found to double the DFS (from 5.9 months to about 11.8 months) when used in combination with paclitaxel. The dose of bevacizumab in breast cancer is 10 mg/kg given days 1 and 15, in combination with weekly paclitaxel 90 mg/m^2 given 3 out of 4 weeks schedule. Side effects include hypertension, proteinuria, headache, cerebrovascular accidents etc. Role of bevacizumab is evolving in the treatment of breast cancer.

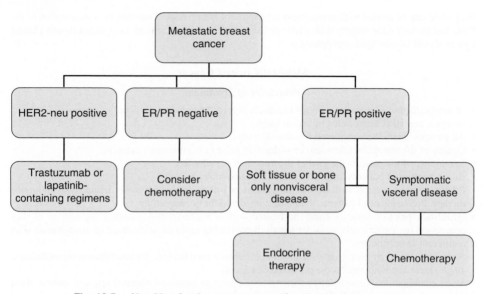

Fig. 12.5. Algorithm for the management of metastatic breast cancer.

Taxanes: Taxanes (docetaxel and paclitaxel) are the two most active agents in the treatment of breast cancer. Both are microtubule-stabilizing agents and are MDR substrates. Almost all the adjuvant and metastatic breast cancer regimen include one of these two drugs.

***nab*-Paclitaxel:** Nanoparticle albumin-bound paclitaxel (nab-paclitaxel) is a novel paclitaxel formulation that does not require Cremophor or polysorbate 80 for solubilization, thus reducing solvent-related toxicity and micelle formation. In a phase 3 randomized clinical trial of paclitaxel, versus nab-paclitaxel, in first-line metastatic breast cancer, nab-paclitaxel is found to have statistically significant superior response rate and improved time to progression. Based on this study, FDA approved nab-paclitaxel 260 mg/m^2 every 3 weeks for the treatment of metastatic breast cancer. The side effects include neutropenia, peripheral neuropathy, nausea, etc. Due to lack of cremophor, nab-paclitaxel do not require premedication with steroids.

Ixabepilone (Ixempra): This drug belongs to a novel class of drugs called epothilones. Epothilones are non-taxane microtubule-stabilizing agents. The tubulin polymerizing activity of ixabepilone is stronger than paclitaxel. It has proven efficacy in taxane-resistant settings. Ixabepilone has low susceptibility to tumor resistance mechanisms such as P-glycoprotein (P-gp) and multidrug-resistance protein-1 (MRP1). The FDA approved ixabepilone in combination with capecitabine in patients with metastatic or locally advanced breast cancer, who are resistant to or refractory to a taxane and anthracycline. Ixabepilone is also approved as a monotherapy in patients who are resistant or refractory to taxane, anthracycline, and capecitabine. The dose is 40 mg/m^2 administered over 3 hours every 3 weeks. Patients should be premedicated with diphenhydramine and cimetidine an hour prior to the infusion with ixabepilone.

Bisphosphonates

Adjuvant

A definite improvement in DFS was seen in a recent study (ABCSG 12) where premenopausal patients were treated with goserelin 3.6 mg every 28 days followed by zometa 4 mg IV every 6 months along with tamoxifen or anastrozole.

Studies have shown that postmenopusal patients who are receiving AIs will experience less osteoporosis, osteopenia, or fractures when treated with upfront zometa (Z-Fast Study).

- Bisphosphonates should be used in patients with bony metastatic disease because they prevent progression of lytic lesions, delay skeletal-related events, and decrease pain. However, the optimal frequency of administration and duration of therapy are not known.
- Zoledronic acid (4 mg by 15-minute infusion) and pamidronate (90 mg by 2-hour infusion) are two available biphosphonates approved for bony metastatic disease.
- Osteonecrosis of the jaw (ONJ) is a very rare but a potential complication of long-term treatment with intravenous bisphosphonates.

Central Nervous System (CNS) Metastasis

CNS metastasis may consist of either parenchymal or leptomeningeal metastasis. The control of systemic disease is crucial in improving the survival of patients with resectable brain metastasis.

The standard treatment for multiple brain lesions remains whole brain radiation (WBR) for symptom control, with no improvement in survival. The therapy for a single brain metastasis remains either surgery or radiosurgery, with conflicting information as to the benefit of prior WBR. Leptomeningeal metastasis is conventionally treated with intrathecal chemotherapy, and may provide short-term symptom control. The superiority of intrathecal versus systemic chemotherapy in leptomeningeal metastasis is controversial. About 30% of HER2/neu positive patients will develop brain metastatic disease and lapatinib-containing regimen is an option in these patients.

LOCALLY RECURRENT BREAST CANCER

After mastectomy:

- Eighty percent of local recurrences occur within 5 years.
- The treatment of choice is surgical excision and radiation therapy.
- Systemic therapy may be considered, although the survival advantage is not clear.

After lumpectomy:

- Mastectomy is the treatment of choice for patients who have only isolated breast cancer recurrence.

FOLLOW-UP FOR PATIENTS WITH OPERABLE BREAST CANCER (BASED ON ASCO GUIDELINES)

1. History and physical examination every 3 to 6 months for the first 3 years, every 6 to 12 months for the next 2 years, and then annually.
2. Monthly breast self-examination.
3. Annual mammogram of the contralateral and ipsilateral (remaining breast after lumpectomy) breast.
4. Annual Papanicolaou smear and pelvic examinations in women who are taking, or who have taken, tamoxifen.
5. Blood tests including a complete blood count, liver function tests, and alkaline phosphatase levels are not routinely recommended.
   - Serum tumor markers (CA 27, 29, and CA 15-3) are not recommended.
   - Bone scan and imaging of the chest, abdomen, pelvis, and brain or PET scans are not recommended routinely, but they are done if symptoms or laboratory abnormalities are present.
6. Rectal examination, occult blood testing, and skin examination must be performed annually or every 2 years.

SUGGESTED READINGS

Bonadonna G, Zambetti M, Valagussa P: Sequential or alternating doxorubicin and CMF regimens in breast cancer with more than three positive nodes. Ten-year results. JAMA 273:542–7, 1995.

Bonadonna G, Valagussa P, Moliterni A, et al: Adjuvant cyclophosphamide, methotrexate, and fluorouracil in node-positive breast cancer: the results of 20 years of follow-up. N Engl J Med 332:901–6, 1995.

Citron ML, Berry DA, Cirrincione C, et al: Randomized trial of dose-dense versus conventionally scheduled and sequential versus concurrent combination chemotherapy as postoperative adjuvant treatment of node-positive primary breast cancer: first report of Intergroup Trial C9741/Cancer and Leukemia Group B Trial 9741. J Clin Oncol 21:1431–9, 2003.

Chia S, Gradishar W, Mauriac L, et al: Double-blind, randomized placebo controlled trial of fulvestrant compared with exemestane after prior nonsteroidal aromatase inhibitor therapy in postmenopausal women with hormone receptor-positive, advanced breast cancer: results from EFECT. J Clin Oncol 26:1664–70, 2008.

Epirubicin-based chemotherapy in metastatic breast cancer patients: role of dose-intensity and duration of treatment. J Clin Oncol 18:3115–24, 2000.

Fisher B, Brown AM, Dimitrov NV, et al: Two months of doxorubicin-cyclophosphamide with and without interval reinduction therapy compared with 6 months of cyclophosphamide, methotrexate, and fluorouracil in positive-node breast cancer patients with tamoxifen-nonresponsive tumors: results from the National Surgical Adjuvant Breast and Bowel Project B-15. J Clin Oncol 8:1483–96, 1990.

Geyer CE, Forster J, Lindquist D, et al: Lapatinib plus capecitabine for HER2-positive advanced breast cancer. N Engl J Med 355:2733–43, 2006.

Henderson IC, Berry DA, Demetri GD, et al: Improved outcomes from adding sequential Paclitaxel but not from escalating Doxorubicin dose in an adjuvant chemotherapy regimen for patients with node-positive primary breast cancer. J Clin Oncol 21:976–83, 2003.

Jones SE, Erban J, Overmoyer B, et al: Randomized phase III study of docetaxel compared with paclitaxel in metastatic breast cancer. J Clin Oncol 23:5542–51, 2005.

Jones SE, Savin MA, Holmes FA, et al: Phase III trial comparing doxorubicin plus cyclophosphamide with docetaxel plus cyclophosphamide as adjuvant therapy for operable breast cancer. J Clin Oncol 24:5381–7, 2006.

Levine MN, Bramwell VH, Pritchard KI, et al: Randomized trial of intensive cyclophosphamide, epirubicin, and fluorouracil chemotherapy compared with cyclophosphamide, methotrexate, and fluorouracil in premenopausal women with node-positive breast cancer. National Cancer Institute of Canada Clinical Trials Group. J Clin Oncol 16:2651–8, 1998.

Martin M, Pienkowski T, Mackey J, et al: Adjuvant docetaxel for node-positive breast cancer. N Engl J Med 352:2302–13, 2005.

Miller K, Wang M, Gralow J, et al: Paclitaxel plus bevacizumab versus paclitaxel alone for metastatic breast cancer. N Engl J Med 357:2666–76, 2007.

Piccart-Gebhart MJ, Procter M, Leyland-Jones B, et al: Trastuzumab after adjuvant chemotherapy in HER2-positive breast cancer. N Engl J Med 353:1659–72, 2005.

Ravdin PM, Cronin KA, Howlader N, et al: The decrease in breast-cancer incidence in 2003 in the United States. N Engl J Med 356:1670–4, 2007.

Romond EH, Perez EA, Bryant J. Trastuzumab plus adjuvant chemotherapy for operable HER2-positive breast cancer. N Engl J Med 353:1673, October 20, 2005.

Romond EH, Perez EA, Bryant J, et al: Trastuzumab plus adjuvant chemotherapy for operable HER2-positive breast cancer. N Engl J Med 353:1673–84, 2005.

Saad A, Abraham J: Role of tumor markers and circulating tumors cells in the management of breast cancer. Oncology (Williston Park) 22:726–31; discussion 734, 739, 743–4, 2008.

Seidman AD, Berry D, Cirrincione C, et al: Randomized phase III trial of weekly compared with every-3-weeks paclitaxel for metastatic breast cancer, with trastuzumab for all HER-2 overexpressors and random assignment to trastuzumab or not in HER-2 nonoverexpressors: final results of Cancer and Leukemia Group B protocol 9840. J Clin Oncol 26:1642–9, 2008.

Sharma M, Abraham J: CNS metastasis in primary breast cancer. Expert Rev Anticancer Ther 7:1561–6, 2007.

Slamon D, Eiermann W, Robert N, et al: BCIRG 006: 2nd interim analysis phase III randomized trial comparing doxorubicin and cyclophosphamide followed by docetaxel (AC→T) with doxorubicin and cyclophosphamide followed by docetaxel and trastuzumab (AC→TH) with docetaxel, carboplatin and trastuzumab (TCH) in Her2neu positive early breast cancer patients, 29th Annual San Antonio Breast Cancer Symposium; December 14–17, 2006. San Antonio, TX, 2006.

Smalley RV, Lefante J, Bartolucci A, et al: A comparison of cyclophosphamide, adriamycin, and 5-fluorouracil (CAF) and cyclophosphamide, methotrexate, 5-fluorouracil, vincristine, and prednisone (CMFVP) in patients with advanced breast cancer. Breast Cancer Res Treat 3:209–20, 1983.

Swayampakula AK, Dillis C, Abraham J: Role of MRI in screening, diagnosis and management of breast cancer. Expert Rev Anticancer Ther 8:811–7, 2008.

SECTION 5

Genitourinary

13

Renal Cell Cancer

Ramaprasad Srinivasan, Inger L. Rosner, and W. Marston Linehan

Renal cell cancer (RCC), a term that includes a variety of cancers arising in the kidney, comprises several histologically, biologically, and clinically distinct entities. Surgical resection for localized disease and immunotherapy for metastatic disease have been the mainstays of therapy for RCC. However, recent advances in our understanding of the molecular mechanisms underlying individual subtypes of the disease have led to newer, more effective, targeted approaches to managing metastatic RCC.

EPIDEMIOLOGY

- An estimated 54,000+ new cases of cancer arising in the kidney and renal pelvis were diagnosed in the United States in 2008, leading to more than 13,000 deaths.
- Incidence is higher in men, with a male:female ratio of 1.6:1.
- Incidence increased approximately 2% to 4% per year between 1975 and 1995. Mortality from RCC also increased during this period, but at a lower rate.
- Largely a disease of adulthood, with peak incidence after the fifth decade of life, RCC may also occur in children and infants.

ETIOLOGY AND RISK FACTORS

Nonhereditary Risk Factors

- Tobacco use. Up to one-third of cases in men and one-fourth of cases in women may be linked to smoking.
- Occupational exposure to trichloroethylene, cadmium, asbestos, and petroleum products
- Obesity, particularly in women
- Acquired cystic disease of the kidney associated with long-term dialysis

Genetic Predisposition/Familial Syndromes

Several familial kidney cancer syndromes have been identified. Although they represent a minority of RCC patients, individuals affected by these heritable disorders have a predisposition for developing kidney cancer, which is often bilateral and multifocal. Systematic evaluation of at-risk families has helped elucidate the molecular mechanisms underlying the origins of several types of kidney cancer. Several forms of sporadic kidney cancer have histologically similar familial counterparts with which they share aberrant oncogenic pathways. The following familial kidney cancer syndromes have been described:

- **Von Hippel-Lindau (VHL) syndrome**
  - VHL is inherited in an autosomal-dominant pattern.
  - Affected individuals have a predilection for developing a variety of tumors, including bilateral, multifocal renal tumors (clear cell RCC), pancreatic neuroendocrine tumors, renal and pancreatic cysts, CNS hemangioblastomas, retinal angiomas, pheochromocytomas, endolymphatic sac tumors, and epididymal/broad ligament cystadenomas.

– Genetic linkage analysis has identified the VHL tumor suppressor gene located on chromosome 3p25. Affected individuals have a mutated/deleted allele of the VHL gene in their germ line. Acquisition of a somatic "second hit" that inactivates the normal copy of VHL leads to tumor formation in the affected organ(s).
- **Hereditary papillary RCC (HPRC)**
  – Affected individuals have bilateral, multifocal type 1 papillary RCC. There are no known extrarenal manifestations of this disease.
  – The underlying defect is an activating germ-line mutation in the c-MET proto-oncogene, located on the long arm of chromosome 7, accompanied by a nonrandom duplication of the aberrant chromosome 7 (resulting in trisomy 7).
  – Patients usually present with renal tumors in or beyond the fifth decade of life, although an early-onset form that presents in the second or third decades has also been described.
- **Birt-Hogg-Dube (BHD) syndrome**
  – Affected individuals are at increased risk of developing cutaneous fibrofolliculomas, pulmonary cysts predisposing to the development of spontaneous pneumothoraces, and renal tumors.
  – Several histologic types of renal tumors have been described in BHD, including chromophobe (34%), hybrid chromophobe-oncocytomas (50%), clear cell, and oncocytomas.
  – The BHD gene, localized to chromosome 17p11, encodes a protein known as folliculin. Identification of somatic "second hit" mutations in BHD/folliculin indicates that this gene may function as a tumor suppressor.
- **Hereditary leiomyomatosis and RCC (HLRCC)**
  – Affected individuals have a predisposition to developing multiple cutaneous and uterine leiomyomas, as well as papillary RCC.
  – Renal tumors are often solitary.
  – Sometimes described as papillary type 2 RCC; may be mistaken for collecting duct RCC. The distinctive histopathologic hallmark of these tumors is the presence of a large nucleus with a prominent orangiophilic nucleolus surrounded by a halo.
  – Tumors tend to metastasize early and have a characteristically aggressive clinical course.
  – The underlying defect is a germ-line mutation in the Krebs cycle enzyme fumarate hydratase, located on chromosome 1.

PATHOLOGIC CLASSIFICATION

Based on histopathologic features, RCC is divided into the following subtypes:

- Clear cell RCC. The most common variety, comprising 70% to 80% of all kidney cancers. Composed predominantly of cells with a clear cytoplasm.
- Papillary RCC. Further divided into type 1 and type 2 based on morphologic appearance. Represents approximately 10% to 15% of all kidney cancers.
- Chromophobe RCC. Represents approximately 5% of all malignant renal neoplasms. Characterized histologically by the presence of sheets of cells with pale or eosinophilic granular cytoplasm.
- Collecting duct RCC. Rare (<1%) variant believed to originate in the collecting system. Medullary RCC, which has some features suggestive of collecting duct RCC, is seen almost exclusively in patients with sickle-cell trait and is characterized by an aggressive clinical course.
- Unclassified. Represents approximately 3% to 5% of renal tumors. Lack distinct features of a particular subtype or variant.
- Renal tumors with sarcomatoid features do not comprise a separate entity. Instead, they represent localized sarcomatoid differentiation of one of the subtypes of RCC. Generally associated with poor prognosis.

MOLECULAR MECHANISMS

Identifying familial kidney cancer syndromes was an important step in unraveling the complex aberrant pathways leading to the development of several types of both hereditary and sporadic RCCs. This has led to the development of therapeutic agents that target pathways critical to the development and growth of these tumors.

Clear Cell RCC

- Germ-line mutations in the VHL gene are the hallmark of VHL syndrome.
- The vast majority of patients with sporadic clear cell RCC show evidence of VHL inactivation in tumor tissue resulting from either mutation or promoter hypermethylation. The absence of functionally active VHL protein has several consequences, the best understood of which is the accumulation of a group of transcription factors called hypoxia-inducible factors (HIF).
- Increased intracellular HIF leads to transcriptional upregulation of several proangiogenic growth and survival factors, such as vascular endothelial growth factor (VEGF), platelet-derived growth factor (PDGF), transforming growth factor-alpha (TGF-α), and the glucose transporter glut-1. This sequence of events appears to be important in the genesis and propagation of clear cell RCC.
- Several components of this pathway are targets for novel therapeutic agents.

Type 1 Papillary RCC

- c-Met is a cell surface receptor normally activated on binding its ligand, hepatocyte growth factor (HGF). HGF/c-Met promotes a variety of biologic functions including cell growth, proliferation, and motility. Activating mutations in the c-Met proto-oncogene (which render the receptor constitutionally active) are responsible for the bilateral, multifocal, type 1 papillary renal tumors seen in patients with HPRC.
- Activating somatic mutations in the tyrosine kinase domain of c-Met have also been identified in 10% to 15% of patients with sporadic papillary RCC. Duplication of chromosome 7, where genes for both c-Met and HGF are located, is seen more frequently in sporadic papillary tumors (approximately 70% in one series) and may represent an alternative mechanism for activation of the HGF/c-Met pathway.
- Agents targeting the c-Met pathway are currently being evaluated in patients with papillary RCC.

Type 2 Papillary RCC

- Includes tumors with papillary architecture but with features inconsistent with type 1 papillary tumors. Patients with HLRCC are at risk for developing renal tumors, which are sometimes described as type 2 papillary RCC.
- The underlying molecular defect in HLRCC-related tumors is inactivation of the Krebs cycle enzyme fumarate hydratase, leading to accumulation of its substrate fumarate. Fumarate interferes with HIF degradation and leads to its accumulation and consequent transcriptional activation of its target genes (VEGF, PDGF, TGF-α, etc.). No sporadic counterpart for this tumor has been described.

Chromophobe RCC

- The precise biochemical aberrations underlying chromophobe RCC are being investigated; however, patients with BHD often present with chromophobe renal tumors.
- The gene for BHD (folliculin) appears to interact with the mTOR and AMPK pathways, which may be important in chromophobe tumors and, potentially, other histologic RCC subtypes seen in BHD.

CLINICAL PRESENTATION

- Many renal masses are found incidentally during evaluation for unrelated medical issues or metastatic foci.
- Only 10% of patients present with the classic triad of hematuria, pain, and flank mass.
- Initial presentation may be a paraneoplastic syndrome or laboratory abnormality, including elevated erythrocyte sedimentation rate, weight loss/cachexia, hypertension from increased renin, anemia, hypercalcemia (release of PTH-like substance), elevated alkaline phosphatase, polycythemia (increased erythropoietin), and Stauffer's syndrome (reversible, nonmetastatic hepatic dysfunction that usually resolves once the primary tumor is removed).

- Approximately 50% of RCC patients present with localized disease, 25% with locally advanced disease, and 25% to 30% with metastatic disease.
- Common sites of metastatic spread include lung (70%–75%), lymph nodes (30%–40%), bone (20%–25%), liver (20%–25%), and CNS.

DIAGNOSIS AND EVALUATION

- Initial workup for a patient with a renal mass includes a history and physical examination, complete blood count with differential, full chemistry panel, and PT/PTT.
- CT scan of the abdomen and pelvis, with and without contrast, is standard for evaluating the renal mass and regional lymph nodes. If CT scan suggests renal vein and/or inferior vena cava involvement, an MRI of the abdomen and chest imaging is warranted.
- Chest x-ray is also recommended. Chest CT is indicated in the presence of an abnormal x-ray, a large primary tumor, or symptoms such as cough or chest pain.
- Bone scan is indicated for elevated alkaline phosphatase, hypercalcemia, pathologic fracture, or bone pain.
- MRI of the brain is usually reserved for patients with clinical features suggesting brain metastases.

STAGING

The most commonly used system for staging RCC is the Tumor–Lymph Node–Metastasis (TNM) staging system outlined by the American Joint Committee for Cancer (AJCC) (Table 13.1).

TABLE 13.1. *TNM staging for renal cell carcinoma*

Primary Tumor (T)

TX	Primary tumor cannot be assessed
T0	No evidence of primary tumor
T1	Tumor ≤7 cm in greatest dimension, limited to kidney
T1a	Tumor ≤4 cm in greatest dimension, limited to kidney
T1b	Tumor >4 cm but <7 cm in greatest dimension, limited to kidney
T2	Tumor >7 cm in greatest dimension, limited to kidney
T3	Tumor extends into major veins or invades adrenal gland or perinephric tissue, but not beyond Gerota's fascia
T3a	Tumor directly invades adrenal gland or perirenal and/or renal sinus fat, but not beyond Gerota's fat
T3b	Tumor grossly extends into renal vein or its segmental (muscle-containing) branches or vena cava below diaphragm
T3c	Tumor grossly extends into vena cava above the diaphragm or invades wall of vena cava
T4	Tumor invades beyond Gerota's fascia

Regional Lymph Nodes (N)*

NX	Regional lymph nodes cannot be assessed
N0	No regional lymph node metastasis
N1	Metastasis in single lymph node
N2	Metastasis in >1 regional lymph node

Distant Metastasis (M)

MX	Distant metastasis cannot be assessed
M0	No distant metastasis
M1	Distant metastasis

(Continued)

TABLE 13.1. *(Continued)*

Stage Groupings			
Stage I	T1	N0	M0
Stage II	T2	N0	M0
Stage III	T1	N1	M0
	T2	N1	M0
	T3	N0	M0
	T3	N1	M0
	T3a	N0	M0
	T3a	N1	M0
	T3b	N0	M0
	T3b	N1	M0
	T3c	N0	M0
	T3c	N1	M0
Stage IV	T4	N0	M0
	T4	N1	M0
	Any T	N2	M0
	Any T	Any N	M1

*Laterality does not affect N classification.
Source: Adapted from *AJCC Cancer Staging Manual*. 6th ed. 2002.

PROGNOSTIC FACTORS

• Several tumor and patient characteristics appear to influence outcome for patients with localized kidney cancer. Nomograms based on factors such as tumor stage and nuclear grade, tumor histology, mode of presentation, and performance status are used to predict risk of disease recurrence following nephrectomy. Several such nomograms are currently available and are gaining acceptance in both clinical practice and clinical trial design as an effective means of risk stratification.

• In patients with metastatic disease, clinical characteristics (performance status, prior nephrectomy, number of metastatic sites, etc.) as well as laboratory parameters (serum lactate dehydrogenase, serum calcium, hemoglobin, etc.) are predictive of survival. A widely used prognostic model based on patients treated with either cytokines or chemotherapeutic agents (Memorial Sloan-Kettering Cancer Center prognostic criteria) implicates the following features with poor outcome:
  – Poor performance status (Karnofsky PS <80)
  – Elevated LDH (>1.5 × upper limit of normal)
  – Elevated corrected calcium (>10 mg/dL)
  – Low hemoglobin (< lower limit of normal)
  – Absence of prior nephrectomy

• The presence or absence of one or more of these prognostic features allows stratification of patients into the following prognostic categories:
  – Favorable: 0 risk factors, median survival 19.9 months
  – Intermediate: 1 or 2 risk factors, median survival 10.3 months
  – Poor: 3 to 5 risk factors, median survival 3.9 months

TREATMENT OF LOCALIZED RCC

Surgery

• For patients with early-stage localized RCC, surgical resection is often curative.
• For tumors >4 cm, radical nephrectomy (open or laparoscopic procedure) is the treatment of choice.
• Smaller lesions may be amenable to nephron-sparing surgery (partial nephrectomy).
• Less invasive techniques such as radiofrequency ablation and cryotherapy are being evaluated and may be effective in eradicating smaller renal tumors; however, long-term outcome data are required before these modalities become standard practice.

Adjuvant Therapy

Although a variety of agents such as cytokines and vaccines have been evaluated in the adjuvant setting, none has proved effective in reducing the risk of recurrence or improving long-term outcome. Ongoing adjuvant trials are evaluating the role of targeted therapeutic agents such as sunitinib and sorafenib in patients with high-risk disease following resection of the primary tumor.

TREATMENT OF METASTATIC RCC

Surgery

- For selected patients with isolated visceral metastases, surgical resection may provide extended disease-free periods.
- Cytoreductive nephrectomy preceding systemic cytokine therapy has been the subject of several studies. At least two randomized phase 3 trials have demonstrated a survival advantage in patients receiving interferon-alpha (IFN-α) following nephrectomy versus patients receiving IFN-α alone. Most centers currently use this approach to manage metastatic RCC. Cytoreductive nephrectomy as a prelude to antiangiogenic targeted therapies is currently under evaluation.
- Cytoreductive nephrectomy can be performed for palliation of intractable hematuria and pain associated with RCC.

Systemic Therapy

- Conventional cytotoxic chemotherapy is ineffective in the vast majority of patients with metastatic RCC (approximately 5%–6% overall response rate with single agent) and is not part of the standard approach for this disease. Its role in patients with sarcomatoid variants bears further study.
- Novel targeted agents directed against the VEGF/PDGF and mammalian target of rapamycin (mTOR) pathways have recently been evaluated in patients with metastatic RCC and have supplanted cytokines as standard first-line agents in the management of clear cell RCC (Table 13.2). The standard initial approach for most patients with metastatic clear cell RCC is treatment with small molecule inhibitors of angiogenesis, although cytokine-based therapy with interleukin (IL)-2 may be appropriate in selected patients.
- There are currently no standard treatments for non–clear cell variants, although several interesting mechanism-based approaches are under investigation.

VEGF Pathway Inhibitors

Up-regulation of proangiogenic factors such as VEGF and PDGF is an important consequence of VHL inactivation and provides the basis for the efficacy of anti-VEGF agents in RCC. Sunitinib and sorafenib, the most widely used agents in this category, are both FDA approved for the treatment of metastatic RCC.

Sunitinib

- An oral tyrosine kinase inhibitor with potent activity against VEGF receptor 2 (VEGFR-2) and PDGF receptor (PDGFR)
- Initial single-arm phase 2 studies have demonstrated a remarkably high overall response rate of 30%–40% in patients with cytokine-refractory disease. A randomized phase 3 study comparing sunitinib with IFN-α in previously untreated clear cell RCC patients has demonstrated a significantly higher response rate (31% vs. 6%), improved progression-free survival (PFS) (median 11 vs. 5 months; Fig. 13.1), and superior overall survival (OS) (26.4 vs. 21.8 months) with sunitinib.
- Dosage is 50 mg/day over 4 weeks, followed by a 2-week rest period.
- Fairly well tolerated by the majority of patients. Common side effects include hypertension, fatigue, cutaneous side effects (rash, hand–foot syndrome), gastrointestinal symptoms (nausea, vomiting, diarrhea, anorexia, constipation), and cytopenia.
- Sunitinib is currently the most widely used first-line agent in metastatic clear cell RCC.

TABLE 13.2. Key studies of targeted agents in metastatic renal cell carcinoma

Agent(s)	Phase	Study population	# of patients	Overall response rate (RECIST)*	Median PFS (mo)*	Median OS (mo)*
First-line therapy						
Sunitinib vs. IFN-α	Randomized phase 3	Previously untreated clear cell	750	**31% vs. 6%**	**11 vs. 5**	**26.4 vs. 21.08**
Tem vs. IFN-α vs. Tem+ IFN-α	Randomized phase 3	Poor prognosis, previously untreated, all histologic subtypes	626	8.6% vs. 4.8% vs. 8.1%	5.5 vs. 3.1 vs. 4.7	**10.9 vs. 7.3** vs. 8.4
Sorafenib vs. IFN-α	Randomized phase 2	Previously untreated clear cell	189	5% vs. 9%	5.7 vs. 5.6	
Bev + IFN-α vs. IFN-α	Randomized phase 3	Previously untreated clear cell	649	**31% vs. 13%**	**102. vs. 5.4**	NR vs. 19.8
Second-line and subsequent therapy						
Sunitinib	Single-arm phase 2	Cytokine-refractory clear cell	63	40%	8.7	
Sunitinib	Single-arm phase 2	Cytokine-refractory clear cell	106	44%	8.1	
Sorafenib vs. placebo	Phase 2 randomized discontinuation	Treatment-refractory, all histologic subtypes	202		**6 vs. 1.5**	
Sorafenib vs. placebo	Randomized phase 3	Cytokine-refractory clear cell	903	10% vs. 2%	**5.5 vs. 2.8**	17.8 vs. 15.2
Bev (10 mg/kg) vs. bev (3 mg/kg) vs. placebo	Randomized, 3-arm phase 2	Cytokine-refractory clear cell	116	10% vs. 0% vs. 0%	**4.8** vs. 3.0 vs. **2.5**	
Everolimus vs. placebo	Randomized phase 3	Clear cell RCC refractory to VEGF-targeted therapy	410	1% vs. 0%	**4.0 vs. 1.9**	NR vs. 8.8

Bev, bevacizumab; IFN-α, interferon-alpha; NR, not reached; OS, overall survival; PFS, progression-free survival; tem, temsirolimus.

*Statistical significance indicated in boldface type.

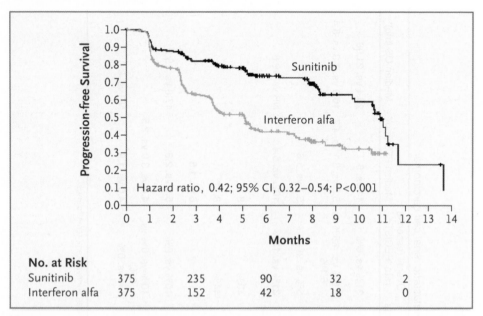

Fig. 13.1. Progression-free survival in untreated metastatic clear cell RCC patients receiving su-nitinib or IFN-α. (From Motzer RJ, Hutson TE, Tomczak P, et al. Sunitinib versus interferon alfa in metastatic renal-cell carcinoma. *NEJM*. 2007;356(2):115–124.)

SORAFENIB

- An oral tyrosine kinase inhibitor with activity against c-Raf, VEGFR-2, and PDGFR
- A randomized phase 2 study showed significant improvement in PFS versus placebo (median 24 vs. 6 weeks) in patients with cytokine-refractory metastatic RCC. This finding was confirmed in a randomized phase 3 trial of sorafenib versus placebo (median PFS 5.5 vs. 2.8 months). OS was similar in the two groups (17.8 vs. 15.2 months) and may have been influenced by the trial's crossover design (patients progressing on placebo could cross over to the sorafenib arm).
- A randomized phase 2 study in metastatic, untreated clear cell RCC failed to demonstrate the drug's superiority over IFN-α.
- Typically administered at a dose of 400 mg twice a day. Adverse events are similar to those of su-nitinib.
- Provides a reasonable option for patients who have failed sunitinib and/or other first-line agents.

BEVACIZUMAB

- A monoclonal antibody against VEGF-A
- A randomized, three-arm phase 2 study comparing two different doses of bevacizumab (10 mg/kg and 3 mg/kg i.v. every 2 weeks) and placebo in cytokine-refractory patients showed a PFS advantage favoring the 10 mg/kg arm (4.8 vs. 2.5 months).
- A multicenter randomized phase 3 study comparing IFN-α alone (9 million IU s.c. 3 times per week) versus the same dose of IFN-α plus bevacizumab (10 mg/kg i.v. every 2 weeks) showed superior PFS in the combination arm (5.4 vs. 10.2 months).

mTOR Pathway Inhibitors

The mTOR inhibitors temsirolimus and everolimus are rapamycin analogs believed to act at least in part by down-regulating mTOR-dependent translation of HIF.

TEMSIROLIMUS

- A prodrug of rapamycin-administered i.v.
- The most convincing evidence for the activity of this drug in RCC comes from a randomized phase 3 trial of 626 patients with previously untreated high-risk metastatic RCC (defined as the presence of three or more poor prognostic criteria). All histologic subtypes of RCC were included in this trial. Patients were randomized to receive temsirolimus 25 mg i.v. per week or temsirolimus 15 mg i.v. per week plus IFN-α (6 million IU 3 times/week) or IFN-α alone (18 million IU 3 times per week as tolerated). Single-agent temsirolimus was associated with significantly prolonged disease-free survival and OS compared to IFN-α alone (median OS 10.9 vs. 7.3 months; Fig. 13.2). An exploratory subgroup analysis suggested that both clear cell and non–clear cell patients benefited from temsirolimus. The combined temsirolimus/IFN-α arm had superior disease-free survival compared to IFN-α alone, but there was no difference in OS between the two groups.
- Common adverse events include rash, fatigue, mucositis, hyperglycemia, hypercholesterolemia, and interstitial pneumonitis. Rapamycin analogs are also associated with a risk of immunosuppression.
- Single-agent temsirolimus is a reasonable first-line option for patients with poor-prognosis RCC. Its activity in non–clear cell variants of RCC and in favorable- and intermediate-risk RCC are under evaluation.

EVEROLIMUS

- An oral rapamycin analog
- In a randomized phase 3 trial of metastatic RCC patients who had progressed on front-line VEGF-targeted therapy, everolimus improved disease-free survival compared to placebo (4 vs. 1.9 months).
- Side effects are similar to those of temsirolimus.
- Both temsirolimus and everolimus are reasonable treatment options for patients who have progressed on sunitinib or other VEGF antagonists.

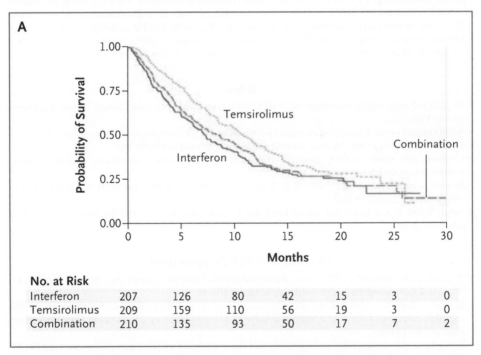

Fig. 13.2. Kaplan-Meier estimate of overall survival in patients receiving temsirolimus alone, IFN-α alone, or the combination. (From Hudes G, Carducci M, Tomczak P, et al. Temsirolimus, interferon alfa, or both for advanced renal-cell carcinoma. *NEJM.* 2007;356(22):2271–2281.)

Cytokines

Until the advent of VEGF-targeted therapy, cytokines were the mainstay of treatment for metastatic clear cell RCC. High-dose IL-2 and IFN-α are the most studied agents in this class.

IL-2

Since the early 1980s, numerous studies have demonstrated the efficacy of IL-2 in patients with metastatic RCC.

- High-dose IL-2 (600,000–720,000 IU/kg every 8 hours as tolerated up to a maximum 15 doses) has shown an overall response rate of 15% to 20%, with complete responses in 7% to 9% of patients. Since only a small subset of patients appears to benefit from this agent, no survival advantage has been demonstrated in randomized trials. However, most complete responses were durable, with very few recurrences noted during long-term follow-up. IL-2 is FDA-approved for treatment of RCC.
- Responses to IL-2 are best characterized in patients with clear cell histology; its role in other subtypes of RCC is unclear.
- The major limitation of IL-2 is toxicity associated with the high-dose regimen. A high incidence of serious and life-threatening but often reversible complications (notably vascular-leak syndrome, hypotension, multiorgan failure, etc.) occurred in early trials, with resultant mortality rates of 1% to 5%. However, further experience with IL-2 has led to better management of side effects. A recent study of over 800 patients treated at the National Cancer Institute reported no treatment-related mortality.
- IL-2 has been evaluated in combination with a variety of other modalities, including cellular therapy with lymphokine-activated killer cells and tumor-infiltrating lymphocytes, chemotherapy, interferon, etc. However, combining any of these therapies with high-dose IL-2 appears to provide no additional benefit.
- Lower doses of either i.v. or s.c. IL-2 have been evaluated to determine if toxicity could be reduced without compromising efficacy. At least two randomized trials have demonstrated that lower-dose IL-2 leads to fewer responses and, more importantly, a decline in durable complete responses.
- Despite the availability of newer, better tolerated, VEGF-targeted agents, high-dose IL-2 remains a reasonable first-line option for selected patients with metastatic clear cell RCC.

IFN-α

- Overall response rate in treatment-naïve RCC patients treated with recombinant IFN-α is approximately 15%.
- Administered s.c. in a variety of dosages (5–18 million IU) and regimens (3–5 times per week)
- Limited long-term follow-up data; durable complete responses relatively rare
- Common side effects include constitutional symptoms, gastrointestinal toxicity, elevated hepatic transaminases, and bone marrow suppression.
- Several studies evaluating combined IL-2 and IFN-α have demonstrated no survival benefit over single-agent cytokine therapy.
- Single-agent IFN-α has fallen out of favor due to associated toxicity and the availability of more effective agents.

Allogeneic Stem Cell Transplantation

- Investigated in metastatic RCC to test the hypothesis that this malignancy may be susceptible to alloimmune donor-mediated graft-versus-solid tumor effects.
- Several groups have reported overall response rates of up to 30% to 40%, including some durable complete responses following nonmyeloablative or reduced-intensity conditioning peripheral blood stem cell transplants.
- Transplant-related morbidity and mortality and the availability of HLA-matched donors are limitations to this current investigational approach.

SUGGESTED READINGS

Atkins MB, Dutcher J, Weiss G, et al. Kidney cancer: the Cytokine Working Group experience (1986–2001): part I. IL-2-based clinical trials. *Med Oncol*. 2001;18(3):197–207.

Childs R, Chernoff A, Contentin N, et al. Regression of metastatic renal-cell carcinoma after non-myeloablative allogeneic peripheral-blood stem-cell transplantation. *N Engl J Med*. 2000;343(11): 750–758.

Dutcher J, Atkins MB, Margolin K, et al. Kidney cancer: the Cytokine Working Group experience (1986–2001): part II. Management of IL-2 toxicity and studies with other cytokines. *Med Oncol*. 2001;18(3):209–219.

Escudier B, Eisen T, Stadler WM, et al. Sorafenib in advanced clear-cell renal-cell carcinoma. *NEJM*. 2007;356(2):125–134.

Escudier B, Pluzanska A, Koralewski P, et al. Bevacizumab plus interferon alfa-2a for treatment of metastatic renal cell carcinoma: a randomised, double-blind phase III trial. *Lancet*. 2007;370(9605): 2103–2111.

Flanigan RC, Salmon SE, Blumenstein BA, et al. Nephrectomy followed by interferon alfa-2b compared with interferon alfa-2b alone for metastatic renal-cell cancer. *NEJM*. 2001;345(23):1655–1659.

Fyfe GA, Fisher RI, Rosenberg SA, Sznol M, Parkinson DR, Louie AC. Long-term response data for 255 patients with metastatic renal cell carcinoma treated with high-dose recombinant interleukin-2 therapy. *J Clin Oncol*. 1996;14(8):2410–2411.

Grubb RL III, Franks ME, Toro J, et al. Hereditary leiomyomatosis and renal cell cancer: a syndrome associated with an aggressive form of inherited renal cancer. *J Urol*. 2007;177(6):2074–2079.

Hudes G, Carducci M, Tomczak P, et al. Temsirolimus, interferon alfa, or both for advanced renal-cell carcinoma. *nejm*. 2007;356(22):2271–2281.

Javidan J, Stricker HJ, Tamboli P, et al. Prognostic significance of the 1997 TNM classification of renal cell carcinoma. *J Urol*. 1999;162(4):1277–1281.

Kammula US, White DE, Rosenberg SA. Trends in the safety of high dose bolus interleukin-2 administration in patients with metastatic cancer. *Cancer*. 1998;83(4):797–805.

Latif F, Tory K, Gnarra J, et al. Identification of the von Hippel-Lindau disease tumor suppressor gene. *Science*. 1993;260(5112):1317–1320.

Linehan WM, Pinto PA, Srinivasan R, et al. Identification of the genes for kidney cancer: opportunity for disease-specific targeted therapeutics. *Clin Cancer Res*. 2007;13(2 Pt 2):671s–679s.

Motzer RJ, Escudier B, Oudard S, et al. Efficacy of everolimus in advanced renal cell carcinoma: a double-blind, randomised, placebo-controlled phase III trial. *Lancet*. 2008;372(9637):449–456.

Motzer RJ, Hutson TE, Tomczak P, et al. Sunitinib versus interferon alfa in metastatic renal-cell carcinoma. *NEJM*. 2007;356(2):115–124.

Motzer RJ, Mazumdar M, Bacik J, Berg W, Amsterdam A, Ferrara J. Survival and prognostic stratification of 670 patients with advanced renal cell carcinoma. *J Clin Oncol*. 1999;17(8):2530–2540.

Motzer RJ, Michaelson MD, Redman BG, et al. Activity of SU11248, a multitargeted inhibitor of vascular endothelial growth factor receptor and platelet-derived growth factor receptor, in patients with metastatic renal cell carcinoma. *J Clin Oncol*. 2006;24(1):16–24.

Motzer RJ, Rini BI, Bukowski RM, et al. Sunitinib in patients with metastatic renal cell carcinoma. *JAMA*. 2006;295(21):2516–2524.

Negrier S, Escudier B, Lasset C, et al. Recombinant human interleukin-2, recombinant human interferon alfa-2a, or both in metastatic renal-cell carcinoma. Groupe Francais d'Immunotherapie. *N Engl J Med*. 1998;338(18):1272–1278.

Ratain MJ, Eisen T, Stadler WM, et al. Phase II placebo-controlled randomized discontinuation trial of sorafenib in patients with metastatic renal cell carcinoma. *J Clin Oncol*. 2006;24(16):2505–2512.

Schmidt LS, Nickerson ML, Angeloni D, et al. Early onset hereditary papillary renal carcinoma: germline missense mutations in the tyrosine kinase domain of the met proto-oncogene. *J Urol*. 2004;172(4 Pt 1):1256–1261.

Schmidt LS, Nickerson ML, Warren MB, et al. Germline BHD-mutation spectrum and phenotype analysis of a large cohort of families with Birt-Hogg-Dube syndrome. *Am J Hum Genet*. 2005;76(6):1023–1033.

Schmidt LS, Warren MB, Nickerson ML, et al. Birt-Hogg-Dube syndrome, a genodermatosis associated with spontaneous pneumothorax and kidney neoplasia, maps to chromosome 17p11.2. *Am
J Hum Genet*. 2001;69(4):876–882.

Yagoda A, Abi-Rached B, Petrylak D. Chemotherapy for advanced renal-cell carcinoma: 1983-1993.
Semin Oncol. 1995;22(1):42–60.

Yang JC, Haworth L, Sherry RM, et al. A randomized trial of bevacizumab, an anti-vascular endothelial
growth factor antibody, for metastatic renal cancer. *NEJM*. 2003;349(5):427–434.

Yang JC, Sherry RM, Steinberg SM, et al. Randomized study of high-dose and low-dose interleukin-2
in patients with metastatic renal cancer. *J Clin Oncol*. 2003;21(16):3127–3132.

Zbar B, Tory K, Merino M, et al. Hereditary papillary renal cell carcinoma. *J Urol*. 1994;151(3):
561–566.

14

Prostate Cancer

James L. Gulley and William L. Dahut

EPIDEMIOLOGY

- Prostate cancer (CaP) is the most common noncutaneous malignancy and the second most frequent cause of cancer-related mortality in men in the United States; 1 in 6 American men will be diagnosed with CaP and 1 in 35 will die from the disease.
- Frequency of clinically aggressive disease varies geographically, but frequency of occult tumors does not, suggesting the influence of environmental factors in the etiology of CaP. Studies of Japanese immigrants to the United States show that incidence of CaP increases after immigration.

RISK FACTORS

- Age: Risk increases progressively with age, with about 70% of cases in men over the age of 65.
- Family history: Risk increases twofold with a first-degree relative diagnosed with CaP, fivefold with two first-degree relatives.
- Race: In the United States, incidence is highest among African Americans, followed by whites, then Asians. African-American men are more likely to be diagnosed with advanced disease and have a greater than twofold risk of death from the disease.
- Geography: Risk is lowest in Asia; high in Scandinavia and the United States.
- Diet: Consumption of red meat and animal fat have been associated with CaP, while eating cruciferous vegetables, soy products, and lycopene-containing tomato products may be protective.

CHEMOPREVENTION TRIALS

Prostate Cancer Prevention Trial

- The Prostate Cancer Prevention trial compared the efficacy of finasteride, a 5-α reductase inhibitor, to placebo in preventing CaP in asymptomatic men older than 50 years who had a normal digital rectal examination (DRE) and a prostate-specific antigen (PSA) of $\leq$3.0 ng/mL.
- Of the more than 9,000 men enrolled, 24.8% in the placebo arm and 18.4% in the finasteride arm developed CaP within 7 years ($P <$0.001).
- The finasteride group showed an increase in Gleason score (GS) of 7 to 10 tumors, with 6.4% being affected compared to 5.1% in the placebo group. However, a pathology review of prostatectomy specimens did not confirm this increase, indicating potential sampling bias in the biopsies, perhaps due to a preferential reduction in normal versus tumor tissue caused by finasteride. Longer follow-up is needed to determine the clinical course of these patients.

Selenium and Vitamin E Cancer Prevention Trial (SELECT)

- Retrospective data from two previous chemoprevention trials have suggested a preventive role for selenium and vitamin E supplementation. SELECT enrolled over 35,000 men at least 50 years old and found that selenium or vitamin E, alone or in combination did not prevent prostate cancer.

SCREENING

- Screening for CaP involves testing for levels of PSA and/or DRE. Screening of asymptomatic men is controversial. Debate centers on whether biologically and clinically significant cancers are being detected early enough to reduce mortality or, conversely, whether cancers detected by screening would cause clinically significant disease if left undetected and untreated. Autopsy series have shown that more men die with, rather than from, CaP, and the rate of occult CaP in men in their eighties is approximately 75%.
- The Prostate, Lung, Colon, and Ovary (PLCO) screening trial and the European Study on Screening for Prostate Cancer are evaluating clinical outcomes based on screening versus no screening. Preliminary data from the PLCO trial reveal that the rate of death from prostate cancer was very low and did not differ significantly between subjects assigned to screening or no screening, with 7 to 10 years of follow-up. One caveat is that a high number of patients (about 50%) in the control arm obtained PSA screening. Preliminary data from the European study suggest that PSA screening was associated with a reduction in rate of death from prostate cancer by 20% after a median follow-up of 9 years. However, 1,410 men would need to be screened and 48 additional cases of prostate cancer would need to be treated to prevent one death from prostate cancer. Final results for these studies are expected in approximately 5 years.
- Despite the controversy, PSA screening in the United States is widespread. Advocates recommend annual screening beginning at age 50 for average-risk men and at age 40 for African-American men and men with a family history of CaP.
- Frank discussions with patients about the risks and potential benefits of screening should be standard practice.

SIGNS AND SYMPTOMS

- With PSA screening now widely practiced, most men are asymptomatic at diagnosis.
- Patients with local or regional disease may be asymptomatic or have lower urinary tract symptoms similar to those of benign prostatic hypertrophy. Men with regional disease occasionally have hematuria.
- Symptoms of metastatic disease include bone pain and weight loss; spinal cord compression is rare.

WORKUP AND STAGING

Biopsy

- Abnormal PSA and/or DRE is followed by transrectal ultrasound with core biopsy (generally 10–12 cores). Historically, a PSA of >4 ng/mL was the threshold for biopsy, but recent data suggest that cancers can be seen with lower PSA levels. A negative biopsy should prompt reassessment in 6 months with repeat biopsy as needed.

Pathology

- 95% of CaPs are adenocarcinomas. Adenocarcinoma arises in the peripheral zone of the prostate in approximately 70% of patients.
- Sarcoma, lymphoma, small cell carcinoma, and transitional carcinoma of the prostate are rare.
- Although visceral or osteolytic bone metastases are found in a few patients with metastatic adenocarcinoma of the prostate, careful pathologic examination should be performed to rule out a nonadenocarcinoma variant, as treatment regimens differ.
- Primary and secondary Gleason grades are determined by the histologic architecture of biopsy tissue. The primary grade denotes the dominant histologic pattern; the secondary grade represents the bulk of the nondominant pattern or a focal high-grade area. Primary and secondary grades range from 1 (well differentiated) to 5 (poorly differentiated). The combined grades comprise the GS (range 2–10).
- There is growing consensus that the highest GS is most predictive of clinical outcome. With current grading practices, scores <6 are very rare. A GS of 8 to 10 represents poorly differentiated CaP that is likely to be clinically aggressive.
- Because of sampling bias, GS may change following radical prostatectomy (RP) (20% of scores are upgraded and up to 10% are downgraded).

- Prostatic intraepithelial neoplasia (PIN), and perhaps proliferative inflammatory atrophy (PIA), are considered precursor lesions.

Baseline Evaluation

- In candidates for local treatment, a bone scan is indicated for bone pain, T3 or T4, GS >7, or PSA >10 ng/mL. There is no clinical evidence that a baseline bone scan improves survival in patients with better prognostic factors.
- In candidates for surgery, computed tomography (CT) or magnetic resonance imaging (MRI) of the abdomen and pelvis is obtained for T3 and T4 lesions, PSA >20 ng/mL, or GS >7 to detect enlarged lymph nodes. Endorectal MRI may help in determining the presence of extraprostatic extension. CT scans aid in treatment planning for radiation therapy (RT).
- Baseline laboratory tests include complete blood count, creatinine level, PSA (if not yet done), and alkaline phosphatase level.

PROGNOSTIC FACTORS

- Stage (Table 14.1)
- Gleason grade/score
- PSA level
- Number of cores and percentage of each core involved
- Age at diagnosis

TABLE 14.1. *Tumor-node-metastasis (TNM) system of classification and staging of prostate cancer*

T1	Tumor not palpable or visible by imaging
T1a	Tumor incidental finding in ≤5% of tissue resected (TURP)
T1b	Tumor incidental finding in >5% of tissue resected (TURP)
T1c	Tumor identified by needle biopsy alone (after PSA is found to be elevated)
T2	Tumor confined to the prostate
T2a	Tumor involves half of a lobe or less
T2b	Tumor involves more than half of a lobe, but not both lobes
T2c	Tumor involves both lobes
T3	Tumor extends through the prostatic capsule
T3a	Extracapsular extension (unilateral or bilateral)
T3b	Tumor invades the seminal vesicle(s)
T4	Tumor is fixed or invades adjacent structures other than seminal vesicles: bladder neck, external sphincter, rectum, levator muscles, and/or pelvic wall
N0	No regional lymph node metastasis
N1	Metastases in regional lymph node(s)
M0	No distant metastases
M1	Distant metastases
M1a	Nonregional LN
M1b	Bone(s)
M1c	Other

Stage grouping

I	T1a	N0	M0	GS 2–4
II	T1a	N0	M0	GS ≥5
	T1b,c	N0	M0	Any GS
	T1/2	N0	M0	Any GS
III	T3	N0	M0	Any GS
IV	T4	N0	M0	Any GS
	Any T	N1	M0	Any GS
	Any T	Any N	M1	Any GS

TURP, transurethral resection of the prostate; PSA, prostate-specific antigen.

TREATMENT OF LOCALIZED DISEASE

Active Surveillance

For men 60 to 75 years of age with a >10-year life expectancy or low-grade (GS ≤6), T1c-T2a tumors, active surveillance is a reasonable alternative to immediate local therapy (Table 14.2). In addition, men 50 to 60 years of age with those same features and low-volume (<3 cores, <50% of any one core involved) tumor may also be candidates for active surveillance. For patients with a <10-year life expectancy, CaP-specific mortality is very low and local definitive therapy may not be appropriate.

Surgery

Radical Prostatectomy

- Approaches include retropubic (RRP), perineal (RPP), or laparoscopic, with the latter often done with robotic assistance (RALP). Typical hospital stays are 1 to 2 days, with 7 to 14 days of urethral catheterization. Surgeries are somewhat longer with RALP, but hospital stays are usually shorter.
- Pelvic lymph node dissection may be performed at the time of RP in patients at high risk of developing positive lymph nodes, but may not be necessary in patients with T1c disease, PSA <10 ng/mL, and GS <7.
- Nerve-sparing RP may conserve potency in men with disease not adjacent to the neurovascular bundles that travel posterior-lateral to the prostate. The bilateral nerve-sparing technique is associated with 60% to 90% of patients recovering spontaneous erections versus only 10% to 50% with the unilateral technique. Both groups, however, may respond to oral therapy for erectile dysfunction.
- There is no role for neoadjuvant androgen-deprivation therapy (ADT) prior to RP.
- Patients with microscopic lymph node metastasis diagnosed following RP may have a longer overall survival (OS) if given ADT immediately than at time of clinical recurrence.
- Salvage RP following RT may be done in select cases where local disease is organ-confined. However, salvage RP is more technically demanding and is associated with higher morbidity.

Surgical Complications

- Immediate morbidity or mortality: 2%
- Impotence: 35% to 60%
- Urinary incontinence: 10% with frank incontinence; up to 60% require protective garments
- Urinary stricture
- Fecal incontinence: retropubic approach, approximately 5%; perineal approach, 18%
- The Prostate Cancer Outcomes Study found statistically significant differences in outcomes following RP or RT. For patients with normal baseline function, RP was associated with inferior urinary function, better bowel function, and similar sexual dysfunction compared with RT.

Cryosurgery

Cryosurgery destroys CaP cells through probes that subject prostate tissue to freezing followed by thawing. This procedure is associated with high rates of erectile dysfunction due to freezing of the

TABLE 14.2. *Treatment by stage/disease state*

Stage/disease state	Suggested treatment options
Localized disease (stage I, II)	RP, RT, primary ADT, or active surveillance
Locally advanced (stage III or T_4) or high risk	RP + ADT
Biochemical progression	Consider ADT
Nonmetastatic castration-sensitive CaP	Clinical trials, second-line ADT
Metastatic castration-sensitive CaP	ADT
Metastatic CRPC	Docetaxel, clinical trials, second-line ADT

RP, radical prostatectomy; RT, radiation therapy; ADT, androgen-deprivation therapy; CaP, prostate cancer; CRPC, castration-resistant prostate cancer.

neurovascular bundle. There are fewer data on long-term outcomes for cryosurgery than for RT or RP, and cryosurgery has no defined role in definitive therapy. Thus, at most centers prostate cryotherapies are largely salvage procedures. Side effects include incontinence, impotence, and injury to the bladder outlet and rectal tissues.

Radiation Therapy

External Beam RT (EBRT)

- EBRT targets the whole prostate, frequently including a margin of extraprostatic tissue, seminal vesicles, and pelvic lymph nodes.
- Higher doses ($\geq$78 Gy) given over approximately 8 weeks are associated with higher PSA control rates; however, survival data are not mature.
- Three-dimensional (3D) conformal RT allows for maximal doses conforming to the treatment field, while sparing normal tissue.
- Intensity-modulated RT is a type of 3D conformal RT that is designed to conform even more precisely to the target.
- Unlike x-rays, which radiate beyond the target volume, proton beam irradiation focuses virtually all its energy within a very small area, thus theoretically minimizing damage to normal tissue.

RT With Adjuvant ADT

At least three randomized controlled trials have shown that combining ADT with RT in patients at high risk for recurrent disease (Table 14.3) improves OS. ADT is usually given during RT and for 2 to 3 years thereafter. It may also be used for 2 months prior to RT to help decrease tumor size and thus the target volume of RT.

Adjuvant RT

Two randomized controlled trials have shown a 50% decrease in PSA relapse in patients with high-risk features at RP who were treated immediately with RT. Survival data are not yet mature.

Salvage RT

For select patients with rising PSA after RP and a high likelihood of organ-confined local recurrence (e.g., PSA <1.5 and slowly rising), salvage RT may be considered. However, there are limited data on which to make recommendations.

Brachytherapy

Interstitial brachytherapy with radioactive palladium or iodine seeds that delivers a much higher dose of radiation to the prostate is used in CaP patients with low-risk tumors and some intermediate patients. Better definition of tumor volume and radiation dosimetry have made this outpatient technique more accurate. CT and/or transrectal ultrasound are used to guide seed placement.

TABLE 14.3. *Risk categories for post-therapy prostate-specific antigen failure*

	Low	Intermediate	High
Stage	T1c, T2a	T2b	T2c
PSA	<10	10–20	>20
Gleason score	$\leq$6	7	$\geq$8
Qualifier	and	or	or
5-year risk of biochemical failure	<25%	25–50%	>50%

Source: Adapted from D'Amico AV, Whittington R, Malkowicz SB, et al. Optimizing patient selection for dose escalation techniques using the prostate-specific antigen level, biopsy Gleason score, and clinical T-stage. *Int J Radiat Oncol Biol Phys.* 1999;45(5):1227–1233.

Combined EBRT and Brachytherapy

EBRT and brachytherapy are increasingly used in combination. A 10-year review of this combination showed a biochemical relapse-free survival of 79% in T3 tumors. However, because no randomized trials have compared this combination with either modality alone, the treatment remains investigational.

Complications of RT

Acute

- Cystitis
- Proctitis/enteritis
- Fatigue

Long-term

- Impotence
- Incontinence (3%)
- Frequent bowel movements (10% more than with RP)
- Urethral stricture (RT delayed 4 weeks after transurethral resection of the prostate)

COMPARISON OF PRIMARY TREATMENT MODALITIES

Comparing treatment modalities in terms of overall and disease-free survival is difficult because of differences in study design, patient selection, and treatment techniques.

- While there have been no satisfactory randomized trials comparing RT with RP, these approaches appear to have equivalent PSA-free survival in appropriately matched patients at 5 years, but differ in type and frequency of side effects. One way to compare the two modalities is by PSA and PSA-free survival (also called biochemical relapse-free survival), provided that patients have reproducible PSA values on repeated measurement before their definitive primary therapy.
- Brachytherapy appears promising, although most studies have been conducted only in patients with early-stage, low-grade disease. One comparison of 3D conformational RT with ^{125}I implants in comparable patients concluded that these modalities had equivalent efficacy, with higher urinary complications in the brachytherapy group.

FOLLOW-UP AFTER DEFINITIVE TREATMENT

- Patients treated with curative intent should have PSA levels checked at least every 6 months for 5 years, then annually. Annual DRE is appropriate for detecting recurrence.
- After RP, a PSA of $\geq$0.3 ng/mL indicates a relapse. PSA failure after RT is defined as 2 ng/mL over the nadir, whether or not the patient had ADT with RT.

TREATMENT FOR MEN WITH RISING PSA AFTER LOCAL THERAPY

Treatment for patients who have rising PSA (biochemical failure) after local therapy has not been standardized, and participation in clinical trials should be encouraged. As previously mentioned, salvage RT, salvage RP, or salvage cryotherapy may be offered to select patients with local recurrence. ADT effectively lowers PSA and can be given intermittently to provide periods of normal testosterone. Based on preliminary results from randomized studies, CaP-specific outcomes with intermittent and continuous ADT appear to be similar. However, there are no data suggesting better survival with ADT than with no ADT. Recent data suggest that on average, men live about 14 years after biochemical failure. Thus a more conservative approach (e.g., treating when symptomatic) is a reasonable option for many men.

TREATMENT OF SYSTEMIC DISEASE

Response Criteria

Only 40% of patients with castration-resistant prostate cancer (CRPC, or progressing disease despite castrate levels of testosterone) have soft tissue disease. Therefore, PSA remains an important tumor marker following response to therapy. PSA response rates (PRRs) are defined as percentage of patients with a PSA decline >50%, a traditionally used criterion. Ranges of PRRs are given when available; confidence intervals are not shown but are generally wide. Because of differences in patient selection, it is difficult to compare clinical trials by PRRs alone. Many trials now include all PSA declines in a "waterfall plot." It is important to note that some agents (particularly cytostatic agents) may up-regulate or down-regulate PSA expression independent of their effect on cancer growth. Definitive studies to date have utilized quality of life and OS for CRPC.

Androgen-Deprivation Therapy

- ADT is the mainstay of treatment for metastatic CaP. However, as discussed previously, it has also been used to treat localized disease and in neoadjuvant and adjuvant settings with RT. CaP cells usually respond to hormonal manipulations that block the production of androgens, producing durable remissions and significant palliation. Duration of response ranges from 12 to 18 months, with 20% of patients having a complete biochemical response at 5 years. However, ultimately, castration-resistant CaP cells emerge and lead to disease progression.
- Bilateral surgical castration and depot injections of GnRH-A (e.g., leuprolide, goserelin, and buserelin) provide equally effective testosterone suppression. Combined androgen blockade can be achieved by adding an oral androgen receptor antagonist (ARA; e.g., nilutamide, flutamide, and bicalutamide). However, this is controversial and provides little if any survival benefit.
- GnRH-A initially increases gonadotropin, causing a transient (~14-day) increase in testosterone that can lead to tumor flare. A lower tumor volume reduces the risk of symptomatic tumor flare. Tumor flare can be prevented by the use of an ARA, which binds to the androgen receptor (AR), effectively stopping the ability of the AR to activate cell growth. An ARA is often given for 1 week prior to GnRH-A in patients at risk for complications (pain, obstruction, and cord compression) associated with tumor flare. For high-risk patients, bilateral orchiectomy or ketoconazole can decrease testosterone more quickly.
- Combined androgen blockade is not currently the standard of care for initial treatment of metastatic disease. In patients initially treated with GnRH-A or surgical castration alone, the addition of an ARA may produce PSA declines or symptomatic improvement in up to 40% of patients.
- Use of estrogens such as diethylstilbestrol has fallen into disfavor due to adverse side effects. Therapeutic doses have been associated with a high incidence of cardiovascular complications and mortality in patients predisposed to cardiovascular disease.
- Continuous testosterone suppression is the current standard of care for patients with metastatic CaP.
- Continuing testosterone suppression after patients develop CRPC is also considered the standard of care. Androgens still play a very important role in driving the growth of CRPC. Levels of AR and intracellular androgens within the tumor cells are significantly elevated in these patients.
- The rationale for combined androgen blockade, ARA withdrawal, and additional ADT (e.g., ketoconazole) are discussed in the section below on second-line hormonal therapy.

Dosages and Side Effects of Hormonal Therapy

- Bilateral orchiectomy: Side effects include tumor flare, impotence, loss of libido, gynecomastia, hot flashes, and osteoporosis.
- GnRH agonists
  - Goserelin acetate (Zoladex): 3.6 mg s.c. every month or 10.8 mg s.c. every 3 months. Side effects: same as orchiectomy plus potential for transient tumor flare
  - Leuprolide acetate (Lupron): 7.5 mg s.c. every month or 22.5 mg i.m. every 3 months, or 30 mg s.c. every 4 months. Comparable efficacy with long-acting formulations. Side effects: same as goserelin

- Oral ARAs
  - Flutamide (Eulexin): 250 mg P.O. 3 times per day. Side effects: diarrhea, nausea, breast tenderness, hepatotoxicity, loss of libido, impotence
  - Bicalutamide (Casodex): 50 mg daily. Side effects: nausea, breast tenderness, hepatotoxicity, hot flashes, loss of libido, impotence
  - Nilutamide (Nilandron): 150 mg P.O. daily. Side effects: pulmonary fibrosis (rare), visual field changes (night blindness or abnormal adaptation to darkness), hepatotoxicity, impotence, loss of libido, hot flashes, nausea, disulfiram-like reaction
- Hot flashes from hormonal therapy can be treated with clonidine (0.1 mg/day), low-dose estrogens, or antidepressants.
- Painful gynecomastia can be prevented with EBRT to the breasts or may be treated with tamoxifen.
- Testosterone-lowering therapy causes a decrease in estradiol, which is needed to maintain bone density. Osteoporosis is increasingly being diagnosed in patients receiving ADT, especially those on long-term ADT or with baseline osteoporosis prior to ADT. Patients receiving ADT should be given daily vitamin D and calcium supplements unless contraindicated. Obtain baseline bone mineral density before starting long-term ADT. Treatment with bisphosphonates should be considered in patients with low bone mineral density.

ARA Withdrawal

- Historically, 20% of patients treated with combined androgen blockade have a PSA decline of $\geq 50\%$ upon discontinuation of oral ARA (range, 15–33%), although these declines generally last only 3 to 5 months. This proportion may be lower with less long-term ARA use.
- Decreases in cancer-related anemia and pain are also reported.
- ARA withdrawal response occurs within 4 to 6 weeks, depending on the ARA's half-life.

Second-Line ADT

Some patients with rising PSA after ARA withdrawal will benefit from switching to other ARAs or initiating treatment with ketoconazole or glucocorticoids. A minimum of 1 month of therapy is required to assess patient response. A substantial minority of patients (35–50%) will have PSA declines with second-line and even third-line ADT.

Adrenal Androgen Inhibitors

Adrenal androgen inhibitors work by achieving a "medical adrenalectomy," which further decreases androgen production. Responses have been seen in patients after ARA withdrawal. Glucocorticoid replacements are important for patients receiving adrenal androgen inhibitors. The usual regimen is hydrocortisone 20 mg every morning and 10 mg every evening, increased to 20 mg p.o. 2 times per day if patients show symptoms of glucocorticoid insufficiency (e.g., fatigue).

Regimens and Toxicities

- Ketoconazole + hydrocortisone (PRR = 35–50%)
  - Ketoconazole (Nizoral): 200 mg p.o. 3 times per day, increasing to 400 mg p.o. 3 times per day + hydrocortisone 20 mg p.o. twice a day
  - Side effects: impotence, pruritus, nail changes, adrenal insufficiency, nausea, emesis, and hepatotoxicity. Liver transaminases need to be monitored. Ketoconazole is absorbed at an acidic pH; therefore, the concomitant use of H_2 blockers, antacids, or proton pump inhibitors should be avoided. Coating agents such as sucralfate may be substituted. Because ketoconazole is a potent inhibitor of CYP3A4, multiple drug interactions, such as with statins, can lead to rhabdomyolysis due to increased concentration of statins. If statins must be used, consider pravastatin.

- Corticosteroids (PRR = 18–22%)
  - Corticosteroids alone have been shown to ease pain in patients with symptomatic bone metastases.
  - Prednisone: 5 mg p.o. every morning and 2.5 mg p.o. every evening, increasing to 5 mg p.o. twice a day. Side effects: same as for any medical use of prednisone

CHEMOTHERAPY FOR CRPC

Patients who develop CRPC have a median survival of about 18 months. Chemotherapy with docetaxel has been shown to improve OS in patients with CRPC.

- Docetaxel (Taxotere) (PRR = 45%)
  - Improved median OS from 16.5 months (mitoxantrone/prednisone) to 18.9 months ($P = 0.0005$) and improved quality of life (Functional Assessment of Cancer Therapy-Prostate, 22% vs. 13%; $P = 0.009$).
  - Docetaxel 75 mg/m^2 i.v.
  - Prednisone 5 mg twice daily
  - Cycle is repeated every 21 days
  - Side effects: grade 3 toxicity: granulocytopenia (32%), infection (5.7%), anemia (4.9%), fatigue (4.5%); any grade of toxicity: anemia (67%), neutropenia (41%), fluid retention (24%), sensory neuropathy (30%), nausea (41%), fatigue (53%), myalgia (15%), alopecia (65%)

- Mitoxantrone (Novantrone) + prednisone (PRR = 33%)
  - Shown to improve quality of life, but not disease-free survival or OS, in two randomized controlled trials versus steroids alone.
  - Prednisone 5 mg p.o. twice on day 1 + mitoxantrone 12 mg/m^2 i.v. on day 21; delayed if not recovered hematologically
  - Mitoxantrone is stopped at a cumulative dose of 140 mg/m^2. Prochlorperazine is used as an antiemetic.
  - Side effects: cardiac abnormalities in 6% of patients in the mitoxantrone-only arm (2% with congestive heart failure), neutropenic fever (1.1%), neutropenia (45%), thrombocytopenia (5%), nausea and vomiting (29%), and alopecia (26%); exacerbation of diabetes in one patient.

- Docetaxel (Taxotere) + carboplatin (PRR = 18%)
  - Single-arm phase 2 trial of patients ($n = 34$) who progressed on docetaxel-based chemotherapy
  - PR in 14%; median progression-free survival: 3 months; median OS: 12.4 months
  - Patients who previously responded to docetaxel are more likely to respond to this combination.

FOLLOW-UP FOR PATIENTS WITH METASTATIC DISEASE

For patients with metastatic disease, type and intensity of follow-up are determined by degree of clinical progression:

- Follow-up at 3 months (with PSA) is reasonable for patients who respond well to hormonal therapy. Interlaboratory variation in PSA levels should be noted.
- Bone scans are indicated based on clinical parameters and should not be routinely ordered.
- Patients with bone metastases are at risk for spinal cord compression; MRI should be ordered when signs or symptoms suggest this complication.

MANAGEMENT OF BONE METASTASES

- RT directed to painful spinal cord metastases provides palliation in approximately 80% of patients. Side effects generally are limited to fatigue and anemia that is usually reversible. Generally, the painful vertebral lesion and the two vertebrae superior to and inferior to the lesion are treated with

30 Gy. The spinal cord can tolerate radiation up to approximately 50 Gy, so retreatment of some lesions may be considered.

- The radioisotope strontium-89 (Metastron), a calcium analog that preferentially localizes in the tumor, can provide palliation for widespread metastases. Strontium relieves bone pain in up to 75% of cases, typically after 1 to 3 weeks of treatment and for several months thereafter. Toxicities include flare (15%), often associated with a later response, and a reversible thrombocytopenia (25%) that usually resolves within 3 months. Strontium can often be readministered. Samarium-153 lexidronam (Quadramet) is a newer radioisotope with treatment indications similar to those of strontium, but a shorter half-life and less marrow toxicity.
- Bisphosphonates inhibit osteoclastic bone resorption and can decrease skeletal-related events in patients with advanced CRPC. Zoledronic acid 4 mg i.v. every 3 to 4 weeks has been approved for this indication. Side effects include infusion-related myalgias, renal dysfunction, and osteonecrosis of the jaw. Dose should be adjusted for renal insufficiency.
- Pain from bone metastases may be treated with narcotics and adjuncts.

Spinal Cord Compression

- Vertebral column metastases impinging on the spinal cord can cause spinal cord compression, an oncologic emergency common in patients with CaP who have widespread bone metastases.
- Pain is an early sign of spinal cord compression in more than 90% of patients. Muscle weakness or neurologic abnormalities are other indicators of spinal cord compression, along with weakness and/or sensory loss corresponding to the level of spinal cord compression, which often indicate irreversible damage. Genitourinary, gastrointestinal, or autonomic dysfunction are late signs; spinal cord compression usually progresses rapidly at this point.
- Diagnosis requires a thorough history and physical, with special attention to musculoskeletal and neurologic examinations. The standard for diagnosing and localizing spinal cord compression is MRI, usually with gadolinium. A myelogram may be used in patients with contraindications to MRI such as a pacemaker.
- High-dose steroids should be started (e.g., dexamethasone 100 mg i.v. followed by 4 mg i.v. or p.o. every 6 hours) as soon as history or neurologic examination suggests spinal cord compression. Neurologic or orthopedic surgeons and/or radiation oncologists should be consulted soon after diagnosis.
- RT is the usual treatment modality, given as 3,000 cGy in 10 fractions to the involved vertebra and the two superior and two inferior vertebrae.
- Surgical resection of the vertebral body should be considered in the following instances:
  - Patient has had previous RT of the involved area or requires spinal stabilization.
  - Patient experiences progression despite treatment with steroids and RT.
  - RT facilities are not locally available.
  - Patient has a rapidly progressive neurologic deficit. A recent randomized trial showed that patients subjected to decompressive surgical resection followed by RT retained the ability to walk significantly longer than those treated with RT alone.

SUGGESTED READINGS

Albertsen PC, Hanley JA, Gleason DF, Barry MJ. Competing risk analysis of men aged 55 to 74 years at diagnosis managed conservatively for clinically localized prostate cancer. *JAMA.* 1998;280(11): 975–980.

Bolla M, Collette L, Blank L, et al. Long-term results with immediate androgen suppression and external irradiation in patients with locally advanced prostate cancer (an EORTC study): a phase III randomised trial. *Lancet.* 2002;360(9327):103–106.

Bolla M, Gonzalez D, Warde P, et al. Improved survival in patients with locally advanced prostate cancer treated with radiotherapy and goserelin. *N Engl J Med.* 1997;337(5):295–300.

Andriole GL, Crawford ED, Grubb RL 3rd, et al. Mortality results from a randomized prostate-cancer screening trial. *N Engl J Med.* 2009;360(13):1310–9.

Bubley GJ, Carducci M, Dahut W, et al. Eligibility and response guidelines for phase II clinical trials in androgen-independent prostate cancer: recommendations from the Prostate-Specific Antigen Working Group. *J Clin Oncol* 1999;17(11):3461–3467.

Crawford ED, Eisenberger MA, McLeod DG, et al. A controlled trial of leuprolide with and without flutamide in prostatic carcinoma. *N Engl J Med.* 1989;321(7):419–424.

Critz FA, Williams WH, Levinson AK, Benton JB, Holladay CT, Schnell FJ Jr. Simultaneous irradiation for prostate cancer: intermediate results with modern techniques. *J Urol.* 2000;164(3 Pt 1): 738–741.

Daniell HW. Osteoporosis after orchiectomy for prostate cancer. *J Urol.* 1997;157(2):439–444.

Dattoli M, Wallner K, True L, Cash J, Sorace R. Long-term outcomes after treatment with external beam radiation therapy and palladium 103 for patients with higher risk prostate carcinoma: influence of prostatic acid phosphatase. *Cancer.* 2003;97(4):979–983.

Eisenberger MA, Blumenstein BA, Crawford ED, et al. Bilateral orchiectomy with or without flutamide for metastatic prostate cancer. *N Engl J Med.* 1998;339(15):1036–1042.

Freedland SJ, Humphreys EB, Mangold LA, et al. Risk of prostate cancer-specific mortality following biochemical recurrence after radical prostatectomy. *JAMA.* 2005;294(4):433–439.

Gleave M, Goldenberg L, Chin JL, et al. Natural history of progression after PSA elevation following radical prostatectomy: update. *J Urol.* 2003;169(4):A690.

Granfors T, Modig H, Damber JE, Tomic R. Combined orchiectomy and external radiotherapy versus radiotherapy alone for nonmetastatic prostate cancer with or without pelvic lymph node involvement: a prospective randomized study. *J Urol.* 1998;159(6):2030–2034.

Hanks GE, Pajak TF, Porter A, et al. Radiation Therapy Oncology Group. Phase III trial of long-term adjuvant androgen deprivation after neoadjuvant hormonal cytoreduction and radiotherapy in locally advanced carcinoma of the prostate: the Radiation Therapy Oncology Group Protocol 92-02. *J Clin Oncol.* 2003;21(21):3972–3978.

Kantoff PW, Halabi S, Conaway M, et al. Hydrocortisone with or without mitoxantrone in men with hormone-refractory prostate cancer: results of the Cancer and Leukemia Group B 9182 study. *J Clin Oncol.* 1999;17(8):2506–2513.

Lawton CA, Winter K, Murray K, et al. Updated results of the phase III Radiation Therapy Oncology Group (RTOG) trial 85-31 evaluating the potential benefit of androgen suppression following standard radiation therapy for unfavorable prognosis carcinoma of the prostate. *Int J Radiat Oncol Biol Phys.* 2001;49(4):937–946.

Lippman SM, Klein EA, Goodman PJ, et al. Effect of selenium and vitamin E on risk of prostate cancer and other cancers: the Selenium and Vitamin E Cancer Prevention Trial (SELECT). *JAMA.* 2009;301(1):39–51.

Medical Research Council Prostate Cancer Working Party Investigators Group. Immediate versus deferred treatment for advanced prostatic cancer: initial results of the Medical Research Council Trial. *Br J Urol.* 1997;79(2):235–246.

Messing E, Manola J, Sarosdy M, et al. Immediate hormonal therapy compared with observation after radical prostatectomy and pelvic lymphadenectomy in men with node positive prostate cancer: results at 10 years of EST 3886. *J Urol.* 2003;169(Suppl 4):A1480.

Penson DF, Mclerran D, Feng Z, et al. 5-year urinary and sexual outcomes after radical prostatectomy; results from the prostate cancer outcomes study. *J Urol.* 2005;173(5):1701–1705.

Petrylak DP, Tangen CM, Hussain MHA, et al. Docetaxel and estramustine compared with mitoxantrone and prednisone for advanced refractory prostate cancer. *N Engl J Med.* 2004;351(15):1513–1520.

Pilepich MV, Caplan R, Byhardt RW, et al. Phase III trial of androgen suppression using goserelin in unfavorable-prognosis carcinoma of the prostate treated with definitive radiotherapy: report of Radiation Therapy Oncology Group Protocol 85-31. *J Clin Oncol.* 1997;15(3):1013–101221.

Pilepich MV, Winter K, Lawton C, et al. Androgen suppression adjuvant to definitive radiotherapy in prostate carcinoma—long-term results of phase III RTOG 85-31. *Int J Radiat Oncol Biol Phys.* 2005 Apr 1;61(5):1285–90.

Potosky AL, Legler J, Albertsen PC. Health outcomes after prostatectomy or radiotherapy for prostate cancer: results from the Prostate Cancer Outcomes Study. *J Natl Cancer Inst.* 2000;92(19)1 582–1592.

Pound CR, Partin AW, Eisenberger MA, Chan DW, Pearson JD, Walsh PC. Natural history of progression after PSA elevation following radical prostatectomy. *JAMA.* 1999;281(17):1591–1597.

Saad F, Gleason DM, Murray R, et al. A randomized, placebo-controlled trial of zoledronic acid in patients with hormone-refractory metastatic prostate carcinoma. *J Natl Cancer Inst.* 2002;94(19): 1458–1468.

Schroder FH, Hugosson H, Roobol MJ, et al. Screening and prostate-cancer mortality in a randomized European study. *N Engl J Med.* 2009;360(13):1320–8.

Talcott JA, Rieker P, Clark JA, et al. Patient-reported symptoms after primary therapy for early prostate cancer: results of a prospective cohort study. *J Clin Oncol.* 1998;16(1):275–283.

Tannock IF, De Wit R, Berry WR, et al. Docetaxel plus prednisone or mitoxantrone plus prednisone for advanced prostate cancer. *N Engl J Med.* 2004; 351(15):1502–1512.

Thompson IM, Goodman PJ, Tangen CM, et al. The influence of finasteride on the development of prostate cancer. *N Engl J Med.* 2003;349(3):215–224.

15

Bladder Cancer

Jeanny B. Aragon-Ching and William L. Dahut

EPIDEMIOLOGY

It is estimated that 67,160 patients were diagnosed with bladder cancer in 2007 and that 13,750 died of the disease. There is a male:female predominant ratio of 3:1, with a peak incidence of occurrence in the seventh decade of life, making bladder cancer the fourth and eighth most commonly diagnosed cancer in men and women, respectively.

ETIOLOGY

- Cigarette smoking: Smoking is the most common cause of bladder cancer, with smokers having twice the risk of developing bladder cancer compared to nonsmokers. There is an association between the duration and amount of cigarette smoking and the development of bladder cancer in both transitional and squamous histology.
- Occupational exposures: Occupational exposures to chemical carcinogens are associated with an increased risk of bladder cancer. Workers exposed to arylamines in the dye, paint, rubber, and leather industries are at increased risk.
- Analgesics: The abuse of analgesics, particularly phenacetin, is associated with an increased risk of urothelial cancers, especially in the renal pelvis.
- Treatment-related risks: Prior treatment with pelvic radiation and cyclophosphamide increases the risk of urothelial cancers.
- Chronic infections or inflammation: In endemic areas, chronic infection with *Schistosoma haematobium* predisposes patients to develop squamous cell cancer (SCC) of the bladder as a result of squamous metaplasia. Individuals with an ongoing source of inflammation (i.e., a spinal cord injury patient with an indwelling catheter) have a higher incidence of bladder cancer, especially SCC, than the general population. Progressive inflammation of the renal parenchyma also occurs in patients with Balkan nephropathy, predisposing patients to low-grade cancers of the upper urinary tracts.
- Other factors: Other less-established and more controversial risk factors include use of artificial sweeteners, coffee consumption, and genetic factors.

PATHOLOGY

Transitional cell carcinoma (TCC) accounts for 90% to 95% of all bladder tumors in the United States. SCC accounts for 5% to 10% of bladder tumors, and adenocarcinomas make up 1% to 2%. Carcinomas in situ (CIS) are flat tumors that usually present as diffuse urothelial involvement in patients with superficial bladder tumors. CIS increases the risk of subsequent invasive disease and recurrence, whether it occurs alone or in association with superficial bladder tumors. Patients with upper-tract urothelial tumors have a 20% to 40% incidence of synchronous or metachronous bladder cancer. Patients with bladder cancer have about a 1% to 4% incidence of synchronous or metachronous upper-tract tumor.

CHAPTER 15

CLINICAL FEATURES

Painless gross or microscopic hematuria occurs in about 85% of patients, and symptoms of bladder irritability are seen in 20% of patients. Patients with invasive disease may present with flank pain due to ureteral obstruction, bladder mass, or lower extremity edema. Constitutional symptoms such as weight loss, abdominal pain, or bone pain may be present in patients with advanced disease.

SCREENING

Hematuria is the most common presenting symptom of patients with bladder cancer. Studies evaluating the role of screening for bladder cancer have examined the utility of conventional Hemastix® testing. However, because hematuria per se is nonspecific, patients who test positive for hematuria need to undergo further tests to determine its etiology. Other noninvasive screening methods have been used, such as urine cytology or urine-based markers. Markers such as nuclear matrix protein 22, bladder tumor antigen, cytokeratins, and many others have widely variable sensitivity and specificity. Therefore, definitive diagnosis can be established only by cystoscopy and biopsy.

DIAGNOSIS AND STAGING WORKUP

Diagnostic workup of a patient with suspected bladder cancer includes intravenous pyelography, urinary cytologic studies, and cystoscopy with full evaluation of the bladder mucosa and urethra. Patients presenting with positive cytology but without gross abnormalities on cystoscopy must undergo examination of the upper tracts; male patients must also have a prostate examination. Computerized tomography scan of the abdomen and pelvis is performed to detect local extension and involvement of abdominal lymph nodes. Chest x-ray is used for initial screening for pulmonary metastases. Bone scan is recommended for patients with elevated alkaline phosphatase level or bone pain. Transurethral resection of the bladder tumor (TURBT) primarily determines clinical staging, with inclusion of muscularis propria in the specimen a must for appropriate diagnosis.

Staging

The staging of bladder cancer (Tables 15.1 and 15.2; Fig. 15.1) is the most important independent prognostic variable for progression and overall survival (OS). Bladder cancers are classified as superficial, muscle-invasive, and metastatic. Superficial bladder cancers are tumors that involve only the mucosa (Ta) or submucosa (T1) and flat CIS (Tis) and account for 75% of bladder cancers. Of the superficial bladder cancers, about 60% are Ta tumors, 30% are T1, and 10% are CIS. Most superficial bladder cancers recur within 6 to 12 months with the same stage, but 10% to 15% of patients may develop invasive or metastatic disease. Low-grade (grade 1 or 2, solitary) and lower stage (Ta) tumors have lower recurrence and progression rates than high-risk disease (T1 associated with CIS, grade 3 or multifocal). Invasive bladder cancers are tumors that invade the muscularis propria (T2), perivesical tissues (T3), or adjacent structures (T4). Patients with muscle-invasive disease have a 50% likelihood of occult distant metastases at the time of diagnosis. The usual sites of metastases are pelvic lymph nodes, liver, lung, bone, adrenal glands, and intestine. Patients with node-positive disease have stage IV bladder cancer.

PROGNOSIS

- The major prognostic factors are tumor stage at the time of diagnosis and degree of tumor differentiation.
- Five-year survival rates for patients with superficial, muscle-invasive, and metastatic bladder cancer are 95%, 50%, and 6%, respectively. Median OS for superficial bladder cancer is 10 years, with a

TABLE 15.1. *Tumor/node/metastasis (TNM) staging of bladder cancer*

Primary tumor (T)

TX	Primary tumor cannot be assessed
T0	No evidence of primary tumor
Ta	Noninvasive papillary carcinoma
Tis*	Carcinoma in situ ("flat tumor")
T1	Tumor invades subepithelial connective tissue
T2	Tumor invades muscle
T2a	Tumor invades superficial muscle (inner half)
T2b	Tumor invades deep muscle (outer half)
T3	Tumor invades perivesical tissue
T3a	Tumor invades perivesical tissue microscopically
T3b	Tumor invades perivesical tissue macroscopically (extravesical mass)
T4	Tumor invades any of the following: prostate, uterus, vagina, pelvic wall, or abdominal wall
T4a	Tumor invades the prostate, uterus, vagina
T4b	Tumor invades the pelvic wall and abdominal wall

Regional lymph nodes (N) (within true pelvis; all others are distant lymph nodes)

NX	Regional lymph nodes cannot be assessed
N0	No regional lymph node metastasis
N1	Metastasis in a single lymph node, ≤2 cm in greatest dimension
N2	Metastasis in a single lymph node, between 2 cm and 5 cm in greatest dimension; or multiple lymph nodes, taken together ≤5 cm in greatest dimension
N3	Metastasis in a single lymph node, >5 cm in greatest dimension

Distant metastasis (M)

MX	Distant metastasis cannot be assessed
M0	No distant metastasis
M1	Distant metastasis

*The suffix "is" may be added to any T to indicate the presence of associated carcinoma in situ. The suffix "m" should be added to the appropriate T category to indicate multiple lesions.

Source: From American Joint Committee on Cancer. *AJCC Cancer Staging Manual.* 6th ed. New York: Springer Science and Business Media; 2002, with permission.

natural history characterized by recurrence of superficial tumor or progression to muscle-invasive disease. Non–muscle-invasive tumors recur in 60% to 70% of cases; about one-third of these progress to a higher stage or grade.

- Other adverse prognostic factors include old age, expression of p53, aneuploidy, tumor multifocality, and palpable mass.

TABLE 15.2. *Stage grouping of carcinoma of the bladder by TNM involvement*

	T1	T2	T3	T4a	T4b
N0	Stage I	Stage II	Stage III	Stage III	
N1					
N2					
N3					
M1					

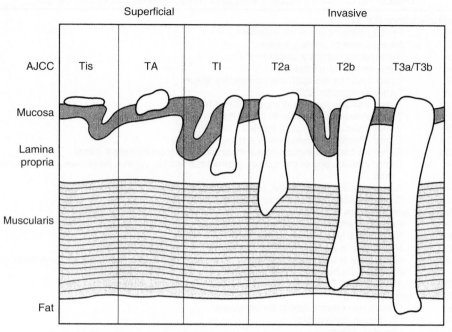

Fig. 15.1. Clinical staging of carcinoma of the bladder.

TREATMENT

Fig. 15.2 shows an algorithm for treatment of bladder cancer.

Superficial or Non–Muscle-invasive Bladder Cancer

- TURBT remains the cornerstone of treatment for grade 1 to 2 Ta and low-risk T1 superficial bladder cancers. In addition to observation after TURBT, intravesical bacillus Calmette-Guerin (BCG) therapy is recommended for high-risk disease (grade 3 Ta, CIS and grade 3 T1).
- Intravesical therapy: Primarily used as an adjunct after TURBT to lower the incidence of disease recurrence.
- Intravesical chemotherapy: Chemotherapeutic agents used for intravesical instillation include thiotepa, doxorubicin, epirubicin, and mitomycin C. Data suggest that currently available intravesical chemotherapeutic agents are equally effective but differ in toxicity. Although no standardized dosing or scheduling have been established as the optimum delivery for intravesical chemotherapy, a meta-analysis showed one dose of cytotoxic chemotherapy reduced the risk of recurrence by 39%. Patients with low-grade solitary papillary tumors particularly benefited. Thus, in addition to observation after TURBT, an option for a grade 1 to 2, clinical stage Ta lesion would be administration of a single dose of intravesical chemotherapy within 24 hours of TURBT.
- Immunotherapy with BCG has shown statistically significant clinical benefits, including induction of complete response (CR) in CIS (70–75%) and reduction of rates of recurrence in non-CIS (20–57%), but has shown no consistent reduction in tumor progression. Maintenance BCG has been shown to reduce recurrence, but optimal dose scheduling and duration have not been determined.
- Intravesical valrubicin is FDA approved for BCG-refractory patients who refuse or are intolerant of cystectomy. Other agents used in this population include gemcitabine and cotreatment with BCG and interferon alpha-2b.

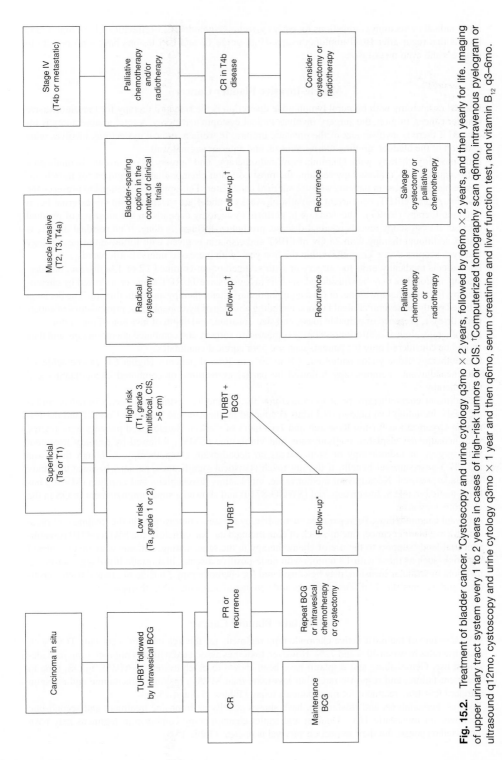

Fig. 15.2. Treatment of bladder cancer. *Cystoscopy and urine cytology q3mo × 2 years, followed by q6mo × 2 years, and then yearly for life. Imaging of upper urinary tract system every 1 to 2 years in cases of high-risk tumors or CIS. †Computerized tomography scan q6mo, intravenous pyelogram or ultrasound q12mo, cystoscopy and urine cytology q3mo × 1 year and then q6mo, serum creatinine and liver function test, and vitamin B_{12} q3–6mo.

• Early radical cystectomy: Indications for early cystectomy include BCG-refractory CIS or high-grade lesions that recur after BCG immunotherapy. High-grade T1 and CIS lesions have a propensity to progress and even metastasize.

Muscle-Invasive Bladder Cancer

• Radical cystectomy with bilateral lymph node dissection is the standard therapy for muscle-invasive bladder cancer. In men, the surgery involves radical cystoprostatectomy. A total urethrectomy is indicated if there is involvement of the prostatic urethra. In women, radical cystectomy involves wide excision of the bladder, urethra, uterus, adnexa, and anterior vaginal wall.

• Multimodality therapy with chemotherapy, radiotherapy, and surgery: Concurrent chemotherapy with cisplatin plus radiotherapy remains the most common chemoradiation regimen for muscle-invasive bladder cancer in patients who are surgical candidates. This approach attempts to preserve the bladder. After TURBT, concurrent cisplatin on weeks 1 and 4 are given with 40 Gy external beam radiation therapy (EBRT). The decision to perform cystectomy depends on the presence of residual disease. If cystoscopy reveals residual disease, prompt cystectomy is done. If no residual disease is found, additional therapy with 25 Gy of EBRT and cisplatin is given with follow-up urine cytology and cystoscopies every 3 months within the first year, with increased intervals afterwards.

• For patients medically unfit for surgery or with selected organ-confined T2 or T3a disease, bladder-sparing approaches may be considered, such as (a) aggressive TURBT alone or followed by chemotherapy, (b) radiotherapy alone, or (c) a combination of chemotherapy and radiotherapy. The decision is based partly on several clinical factors, including absence of hydronephrosis, prior history of superficial disease, presence of palpable mass, and size, location, and depth of invasion of the tumor.

• Radiotherapy alone has inferior outcomes compared to surgery and combined chemotherapy and thus should be considered only for patients who are poor surgical candidates.

• Chemotherapy alone yields pathologic CR in 20% to 30% of patients. Higher CR can be achieved with neoadjuvant chemotherapy followed by partial cystectomy or combined chemotherapy and radiotherapy.

• Neoadjuvant chemotherapy prior to cystectomy for T2 and T3 lesions has been studied in multiple trials, including two randomized trials conducted by the Medical Research Council and the European Organization for the Research and Treatment of Cancer. Randomized patients were treated with neoadjuvant cisplatin, methotrexate, and vinblastine (CMV), followed by primary treatment with surgery or radiotherapy or both, versus no neoadjuvant chemotherapy. Although there was a 5.5% 3-year survival benefit, it did not reach statistical significance, perhaps because the study was underpowered. Neoadjuvant methotrexate, vinblastine, doxorubicin, and cisplatin (MVAC) has been studied in a U.S. Intergroup trial (SWOG-8710) and showed a small improvement in OS in the chemotherapy arm.

• Adjuvant chemotherapy: Postoperative chemotherapy remains controversial in the treatment of muscle-invasive bladder cancer due to a lack of convincing data. Nevertheless, the SWOG-8710 neoadjuvant trial lends support to the use of chemotherapy in the same setting. Patients who are considered high risk, such as those with T2 tumors with node-positive disease, high-grade histology, transmural invasion, or vascular invasion, may be considered for chemotherapy. Outside of clinical trials, physicians and patients should discuss the risks and benefits of adjuvant chemotherapy.

Metastatic Bladder Cancer

• MVAC is one of the most active chemotherapy regimens for the treatment of metastatic TCC, with response rates between 40% and 72%. However, toxicities associated with this regimen limit its widespread use. Gemcitabine and cisplatin have been shown to be equivalent to MVAC in OS, time to treatment failure, and response rates, but less toxic than MVAC, making gemcitabine and cisplatin standard first-line treatment for most patients today (Tables 15.3 and 15.4).

• Taxanes, gemcitabine, and ifosfamide, have shown activity as front-line treatment and second-line treatment for metastatic TCC. Doublet and triplet chemotherapy combination regimens may have increased response, but their impact on survival is unclear (Table 15.5).

TABLE 15.3. *Combination chemotherapy regimens in advanced urothelial carcinoma*

Regimen	Dosing	Duration	Comments
CISCA	• Cyclophosphamide, 650 mg/m² i.v. d 1 (total dose/cycle, 650 mg/m²). • Doxorubicin, 50 mg/m² i.v. d 2 (total dose/cycle, 50 mg/m²). • Cisplatin, 100 mg/m² i.v. d 2 (total dose/cycle, 100 mg/m²).	21–28 d	
CMV	• Methotrexate, 30 mg/m² i.v. d 1 and 8 (total dose/cycle, 60 mg/m²). • Vinblastine, 4 mg/m² i.v. d 1 and 8 (total dose/cycle, 8 mg/m²). • Cisplatin, 100 mg/m² i.v. infusion over 4 h on d 2, ≥12 h after methotrexate and vinblastine (total dose/cycle, 100 mg/m²).	21 d	
Docetaxel + cisplatin[a]	• Docetaxel, 75 mg/m² slow i.v. infusion over 1 h d 1(total dose/cycle, 75 mg/m²). • Cisplatin, 75 mg/m² i.v. d 1 (total dose/cycle, 75 mg/m²)	21 d	
Gemcitabine + cisplatin	• Gemcitabine, 1,000 mg/m² i.v. d 1, 8, and 15 (total dose/cycle, 3,000 mg/m²). • Cisplatin, 70 mg/m² i.v. d 1 (total dose/cycle, 70 mg/m²)	28 d	
ITP[a]	• Ifosfamide, 1,500 mg/m²/d i.v. for d 1–3 (total dose/cycle, 4,500 mg/m²). • Mesna, 300 mg/m² i.v. 30 min before ifosfamide, then 300 mg/m² i.v. 4 and 8 h after ifosfamide; 600 mg/m² p.o. 4 and 8 h after ifosfamide. • Paclitaxel, 200 mg/m² i.v. infusion over 3 h d 1 (total dose/cycle, 200 mg/m²). • Cisplatin, 70 mg/m² i.v. d 1 (total dose/cycle, 70 mg/m²).	28 d	Regimen includes primary hematopoietic growth factor support with filgrastim, 5 μg/kg or per d s.c. given per cycle.
MVAC	• Methotrexate, 30 mg/m² i.v. d 1, 15, and 22 (total dose/cycle, 90 mg/m²). • Vinblastine, 3 mg/m² i.v. d 2, 15, and 22 (total dose/cycle, 9 mg/m²). • Doxorubicin, 30 mg/m² i.v. d 2 (total dose/cycle, 30 mg/m²). • Cisplatin, 70 mg/m² i.v. d 2 (total dose/cycle, 70 mg/m²).	28 d	Cycles not initiated unless WBC count ≥3 × 10⁹/L and platelets ≥100 × 10⁹/L
Paclitaxel + carboplatin[a]	• Paclitaxel, 200 mg/m² i.v. infusion over 3 h d 1 (total dose/cycle, 200 mg/m²). • Carboplatin i.v. after paclitaxel; dosage calculated by Calvert formula to achieve target AUC of 5 mg/mL/min.[b]	21 d	Premedicated with dexamethasone p.o. 12 and 6 h before paclitaxel and i.v. antihistamines 30 min prior to paclitaxel

AUC, graphically represented area under the plasma concentration versus time curve for carboplatin; i.v., intravenously; p.o., orally; s.c., subcutaneously; WBC, white blood cell.

[a]Regimen includes primary prophylaxis with antihistamines and corticosteroids against hypersensitivity reactions before taxoid administration.

[b]Calvert formula: Total dose (mg) = [target AUC (mg/mL/min)] × [GFR (mL/min) + 25]. GFR = glomerular filtration rate (urinary cretatinine clearance/24 h).

Source: From Calvert AH, Newell DR, Gumbrell LA, et al. Carboplatin dosage: prospective evaluation of a simple formula based on renal function. *J Clin Oncol* 1989;7:1748–56, with permission.

TABLE 15.4. *Selected randomized phase 3 trials in patients with advanced urothelial carcinoma*

Randomized trial (ref.)	Overall response rate	Median survival
MVAC vs. cisplatin (Loehrer et al.)	39% vs. 12%	12.5 vs. 8.2 mo
MVAC vs. CISCA (Logothetis et al.)	65% vs. 46%	48.3 vs. 36.1 wk
MVAC vs. gemcitabine + cisplatin (von der Maase et al.)	46% vs. 49%	15.2 vs. 14 mo

TABLE 15.5. *Agents used in phase 2 trials for untreated advanced urothelial carcinoma*

Phase 2 trials (ref.)	Evaluable patients	Overall response rate (%)
Docetaxel + cisplatin (Sengelov et al.)	25	60
Gemcitabine + paclitaxel (Meluch et al.)	54	54
Ifosfamide + paclitaxel + cisplatin (Bajorin et al.)	44	68
Paclitaxel + carboplatin (Redman et al.)	35	51.5
Paclitaxel + cisplatin + gemcitabine (Bellmunt et al.)	49	78

- There are no data showing that carboplatin can be efficaciously substituted for cisplatin. Before it closed prematurely due to poor accrual, an ECOG phase 3 study comparing MVAC with carboplatin and paclitaxel demonstrated a nonstatistically significant difference in median OS of 15.4 months for the MVAC arm versus 13.8 months for the carboplatin-paclitaxel arm ($P = 0.65$), with toxicity profiles favoring the carboplatin-paclitaxel arm (Table 15.4). Therefore, carboplatin should be substituted for cisplatin only in patients deemed cisplatin-intolerant, such as those with significant renal dysfunction.

REFERENCES

Bajorin DF, McCaffrey JA, Dodd PM, et al. Ifosfamide, paclitaxel, and cisplatin for patients with advanced transitional-cell carcinoma of the urothelial tract: final report of a phase II trial evaluating two dosing schedules. *Cancer.* 2000;88(7):1671–1678.

Bellmunt J, Guillem V, Paz-Ares L, et al. Spanish Oncology Genitourinary Group. Phase I-II study of paclitaxel, cisplatin, and gemcitabine in advanced transitional-cell carcinoma of the urothelium. *J Clin Oncol.* 2000;18(18):3247–3255.

Loehrer PJ Sr, Einhorn LH, Elson PJ, et al. A randomized comparison of cisplatin alone or in combination with methotrexate, vinblastine, and doxorubicin in patients with metastatic urothelial carcinoma: a cooperative group study. *J Clin Oncol.* 1992;10:1066–1073.

Logothetis CJ, Dexeus FH, Chong C, et al. Cisplatin, cyclophosphamide and doxorubicin chemotherapy for unresectable urothelial tumors: the MD Anderson experience. *J Urol.* 1989;141:33–37.

Logothetis CJ, Dexeus FH, Finn L, et al. A prospective randomized trial comparing MVAC and CISCA chemotherapy for patients with metastatic urothelial tumors. *J Clin Oncol.* 1990;8:1050–1055.

Meluch AA, Greco FA, Burris HA III, et al. Paclitaxel and gemcitabine chemotherapy for advanced transitional-cell carcinoma of the urothelial tract: a phase II trial of the Minnie Pearl cancer research network. *J Clin Oncol.* 2001;19(12):3018–3024.

Redman BG, Smith DC, Flaherty L, Du W, Hussain M. Phase II trial of paclitaxel and carboplatin in the treatment of advanced urothelial carcinoma. *J Clin Oncol.* 1998;16:1844–1848.

Sengelov L, Kamby C, Lund B, Engelholm SA. Docetaxel and cisplatin in metastatic urothelial cancer: a phase II study. *J Clin Oncol.* 1998;16:3392–3397.

von der Maase H, Hansen SW, Roberts JT, et al. Gemcitabine and cisplatin versus methotrexate, vinblastine, doxorubicin, and cisplatin in advanced or metastatic bladder cancer: results of a large, randomized, multinational, multicenter, phase III study. *J Clin Oncol.* 2000;18(17):3068–3077.

von der Maase H, Sengelov L, Roberts JT, et al. Long term survival results of a randomized trial comparing gemcitabine plus cisplatin, with methotrexate, vinblastine, doxorubicin, plus cisplatin in patients with bladder cancer. *J Clin Oncol.* 2005;23(21):4602–4608.

SUGGESTED READINGS

Advanced Bladder Cancer Meta-analysis Collaboration. Neoadjuvant chemotherapy in invasive bladder cancer: a systematic review and meta-analysis. *Lancet.* 2003;361(9373):1927–1934.

American Urological Association Guideline for the Management of Nonmuscle Invasive Bladder Cancer: 2007 Update. Available at: http://www.auanet.org/guidelines/main_reports/bladcan07/cover.pdf. Accessed February 2008.

Calvert AH, Newell DR, Gumbrell LA, et al. Carboplatin dosage: prospective evaluation of a simple formula based on renal function. *J Clin Oncol* 1989;7:1748–56.

Garcia JA, Dreicer R. Systemic chemotherapy for advanced bladder cancer: update and controversies. *J Clin Oncol.* 2006;24:5545–5551.

Greene FL, Page DL, Fleming ID, et al. *AJCC Cancer Staging Manual.* 6th ed. New York: Spring Science and Business Media; 2002.

Grossman HB, Natale RB, Tangen CM, et al. Neoadjuvant chemotherapy plus cystectomy compared with cystectomy alone for locally advanced bladder cancer. *N Engl J Med.* 2003;349:859–866.

Harker WG, Meyers FJ, Freiha FS, et al. Cisplatin, methotrexate, and vinblastine (CMV): an effective chemotherapy regimen for metastatic transitional cell carcinoma of the urinary tract: a Northern California Oncology Group study. *J Clin Oncol.* 1985;3:1463–1470.

Levin RM, Crawford DE. Bladder, renal pelvis, and ureters. In: Haskell CM, ed. *Cancer Treatment.* 4th ed. Philadelphia: WB Saunders; 1995:567–588.

National Cancer Comprehensive Network (NCCN) Bladder Cancer Practice Guidelines. Available at: http://www.nccn.org/professionals/physician_gls/PDF/bladder.pdf. Accessed February 2008.

Parekh DJ, Bochner BH, Dalbagni G. Superficial and muscle-invasive bladder cancer: principles of management for outcomes assessment. *J Clin Oncol.* 2006;24:5519–5527.

Shipley WU, Kaufman DS, McDougal WS, et al. Cancer of the bladder, ureter and renal pelvis. In: DeVita VT Jr, Hellman S, Rosenberg SA, eds. *Cancer: Principles and Practice of Oncology.* 7th ed. New York: Lippincott–Raven Publishers; 2005:1168–1192.

16

Testicular Carcinoma

Ravi A. Madan and Barnett S. Kramer

Testicular carcinoma is the most common malignancy in men between the ages of 20 and 35, but represents only 1% of all malignancies in males. The disease is believed to originate from the malignant transformation of primordial germ cells that may occur early in embryonic development. As late as the 1970s, testicular carcinoma was generally fatal, but can now usually be cured. Effective treatment paradigms have been developed to help manage acute disease and follow-up. Given the high cure rate and resulting improved life expectancy, special considerations must be given to the side effects of therapy, especially in early-stage disease where even conservative interventions yield a cure in over 98% of patients. Whatever the therapeutic intervention, all patients should be monitored closely in ensuing years for both recurrent disease and long-term sequelae of therapy.

CLINICAL FEATURES

Epidemiology

- In 2007, there were an estimated 7,920 new cases of testicular carcinoma, with 380 deaths.
- Testicular cancer accounts for 1% of all malignancies in men.
- Whites are 5 times more likely than African Americans to have testicular carcinoma.
- For unclear reasons, the incidence of testicular cancer has been increasing over the last 4 to 5 decades.
- The greatest incidence occurs between the ages of 20 and 35.
- Testicular cancer is rare after the age of 40.

Risk Factors

- Cryptorchid testes, with intra-abdominal testes having a higher risk than inguinal testes. There is also increased risk in the normally descended contralateral testis.
- Testicular carcinoma in the contralateral testis; 1% to 5% of patients have bilateral disease.
- Intratubular germ cell neoplasia, a premalignant condition seen in 90% of testicular carcinomas
- Family history (eightfold increase for brothers with testicular carcinoma; fourfold increase if father had the disease)
- Klinefelter syndrome (increased risk of mediastinal germ cell tumors)
- Peutz-Jeghers syndrome (increased risk of Sertoli cell tumors)
- Human immunodeficiency virus infection
- There is an association between testicular cancer and sarcoidosis.

History and Signs and Physical Examination

- Asymptomatic testicular nodule or swelling (painful in 10–20% of patients)
- Feeling of testicular heaviness, dull ache, and/or hardness (up to 40% of patients)

- Disease at extragonadal site (5–10% of patients; symptoms vary with site):
  – Dyspnea, cough, or hemoptysis (pulmonary metastases)
  – Weight loss, anorexia, nausea, abdominal or back pain (retroperitoneal adenopathy)
  – Mass or swelling in neck (supraclavicular lymphadenopathy)
  – Superior vena cava syndrome due to mediastinal disease
- Rare presentations:
  – Urinary obstruction
  – Headaches, seizures, or other neurologic complaints due to brain metastases
  – Bone pain due to bone metastases
  – Gynecomastia due to elevated β-human chorionic gonadotropin (β-HCG).

DIFFERENTIAL DIAGNOSIS

- Epididymitis (initial diagnosis and treatment in 18% to 33% of testicular cancer patients)
- Orchitis, hydrocele, varicocele, or spermatocele
- Lymphoma or leukemia
- Metastasis from other tumors including melanoma or lung cancer
- Infectious diseases including tuberculosis and gumma

DIAGNOSIS

The diagnostic workup for testicular carcinoma is outlined in Fig. 16.1.

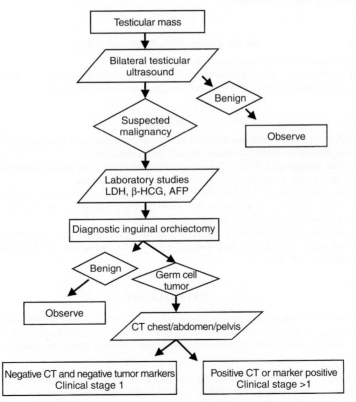

Fig. 16.1. Diagnostic workup for testicular carcinoma.

Goals

- Every testicular mass requires a timely workup to exclude testicular carcinoma.
- Histologic determination of tumor type and stage have prognostic and therapeutic significance.
- Testicular cancer is highly curable, with 5-year survival >95%.
- Long-term sequelae of therapy should be considered and minimized when possible.

Laboratory

Serum α-Fetoprotein (AFP)

- Half-life of approximately 4 to 6 days
- Commonly produced by the fetal yolk sac, liver, and gastrointestinal tract
- Should not be elevated in serum of healthy patient
- Not present in patient with pure seminoma. Elevated serum AFP levels indicate a nonseminomatous component to the patient's testicular cancer.

Serum β-Human Chorionic Gonadotropin (β-HCG)

- Secreted by syncytiotrophoblasts; half-life of 0.5 to 1.5 days
- Most commonly elevated tumor marker in patients with testicular cancer
- Present in choriocarcinomas; may be modestly elevated in pure seminomas
- High levels may lead to gynecomastia

Serum Lactate Dehydrogenase (LDH)

- Nonspecific tumor marker in testicular cancer
- Elevated in 80% of metastatic seminomas and 60% of advanced nonseminomatous tumors
- Reflects overall tumor burden, tumor growth rate, and cellular proliferation

Imaging

- Ultrasound: Ultrasound detects the presence of testicular parenchymal abnormality in both testes.
- Chest x-ray: PA and lateral film evaluate for pulmonary metastases.
- Computerized tomography (CT): CT scans of chest, abdomen, and pelvis determine extragonadal metastasis and are the most effective modality for staging the disease.
- Magnetic resonance imaging (MRI): MRI may provide additional information if ultrasound is indeterminate. MRI of the brain is necessary only when there are symptoms involving the central nervous system (e.g., headache, neurologic deficit, seizure).
- Positron emission tomography (PET) scan: PET scans are not indicated in primary staging, but may have limited utility for characterizing residual masses. The routine use of PET scans has not been shown to improve outcome.

PATHOLOGY

Patients with testicular masses should have surgical exploration, with complete removal of the testis and spermatic cord through the inguinal ring. Trans-scrotal testicular biopsy is not recommended due to the risk of local and nodal dissemination of tumor, although empirical evidence supporting this is weak.

- Germ cell tumors are frequently aneuploid and display an array of histopathology (Table 16.1).
- Several genes (either deleted or amplified) located on isochromosome 12p have been implicated in the malignant transformation of primordial germ cells.

TABLE 16.1. *Histopathologic characteristics of germ cell tumors*

Tumor type	Percentage	Pathologic feature(s)	Percentage
Germ cell tumors	95	Seminomas	40–50
Single cell–type tumors	60	Primordial germ cell	
Combination tumors	40	Nonseminomas	50–60
		Embryonal cell tumors	
		Yolk sac tumors	
		Teratomas	
		Choriocarinomas	
Tumors of gonadal stroma	1–2	Leydig cell	
		Sertoli cell	
		Primitive gonadal structures	
Gonadoblastoma	1	Germ cell + stromal cell	

STAGING

Tables 16.2 and 16.3 contain the tumor/node/metastasis (TNM) classification and staging criteria of the American Joint Committee for Cancer.

TABLE 16.2. *Tumor/node/metastasis (TNM) classification and staging of testicular carcinoma*

Primary Tumor (extent classified after radical orchiectomy)
TX   Primary tumor cannot be assessed (no radical orchiectomy has been performed)
T0   No evidence of primary tumor (e.g., histologic scar in testis)
Tis   Intratubular germ cell neoplasia (carcinoma in situ)
T1   Tumor limited to testis and epididymis without lymphatic or vascular invasion; may invade into the tunica albuginea but not the tunica vaginalis
T2   Tumor limited to testis and epididymis with vascular or lymphatic invasion, or tumor extending through the tunica albuginea with involvement of the tunica vaginalis
T3   Tumor invades the spermatic cord with or without vascular or lymphatic invasion
T4   Tumor invades the scrotum with or without vascular or lymphatic invasion
Regional Lymph Nodes (N)
NX   Regional lymph nodes cannot be assessed
N0   No regional lymph node metastasis
N1   Metastasis in a single lymph node, ≤ 2 cm in greatest dimension; or multiple lymph nodes, none >2 cm in greatest dimension
N2   Metastasis in a single lymph node mass between 2 and <5 cm in greatest dimension; or multiple lymph nodes, any one mass >2 cm but none >5 cm in greatest dimension
N3   Metastasis in a lymph node mass >5 cm in greatest dimension
Pathologic Lymph Nodes (pN)
pNX   Regional lymph nodes cannot be assessed
pN0   No regional lymph node metastasis
pN1   Metastasis with a lymph node mass ≤ 2 cm in greatest dimension and ≤ 5 nodes positive, none >2 cm in greatest dimension
pN2   Metastasis with a lymph node mass between 2 and <5 cm in greatest dimension; or more than 5 nodes positive, none >5 cm; or evidence of extranodal extension of tumor
pN3   Metastasis with a lymph node >5 cm in greatest dimension

(Continued)

TABLE 16.2. *(Continued)*

Distant Metastasis (M)

MX	Presence of distant metastasis cannot be assessed
M0	No distant metastasis
M1	Distant metastasis
M1a	Nonregional nodal or pulmonary metastasis
M1b	Distant metastasis other than to nonregional nodes and lungs

Serum Tumor Markers (S)

SX	Marker studies not available or not performed
S0	Marker studies within normal limits
S1	LDH <1.5 × ULN and β-HCG <5,000 mIU/mL and AFP <1,000 ng/mL
S2	LDH 1.5–10 × ULN or β-HCG 5,000–50,000 mIU/mL or AFP 1,000–10,000 ng/mL
S3	LDH >10 × ULN or β-HCG >50,000 mIU/mL or AFP >10,000 ng/mL

LDH, lactate dehydrogenase; HCG, human chorionic gonadotropin; AFP, α-fetoprotein; ULN, upper limit of normal.

TABLE 16.3. *American Joint Committee for Cancer stage groupings*

Stage 0	pTis N0 M0 S0
Stage I	pT1–4 N0 M0 SX
Stage IA	pT1 N0 M0 S0
Stage IB	pT2–4 N0 M0 S0
Stage IS	Any pT/Tx N0 M0 S1–S3
Stage II	Any pT/Tx N1–N3 M0 SX
Stage IIA	Any pT/Tx N1 M0 S0–S1
Stage IIB	Any pT/Tx N2 M0 S0–S1
Stage IIC	Any pT/Tx N3 M0 S0–S1
Stage III	Any pT/Tx any N M1 SX
Stage IIIA	Any pT/Tx any N M1a S0–S1
Stage IIIB	Any pT/Tx N1–3 M0 S2
	Any pT/Tx any N M1a S2
Stage IIIC	Any pT/Tx N1–3 M0 S3
	Any pT/Tx any N M1a S3
	Any pT/Tx any N M1b any S

PROGNOSIS

Table 16.4 outlines the International Consensus Risk Classification for germ cell tumors; Table 16.5 discusses expected survival.

TREATMENT MODALITIES

Treatments vary depending on tumor histology and stage. The need for aggressive therapy with early-stage disease is currently controversial.

Seminomas

Adjuvant treatment options for seminoma are outlined in Fig. 16.2.

Stage I

Seminomas are sensitive to both radiation and chemotherapy. For stage I seminomas, active surveillance following radical orchiectomy is an option, with a recurrence rate of up to 20%. When disease

TABLE 16.4. *International Consensus Risk Classification for germ cell tumors*

Prognosis	Nonseminoma	Seminoma
Good	Testis/retroperitoneal primary. No non-pulmonary visceral metastases. AFP <1,000 mg/mL; HCG <5,000 IU/L (1,000 mg/mL); LDH <1.5 × ULN; (56–61% of all nonseminomas)	Any primary site. No nonpulmonary visceral metastases. Normal AFP <1,000; any concentration of HCG; any concentration of LDH; (90% of all seminomas)
Intermediate	Testis/retroperitoneal primary. No non-pulmonary visceral metastases. AFP ≥1,000 and ≤10,000 ng/mL or HCG ≥5,000 IU/L and ≤50,000 IU/L or LDH ≥1.5 × NL and ≤10 × NL; (13–28% of all nonseminomas)	Any primary site. No nonpulmonary visceral metastases. Normal AFP; any concentration of HCG; any concentration of LDH; (10% of all seminomas)
Poor	Mediastinal primary or nonpulmonary visceral metastases or AFP >10,000 ng/mL or HCG >50,000 IU/L (10,000 ng/mL) or LDH >10 × ULN; (16–26% of all nonseminomas)	No patients classified as poor prognosis

LDH, lactate dehydrogenase; HCG, human chorionic gonadotropin; AFP, α-fetoprotein; ULN, upper limit of normal; NL, normal limit.

TABLE 16.5. *Expected survival*

	5-year progression-free survival (%)		5-year overall survival (%)	
Prognosis	Seminoma	Nonseminoma	Seminoma	Nonseminoma
Good	82	89	86	92–94
Intermediate	67	75	72	80–83
Poor*	—	41	—	71

*There is no poor prognosis category for seminoma.

does recur, nearly all patients can be cured with radiation therapy or chemotherapy. Low-dose radiation therapy to regional lymph nodes after surgical resection results in cure over 90% of the time. A single cycle of carboplatin has also proven to be equivalent to radiation in producing a high rate of relapse-free survival (RFS) and overall survival (OS) at 4 years. Regardless of initial therapy, over 98% of patients will ultimately be cured. Physicians and patients must discuss the short-term and long-term advantages and disadvantages of more aggressive therapies in this stage of disease. Regardless of the treatment chosen, the patient must understand the need for frequent visits and imaging during follow-up.

Stage II

For stage IIA/B, or nonbulky disease (<5 cm), radical inguinal orchiectomy followed by radiation therapy (30 Gy) to ipsilateral and retroperitoneal lymph nodes results in cure 90% of the time. For stage IIC or bulky disease cisplatin-based chemotherapy is required after radical orchiectomy. There is no evidence that the combination of both radiation and chemotherapy increases RFS or OS.

Stage III

Stage III disease is usually still curable. Chemotherapy is required for patients following radical orchiectomy. Patients with good prognosis may be treated with 3 cycles of BEP; all other patients should be treated with 4 cycles of BEP.

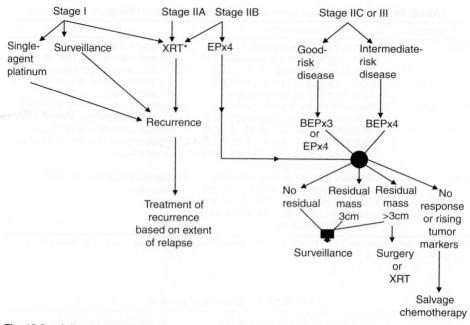

Fig. 16.2. Adjuvant treatment options for seminoma. XRT, radiation therapy to para-aortic lymph nodes.

Nonseminomas

Adjuvant treatment options for stage I, II, and III nonseminoma are outlined in Figs.16.3 and 16.4.

Stage I

Stage I nonseminomatous disease (including tumors appearing to be seminomas but with elevated levels of serum AFP) is also highly curable, with several effective treatment options after radical orchiectomy. Retroperitoneal lymph node dissection (RPLND) has long been the mainstay of therapy in this disease and reports of cure are as high as 99%. After RPLND, 30% to 50% patients will be found to have pathologic stage II disease, although it is important to note that up to 10% of patients will have occult distant metastasis elsewhere (primarily in the lungs) that will not be detected by RPLND. While extremely effective, up to 70% of patients will be overtreated with RPLND and 10% may still require chemotherapy because of metastatic disease elsewhere. Adjuvant cisplatin-based chemotherapy for two cycles reduces the risk of recurrence to <2%, but is similar to RPLND in that patients may be overtreated. Active surveillance is again an option, with 30% of all patients expected to relapse (95% within 2 years; 99% within 4 years). Regardless of recurrence, if patient follow-up is appropriate and subsequent therapy is given as indicated, OS is still >98%. Several considerations must be taken into account before choosing active surveillance, including the patient's anxiety, compliance, and access to a facility with experienced physicians, radiologists, and CT scanners to detect recurrence.

Stage II

Patients who have a radical orchiectomy followed by RPLND have an expected recurrence rate of 20% to 30%, with >95% of all patients being cured. Platinum-based chemotherapy after RPLND may improve RFS in patients with lymphatic or venous invasion by tumor, although studies indicate

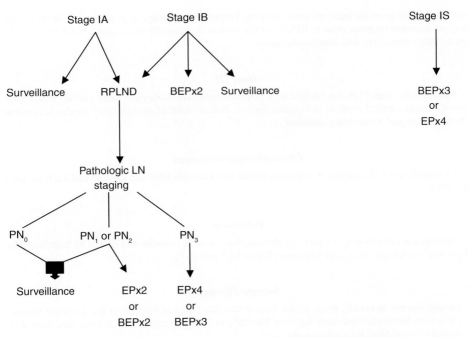

Fig. 16.3. Adjuvant treatment options for stage I nonseminoma.

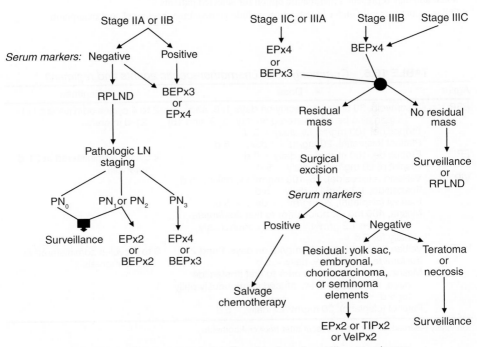

Fig. 16.4. Adjuvant treatment options for stage II and III nonseminoma.

equivalent cure rates for adjuvant chemotherapy versus chemotherapy at recurrence. Chemotherapy may occasionally be given prior to RPLND if the disease is especially bulky and it is felt that smaller preoperative tumor size will improve outcome.

Stage III

Patients with stage III disease should have platinum-based chemotherapy; some patients will require post-treatment surgical removal of residual masses. Patients with brain metastasis require concurrent chemotherapy and whole-brain radiation.

Chemotherapy Regimens

Commonly used chemotherapy regimens (Table 16.6) include BEP and EP. VIP and VeIP are used less often.

Follow-up

Appropriate surveillance of patients with testicular cancer is essential and should be determined by the tumor's histology, stage, and treatment (Tables 16.7 and 16.8).

Salvage Therapy

- Salvage therapy is usually reserved for disease that has failed to respond or has persisted through a platinum-based chemotherapy regimen. The 20% to 30% of patients who achieve long-term RFS should be considered for clinical trials.
- VIP is commonly used as an initial salvage therapy.
- High-dose chemotherapy with autologous bone marrow or peripheral stem cell support is investigational and may represent a therapeutic option for selected patients.
- Other agents currently under investigation include gemcitabine, paclitaxel, and oxaliplatin.

TABLE 16.6. *Commonly used chemotherapeutic agents and regimens*

Agent	Dose	Regimen
BEP	Bleomycin, 30 units i.v. weekly on days 1, 8, and 15 (can also be administered on days 2, 9, and 16) Etoposide, 100 mg/m^2 i.v. daily × 5 d Platinol (cisplatin), 20 mg/m^2 i.v. daily × 5 d	2 to 4 cycles administered at 21-d intervals
EP	Etoposide, 100 mg/m^2 i.v. daily × 5 d Cisplatin, 20 mg/m^2 i.v. daily × 5 d	4 cycles administered at 21-d intervals
VIP*	VePesid (etoposide), 75–100 mg/m^2 i.v. daily × 5 d Ifosfamide, 1.2 g/m^2 i.v. daily × 5 d Platinol (cisplatin), 20 mg/m^2 i.v. daily × 5 d Mesna, 400 mg i.v. bolus prior to first ifosfamide dose, then 1.2 g/m^2 i.v. infused continuously daily for 5 d	
VeIP[a]	Velban (vinblastine), 0.11 mg/kg on days 1 and 2 Ifosfamide, 1.2 g/m^2 i.v. daily × 5 d Mesna, 400 mg i.v. bolus prior to first ifosfamide dose, then 1.2 g/m^2 i.v. infused continuously daily for 5 d Platinol (cisplatin), 20 mg/m^2 i.v. daily × 5 d	3 to 4 cycles administered at 21-d intervals

[a]Generally reserved for tumors that recur after prior chemotherapy.

TABLE 16.7. *Surveillance schedule for seminoma*

Year	H&P, CXR, markers (monthly interval)	ABD/pelvic CT (monthly interval)
Stage IA, IB, IS (active surveillance)		
1–3	3–4	3–4
4–7	6	6
8–10	12	12 (only third year)
Stage IA, IB, IS (postradiation)		
1	3	12
2	4	12
3–5	6	12 (only third year)
Stage IIA, *IIB (postradiation) or IIC, III (postchemotherapy)*		
1	2	After 4 months, then every every
2	3	3 months until stable
3	4	
4	6	
5+	12	

H&P, history and physical; CXR, chest x-ray; ABD, abdomen; CT, computed tomography.

Based on National Comprehensive Cancer Network (NCCN) guidelines. There is considerable interinstitutional variation in the standard of follow-up care, with little evidence that different schedules lead to different outcomes.

Therapy-Related Toxicity

Complications of RPLND

- 1% to 2% of patients will have bowel perforation, chylous ascites, lymphocele, vascular injuries, pancreatitis, and ejaculatory dysfunction or retrograde ejaculation.

Fertility

- Even though 80% of patients treated with chemotherapy may recover sperm production within 5 years, sperm banking should be offered to all patients desiring to father children after therapy.

TABLE 16.8. *Surveillance schedule for nonseminoma*

Year	H&P, CXR, markers (monthly interval)	ABD/pelvic CT (monthly interval)
Stage IA, IB		
1	1–2	2–3
2	2	3–4
3	3	4
4	4	6
5	6	12
6+	12	12
After complete response to chemotherapy and/or retroperitoneal lymph node dissection (RPLND)		
1	1–2	6
2	2	6
3	3	12
4	4	12
5	6	12
6+	12	12

H&P, history and physical; CXR, chest x-ray; ABD, abdomen; CT, computed tomography.

Based on National Comprehensive Cancer Network (NCCN) guidelines. There is considerable interinstitutional variation in the standard of follow-up care, with little evidence that different schedules lead to different outcomes.

- Approximately 25% of patients have oligospermia, sperm abnormalities, or altered follicular stimulating hormone levels prior to therapy.
- Almost all patients become azospermic or oligospermic during chemotherapy.
- Children of treated patients do not appear to have an increased risk of congenital abnormalities.

Pulmonary Toxicity

- Chronic lung damage that can lead to pulmonary fibrosis is associated with bleomycin.
- Toxicities are rarely fatal. More frequently, asymptomatic decreases in pulmonary function resolve after completion of bleomycin therapy.
- Bleomycin should be discontinued if early signs of pulmonary toxicity develop or if a 40% to 60% decrease in diffusing capacity of lung for carbon monoxide is noted.
- Routine pulmonary function tests are rarely indicated and should be reserved for patients with signs and symptoms of pulmonary toxicity (e.g., dry rales on physical examination and shortness of breath or dyspnea on exertion).
- Corticosteroids may be used to reduce lung inflammation if pulmonary toxicity occurs.
- Smokers treated with bleomycin should be particularly discouraged from tobacco use.
- Supplemental oxygen should be used with caution and at low fraction of inspired oxygen (F_{IO_2}) settings.
- If fluids are indicated, i.v. colloids rather than crystalloids are preferred.

Nephrotoxicity

- Cisplatin-based chemotherapy may result in decreased glomerular filtration rate, which can be permanent in 20% to 30% of patients.
- Hypokalemia and hypomagnesemia are also frequent manifestations of altered kidney function in these patients.

Neurologic Toxicity

- Cisplatin-based chemotherapy may result in persistent peripheral neuropathy in 20% to 40% of patients.
- Peripheral digital dysesthesias and paresthesias are the most common manifestations.
- A small proportion of patients will have tinnitus or high-frequency hearing loss, usually outside the frequency of spoken language.

Cardiovascular Toxicity

- Bleomycin, cisplatin, and radiation alone or in combination can increase the risk of cardiovascular disease in patients who have completed therapy.
- Angina, myocardial infarction, and sudden cardiac death are increased by up to twofold.
- Hypertension, hypercholesterolemia, and Raynaud's phenomenon are also increased in patients who have completed therapy.

Secondary Malignancies

- Secondary malignancies are associated with the use of cisplatin, etoposide, and radiation. Patients treated for testicular cancer with these agents reportedly have a 1.7-fold increase in their risk of developing a secondary malignancy.
- Alkylating agents such as cisplatin may lead to a myelodysplastic syndrome within 5 to 7 years that can eventually progress to leukemia. Topoisomerase inhibitors such as etoposide may cause secondary leukemias within 3 years.
- There is an increased incidence of solid tumors in potential radiation fields, including the bladder, stomach, pancreas, and kidney.

Disclaimer: The opinions expressed in this chapter represent those of the authors and do not necessarily represent official positions or opinions of the U.S. government or of the U.S. Department of Health and Human Services.

SUGGESTED READINGS

Albers P, Albrecht W, Algaba F, et al. Guidelines on testicular cancer. *Eur Urol.* 2005;48:885–894.

Bosl GJ, Steinfeld J, Barjorin DF, et al. Cancer of the testis. In: DeVita VT, Hellman S, Rosenberg SA, eds. *Cancer, Principles and Practice of Oncology.* 7th ed. Philadelphia, PA: Lippincott Williams & Wilkins; 2005.

Bridges B, Hussain A. Testicular germ cell tumors. *Curr Opin Oncol.* 2007;19:222–228.

Carver BS, Sheinfeld J. Germ cell tumors of the testis. *Ann Surg Oncol.* 2005;12:871–880.

de Wit R, Fizazi K. Controversies in the management of clinical stage I testis cancer. *J Clin Oncol.* 2006;24:5482–5492.

Farmakis D, Pectasides M, Pectasides D. Recent advances in conventional-dose salvage chemotherapy in patients with cisplatin-resistant or refractory testicular germ cell tumors. *Eur Urol.* 2005;48: 400–407.

Horwich A, Shipley J, Huddart R. Testicular germ-cell cancer. *Lancet.* 2006;367:754–765.

Huddart RA, Norman A, Shahidi M, et al. Cardiovascular disease as a long-term complication of treatment for testicular cancer. *J Clin Oncol.* 2003;21:1513–1523.

Jemal A, Siegel R, Ward E, et al. Cancer statistics, 2007. *CA Cancer J Clin.* 2007;57:43–66.

Kaufman MR, Chang SS. Short- and long-term complications of therapy for testicular cancer. *Urol Clin North Am.* 2007;34:259–268.

Kopp HG, Kuczyk M, Classen J, et al. Advances in the treatment of testicular cancer. *Drugs.* 2006;66:641–659.

National Comprehensive Cancer Network (NCCN) Guidelines: Testicular Cancer. Available at: http://www.nccn.org/professionals/physician_gls/PDF/testicular.pdf.

Oliver T. Conservative management of testicular germ-cell tumors. *Nat Clin Pract Urol.* 2007;4: 550–560.

Testicular Cancer Treatment (PDQ)—National Cancer Institute. Available at: http://www.cancer.gov/cancertopics/pdq/treatment/testicular/HealthProfessional.

van den Belt-Dusebout AW, de Wit R, Gietema JA, et al. Treatment-specific risks of second malignancies and cardiovascular disease in 5-year survivors of testicular cancer. *J Clin Oncol.* 2007;25: 4370–4378.

SECTION 6

Gynecologic

17

Ovarian Cancer

Nilofer S. Azad, David Adelberg, and Elise C. Kohn

BACKGROUND

- Ovarian cancer is the leading cause of gynecologic cancer death.
- 90% of all cases of ovarian cancer are of epithelial origin, most often papillary serous histology.
- 10% are stromal or germ-cell histology.
- Fallopian tube and peritoneal carcinoma are generally treated as epithelial ovarian cancer.
- In 2007, approximately 22,000 cases were diagnosed, resulting in 15,000 deaths.
- Median age at diagnosis is 61.
- 70% of cases are diagnosed at stage III or IV (Table 17.1).
- 5-year survival of advanced-stage disease is <35%.

PATHOLOGY

- Epithelial histologies account for about 90% of all ovarian cancers.
- Papillary serous, mucinous, endometrioid, transitional, and clear cell carcinoma are considered epithelial.
- Fallopian tube and primary peritoneal adenocarcinoma occur exclusively in women. They are clinically similar to epithelial ovarian cancer, and staging and treatment are the same as for ovarian cancer.
- Recent data indicate that the fimbria of the fallopian tubes may be the source of epithelial ovarian cancer in sporadic as well as BRCA1/2-associated cancers.

TABLE 17.1. *Ovarian cancer staging*

Stage I	Confined to the ovaries
IA	Single ovary only
IB	Both ovaries only
IC	Malignant ascites, capsular involvement or rupture preoperatively or intraoperatively
Stage II	One or both ovaries with pelvic extension
IIA	Metastases to uterus or fallopian tube
IIB	Other pelvic organs
IIC	Stage II disease with malignant ascites, capsular involvement or rupture preoperatively or intraoperatively
Stage III	Peritoneal disease
IIIA	Microscopic abdominoperitoneal disease
IIIB	Visible abdominal disease <2 cm diameter
IIIC	Visible abdominal disease ≥2 cm diameter and/or lymph node metastases
Stage IV	Distant metastases, including malignant pleural effusion, parenchymal organ disease, transmural serosal disease

- Mixed müllerian tumors, also known as carcinosarcomas, are epithelial tumors with metaplastic sarcomatous change. They are relatively chemoresistant.
- Clear cell carcinoma has a poorer prognosis than other subtypes at every stage of disease.
- Tumors of low malignant potential (borderline tumors) may exist alone or within the above histologic types, excluding clear cell carcinoma.
- Poorly differentiated histology predicts a worse prognosis.
- Germ cell tumors are classified as dysgerminoma, endodermal sinus tumor, malignant teratoma, embryonal carcinoma, or primary choriocarcinoma.
- Germ cell tumors are treated similarly to testicular cancer.
- Stromal tumors are mesenchymal in origin and consist of granulosa tumors or Sertoli-Leydig cell tumors.

SCREENING

- There are no level 1 or 2 data to support screening of the general or high-risk population. However, CA125 and transvaginal ultrasonography are commonly used in follow-up of high-risk individuals.
- There are no validated screening tools to identify ovarian cancer. Use of CA125, alone or in combination with imaging or other modalities, has not been shown to identify disease earlier or to have an impact on survival.
- CA125 and transvaginal ultrasound are being studied in a randomized controlled trial in the general population.
- Novel screening techniques, including alternate biomarkers and serum proteomics, are being explored.

RISK FACTORS AND PREVENTION

Increased Risk

- Age
- Family history of breast or ovarian cancer
- Personal history of breast or ovarian cancer
- Genetic syndromes including BRCA1/2 and hereditary nonpolyposis colorectal cancer (HNPCC)
- Nulliparity
- Primary and secondary infertility

Decreased Risk

- Use of oral contraceptives for >5 years
- Multiparity
- Oophorectomy
- Lactation

In the general population, use of oral contraceptives has a documented protective benefit, especially if used for >5 years and in later reproductive years. This benefit may last up to 15 years. It is controversial if oral contraceptives reduce the risk associated with BRCA1/2 mutations. Prophylactic bilateral salpingo-oophorectomy can reduce the predicted occurrence of ovarian cancer in >90% of women with BRCA1/2 mutations.

CA125

- CA125 is a high molecular-weight glycoprotein.
- CA125 is elevated in up to 50% of stage I tumors and in 80% to 90% of stage II to IV tumors.

- Elevated CA125 concentrations may be seen in other benign and malignant pathologies of the gynecologic tract and peritoneal cavity, including endometrial and breast cancers and benign conditions such as endometriosis, uterine fibroids, and pregnancy.
- CA125 concentration >2,000 should be considered epithelial ovarian cancer until proven otherwise.
- CA125 is an FDA-approved marker for monitoring disease recurrence and response to treatment, if abnormal at diagnosis.
- The utility of following CA125 levels with molecularly targeted therapy is unknown.

DIAGNOSIS AND WORKUP

- >70% of ovarian cancer presents in advanced stage (i.e., III or IV)
- Common symptoms of epithelial ovarian cancer are pelvic/abdominal discomfort, bloating, increased abdominal size, early satiety, and difficulty eating.
- Stromal tumors can produce virilization, precocious puberty, amenorrhea, or postmenopausal bleeding, depending on the age of the patient.
- Approximately 50% of postmenopausal women who have surgery for a pelvic mass will have a malignant neoplasm. This risk does not increase further with age.
- Preoperative workup of a patient with a suspected ovarian mass should include the following (Table 17.2):
  – Blood chemistries
  – Liver function tests
  – Complete blood count
  – Ultrasonography
  – CA125 measurement
  – Computerized tomography (CT) scan of the chest, abdomen, and pelvis
  – α-fetoprotein and β-human chorionic gonadotropin (β-HCG) for patients <30 years old
- Surgery should be performed by a gynecologic oncologist in cases highly suspicious for malignancy.
- The extent and quality of surgical debulking has important prognostic value and is an integral part of the upfront management of an epithelial ovarian cancer patient.
- Favorable prognostic factors include:
  – Age <65 years
  – Good performance status
  – Non–clear cell histology

TABLE 17.2. *Workup for patient with a pelvic mass and/or suspected ovarian cancer*

Labwork
    Complete blood count
    Chemistries including renal function
    Liver function tests
    Coagulation tests
    CA125
    β-HCG (depending upon age and presentation; should also be used to rule out pregnancy in women of childbearing potential)
    AFP (depending upon age and presentation)
Imaging[a]
    Transvaginal/abdominal ultrasound
    CT abdomen/pelvis
    Chest x-ray (chest CT if abnormal)
Family history
Particular emphasis on breast, ovarian colon, pancreatic, and prostate cancers

[a]Value of PET and MRI uncertain.

– Early-stage disease
– Well-differentiated tumor
– Diploid tumors
– No overexpression of HER2
– Low vascular endothelial growth factor (VEGF) expression
– Optimal tumor debulking during surgery to <1 cm for any single lesion
• Patients with germ-line mutations of BRCA1 may have better survival after chemotherapy.

STAGING

• Ovarian cancer can present as stage I to stage IV (see Table 17.1).
• Incidence at diagnosis is 20% for stage I, 5% for stage II, 58% for stage III, and 17% for stage IV.

TREATMENT

Surgery

• Surgery is a pivotal part of the treatment of ovarian cancer.
• Proper ovarian cancer staging requires laparotomy, abdominal fluid sampling, complete debulking to <1 cm diameter for any single residual lesions. Unilateral salpingo-oophorectomy can be considered in women with stage I unilateral well-differentiated tumors who wish to conserve fertility.
• The primary goal of ovarian cancer surgery is to remove all visible disease. Data show that patients receiving debulking and staging surgery by a gynecologic oncologist will have a better outcome.
• Optimal debulking has positive prognostic value and is now considered to be no residual disease, but includes <1 cm maximal diameter residual.
• Stage I disease with favorable prognostic features (well-differentiated histology, nonclear-cell histology, and stage IA or IB disease) can be treated by surgery alone.
• Stage IC disease with favorable prognostic features can be treated by surgery followed by a limited course (3 cycles) of platinum-based chemotherapy.
• All other settings of ovarian cancer of epithelial histology require debulking surgery as detailed previously, followed by six cycles of paclitaxel and carboplatin chemotherapy.
• Second-look laparoscopy/laparotomy is not recommended except as part of a clinical trial.

Chemotherapy for Initial Disease Presentation

• Intraperitoneal (IP) therapy is now an important part of upfront therapy for patients with good performance status who are optimally debulked and can tolerate the treatment.
• A recent randomized phase 3 trial showed a survival advantage, but increased toxicity, for IP therapy in optimally debulked stage III epithelial ovarian cancer patients randomly assigned to i.v. paclitaxel/cisplatin versus a combination of i.v. paclitaxel plus IP cisplatin/paclitaxel.
• Various advisory boards have recommended IP chemotherapy as first-line treatment for women with small-volume residual tumor after maximal surgical cytoreduction for stage III disease, taking into consideration the risk of more severe side effects.
• The standard of care for suboptimally debulked stage III or any stage IV disease and patients who cannot tolerate IP chemotherapy is, after appropriate surgery, 6 cycles every 3 weeks of i.v. carboplatin (area under the exposure-time curve [AUC] of 5 or 6) and paclitaxel at 175 mg/m^2 every 21 days.
• Carboplatin and cisplatin are equally effective in this disease, but carboplatin does not cause the renal or auditory toxicities of cisplatin.
• Paclitaxel and docetaxel have been shown to be similar in initial therapy outcomes.
• Carboplatin dosing should be based on the Calvert formula for calculating AUC; mg dosage of carboplatin = AUC × (GFR + 25), where GFR is glomerular filtration rate.
• Patients can develop hypersensitivity to paclitaxel with the very first treatment doses due to an anaphylactoid reaction to either the paclitaxel or the vehicle.

- Platinum sensitivity usually presents in subsequent cycles as an anaphylactic, true allergic reaction. Cisplatin can be substituted for carboplatin, depending on the severity of the reaction, but the two agents can have cross-sensitivity.
- Desensitization can be attempted for both paclitaxel and platinum-based therapy.
- Several desensitization regimens have been published; they generally meet with variable success.
- In patients with stromal tumors with poor prognostic features, chemotherapy with etoposide and carboplatin (with or without doxorubicin) should be considered after surgery.

Radiation

Epithelial, stromal, and germ cell ovarian cancer are sensitive to external beam radiation therapy (EBRT). EBRT is useful for several manifestations of this illness:

- Metastases to the brain (uncommon)
  - Gamma-knife approaches to single, clinically problematic lesions
  - Standard whole-brain radiotherapy
- Radiation to single clinically problematic lesions, such as impending obstruction

Maintenance Chemotherapy

- In a clinical study of maintenance chemotherapy after initial chemotherapy, monthly maintenance paclitaxel for 3 versus 12 months after completion of initial chemotherapy showed progression-free survival (PFS). No overall survival (OS) benefit was observed, but the study was not powered for this endpoint.
- Initial data from the AFTER-6 trial showed no PFS or OS benefit of 0 versus 6 cycles of monthly maintenance paclitaxel after completion of initial chemotherapy.
- There is no role for maintenance chemotherapy at this time, though ongoing studies are evaluating its use.

Chemotherapy for Recurrent or Persistent Disease

- 80% to 90% of stage III to IV patients will recur.
- Recurrence within 6 months of initial platinum-based chemotherapy is platinum-resistant disease.
- Recurrence/progression while on initial chemotherapy is platinum-refractory disease.
- Platinum-sensitive patients may be retreated with platinum ($\pm$taxane) therapy; 70% of patients $\geq$2 years from initial treatment will respond to retreatment.
- Recurrence within 6 to 12 months from initial therapy is considered a gray zone but is generally treated according to a platinum-resistant paradigm.
- Recurrent ovarian cancer is not curable.
- There is no known benefit to treating a chemical recurrence defined as a rise in CA125 alone.
- Single-agent therapy is usually recommended in the treatment of recurrent disease, with this caveat: Gemcitabine/cisplatin has been shown to improve survival in both platinum-sensitive and platinum-resistant disease, albeit with markedly increased toxicity.
- Single agents commonly used include:
  - Pegylated liposomal doxorubicin
  - Topotecan
  - Gemcitabine
  - Taxotere
  - Oral etoposide
  - Weekly paclitaxel
  - Hexamethylmelamine
  - Consideration of hormone ablation with letrozole/anastrazole or tamoxifen
- There has been increasing interest in the use of molecularly targeted therapy, particularly antiangiogenic therapy.

– Bevacizumab, an anti-VEGF antibody, has modest activity in relapsed ovarian cancer, both platinum-sensitive and platinum-resistant, but is not currently approved for use.
– Bevacizumab is presently being tested in combination with other agents in both the upfront (with carboplatin/paclitaxel) and relapsed settings (e.g., with sorafenib).

Experimental Therapy

Patients with ovarian cancer should be encouraged to participate in controlled clinical trials approved by the NCI and/or the FDA. Cooperative groups and individual institutions such as the Gynecologic Oncology Group have trials for patients at first diagnosis, follow-up in remission, and in recurrence. Phase 1 clinical trials are reasonable treatment options for some patients.

SUPPORTIVE CARE

Common Toxicities From Treatment

• Table 17.3 lists a range of toxicities that commonly occur with chemotherapy regimens for ovarian cancer.
• Myelosuppression
  – Initial prophylaxis for myelosuppression is not recommended with current therapy.
  – Erythropoietin and granulocyte colony-stimulating factor (G-CSF) are effective treatments.
  – Platelet count should be followed carefully in patients receiving carboplatin.
  – In upfront therapy, the dosage of carboplatin should be reduced only if patients are refractory to growth factor support and cannot be switched to cisplatin, as this is potentially curative treatment.

TABLE 17.3. *Toxicities of ovarian cancer treatment*

Myelosuppression	More common with carboplatin than cisplatin
	Can be treated with growth factors
Nausea/vomiting	More common with cisplatin than carboplatin
	Every attempt should be made to aggressively premedicate patients
	Anticipatory nausea is also common and responds best to benzodiazeipines
Renal dysfunction	More common with cisplatin than carboplatin
	Can be irreversible
	Usually nonoliguric—vigilance is required
Neurotoxicity	Subjective sensory neuropathy can occur without objective findings
	Common distribution is peripheral neuropathy (fingers/toes)
	More common with cisplatin than carboplatin
Fatigue	Common postoperatively and with chemotherapy
	No effective intervention
	Patient should be evaluated for anemia and hypothyroidism (side effect of some of the novel targeted agents)
Altered sexual function	Combination etiologies of oophorectomy and chemotherapy
	Should be queried regularly
	Uncertain benefit of hormonal therapy and uncertain effect on disease
Depression	Can be chemotherapy-related as well as situational
	Antidepressants can help, and may help other side effects such as hot flashes (i.e., venlafaxine)
	Psychiatric referral should be considered
Rare toxicities	Ototoxicity, hypersensitivity reactions, perforation with bevacizumab, acute myelogenous leukemia

- Nausea/vomiting
  - Patients should be aggressively premedicated due to the emetogenic potential of platinum therapy.
  - 5HT-3 receptor antagonists, phenothiazines, benzodiazepines, and corticosteroids are appropriate choices.
  - Neurokinin 1 receptor antagonists should be considered standard with cisplatin treatment and may be effective in refractory patients treated with other agents.
- Renal dysfunction
  - In patients treated with platinums, serum creatinine underestimates renal dysfunction.
  - Great care should be taken in patients with borderline or abnormal renal function.
- Neurotoxicity
  - Both platinums and taxanes cause neuropathy.
  - Grade 1 to 2 neuropathy generally resolves by 1 year after treatment.
  - Grade 3 to 4 neuropathy can have long-term effects and may require substitution or discontinuation of the offending agent(s).
- Perforation
  - Bevacizumab has been associated with a risk of gastrointestinal perforation in ovarian cancer patients (5–11%).
  - Possible risk factors for perforation include previous irradiation, tumor involving bowel, and early tumor response.
- Sexual dysfunction/depression
  - Sexual dysfunction and depression are commonly overlooked side effects of surgery and chemotherapy.
  - Depression can seriously compromise patients' quality of life and adherence to cancer therapy.
  - Patients should be regularly questioned about symptoms.
  - There are no solid data regarding the effects of hormonal treatment for sexual dysfunction on disease behavior.
  - Antidepressant therapy may be a reasonable option for many patients.
  - Participation in cancer support groups can be very helpful to patients and their families.

Obstruction

- Patients can present with both bowel and urinary tract obstruction.
- Initial treatment for bowel obstruction may be conservative, with bowel rest and nasogastric suction.
- Many patients will require surgical correction of the obstruction.
- The aggressiveness of intervention should be balanced with patient prognosis, understanding that recurrent ovarian cancer is a chronic disease that may respond to many agents.
- Systemic therapy should follow surgery.
- Urinary obstruction may be relieved with nephrostomies or ureteral stents, depending on the location of the obstruction.
- Occasionally, radiation therapy to a particular tumor causing obstruction may be appropriate.

SUGGESTED READINGS

Armstrong DK, Bundy B, Wenzel L, et al. Intraperitoneal cisplatin and paclitaxel in ovarian cancer. *N Engl J Med.* 2006;354:34–43.

Berek JS. Epithelial ovarian cancer. In: Berek JS, Hacker NF, eds. *Practical Gynecologic Oncology.* 3rd ed. Philadelphia, PA: Lippincott Williams & Wilkins; 2000:457–522.

Burger RA, Sill MW, Monk BJ, et al. A phase II trial of bevacizumab in persistent or recurrent epithelial ovarian cancer or primary peritoneal cancer: a Gynecologic Oncology Group study. *J Clin Oncol.* 2007;25:5165–5171.

Calvert AH, Newell DR, Gumbrell LA, et al. Carboplatin dosage; prospect of evaluation of a simple formula based on renal function. *J Clin Oncol.* 1989;7:1748–1756.

Cornelison TL, Reed E. Nephrotoxicity and hydration management for cisplatin, carboplatin, and ormaplatin: a review. *Gynecol Oncol.* 1993;50:147–158.

Goff BA, Mandel LS, Drescher CW, et al. Development of an ovarian cancer symptom index. *Cancer.* 2006;109:221–227.

Hoskins WJ, McGuire WP, Brady MF, et al. The effect of diameter of largest residual disease on survival after primary cytoreductive surgery in patients with suboptimal residual epithelial ovarian carcinoma. *Am J Obstet Gynecol.* 1994;170:974–979.

Jacobs I, Skates SJ, MacDonald N, et al. Screening for ovarian cancer: a pilot randomized controlled trial. *Lancet.* 1999;353:1207–1210.

Link C, Bicher A, Kohn E, et al. Flexible G-CSF dosing in ovarian cancer patients receiving dose intense taxol therapy. *Blood.* 1994;83:1188–1192.

McGuire WP, Hoskins WJ, Brady MF, et al. Taxol and cisplatin improve outcome in patients with advanced ovarian cancer as compared to cytoxan/cisplatin. *N Engl J Med.* 1996;334:1–6.

NCCN Practice Guidelines. Ovarian Cancer.v.1. 2008. Available at: http://www.nccn.org/professionals/physician_gls/f_guidelines.asp. Accessed February 2008.

Ozols RF, Bundy BN, Greer BE, et al. Gynecologic Oncology Group. Phase III trial of carboplatin and paclitaxel compared with cisplatin and paclitaxel in patients with optimally resected stage III ovarian cancer: a Gynecologic Oncology Group study. *J Clin Oncol.* 2003;21:3194–3200.

Ozols RF, Schwartz PE, Eifel PJ. Ovarian cancer, fallopian tube carcinoma, and peritoneal carcinoma. In: DeVita VT Jr, Hellman S, Rosenberg SA, eds. *Cancer Principles and Practice of Oncology.* 6th ed. Philadelphia, PA: Lippincott Williams & Wilkins; 2001:1597–1532.

Reed E. Cisplatin and analogs. In: Chabner BA, Longo D, eds. *Cancer Chemotherapy and Biotherapy Principles and Practice.* 3rd ed. Philadelphia, PA: Lippincott Williams & Wilkins; 2001:447–465.

Reed E, Jacob J. Carboplatin and renal dysfunction. *Ann Intern Med.* 1989;110:409.

Reed E, Zerbe CS, Brawley OW, et al. Analysis of autopsy evaluations of ovarian cancer patients treated at the National Cancer Institute, 1972–1988. *Am J Clin Oncol.* 2000;28:107–116.

Simpkins FA, Devoogdt NM, Rasool N, et al. The alarm anti-protease, secretory leukocyte protease inhibitor, is a proliferation and survival factor for ovarian cancer cells. *Carcinogenesis.* 2008;29(3):466–472.

18

Endometrial Cancer

Christina M. Annunziata and Michael J. Birrer

EPIDEMIOLOGY

- Endometrial cancer is the most common pelvic gynecologic malignancy in women, comprising 6% of all cancers in women.
- In 2008, 40,100 new cases were projected. The current incidence of endometrial cancer is 10 to 20 cases per 100,000 population and has stayed constant since the 1980s.
- An estimated 7,470 deaths occurred in 2008 due to this malignancy, accounting for 3% of all cancer deaths in women.
- The mortality rate continues to decline, likely because of increased awareness of symptoms including abnormal vaginal bleeding.
- Although incidence is 1.4 times higher in white women than in African-American women, the 5-year survival rate is lower in African American women than in white women (60% vs. 85%).
- Peak incidence is in the sixth and seventh decades of life; 5% of cases are diagnosed before the age of 40; 20% to 25% of patients are diagnosed before menopause.

RISK FACTORS

- Endogenous estrogen excess:
  - Polycystic ovary disease
  - Anovulatory menstrual cycles
  - Obesity: being overweight by 20 to 50 pounds increases risk threefold and being overweight by >50 pounds increases risk 10-fold.
  - Granulosa cell tumor of the ovary, or other estrogen-secreting tumors
  - Advanced liver disease
- Endogenous prolonged estrogen exposure:
  - Early menarche and late menopause: menopause in women older than 52 years increases risk by 2.4-fold.
  - Irregular menses, infertility, and nulliparity: Nulliparous women have twice the risk of developing uterine cancer compared to women with one child and thrice the risk compared to women who give birth to five or more children.
- Exogenous unopposed estrogen sources: of note, tamoxifen (TAM) acts as a weak estrogen, increasing the relative risk (RR) of developing endometrial cancer by twofold to eightfold depending on length of exposure to the drug.
- Type 2 diabetes mellitus (DM), possibly related to the effects of hyperinsulinemia
- Hypertension
- Personal or family history:
  - Personal history of breast, ovarian, or colorectal cancer
  - Personal or family history consistent with hereditary nonpolyposis colorectal cancer (HNPCC) (Lynch II syndrome)
  - History of endometrial cancer in a first-degree relative increases risk threefold.
  - History of colorectal cancer in a first-degree relative increases risk of endometrial cancer twofold.

PROTECTIVE FACTORS

- Oral contraceptives:
  - There is a 50% decrease in RR when oral contraceptives that include a progestin are used for at least 12 months.
  - Protection lasts for at least 10 years after discontinuation of oral contraceptive.
  - Similar protection has been observed with hormone replacement therapy that includes daily progestin.
- Physical activity: Epidemiologic evidence suggests lower incidence of endometrial cancer with increased physical activity.
- Cigarette smoking appears to have a modest protective role. However, this is strongly outweighed by the significantly increased risk of lung cancer and other major health hazards.

DIAGNOSIS AND SCREENING

- Routine screening for endometrial cancer is not required in asymptomatic women, except those with HNPCC. ACS recommendation for women with HNPCC is annual endometrial biopsy after age 35.
- Women taking TAM should have a gynecologic evaluation according to the same guidelines for women not taking TAM.
- Endometrial biopsy is the preferred diagnostic test for symptomatic patients (vaginal bleeding or spotting).

Signs and Symptoms

Abnormal vaginal bleeding is a common symptom of endometrial cancer, seen in approximately 90% of cases.

- Premenopausal women with prolonged and/or heavy menses or intermenstrual spotting should undergo endometrial biopsy.
- All postmenopausal women with vaginal bleeding should be evaluated for endometrial cancer (20% of these patients will ultimately be diagnosed with the malignancy).
- Biopsy is also recommended for women taking estrogen therapy for menopausal symptoms who may have withdrawal bleeding.

Asymptomatic patients with abnormal glandular tissue on Pap smear should be evaluated for endometrial cancer.

- All postmenopausal women with endometrial cells on Pap smear should be evaluated for malignancy.
- Approximately 10% of uterine cancer cases are detected by Pap smear. Pap smear alone, however, is not an adequate tool for detecting endometrial malignancy.

Palpable, locally advanced tumor detected on pelvic examination is suggestive of endometrial cancer. Signs and symptoms of advanced disease, manifested in <10% of cases, include:

- Bowel obstruction
- Jaundice
- Ascites
- Pain

Procedures

- Endocervical curettage and endometrial biopsy are well-tolerated outpatient procedures.
- Pap smear is of limited value (see previous section).
- Fractional curettage under anesthesia involves scraping of the endocervical canal, followed by the uterine walls, in a set sequence. This is standard procedure for the diagnosis of endometrial cancer in symptomatic women with negative or inadequate endometrial biopsy.

- Available data on transvaginal ultrasound suggest a correlation between endometrial stripe thickness, as seen on ultrasound, and subsequent risk of endometrial cancer. An endometrial stripe cutoff of <4 to 5 mm has been used as a diagnostic criterion; however, cases of endometrial cancer could occasionally be missed. Patients taking TAM tend to have thicker endometrium than women who do not take TAM. There is therefore no consensus on the cutoff thickness of endometrial stripe that would indicate a need for endometrial biopsy.

HISTOLOGY

Subtypes

Subtypes of endometrial cancer include endometrioid (75–80%), uterine papillary serous (5–10%), clear cell (1–5%), mucinous (1%), squamous cell (<1%), and uterine sarcoma (<10%). Endometrial carcinoma may also be divided into types 1 and 2, according to estrogen dependence:

- Type 1 (estrogen-related), the more common type of endometrial carcinoma, is associated with DM and obesity and tends to have better prognosis. Characteristics include the following:
  - Endometrioid histology
  - More differentiated, lower grade, higher progesterone receptor (PR) levels
  - Less myometrial invasion, lower stage at presentation
  - Younger patients
  - Genetic aberrations: mutations in K-ras, b-catenin, PI3K, and PTEN, microsatellite instability, DNA mismatch repair defects
- Type 2 (unrelated to estrogen stimulation and endometrial hyperplasia):
  - Nonendometrioid histology (serous, clear cell)
  - Commonly associated with p53 mutations (serous)
  - Aneuploid
  - Her2/neu overexpressed
- Adenomatous hyperplasia is an estrogen-dependent lesion that could be seen along with type 1 but not type 2 endometrial carcinoma.

PRETHERAPY EVALUATION

- Physical examination
- Chest x-ray
- Urinary imaging studies (i.v. pyelogram or renal scan), cystoscopy, and proctoscopy (very rarely done)
- Routine blood and urine studies
- CA125 >65 can predict extrauterine and/or lymph node metastasis.
- Routine age-appropriate health maintenance; if HNPCC is suspected, colonoscopy should be performed before planning treatment.
- Evaluation of specific symptoms or physical examination findings as indicated
- Routine use of ultrasound, computerized tomography (CT) scan, and magnetic resonance imaging (MRI) are NOT recommended; bone scan rarely yields useful information.

STAGING

- Staging for endometrial carcinoma is surgical (Table 18.1) and is based on information from hysterectomy, bilateral salpingo-oophorectomy (BSO), peritoneal cytology, and pelvic and periaortic lymph node (LN) dissection.
- Endometrial cancer distribution by stage:
  - Stage I: 70% to 75%
  - Stage II: 10% to 15%
  - Stage III: 5% to 10%
  - Stage IV: <5%

TABLE 18.1. *Staging for endometrial cancer*

Stage IA G123	Tumor limited to endometrium
Stage IB G123	Invasion to <50% of the myometrium
Stage IC G123	Invasion to >50% of the myometrium
Stage IIA G123	Endocervical glandular involvement only
Stage IIB G123	Cervical stromal invasion
Stage IIIA G123	Tumor invades serosa and/or adnexa, and/or positive peritoneal cytology
Stage IIIB G123	Vaginal metastases
Stage IIIC G123	Metastases to pelvic and/or para-aortic lymph nodes
Stage IVA G123	Tumor invasion of bladder and/or bowel mucosa
Stage IVB	Distant metastases including intra-abdominal and/or inguinal lymph nodes

Histopathology—degree of differentiation:
Cases of carcinoma of the corpus should be classified (or graded) according to the degree of histologic differentiation, as follows:
  G1: 5% of a nonsquamous or nonmorular solid growth pattern
  G2: 6% to 50% of a nonsquamous or nonmorular solid growth pattern
  G3: >50% of a nonsquamous or nonmorular solid growth pattern
Notes on pathologic gradings;
1. Notable nuclear atypia, inappriopriate for the architectural grade, raises the grade of a grade 1 or grade 2 tumor by 1.
2. In serous adenocarcinomas, clear cell adenocarcinomas, and squamous cell carcinomas, nuclear grading takes precedence.
3. Adenocarcinomas with squamous differentiation are graded according to the nuclear grade of the glandular component.
Rules related to staging:
1. Because corpus cancer is now staged surgically, procedures previously used for determining stages are no longer applicable, such as findings from fractional dilation and curettage to differentiate between stage I and II.
2. A small number of patients with corpus cancer may be treated primarily with RT. In that case, the clinical staging adopted by FIGO (Federation Internationale de Gynecogie et d'Obstetrique) in 1971 should still apply, but designation of that staging system should be noted.
3. Ideally, the width of the myometrium should be measured along with the width of tumor invasion.

Source: From DiSaia PJ, Creasman WT. *Clinical Gynecologic Oncology.* 5th ed. St. Louis: Mosby; 1997: 140–141, with permission.

PROGNOSTIC FACTORS

Uterine

- Histologic type
- Histologic differentiation
- Tumor hormone-receptor status: the presence and levels of estrogen receptor (ER)/PR are inversely proportional to histologic grade and are associated with longer survival.
- Five-year survival (%) distribution by stage:
  - Stage I: 81% to 91%
  - Stage II: 71% to 79%
  - Stage III: 30% to 60%
  - Stage IV: 14% to 17%
- Tumor size: tumors >2 cm have worse prognosis.
- Vascular-space invasion: rate of disease recurrence is approximately 25%.

Extrauterine

- Positive peritoneal cytology: rate of disease recurrence is approximately 15%.
- LN metastasis:
  - Involvement of pelvic LN or peritoneal metastases: approximately 25% risk of recurrence
  - Metastasis to para-aortic LN: risk increases to 40%

- Adnexal metastasis: approximately 15% risk of recurrence
- Myometrial invasion

MANAGEMENT

Total abdominal hysterectomy (TAH) or BSO is the treatment of choice for patients with persistent endometrial hyperplasia after failure of adequate therapy with progestin.

Therapy should be individualized for endometrial carcinoma. However, the following guidelines may be generally employed:

- Low risk: TAH/BSO (selected pelvic LN may be removed). This can considered adequate for certain patients with:
  - Well-differentiated or moderately differentiated tumors
  - Negative peritoneal cytology. If no peritoneal fluid is found during surgery, peritoneal washing with normal saline should be done.
  - No vascular-space invasion
  - <50% myometrial invasion
- Intermediate risk: TAH/BSO combined with para-aortic and selective pelvic LN sampling or dissection. If there are no medical or technical contraindications (e.g., morbid obesity), this should be done in patients with:
  - Grade 1 or 2 tumors involving >50% of myometrium (stage IC)
  - Tumor presence in cervical isthmus (stage II)
  - Nonendometrioid histology
  - Visible or palpable LN enlargement
- High risk: Adjuvant therapy is recommended. Adjuvant radiation reduces the risk of local recurrence; adjuvant chemotherapy has shown a survival advantage (see following section). Adjuvant therapy is recommended for patients with:
  - Grade 3 with any myometrial invasion
  - Grade 2 with >50% myometrial invasion or cervical/vaginal involvement
  - Adnexal or pelvic metastasis
  - Lymphovascular-space involvement

Adjuvant Therapies

Chemotherapy

Chemotherapy is recommended for women with advanced extrauterine disease. Regimens of choice include:

- TAP (doxorubicin 45 mg/m^2, cisplatin 50 mg/m^2 on day 1; paclitaxel 160 mg/m^2 on day 2) for six cycles with G-CSF support
- TC (paclitaxel 175 mg/m^2 and carboplatin AUC 5) for six cycles

Chemotherapy has shown a survival advantage over whole abdominal irradiation (WAI) in advanced endometrial carcinoma (Trial GOG 122 by the Gynecologic Oncology Group).

- AP (doxorubicin 60 mg/m^2, cisplatin 50 mg/m^2 for seven cycles, plus one additional cycle of cisplatin alone) was compared to WAI (30 Gy in 20 fractions with a 15-Gy boost to pelvic and para-aortic nodes).
- Better progression-free and overall survival were seen in the chemotherapy arm.

Radiation Therapy

Radiation therapy (RT) may be used alone in women with high-risk cancer confined to the endometrium. It may be considered in patients with extrauterine disease confined to the pelvic lymph nodes. RT reduces risk of local recurrence. Strategies include the following:

- Whole pelvic RT: 45 to 50 Gy external beam radiation (EBRT) along with vaginal irradiation with vaginal cylinder or colpostats to bring the vaginal surface dose to 80 to 90 Gy (5-year disease-free survival of 80% and locoregional control of 90% seen with this treatment).

- Vaginal brachytherapy: may be administered alone if patient has undergone complete surgical staging to confirm that disease is confined to the uterus.
- WAI (falling out of favor)
- Preoperative intracavitary radiation plus EBRT: This method is a combination of preoperative intracavitary radiation (consisting of uterine tandem and vaginal colpostat insertions with a standard Fletcher applicator delivering 20 to 25 Gy to a point A) and EBRT (40–45 Gy with standard fractionation delivered to multiple fields). In patients with extensive cervical involvement precluding initial hysterectomy, EBRT should be followed in 4 to 6 weeks by hysterectomy and BSO with periaortic LN sampling. This approach can provide 5-year disease-free survival of 70% to 80%.

Combined Chemotherapy and RT

- May decrease local recurrence rate, which can be as high as 50% with chemotherapy alone.
- Clinical trials are currently underway to address concomitant (GOG 9907) or sequential (GOG 9908) administration of chemotherapy and RT.

Special Considerations

- Low-risk, low-grade patients who still desire fertility can be managed with progestational agents such as Mirena IUD, with appropriate follow-up to ensure a response to therapy.
- Low-risk patients who are not surgical candidates can be treated with RT alone; however, this may achieve a lower cure rate than surgery.
- Combined surgery and EBRT has a higher complication rate than either treatment alone (e.g., bowel complications, 4%). Therefore, special attention should be given to appropriate patient selection and choice of surgical techniques. Fewer complications are seen with retroperitoneal approach and with LN sampling versus LN dissection.
- Pelvic surgery has an increased risk for thrombophlebitis in the pelvis and lower extremities; hence, low-dose heparin or Venodyne compression stockings should be used.
- The subgroup of women with isolated ovarian metastasis has a relatively better prognosis. However, some believe that this represents double primary tumors rather than true metastasis from primary endometrial cancer. Five-year disease-free survival ranges between 60% and 82%, depending on histologic grade and depth of myometrial invasion. Pelvic radiation doses of 45 to 50 Gy are given in standard fractionation, with vaginal boost with cylinder or colpostats adding 30 to 35 Gy to the vaginal surface.
- If tumor extends to the pelvic wall, patients should be considered inoperable and treated with RT.
- When parametrial extension is present, preoperative RT (external and intracavitary) is applied.
- Patients who are not candidates for either surgery or RT are treated with progestational agents (see subsequent text).

Stage IVB and Recurrent Disease

Therapy recommendations depend on sites of metastasis or recurrent disease and disease-related symptoms. All patients should be considered for clinical trials.

Local Recurrence

- Pelvic exenteration: This method can be considered for patients with disease extending only to the bladder or rectum or for isolated central recurrence after irradiation. Occasional long-term survival has been reported.
- Palliative radiation: Radiation is applied for localized recurrences, for example, pelvic LN (EBRT together with brachytherapy boost), para-aortic LN, or distant metastases. For isolated vaginal recurrence, irradiation may be curative if not previously administered.

Distant Metastasis—Systemic Therapy

Hormonal therapy produces responses in 15% to 30% of patients and is associated with survival twice as long as in nonresponders. On average, responses last for 1 year. Tumor tissue should be checked for ER and PR levels, since hormone-receptor levels and degree of tumor differentiation correlate well with response. Hormonal therapy is preferred as first-line intervention for recurrent or metastatic endometrial cancer due to its lower toxicity profile and response rate similar to chemotherapy. Options include the following:

- Megestrol acetate (Megace), 160 to 320 mg daily is the preferred initial regimen.
- Medroxyprogesterone acetate (Depo-Provera), 400 to 1,000 mg i.m. weekly for 6 weeks and then monthly, or oral medroxyprogesterone (Provera), 150 mg PO daily.
- TAM, 20 mg PO daily, may be given as second-line with or without a progestin (addition of progestin may improve response rate).
- Aromatase inhibitors (e.g., anastrozole, letrozole) have limited activity.

CHEMOTHERAPY

- Single-agent therapy
  - Response rates 17% to 28%; partial responses of short duration (<6 months); overall survival 9 to 12 months
  - Options include doxorubicin, cisplatin, carboplatin, docetaxel, topotecan.
  - Paclitaxel: response rate 27% to 37%
- Combination chemotherapy
  - Response rates 36% to 67%; partial responses of short duration (4–8 months)
  - Overall survival not improved over single-agent therapy.
  - Combinations may include doxorubicin with cisplatin and/or cyclophosphamide; carboplatin with liposomal doxorubicin; cyclophosphamide, doxorubicin, and 5-FU.
  - Paclitaxel-containing regimens may improve response, progression-free intervals, and overall survival. Such regimens may include TAP (doxorubicin 45 mg/m^2, cisplatin 50 mg/m^2 on day 1; paclitaxel 160 mg/m^2 on day 2) or TC.
- Chemotherapy in conjunction with hormonal therapy
  - Response rates may be slightly higher than with either therapy alone.
  - Overall survival may also be improved.
- The addition of medroxyprogesterone (200 mg daily) to cyclophosphamide, doxorubicin, and 5-FU, followed by TAM 20 mg daily for 3 weeks was tested in a small clinical trial of 46 women. Overall survival was 14 months compared to 11 months with chemotherapy alone.

Estrogen-Replacement Therapy

Estrogen-replacement therapy for patients with endometrial cancer remains controversial.

Post-therapy Surveillance

- Most recurrences are seen in the first 3 years after primary therapy.
- NCCN guidelines for post-therapy surveillance of endometrial cancer include:
  - History and physical examination, including CA125 level, every 3 to 6 months for 2 years, then annually. Up to 70% of patients will report symptoms of vaginal bleeding, pain, cough, weight loss, etc.
  - Vaginal cytology every 6 months for 2 years, then annually

SUGGESTED READINGS

Chen L-M, Berek JS. Endometrial cancer: clinical features, diagnosis and screening. Available at: http://www.uptodateonline.com/utd/content/topic.do?topicKey=gyne_onc/9015&selectedTitle=2~150&source=search_result. Accessed February 2008.

NCCN Clinical Practice Guidelines in Oncology: Uterine Cancers. Available at: http://www.nccn.org/professionals/physician_gls/PDF/uterine.pdf. Accessed February 2008.

Plaxe SC, Mundt AJ. Staging, treatment, and follow-up of endometrial cancer. Available at: http:// www.uptodateonline.com/utd/content/topic.do?topicKey=gyne_onc/9499&selectedTitle= 3~150&source=search_result. Accessed February 2008.

Plaxe SC, Mundt AJ. Treatment of locally recurrent or advanced endometrial cancer. Available at: http://www.uptodateonline.com/utd/content/topic.do?topicKey=gyne_onc/13394&selectedTitle= 1~150&source=search_result. Accessed February 2008.

Prat J, Gallardo A, Cuatrecasas M, Catasus L. Endometrial carcinoma: pathology and genetics. *Pathology.* 2007;39(1):72–87.

Trope CG, Alektiar KM, Sabbatini P, Zaino RJ. Corpus: epithelial tumors. In: Hoskins WJ, Perez CA, Young RC, Barakat RR, Markman M, Randall ME, eds. *Principles and Practice of Gynecologic Oncology.* 4th ed. Philadelphia: Lippincott Williams and Wilkins; 2005:823–872.

19

Cervical Cancer

Alyssa C. Perroy and Herbert L. Kotz

EPIDEMIOLOGY

- Worldwide, cervical cancer is the second most common cancer and the second leading cause of cancer death in women.
- In 2002, more than 493,200 new cases were diagnosed worldwide; an estimated 273,500 women die each year of this disease.
- In the United States, cervical cancer is the third most common cancer of the female reproductive tract, with more than 11,000 new cases and 3,600 deaths estimated in 2007.
- Introduction of Papanicolaou (Pap) smear screening has reduced the incidence and mortality of invasive cervical cancer by almost 75% over the last 50 years; still, 10,000 to 15,000 new cases and 3,500 to 5,000 deaths occur annually in the United States.
- Only about one-third of women at risk for cervical cancer receive appropriate screening. With screening, the lifetime risk for developing cervical cancer is 0.83%; the lifetime risk of dying from the disease is 0.27%.

RISK FACTORS

Human Papillomavirus

- Women who have never had human papillomavirus (HPV) infection are not at risk for cervical cancer.
- More than 99% of all cervical cancers harbor HPV DNA and more than 200 types of HPV have been recognized on the basis of DNA sequence. Approximately 40 distinct HPV types are known to infect the genital tract, and at least 15 types have been associated with cancer.
- HPV viruses of high oncogenic potential that are associated with cervical cancer include types 16, 18, 31, 33, 35, 39, 45, 51, 52, 56, 58, 59, 68, 73, and 82. HPV types 26, 53, and 66 have been identified as probable high-risk types.
- The oncogenic effect of the high-risk HPV subtypes appears to be mediated by E6 and E7 proteins, which have been shown to inactivate tumor-suppressor genes p53 and pRb, respectively. The subsequent loss of the cell-cycle regulatory mechanism leads to malignant transformation.
- Current clinical data show no evidence that determining whether an invasive cervical cancer harbors HPV influences clinical outcome or management. Therefore, routine HPV typing is not recommended except in clinical trials. For patients with cervical intraepithelial neoplasia (CIN), the presence of high-risk HPV serotypes increases the risk of invasive disease.

Demographic Risk Factors

- Race: higher incidence among Latin American, African American, and Native American women
- Socioeconomic status: more prevalent in lower socioeconomic classes
- Education: higher incidence among undereducated
- Age: more common in older women

Personal or Sexual Risk Factors

- Penile cancer in a male sexual partner places a woman at higher risk for cervical cancer.
- Among males with multiple sex partners (a known risk factor for HPV infection), there is a significant inverse association between penile circumcision and risk of cervical cancer for their female partners.
- Smoking increases relative risk (RR) of squamous cell cervical cancer twofold and has been shown to accelerate progression of dysplasia to invasive carcinoma twofold.
- Use of oral contraceptives for more than 5 years results in RR of 2.7.
- HIV-positive women have an RR of 2.5 (standardized incidence ratio = 12.5).

Medical and Gynecologic Risk Factors

- Incidence of cervical cancer is higher in multiparous versus nulliparous women (RR = 3.8).
- Prior abnormal Pap smear or documented dysplasia is associated with increased risk.
- Renal transplantation (RR = 5.7) and HIV infection increase the risk of cervical cancer. (AIDS in HIV-positive women with cervical cancer is defined according to the 1993 Centers for Disease Control and Prevention criteria.)

SCREENING

The American College of Obstetricians and Gynecologists recommends the following:

- Women should begin screening 3 years after the onset of sexual activity or at age 21, whichever is earlier.
- Women under age 30 should have an annual liquid-based Pap test until the age of 30. After age 30, if a woman has had three consecutive normal Pap tests, screening can be performed every 2 to 3 years.
- Alternatively, women over 30 can undergo a combination of cytology and DNA testing. If both are negative, repeat screening should resume no more frequently than every 3 years.
- Cervical cytology should be described using the 2001 Bethesda System (Table 19.1), detailing specimen adequacy and interpretation.
- Interpretation is divided into nonmalignant findings and epithelial cell abnormalities including atypia, low-grade and high-grade intraepithelial lesions, glandular lesions, and squamous cell carcinoma.
- Screening should end at age 70. It may end earlier for women who have had a complete hysterectomy and no prior history of grade 2 or 3 CIN.

PRECURSOR LESIONS

- Mild, moderate, and severe cervical dysplasias are categorized as CIN 1, 2, and 3, respectively.
- Mild to moderate dysplasias are more likely to regress than progress. Nevertheless, the rate of progression of mild dysplasia to severe dysplasia is 1% per year; the rate of progression of moderate dysplasia to severe dysplasia is 16% within 2 years and 25% within 5 years.
- In more than 30% of cases, untreated carcinoma in situ will progress to invasive cancer within 10 years.

SIGNS AND SYMPTOMS

- Abnormal vaginal bleeding (i.e., postcoital, intermenstrual, or menorrhagia) is usually the first manifestation of CIN.
- Vaginal discharge (serosanguineous or yellowish, sometimes foul smelling) usually represents a more advanced lesion.

TABLE 19.1. *The 2001 Bethesda system of terminology for reporting results of cervical cytology*

Specimen adequacy
- Satisfactory for evaluation (note presence/absence of endocervical/transformation zone component)
- Unsatisfactory for evaluation (specify reason)
  - Specimen rejected/not processed (specify reason)
  - Specimen processed and examined, but unsatisfactory for evaluation of epithelial abnormality because of (specify reason)

General categorization (optional)
- Negative for intraepithelial lesions or malignancy
- Epithelial cell abnormality
- Other

Interpretation/result
- Negative for intraepithelial lesions or malignancy
  - Organisms
    - Trichomonas vaginalis
    - Fungal organisms morphologically consistent with *Candida* species
    - Shift in flora suggestive of bacterial vaginosis
    - Bacteria morphologically consistent with *Actinomyces* species
    - Cellular changes consistent with herpes simplex virus
  - Other non-neoplastic findings (optional to report; list not comprehensive)
    - Reactive cellular changes associated with
      - Inflammation (includes typical repair)
      - Radiation
      - Intrauterine contraceptive device
    - Glandular cells status post-hysterectomy
    - Atrophy
- Epithelial cell abnormalities
  - Squamous cell
    - Atypical squamous cell (ASC)
      - Undetermined significance (ASC-US)
      - Cannot exclude high-grade squamous intraepithelial lesion (ASC-H)
    - Low-grade squamous intraepithelial lesion (LSIL)
      - Encompassing human papillomavirus/mild dysplasia/cervical intraepithelial neoplasia 1 (CIN1)
    - High-grade squamous intraepithelial lesion (HSIL)
      - Encompassing moderate and severe dysplasia, carcinoma in situ (CIN2 and CIN3)
    - Squamous cell carcinoma
  - Glandular cell
    - Atypical glandular cells (AGC) (specify endocervical, endometrial, or not otherwise specified)
    - AGC, favor neoplastic (specify endocervical or not otherwise specified)
    - Endocervical adenocarcinoma in situ (AIS)
    - Adenocarcinoma
- Other (list not comprehensive)
- Endometrial cells in a woman ≥40 years of age

Source: From Solomon D, Davey D, Kurman R, et al. The 2001 Bethesda System: terminology for reporting results of cervical cytology. *JAMA.* 2002;287:2114–2119, with permission.

- Fatigue and anemia-related symptoms: common in patients with chronic bleeding
- Pain in the lumbosacral or gluteal area: may suggest hydronephrosis caused by tumor, or tumor extension to lumbar roots
- Urinary or rectal symptoms (hematuria, rectal bleeding, etc.): indicates bladder or rectal involvement
- Persistent, unilateral, or bilateral edema in legs: indicates lymphatic and venous blockage caused by extensive pelvic-wall disease
- Leg pain, edema, and hydronephrosis: characteristic of advanced-stage disease (IIIB)

DIAGNOSTIC WORKUP

- History and physical exam should include bimanual pelvic and rectal examinations. These are usually normal with stage IA disease (microscopic invasion only).
- Most frequent findings include visible cervical lesion or abnormal bimanual pelvic examination

Standard Diagnostic Procedures

- Pap smear in absence of gross lesion
- Colposcopic biopsy
- Conization (subclinical tumor)
- Punch biopsies (edge of gross tumor)
- Dilation and curettage
- Cystoscopy and rectosigmoidoscopy for symptoms referable to the bladder, colon, or rectum

Radiologic Studies

- Chest x-ray
- Intravenous pyelography (IVP) or CT scan with i.v. contrast. In the current Federation of Gynecology and Obstetrics (FIGO) system, information obtained from CT scan beyond that which would be apparent from IVP cannot be used for staging.
- Barium enema (stages III, IVA; used in earlier stages if there are symptoms referable to colon or rectum)
- MRI if required for better disease evaluation
- FDG-PET (most accurate nonsurgical means of detecting involved lymph nodes)

Laboratory Studies

- Complete blood count
- Blood chemistries
- Urinalysis

HISTOLOGY

- Cervical carcinoma originates at the squamous-columnar junction, or transformation zone, of the cervix.
- 75% to 80% of cervical cancers are of squamous cell histology; the remaining 20% to 25% are mostly adenocarcinomas or adenosquamous carcinomas.

STAGING

- Unlike other gynecologic malignancies, cervical cancer is clinically staged (Table 19.2). Laparoscopy, lymphangiography, CT, MRI, FDG-PET, and major surgical procedures are not used for the purpose of staging.
- While surgical staging is more accurate than clinical staging and would therefore seem preferable, there is no definitive evidence that it improves overall survival (OS). Surgical staging should thus be reserved for clinical trials.

PROGNOSTIC FACTORS

- Multivariate analysis by the Gynecologic Oncology Group (GOG) determined that para-aortic lymph node (LN) involvement is the most significant negative prognostic factor, followed by pelvic LN involvement, larger tumor size, younger age, and advanced tumor stage.

TABLE 19.2. *Staging of cervical cancer*

Stage	Definition
0	Carcinoma in situ; confined to cervix
IA	Microscopic evidence of cancer
IA1	Measured stromal invasion ≤3.0 mm deep and extension ≤7.0 mm wide
IA2	Measured stromal invasion >3.0 mm deep and ≤5.0 mm; extension ≤7.0 mm wide
IB	Clinically visible lesion limited to cervix uteri
IB1	Clinically visible lesions ≤4.0 cm
IB2	Clinically visible lesions >4.0 cm
II	Carcinoma invades beyond uterus but not to pelvic wall or lower third of vagina
IIA	No obvious parametrial involvement
IIB	Obvious parametrial involvement
III	Extension to pelvic wall
IIIA	Tumor involves lower third of vagina, with no extension to pelvic wall
IIIB	Extension to pelvic wall and/or hydronephrosis or nonfunctioning kidney
IV	Extension beyond true pelvis or has clinically involved mucosa of bladder or rectum
IVA	Spread to adjacent organs
IVB	Spread to distant organs

Source: From International Federation of Gynecology and Obstetrics. Benedet JL, Odicino F, Maisonneneuve P, et al. Carcinoma of the cervix uteri. *J Epidemiol Biostat.* 2001;6:5–44, with permission.

- Uterine-body invasion, determined by MRI, is a proven negative prognostic factor for OS.
- Lymphovascular invasion and tumor grade are significant prognostic factors.
- In one series of advanced cervical cancer patients, adenocarcinoma was a negative prognostic factor for OS, but whether adenocarcinoma histology is a more negative prognostic factor than squamous cell histology remains controversial.
- Five-year survival based on extent of tumor at diagnosis:
  - Localized: 92%
  - Regional: 56%
  - Distant spread: 16.5%
  - Unstaged at diagnosis: 60%

MODE OF SPREAD

- Spread is usually orderly along lymphovascular planes into the parametria. It may extend to the vaginal mucosa or endomyometrium, or by direct extension into adjacent structures.
- Lymphatic spread most commonly involves pelvic and para-aortic LNs.
- Hematogenous spread most commonly involves lung, liver, and bone.

TREATMENT

Stage 0 (Carcinoma In Situ)

- Noninvasive lesions can be eradicated by electrocautery, cryotherapy, laser therapy, or surgical procedure.
- A one-step diagnostic and therapeutic option is the loop electrosurgical excision procedure (LEEP), which allows excision of the entire transformation zone of the cervix with a low-voltage diathermy loop. In select situations, LEEP may be an acceptable alternative to cold-knife conization because it is a quick, outpatient procedure requiring only local anesthesia. However, current data do not support LEEP as an adequate replacement for conization in all clinical situations.
- Management of adenocarcinoma in situ remains unsettled, but hysterectomy is preferred in women who have completed childbearing. If preservation of fertility is desired, conservative management is acceptable if cone margins are negative.

Invasive Cervical Cancer

- Treatment in each stage may vary depending on the size of the tumor.
- Results from five randomized phase 3 trials demonstrated an OS advantage for cisplatin-based chemotherapy given concurrently with radiation therapy. These trials have demonstrated a 30% to 50% overall reduction in risk of death in patients with FIGO stage IB2 to IVA tumors and in patients with FIGO I to IIA tumors with poor prognostic factors (i.e., pelvic LN involvement, parametrial disease, and positive surgical margins). Therefore, chemoradiation is the current standard of care for patients with more advanced disease requiring radiation therapy.
- The current standard of care is once-weekly cisplatin, 40 mg/m^2 i.v. (maximum 70 mg) for six doses, concurrent with radiation.

Stage IA1

- For patients with no lymphovascular invasion who have completed childbearing, a simple hysterectomy is indicated.
- For those who wish to preserve fertility, a conization with negative margins is adequate therapy.

Stage IA2, IB1, IIA (Early-Stage Disease)

Minimally Invasive Laparoscopic Surgery

- Shortened recovery time makes this an option whenever surgery is the chosen treatment modality, even in the case of radical vaginal hysterectomy.

Radical Trachelectomy

- This fertility-preserving surgery may be an option for small-volume, early-stage disease.

Para-aortic LN Sampling

- May be indicated in patients with positive pelvic nodes, clinically enlarged nodes, or patients with larger-volume disease.

Radiation Therapy

- Pelvic external beam radiation therapy (EBRT) followed by intracavitary applications may be considered. Pelvic inflammatory disease, inflammatory bowel disease, and pelvic kidney are relative contraindications to pelvic radiation.
- Higher central primary tumor doses of radiation can be delivered with the combination of EBRT and intracavitary irradiation than with EBRT alone. This strategy also leads to improved pelvic control and OS.
- Both high-dose rate (200–300 cGy/minute) and low-dose rate (50–60 cGy/hour) brachytherapy are currently being used. The relative merits of each are under evaluation.
- When necessary, radioactive isotopes (e.g., cesium 137) are introduced to the uterine cavity and vaginal fornices with special applicators such as the Fletcher-Suit intrauterine tandem and vaginal ovoid.
- Determining maximum effective dose to the primary tumor, as well as to the bladder and rectum, is of primary importance. A typical regimen of EBRT is 40 to 50 Gy, followed by 40 to 50 Gy to point A with brachytherapy for a total dose of 80 to 90 Gy to point A. (Point A is located 2 cm cephalad and 2 cm lateral to the cervical os. Anatomically, it correlates with the medial parametrium or lateral cervix, the point where the ureter and uterine artery cross.)
- Depending on the extent of disease, a parametrial boost with EBRT to a total dose of 60 Gy may be applied to point B (3 cm lateral to point A, corresponding to the pelvic-wall nodes).
- Radiation treatment is equivalent to surgery for stages IB and IIA, with identical 5-year OS and disease-free survival. Expected cure rate is 75% to 80% (85–90% in small-volume disease).

- In one series of patients with bulky stage IB2 or IIA disease treated with radiation alone, pelvic control was 70% compared to 89% for patients with nonbulky (<4 cm) tumors. Survival rate was also lower in patients with bulky tumors treated with radiation alone.
- A study by the Radiation Therapy Oncology Group (RTOG) showed an 11% 10-year survival advantage for patients with IB2, IIA, and IIB disease treated with prophylactic para-aortic nodal and total pelvic irradiation compared to those treated with pelvic irradiation alone.

Surgery

- The choice of surgery versus radiation depends on many factors, including size of tumor, age of patient, availability of local expertise, presence of other comorbid conditions, and patient's desire to preserve ovarian function.
- Postradiation (adjuvant) surgery may be considered in patients with residual tumor confined to the cervix or in patients with suboptimal brachytherapy because of vaginal anatomy.

Postoperative Pelvic Chemoradiation

- Pelvic chemoradiation following radical hysterectomy and bilateral pelvic LN dissection has been shown to reduce recurrence and improve survival among patients with negative pelvic nodes who are at risk for pelvic failure. Pelvic failure is characterized by a primary tumor >4 cm, outer third cervical stromal invasion, lymphovascular space invasion, and close vaginal margins (<0.5 cm).
- This treatment approach is also recommended for patients with positive pelvic nodes or positive surgical margins.
- Radiation doses are 45 to 50 Gy by external pelvic radiation, with boosts to specific sites as needed using external beam, intracavitary, or interstitial radiation.

Special Considerations

- Recent studies have clearly demonstrated the deleterious effect of radiotherapy on patients with anemia. Hemoglobin <12 g/dL at the time of radiation therapy results in increased local recurrence and decreased survival.
- Patients with suspected or confirmed para-aortic nodal disease should receive extended-field radiation encompassing pelvic and para-aortic areas. RTOG 79-20 demonstrated a survival advantage in stage IB2, IIA, and IIB disease with the addition of external beam para-aortic radiation over external beam pelvic radiation alone. Some patients with small-volume disease in para-aortic LNs and controllable pelvic disease can potentially be cured. However, radiation is of little use in gross para-aortic disease because surrounding organs (bowel, kidney, spinal cord, etc.) cannot tolerate the high doses of radiation required. For this reason, removal of grossly involved nodes prior to radiotherapy is indicated.
- Toxicity from standard para-aortic LN radiation is greater than from pelvic radiation alone, but is seen mostly in patients with prior abdominopelvic surgery.
- Different surgical techniques affect the incidence of complications secondary to para-aortic LN radiation. For example, extraperitoneal LN sampling leads to fewer postradiation complications than transperitoneal sampling.
- Intensity-modulated radiation therapy is also likely to reduce sequelae of para-aortic nodal irradiation.

Stages IIB, III, IVA

The role of surgery as a curative treatment decreases when tumor spreads beyond the cervix and vaginal fornices. Patients presenting with tumors at stages IIB, III, and IVA have the following treatment options:

- Chemoradiation: Single-agent weekly cisplatin is the most commonly utilized chemosensitizer. Other agents have been proposed, but are still in clinical trials.

• Radiation therapy: for patients with no para-aortic LN involvement, external beam pelvic radiation of 45 to 50 Gy, followed by brachytherapy with 40 to 50 Gy to point A, for a total dose of 80 to 90 Gy (applies to stages IB2 to IVA). Patients with para-aortic LN involvement benefit from extended-field radiation.

Special Considerations

Multivariate analysis has shown that a total dose of >8,500 cGy intracavitary radiation to point A (advanced stage only), use of chemosensitizers, and overall treatment time of <8 weeks are associated with improved pelvic tumor control and survival in cervical cancer patients.

Stage IVA

Treatment options include radical surgery (anterior, posterior, or total pelvic exenteration) and chemoradiation.

Stage IVB

Radiation, chemoradiation, or chemotherapy for palliation of central disease or distant metastases.

Palliative Chemotherapy

• No standard chemotherapy regimen has been shown to produce prolonged complete remissions.
• All patients are appropriate candidates for clinical trials.
• The most active single agents include:
  – Cisplatin: usual dose as a single agent or in combination regimens is 50 mg/m2 i.v. once every 3 weeks for a maximum of six cycles. A response rate of 18% to 31% has been documented. Higher doses (e.g., 100 mg/m2 i.v. once every 3 weeks) produce higher response rates, but toxicity is greater and response duration, survival, and progression-free survival were similar to those seen with the lower dose.
  – Carboplatin: 15% to 28% response rate, with less nephrotoxicity and neurotoxicity than cisplatin. May be considered an alternative to cisplatin in select patients.
  – Ifosfamide: 16% to 33% response rate in advanced disease; 15% response rate in recurrent disease.
  – Paclitaxel: 17% to 25% response rate, depending upon dose.
  – Irinotecan, vinorelbine, and gemcitabine.
  – In 2008 the GOG reported a comparison of cisplatin/taxol, cisplatin/topotecan, cisplatin/gemzar, and cisplatin/vinorelbine. Cisplatin/taxol had the best response rate, 29.1%. Also reported in 2008 was a small trial of bevicizumab as second- or third-line chemotherapy with an objective response rate of 11%.
• Responses to chemotherapy are of brief duration but ongoing GOG trials continue to assess combination regimens.
• The benefit of chemotherapy with or without radiation versus best supportive care in this patient population has not yet been established.

Recurrent Disease

• A 10% to 20% recurrence rate has been reported following primary surgery or radiotherapy in patients with stage IB to IIA disease with negative nodes; up to 70% of patients with more advanced-stage disease with or without positive nodes exhibit recurrences. As tumor volume at the primary disease site increases, local recurrence in the pelvis becomes more likely than the development of distant metastases.
• No curative therapy is available for recurrent disease outside previous surgical or radiation fields.

- For patients with recurrence in the pelvis after radical surgery, radiation combined with cisplatin has a 40% to 50% cure rate.
- Pelvic exenteration (resection of the bladder, rectum, vagina, uterus/cervix) is the preferred treatment for centrally located recurrent disease after radiation, with a 32% to 62% 5-year survival in select patients. Reconstructive procedures include continent urinary conduit, end-to-end rectosigmoid re-anastomosis, and myocutaneous graft for a neovagina. High-dose intraoperative radiation therapy combined with surgical resection is offered by some centers for patients whose tumors extend close to the pelvic sidewalls.
- Chemotherapy for recurrent disease is palliative, not curative, demonstrating low response rates, short response duration, and low OS rates (see Palliative Chemotherapy). Cisplatin is the most active single agent, with a response rate of 20% to 30% and a median survival of 7 months.

TREATMENT DURING PREGNANCY

- Cervical cancer is the most common gynecologic malignancy associated with pregnancy, ranging from 1 in 1,200 to 1 in 2,200 pregnancies.
- No therapy is warranted for preinvasive lesions; colposcopy is recommended to rule out invasive cancer.
- Conization is reserved for suspicion of invasion or for persistent cytologic evidence of invasive cancer in the absence of colposcopic confirmation. Management of dysplasia is usually postponed until postpartum.
- Treatment of invasive cancer depends on tumor stage and the fetus's gestational age. If cancer is diagnosed before fetal maturity, immediate appropriate cancer therapy for the relevant stage is recommended. However, with close surveillance, delay of therapy to achieve fetal maturity is a reasonable option for patients with stage IA and early IB disease. For more advanced disease, delaying therapy is not recommended unless diagnosis is made in the final trimester. When the fetus reaches acceptable maturity, a caesarean section precedes definitive treatment.

TREATMENT OF HIV-POSITIVE PATIENTS

- Cervical cancer patients who are HIV-positive have more aggressive and more advanced disease and poorer prognosis than HIV-negative patients.
- Treatment of preinvasive lesions and cervical cancer in HIV-positive patients is the same as in HIV-negative patients, though response to therapy is usually poorer.
- HIV alters the natural history of HPV infections, with decreased regression rates and more rapid progression to high-grade and invasive lesions.
- Data from Africa show that cervical cancer is the most common AIDS-defining neoplasm in women.

FOLLOW-UP AFTER PRIMARY THERAPY

In the first 2 years following therapy, 80% to 90% of tumors recur, indicating a need for frequent surveillance. Follow-up visits are recommended every 3 to 4 months in the first year post-treatment, every 4 months for the next year, every 6 months for the following 3 years, then annually to detect any potentially curable recurrences.

PREVENTION

The efficacy of vaccination against HPV-16 and -18 to prevent high-grade CIN has been demonstrated in multiple studies since 2002. The Centers for Disease Control and Prevention now recommend that American females between the ages of 11 and 26 be vaccinated.

SUGGESTED READING

ACOG Committee on Practice Bulletins. ACOG Practice Bulletin: clinical management guidelines for obstetrician-gynecologists. Number 45, August 2003. Cervical cytology screening (replaces committee opinion 152, March 1995). *Obstet Gynecol.* 2003;102:417–427.

Atahan IL, Onal C, Ozyar E, Yiliz F, Selek U, Kose F. Long-term outcome and prognostic factors in patients with cervical carcinoma: a retrospective study. *Int J Gynecol Cancer.* 2007;17:833–842.

Beriwal S, Gan GN, Heron DE, et al. Early clinical outcome with concurrent chemotherapy and extended-field, intensity-modulated radiotherapy for cervical cancer. *Int J Radiol Oncol Biol Phys.* 2007;68:166–171.

Blythe J, Edwards E, Heimbecker P. Paraaortic lymph node biopsy: a twenty-year study. *Am J Obstet Gynecol.* 1997;176:1157–1162.

Bosch FX, de Sanjose S. The epidemiology of human papillomavirus infection and cervical cancer. *Dis Markers.* 2007;23:213–227.

Bosch FX, Manos MM, Munoz N, et al. Prevalence of human papillomavirus in cervical cancer: a worldwide perspective. International Biological Study on Cervical Cancer (IBSCC) Study Group. *J Natl Cancer Inst.* 1995;87796–87802.

Burd EM. Human papillomavirus and cervical cancer. *Clin Microbiol Rev.* 2003;161–17.

Castellsague X, Bosch FX, Munoz M, et al. Male circumcision, penile human papillomavirus infection, and cervical cancer in female partners. *N Engl J Med.* 2002;346:1105–1112.

Clarke B, Chetty R. Postmodern cancer: the role of human immunodeficiency virus in uterine cervical cancer. *Mol Pathol.* 2002;55(1):19–24.

Friedlander M, Grogan M; U.S Preventative Services Task Force. Guidelines for the treatment of recurrent and metastatic cervical cancer. *Oncologist.* 2002;7342–7347.

FUTURE II Study Group. Quadrivalent vaccine against human papillomavirus to prevent high-grade cervical lesions. *N Engl J Med.* 2007;356:1915–1927.

Greer BE, Koh WJ, Stelzer KJ, Goff BA, Comsia N, Tran A. Expanded pelvic radiotherapy fields for treatment of local-regionally advanced carcinoma of the cervix: outcome and complications. *Am J Obstet Gynecol.* 1996;174:1141–1150.

Grigsby PW, Herzog TJ. Current management of patients with invasive cervical carcinoma. *Clin Obstet Gynecol.* 2001;44531–44537.

Hertel H, Kohler C, Grund D, et al. Radical vaginal trachelectomy (RVT) combined with laparoscopic pelvic lymphadenectomy: prospective multicenter study of 100 patients with early cervical cancer. *Gynecol Oncol.* 2006;103:506–511.

Hertel H, Kohler C, Michels W, Possover M, Tozzi R, Schneider A. Laparoscopic-assisted radical vaginal hysterectomy (LARVH): prospective evaluation of 200 patients with cervical cancer. *Gynecol Oncol.* 2003;90:505–511.

Holowaty P, Miller AB, Rohan T, To T. Natural history of dysplasia of the uterine cervix. *J Natl Cancer Inst.* 1999;91:252–258.

Kim H, Kim W, Lee M, Song E, Loh JJ. Tumor volume and uterine body invasion assessed by MRI for prediction of outcome in cervical carcinoma treated with concurrent chemotherapy and radiotherapy. *Jpn J Clin Oncol.* 2007;37:858–866.

Koutsky LA, Ault KA, Wheeler CM, et al. A controlled trial of a human papillomavirus type 16 vaccine. *N Engl J Med.* 2002;347(21):1645–1651.

Landoni F, Maneo A, Colombo A, et al. Randomised study of radical surgery versus radiotherapy for stage IB-IIA cervical cancer. *Lancet.* 1997;350:535–540.

Maiman M, Fruchter RG, Serur E, Remy JC, Feuer G, Boyce J. Human immunodeficiency virus infection and cervical neoplasia. *Gynecol Oncol* 1990;38:377–382.

Markowitz LE, Dunne EF, Saraiya M, et al. Quadrivalent human papillomavirus vaccine: recommendations of the Advisory Committee on Immunization Practices (ACIP). *MMWR Recomm Rep.* 2007;56(RR-2):1–24.

McDonald SD, Faught W, Gruslin A. Cervical cancer during pregnancy. *J Obstet Gynaecol Can.* 2002;24:491–498.

Munoz N, Bosch FX, de Sanjose S, et al. Epidemiologic classification of human papillomavirus types associated with cervical cancer. *N Engl J Med.* 2003;348:518–527.

Munoz N, Franceschi S, Bosetti C, et al. Role of parity and human papillomavirus in cervical cancer: the IARC multicentric case-control study. *Lancet.* 2002;359:1093–1101.

Murthy NS, Mathew A. Risk factors for pre-cancerous lesions of the cervix. *Eur J Cancer Prev.* 2000; 9(1):5–14.

National Cancer Institute. SEER: Surveillance Epidemiology and End Results. Cancer of the Cervix Uteri. Available at: http://seer.cancer.gov/statfacts/html/cervix.html?statfacts_page=cervix. html&x=16&y=18

Nguyen C, Montz FJ, Bristow RE. Management of stage I cervical cancer in pregnancy. *Obstet Gynecol Surv.* 2000;55:633–643.

Parkin DM, Bray F, Ferlay J, Pisani P. Global cancer statistics, 2002. *CA Cancer J Clin.* 2005;55: 74–108.

Plummer M, Herrero R, Franceschi S, et al. Smoking and cervical cancer: pooled analysis of the IARC multi-centric case-control study. *Cancer Causes Control.* 2003;14:805–814.

Rotman M, Pajak TF, Choi K, et al. Prophylactic extended-field irradiation of para-aortic lymph nodes in stages IIB and bulky IB and IIA cervical carcinomas. Ten-year treatment results of RTOG 79-20. *JAMA.* 1995;274(5):387–393.

Serraino D, Carrieri P, Pradier C, et al. Risk of invasive cervical cancer among women with, or at risk for, HIV infection. *Int J Cancer.* 1999;82(3):334–337.

Solomon D, Davey D, Kurman R, et al. The 2001 Bethesda System: terminology for reporting results of cervical cytology. *JAMA.* 2002;287:2114–2119.

Spriggs AI, Boddington MM. Progression and regression of cervical lesions. Review of smears from women followed without initial biopsy or treatment. *J Clin Pathol.* 1980;33:517–522.

Wright JD, Herzog TJ. Human papillomavirus: emerging trends in detection and management. *Curr Womens Health Rep.* 2002;2(4):259–265.

Wright TC Jr, Massad LS, Dunton CJ, et al. 2006 consensus guidelines for the management of women with cervical intraepithelial neoplasia or adenocarcinoma in situ. *Am J Obstet Gynecol.* 2007;197:340–345.

20

Vulvar Cancer

Christina M. Annunziata and Michael J. Birrer

EPIDEMIOLOGY

- Vulvar cancer accounts for 4% of all female genital malignancies.
- 3,460 new cases and 870 deaths from vulvar cancer were projected for 2008.
- It is most frequent in women in the seventh decade of life, but is occasionally diagnosed in women younger than 40 years.

ETIOLOGY AND RISK FACTORS

The etiology of vulvar cancer remains unclear, but potentially involves two distinct diseases associated with the following:

- Human papillomavirus (HPV) DNA, especially type 16
  - Can be detected in 80% of intraepithelial lesions
  - Found in 10% to 15% of invasive vulvar cancers (especially squamous cell)
- Chronic inflammation
  - Venereal or granulomatous lesions
  - Lichen sclerosus (coexists with up to 25% of vulvar cancers)
  - Paget's disease (preinvasive)

Risk Factors

- Vulvar intraepithelial neoplasia (VIN), especially high-grade (VIN III), increases risk for development of invasive vulvar cancer.
- Other risk factors include prior history of cervical cancer, immunodeficiency disorders, and cigarette smoking.
- Classic risk factors such as hypertension, diabetes mellitus, and obesity are probably associated with aging and are not truly independent risk factors for this malignancy.

HISTOLOGY

- Squamous cell carcinomas (SCCs) constitute >90% of cases.
- Melanomas constitute <10% of cases.
- The remainder of tumor types include adenocarcinoma, basal cell carcinoma, verrucous carcinoma, sarcoma, and other rare tumors.

VULVAR SQUAMOUS CELL CARCINOMA

Vulvar squamous cell carcinoma (SCC) is commonly indolent, with slow extension and late metastases. Signs and symptoms in order of decreasing frequency are pruritus, mass, pain, bleeding, ulceration, dysuria, and discharge. Many patients are asymptomatic.

Diagnostic Workup

- Biopsy must include adequate tissue to determine histology and grade, depth of invasion, and stromal reaction present.
- Colposcopy using 5% acetic acid solution may be necessary to delineate suspected multifocal lesions.
- Cystoscopy, proctoscopy, chest x-ray, and intravenous urography should be performed as needed based on the extent of disease.
- Suspected bladder or rectal involvement must be biopsied.

Indications for Excisional Biopsy of Vulvar Lesions

- Any gross lesion
- Red, white, dark brown, or black skin patches
- Areas firm to palpation
- Pruritic, tingling, or bleeding lesions
- Any nevi in the genital tract
- Enlarged or thickened areas of Bartholin glands, especially in postmenopausal women

Location and Metastatic Spread Pattern of Vulvar SCC

- Vulvar SCC is found on:
  - The labia majora in 50% of cases
  - The labia minora in 15% to 20% of cases
  - The clitoris and perineum in rare cases
- Vulvar SCC tends to grow locally, with subsequent spread to inguinal, femoral, and pelvic lymph nodes (LNs).
- Hematogenous spread rarely occurs without LN involvement.

Staging, Prognosis, and Survival

- Vulvar cancer is a surgically staged disease (Table 20.1).
- Survival depends on stage, LN involvement, depth of invasion, structures involved, and tumor location.
- LN metastases are related to tumor size, clinical stage, and depth of invasion.

TABLE 20.1. *Tumor/node/metastasis (TNM) classification and staging of vulvar carcinoma*

Primary tumor (T)	
Tis/Stage 0	Preinvasive carcinoma in situ; intraepithelial carcinoma (VIN).
T1/Stage I	Tumor confined to the vulva and/or perineum; $\leq$2 cm in greatest dimension
T2/Stage II	Tumor confined to the vulva and/or perineum; >2 cm in greatest dimension
T3/Stage III	Tumor of any size, with adjacent spread to the urethra, vagina, and/or anus
T4/Stage IV	Tumor of any size infiltrating the bladder or rectal mucosa or both, the upper part of the urethral mucosa, or fixed to the anus
	Stage IVA: any T; any N
	Stage IVB: any T; any N; M1
Regional lymph nodes (N)	
N0	No palpable lymph node metastases
N1	Unilateral regional lymph node metastases
N2	Bilateral regional lymph node metastases
Distant metastases (M)	
M0	No distant metastases.
M1	Distant metastases (including pelvic lymph node metastases)

Source: From Creasman WT. New gynecologic cancer staging. *Obstet Gynecol.* 1990;75(2):287–288, with permission.

- Statistics based on the pathologic status of the inguinal LNs and the size of the primary lesion:
  - Lesions <2 cm in greatest dimension without LN involvement (stage I): 77% 5-year survival.
  - Lesions of any size with unilateral LN[1] (stage III): 31% 5-year survival.

Management

Stage 0 (VIN)

Therapeutic options are based on individual patient need.

- Wide local excision, laser ablation, or both
- Skinning vulvectomy with or without grafting
- Topical treatments include:
  - 5-FU cream: response rate (RR) 40% to 75%
  - Imiquimod: RR approximately 50%

Recurrences are seen in up to 35% of women regardless of type of initial treatment. The most common sites of recurrence are perineal skin and clitoral hood.

Stage I

- <1-mm invasion (stage IA): wide local excision
  - Excise down to inferior fascia of urogenital diaphragm.
  - Strive for 2-cm clear margins to minimize risk of local recurrence.
- >1-mm invasion (stage IB):
  - Modified radical vulvectomy with ipsilateral superficial inguinal lymphadenectomy for lesions located laterally
  - Bilateral inguinofemoral node dissection for centrally located lesions
  - Sentinel LN biopsy is an emerging technique in early-stage vulvar cancer and may obviate the need for full nodal dissections in many women.

SPECIAL CONSIDERATIONS

- Poor surgical candidates can be treated with radiation therapy, achieving long-term survival.
- Surgical complications include mortality (2–5%), wound breakdown or infection, sepsis, thromboembolism, chronic leg lymphedema (use of separate incision for the groin LN dissection reduces wound breakdown and leg edema), urinary tract infection, stress urinary incontinence, and poor sexual function.

Stage II

- Modified radical vulvectomy and bilateral inguinofemoral lymphadenectomy can be used if ≥1 cm of negative margins can be achieved with preservation of midline structures.
- Adjuvant radiation therapy is recommended for women with more than one positive lymph node or surgical margins <1 cm.

Stages III and IV

The management of stage III and IV disease is shown in Fig. 20.1.

SPECIAL CONSIDERATIONS

- Management of positive groin nodes: one LN requires no further therapy. Two or more LNs can be treated with groin and pelvic radiation therapy, based on data from GOG randomized trial in which improved survival was documented with this therapy compared to pelvic LN dissection.
- Suggested doses of localized adjuvant radiation are 45 to 50 Gy.

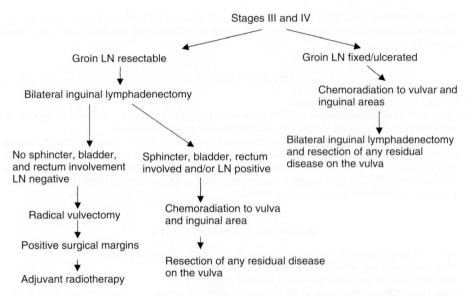

Fig. 20.1. Management algorithm for stages III and IV disease. (Used with permission from Di-Saia PJ, Creasman WT. *Clinical Gynecologic Oncology*. 5th ed. St. Louis: Mosby; 1997:222.)

- Neoadjuvant chemoradiation can be used in stage III and IV disease to improve the operability of the tumor. Recent GOG trials have successfully used cisplatin and 5-FU concurrently with radiation.
- Patients with inoperable disease can achieve long-term survival with radical radiation therapy.
- When radiation is given as primary definitive treatment, it is suggested that the addition of 5-FU with cisplatin or mitomycin C be considered.
- Radiation fraction size of ≤180 cGy has been proven to minimize the radiation complication rate (i.e., late fibrosis, atrophy, telangiectasia, and necrosis). Total doses of 54 to 65 Gy should be used.
- Radical vulvectomy and pelvic exenteration are not commonly used due to extensive morbidity and uncertain survival benefit.

Recurrent and Metastatic Disease

Treatment and outcome depend on site (local, inguinal, or distant) and extent of recurrence.

- Local recurrence can be treated with:
  - Wide local re-excision with or without radiation (5-year survival of 56% if regional LNs are negative).
  - In cases with small, localized recurrence, radiation with or without 5-FU can be curative.
- Inguinal nodes can be subjected to radiation and surgery.
- Distant recurrence: no standard systemic chemotherapy is available for metastatic disease. These patients are appropriate candidates for clinical trials. Agents such as cisplatin, methotrexate, cyclophosphamide, bleomycin, and mitomycin C have shown a partial RR of only 10% to 15% and are of short duration (a few months). Trials evaluating the efficacy of paclitaxel in vulvar cancer are ongoing.

VERRUCOUS CARCINOMA

- Verrucous carcinoma is very rare and can be confused with condyloma acuminatum because of exophytic growth pattern.
- It is locally destructive and rarely metastasizes.
- It is associated with HPV type 6.

- The main treatment is surgery. LN dissection is of questionable value unless LNs are obviously involved. Radiation therapy is contraindicated because it is ineffective and can potentially lead to more aggressive disease.

PAGET'S DISEASE

- Characterized by preinvasive lesions.
- Most frequent symptoms include pruritus, tenderness, or vulvar lesions (i.e., "red velvet," hyperemic, well-demarcated, thickened lesions with areas of induration and excoriation).
- Can be associated with underlying adenocarcinoma of the vulva (1%–2%). Although Paget's disease is histologically a preinvasive disease locally, it should be treated with radical wide local excision, as with other vulvar malignancies. Patients require radical excision, often with intraoperative frozen section confirmation of clear margins, because microscopic disease often extends beyond the gross visual margin observed by the operating surgeon.

MALIGNANT MELANOMA

- Malignant melanoma of the vulva is a rare tumor (5% of all melanoma cases).
- Most melanomas are located on the labia minora and clitoris.
- Prognosis depends on size of lesion and depth of invasion.
- Staging of malignant melanoma is the same as for skin melanoma.
- Suggested therapy is radical vulvectomy with inguinal and pelvic lymphadenectomy, although there is a current trend toward a more conservative approach. For most well-demarcated lesions, 2-cm margins are suggested for thin (up to 7 mm) lesions and 3- to 4-cm margins for thicker lesions.

BARTHOLIN GLAND

Adenocarcinoma

- Adenocarcinoma of the Bartholin gland is a very rare tumor (1% of all vulvar malignancies).
- Peak incidence is in women in their mid-60s.
- Enlargement of the Bartholin gland area in postmenopausal women requires evaluation for malignancy.
- Therapy includes radical vulvectomy with wide excision to achieve adequate margins and inguinal lymphadenectomy.

Adenoid Cystic Carcinoma

- Adenoid cystic carcinoma is a very rare tumor.
- It is characterized by frequent local recurrences and very slow progression.
- Recommended therapy is wide local excision with ipsilateral inguinal lymphadenectomy.

Basal Cell Carcinoma

- The natural history and therapeutic approach for basal cell carcinoma are similar to those for primary tumors seen in other sites (i.e., wide local excision).

SUGGESTED READING

DiSaia PJ, Creasman WT. *Clinical Gynecologic Oncology*. 5th ed. St. Louis: Mosby; 1997.

Elkas JC, Berek JS. Clinical manifestations, diagnosis, pathology, and staging of vulvar cancer. Available at: http://www.uptodateonline.com/utd/content/topic.do?topicKey=gyne_onc/5385&selectedTitle=1~18&source=search_result.

Elkas JC, Berek JS. Treatment and prognosis of vulvar cancer. Available at: http://www.uptodateonline. com/utd/content/topic.do?topicKey=gyne_onc/8776&selectedTitle=2~18&source=search_result.

Moore DH, Koh WJ, McGuire WP, Wilkinson EJ. Vulva. In: Hoskins WJ, Perez CA, Young RC, Barakat RR, Markman M, Randall ME, eds. *Principles and Practice of Gynecologic Oncology.* 4th ed. Philadelphia: Lippincott Williams and Wilkins; 2005:665–705.

Nash JD, Curry S. Vulvar cancer. *Surg Oncol Clin N Am.* 1998;7(2):335–346.

SECTION 7

Musculoskeletal

21

Sarcomas and Malignancies of the Bone

Patrick J. Mansky and Lee J. Helman

EPIDEMIOLOGY

- Malignancies of the soft tissue (6.1%) and bones (4.7%) account for more than 10% of newly diagnosed cancers in children, adolescents, and young adults.
- Median age at diagnosis of rhabdomyosarcoma (RMS) is 5 years, with a male preponderance.
- Osteosarcomas account for approximately 60% of malignant bone tumors in the first two decades of life.
- Most of the remaining bone malignancies in children and adolescents are Ewing sarcomas and the histologically similar and genetically identical peripheral primitive neuroectodermal tumors (PNETs). Together, these tumors are often called the Ewing family of tumors (EFT).
- Identification of specific, recurrent genetic alterations in RMS and Ewing sarcoma has improved diagnosis by clarifying pathogenesis. Better supportive care and systematic application of effective multimodality treatment have dramatically improved survival during the last 30 years (Fig. 21.1 and Table 21.1).

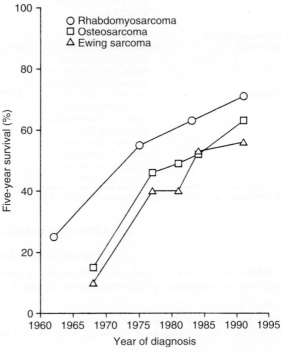

Fig. 21.1. Five-year survival rates among children and adolescents with rhabdomyosarcoma, osteosarcoma, and Ewing sarcoma. (Used with permission from Arndt CA, Crist WM. Common musculoskeletal tumors of childhood and adolescence. *N Engl J Med.* 1999;341:342–52.)

TABLE 21.1. *Outcome of therapy for musculoskeletal tumors of childhood and adolescence*

Tumor type	Commonly used chemotherapy agents	Duration of therapy (mo)	Long-term survival[a] (%)	Additional treatment
Rhabdomyosarcoma				
Low-risk (pts with group I or II embryonal tumors at sites with favorable outcome or group III orbital tumors)	Vincristine, dactinomycin	8–12	90–95	Resection of primary tumor for all except orbital tumors; irradiation of group II or III tumors
Intermediate-risk	Vincristine, dactinomycin, cyclophosphamide	8–12	70–80	Irradiation of primary tumor and any metastases
High-risk [pts with metastases (group IV), except pts <10 yr old who have embryonal tumors]	Vincristine, dactinomycin, cyclophosphamide; new agents; high-dose therapy with hematopoietic stem-cell transplantation	8–12	20	Irradiation of primary tumor and all metastatic lesions
Osteosarcoma				
Localized to limb	Doxorubicin, high-dose methotrexate, ifosfamide, cisplatin	8–12	58–76	Surgery for control of tumor
Metastatic	Doxorubicin, methotrexate, ifosfamide, cisplatin	8–12	14–50	Resection of primary tumor and any metastases
Ewing sarcoma				
Localized	Vincristine, doxorubicin, cyclophosphamide, dactinomycin, etoposide-ifosfamide	8–12	50–70	Surgery, radiation, or both for local control of tumor
Metastatic	Vincristine, doxorubicin, cyclophosphamide, dactinomycin, etoposide-ifosfamide; high-dose therapy with hematopoietic stem cell transplantation	8–12	19–30	Surgery, radiation, or both for local control of tumor

[a]Estimated progression- or relapse-free survival at 3 to 5 years.

RHABDOMYOSARCOMA

Clinical Presentation

RMS, which can occur in almost any anatomic site, is associated with development of a mass, along with signs and symptoms typically related to the anatomic location (Fig. 21.2):

- Orbit: proptosis
- Nasopharynx: nasal discharge and obstruction
- Basal skull and posterior orbit: cranial nerve palsies and visual loss

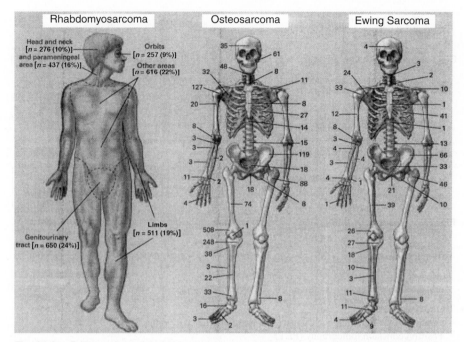

Fig. 21.2. Primary sites of rhabdomyosarcoma, osteosarcoma, and Ewing sarcoma, showing numbers of patients with primary tumors at specific sites.

- Parameninges: headache and meningism
- Vagina or uterus: vaginal polyp/discharge
- Bladder or prostate: urinary obstruction
- Male genitals: paratesticular scrotal mass

Pathophysiology

RMS is of mesenchymal origin and is characterized by myogenic differentiation. There are two main histological subtypes, embryonal (80%) and alveolar (15%–20%), with characteristic genetic differences (Table 21.2 and Fig. 21.3). Botryoid RMS and spindle cell sarcoma are both morphologic variants of embryonal RMS. Numerous environmental and genetic factors have been associated with an increased risk of RMS (Table 21.3).

TABLE 21.2. *Histologically distinguished subtypes of rhabdomyosarcoma (RMS)*

Embryonal RMS
Characteristic loss of heterogenicity (LOH) 11p15.5 (IGH-II gene)
Hyperdiploid DNA
Alveolar RMS
Characteristic translocations:
    PAX3/FKHR t(2,13)(q35;q14)
    PAX7/FKHR t(1;13)(p36;q14)
Tetraploid DNA

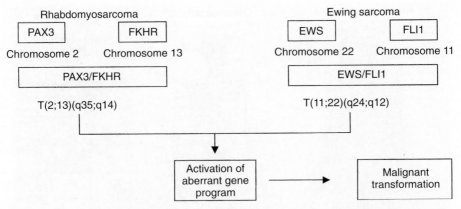

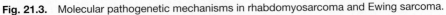

Fig. 21.3. Molecular pathogenetic mechanisms in rhabdomyosarcoma and Ewing sarcoma.

Diagnosis

Radiologic

Comprehensive radiologic evaluation includes the following:

- **Tumor localization**
  - Computerized tomography (CT) and magnetic resonance imaging (MRI)
  - Positron emission tomography (PET)
- **Assessment of metastatic spread**
  - CT of chest/lungs
  - Technetium bone scan for bone or bone marrow involvement
  - PET

Pathologic

Open biopsy is the preferred approach for tissue diagnosis and should be undertaken at an oncology center, where diagnostic material can be optimally used and the initial surgical approach can be determined by a multidisciplinary team responsible for the patient's subsequent treatment. Needle biopsy may restrict access to fresh and frozen tissue for cytogenetic and molecular genetic investigations.

1. Tumor characterization
   - Histopathology
     - Immunohistochemistry (desmin and myoD1)

TABLE 21.3. *Risks factors for rhabdomyosarcoma in children and adolescents*

Genetic
Familial cancer[a]
Germline mutant p53
Congenital abnormalities
Neurofibromatosis type I
Li-Fraumeni syndrome
Parental behaviors
Smoking
Use of recreational drugs
Prenatal consumption of alcohol
Chemical exposure at workplace

[a]Particularly breast cancer in a female relative.

– Genetics
  ▪ RT-PCR for presence of PAX/FKHR translocation
  ▪ Cytogenetics
2. Metastatic spread
  – Cerebrospinal fluid PCR for PAX/FKHR translocation
  – Bone marrow aspirate cytology
  – Bone marrow biopsy for histochemistry and PCR

Treatment

The diversity of primary sites, distinctive surgical approaches and radiotherapies for each primary site, subsequent site-specific rehabilitation, and potential treatment-related sequelae (Table 21.4)

TABLE 21.4. *Treatment options, local control, and potential sequelae in rhabdomyosarcoma*

Tumor site	Treatment options	Local control	Sterility	Renal toxicity	On growth	Esthetics
Orbit	Radical surgery then VA ± C	++	−	−	±	±
	Biopsy then radiation + V ± C	++	±	−	++	++
	Biopsy then IVA/VAC	±	±	±	−	−
	No CR: radical surgery	−	−	−	++	++
	or radiation	−	−	−	++	++
Paratesticular	Surgery + VA	±	−	−	−	−
	Surgery + VAC/IVA	++	±	±	−	−
Limbs	Surgery + VA	±	−	−	−	±
	Surgery + IVA	++	±	±	−	±
Vagina	IVA/VAC, then monitoring if CR	±	±	±	−	−
	IVA then elective surgery or interstitial radiation	++	±	±	±	±
Bladder/prostate	Radical surgery then IVA/VAC with/without selective radiation	++	±	±	±	±
	IVA/VAC then local surgery	±	±	±	−	±
	No CR: radiation	±	−	−	−	−
Thorax/abdomen/pelvis	IVA/VAC then radiation then IVA/VAC	−	++	±	±	±
	IVA/VAC, CR with/without surgery then IVA/VAC	±	±	±	±	−
Parameningeal	IVA/VAC then extensive early radiation then IVA/VAC	++	±	±	++	−
	IVA/VAC then delayed limited radiation then IVA/VAC	±	±	±	±	−
Nonparameningeal head/neck	Radical surgery then VA	++	−	−	−	++
	Biopsy then IVA/VAC	±	±	±	−	−
	No CR: radiation *or*	−	−	−	++	±
	surgery	−	−	−	−	±

A, actinomycin D; C, cyclophosphamide; CR, complete remission; I, ifosfamide; V, vincristine; ++, yes; ±, possible; −, no.

underscore the importance of treating children and young adults with RMS in the context of a clinical trial at a major medical center that has appropriate experience in all therapeutic modalities.

Surgery

Local tumor control is the cornerstone of therapy, especially for patients with nonmetastatic disease. Primary tumor resection should be undertaken only if there is no evidence of lymph node or metastatic disease and if the tumor can be excised with good margins without functional impairment or mutilation. Surgery has minimal, if any, role in the primary management of orbital tumors and a limited role in local control of head and neck tumors. To achieve local control of pelvic tumors in very young children, the risks of radical surgery may be more acceptable than those of pelvic irradiation.

Radiotherapy

Radiotherapy after initial surgical resection or chemotherapy is recommended in the following instances:

- Completely resected tumor (clinical group I) with unfavorable histology (alveolar RMS)
- Microscopic residual disease (clinical group II: up to 4,100 cGy)
- Gross residual disease (clinical group III: up to 5,040 cGy)

Treatment volume
- Volume is determined by extent of disease at diagnosis
- Radiation field should extend 2 cm beyond tumor margin
- Whole-brain irradiation of 2,340 to 3,060 cGy for parameningeal disease with intracranial extension

Chemotherapy

Neoadjuvant combination, multiagent chemotherapy for extensive, primarily unresectable tumors is known to reduce the extent of subsequent surgery or radiotherapy. (Fig. 21.4 outlines this multidisciplinary approach for osteosarcoma.)

OSTEOSARCOMA

Osteosarcoma is a primary bone malignancy with peak incidence in the pubescent growth spurt (15–19 years) in the metaphyses of the most rapidly growing bones. Risk factors are listed in Table 21.5; clinical presentation in Table 21.6.

Clinical Presentation

- Bone pain
- Swelling
- Mass in metaphyseal area of bone, most commonly femur or tibia

Diagnosis and Staging

Radiologic

1. Tumor assessment: Plain radiographs
    - Destruction of bone with consequent loss of normal trabeculae and appearance of radiolucent areas
    - New bone formation
    - Lytic or sclerotic appearance
    - "Sunburst sign": periosteal elevation from tumor penetrating cortical bone

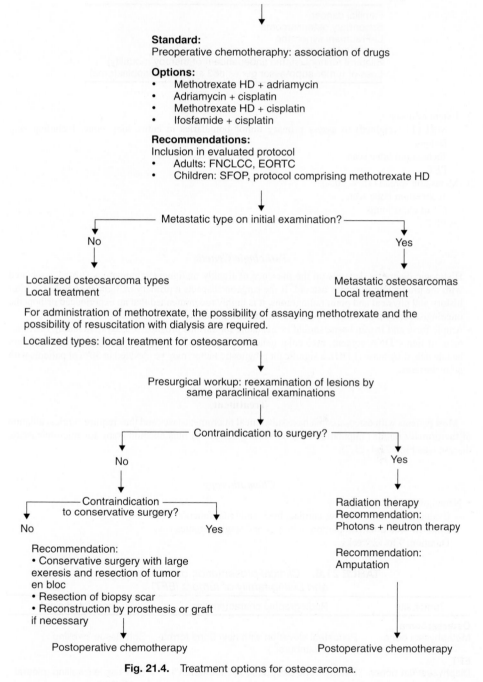

Fig. 21.4. Treatment options for osteosarcoma.

TABLE 21.5.   *Risk factors for osteosarcoma*

Familial cancer
Secondary osteosarcoma
Li-Fraumeni syndrome
Irradiated bones
Bilateral retinoblastoma (independent of therapy modality)
Loss of tumor-suppressor genes p53 and Rb (retinoblastoma)

2. Extent of disease
   – MRI (T1-weighted) to assess primary tumor boundaries in entire long bone, including skip lesions
   – Technetium bone scan
   – PET
3. Metastatic spread (15%–20%)
   – Technetium bone scan
   – CT of chest/lungs
   – PET

Pathologic/Genetic

- Histologic diagnosis depends on the presence of frankly malignant sarcomatous stroma associated with the production of tumor osteoid. If the surgeon suspects a primary malignant bone lesion after history and physical and plain radiographs, it is highly recommended that an experienced orthopedic oncologist perform all invasive procedures, including biopsy.
- Ample fresh and frozen tissue should be available for various prognostic assays, including measurement of tumor DNA content, molecular genetic evaluations, and P-glycoprotein estimation. Serum lactate dehydrogenase (LDH), a significant prognostic factor, may be elevated in 30% of patients with no metastases.

Treatment

Most patients with osteosarcoma have subclinical micrometastases and thus require surgical ablation of the primary tumor (amputation or limb-sparing resection) plus chemotherapy for micrometastatic disease (see Figs. 21.4–21.7).

Chemotherapy

- Neoadjuvant
  – Evaluation of bone marrow, cardiac, liver, and renal function
  – Initiated soon after completion of biopsy and staging studies
  – Duration: 9 to 12 weeks

TABLE 21.6.   *Clinical presentation of osteosarcoma and Ewing family of tumors (EFT)*

Tumor site	Radiographic characteristics	Associated signs
Ostersarcoma		
Metaphyseal bone	Periosteal elevation with new bone formation ("sunburst")	Soft-tissue swelling
EFT		
Diaphyseal/flat bones	Patchy bone destruction ("motheaten")	Soft-tissue swelling, pleural effusion
	Periosteal lamellation ("onion skin")	

Metastasized types: local treatment

↓

Presurgical workup:
Reexamination of lesions by
same paraclinical examinations

↓

Standard surgery of primary tumor and metastases

Recommendations:

• Conservative surgery with large exeresis and resection
  of tumor en bloc
• Resection of biopsy scar
• Amputation must remain the exception
• Surgery of metastases according to localization

↓

Fig. 21.5. Treatment options for
metastatic osteosarcoma.

Postoperative chemotherapy

Metastatic types after surgery

↓

Good responder:
Grades III and IV according to Huvos grading system
of tumor and metastases?

Yes   No

Standard: **Standard:**
Postoperative chemotherapy: Postoperative chemotherapy:
Same protocol as in preoperative   Other drugs effective in
                                                 osteosarcoma

                                                 Options:
                                                 If methotrexate and adriamycin in preoperative:
                                                 • Ifosfamide + VP16 or
                                                 • Ifosfamide + cisplatin

                                                 Recommendation:
                                                 Protocol evaluated:
                                                 • Adults: FNCLCC, EORTC
                                                 • Children: SFOP
                                                 • Adults and children: phase 2 trial

Fig. 21.6. Treatment options for postoperative metastatic osteosarcoma.

Localized types: postoperative chemotherapy

Good responder:
Grades III and IV according to Huvos

Yes

Standard:
Postoperative chemotherapy:
Same protocol as in preoperative

No

Standard:
Postoperative chemotherapy:
Other drugs effective in osteosarcoma

Options:
If methotrexate and adriamycin in preoperative:
• Ifosfamide + VP16 or
• Ifosfamide + cisplatin

Recommendation:
Protocol evaluated:
• Adults: FNCLCC, EORTC
• Children: SFOP

Fig. 21.7. Treatment options for postoperative localized osteosarcoma.

• Adjuvant
  – Evaluation of extent of tumor necrosis in surgical specimen as predictor of disease-free and overall survival
  – Initiated soon after definitive surgery for primary tumor
  – Duration: 35 to 40 weeks

Surgery

Amputation and limb-sparing resection incorporate wide en bloc excision of the tumor and biopsy site through normal tissue planes, leaving a cuff of normal tissue around the periphery of the tumor. Limb-sparing surgery is now the preferred approach for 70% to 90% of patients with osteosarcoma due to improved functional outcome. Reconstruction involves allografts, customized endoprosthetic devices, modular endoprosthetic devices, or combinations of these methods. This approach requires a multidisciplinary team and close cooperation between the chemotherapist and orthopedic oncologist.

Follow-up

Patients with osteosarcomas should have frequent radiographic monitoring for metastases for at least 5 years after completion of therapy. Most first recurrences appear asymptomatically in the lungs. Durable salvage has been reported in 10% to 20% of such patients; thus, all patients with recurrent disease should be treated with curative intent.

EWING FAMILY OF TUMORS

• The EFT comprises Ewing sarcoma of the bone, PNETs, Askin-Rosai tumor (PNET of the chest wall), and extraosseous Ewing sarcoma. Studies using immunohistochemical markers, cytogenetics, and tissue culture indicate that these tumors all derive from the same primordial stem cell and are distinguished only by the degree of neural differentiation.
• Ewing sarcoma accounts for 10% to 15% of all malignant bone tumors, with peak incidence between 10 and 15 years of age.

- Incidence in African American and Chinese populations is remarkably low.
- Nearly 12% of patients with Ewing sarcoma also have associated urogenital anomalies such as cryptorchidism, hypospadias, and ureteral duplication.

Clinical Presentation

- Persistent and increasing pain, local swelling, and functional impairment of affected area (see Table 21.6)
- Fever
- Associated neurologic symptoms, including paraplegia and peripheral nerve abnormalities
- Uncommon symptoms:
  - Lymph node involvement
  - Meningeal spread
  - Central nervous system disease

Diagnosis and Staging
Radiologic

1. Evaluation of primary tumor
   - CT and MRI of primary lesion
   - PET
2. Metastatic spread
   - CT of chest/lungs
   - Technetium bone scan for tumor extent and bone marrow involvement
   - PET

Approximately 20% of patients have visible metastases at diagnosis. Of these patients, about 50% have lung metastases and about 40% have multiple bone involvement and diffuse bone marrow involvement.

Biopsy and Laboratory Investigations

Open biopsy is preferred for tissue diagnosis. It should be undertaken at an oncology center where the diagnostic material can be optimally used and the initial surgical approach can be determined by a multidisciplinary team responsible for the patient's subsequent treatment. Needle biopsy may restrict access to fresh and frozen tissue for cytogenetic and molecular genetic investigations.

- Serology
  - LDH: prognostic indicator reflecting disease burden
- Histopathology
  - "Small blue round cell tumor"
  - Immunohistochemistry: NSE, vimentin, S-100, HBA-71
- Cytogenetics/molecular genetics
  - t(11;22)(q24;q12) translocation in 85% of tumors
  - RT-PCR of EWS/FLI-1 transcripts

The t(11;22)(q24;q12) translocation results in the formation of a chimeric gene between EWS (Ewing sarcoma gene), a novel putative RNA-binding gene located on chromosome 22q12, and FLI-1, a member of the erythroblastosis virus-transforming sequence family of transcription factors located on chromosome 11q24. It has been fully characterized at the molecular genetic level. RT-PCR of fusion transcripts from the tumor can identify patients with favorable prognosis.

Treatment

Most patients with apparently localized disease at diagnosis have subclinical micrometastases. Thus, a multidisciplinary approach including local disease control with surgery and/or radiation as well as systemic chemotherapy is indicated (Fig. 21.8).

Treatment Schema

iii c	iii c	iii c	SR	V	V	V	V	V	V	I	C
eee a	eee a	eee a	RAD	Dac	Dac		Dac		Dac	E	A
0	3	6	9	11			15		17	20	23

I	C	I	C	I	C
E	A	E	A	E	A
26	29	32	35	138	41	44

Induction (week 0–6)
i = ifosfamide 2 g/m^2/day × 3
e = etoposide 150 mg/m^2/day × 3
c = cyclophosphamide 1.5 g/m^2 day 5
a = doxorubicin 45 mg/m^2 day 5

Local control (weeks 9–17)
SR = surgical resection
V = vincristine 1.5 mg/m^2
Dac = dactinomycin 1.5 mg/m^2
RAD = start radiotherapy

Maintenance (weeks 20–44)
I = ifosfamide 2 g/m^2/day × 5
E = etoposide 150 mg/m^2/day × 5
C = cyclophosphamide 1.0 OR 1.5 g/m^2/day × 2
A = doxorubicin 60 mg/m^2 continous infusion over 24 hours

Fig. 21.8. Dose-intensive chemotherapy for children with Ewing family of tumors. (Used with permission from Marina NM, Pappo AS, Parham DM, et al. Chemotherapy dose-intensification for pediatric patients with Ewing's family of tumors and desmoplastic small round-cell tumors: a feasibility study at St. Jude Children's Research Hospital. *J Clin Oncol.* 1999;17(1):180–90.)

Surgery

Generally, surgery is the preferred approach for resectable tumors.

Radiotherapy

Radiotherapy is indicated for patients with no function-preserving surgical option or whose tumors have been excised with inadequate margins. Radiotherapy for EFT requires stringent planning and delivery by a team experienced in the treatment of this disease. Recommendations of the Intergroup Ewing's Sarcoma Study (IESS) include the following:

- Gross residual disease: 4,500 cGy plus 1,080 cGy boost to tumor site
- Microscopic residual disease: 4,500 cGy plus 5,400 cGy boost
- Pulmonary metastasis: whole-lung irradiation of 1,200 to 1,500 cGy even if complete resolution of pulmonary metastatic disease is possible with chemotherapy
- Metastasis to bone and soft tissues: 4,500 to 5,600 cGy

Chemotherapy

- The most effective agents are cyclophosphamide and doxorubicin, but vincristine and dactinomycin are also active. Recent dose-intensification studies of ifosfamide and etoposide have shown significant promise.
- Prognosis was poor before the advent of effective multiagent chemotherapy (5-year survival: 10%–20% despite good local control) and is still dismal for patients with metastatic disease. A recent study reported a 3-year event-free survival of only 26.7% ± 13.2%.

FUTURE DIRECTIONS

Characterization of chromosomal translocations associated with RMS and Ewing sarcoma could elucidate the molecular pathogenesis of these tumors and lead to novel therapeutic strategies. Some current investigational approaches include:

- Biologic response modifiers
- Cell-cycle signaling pathway inhibitors (i.e., IGF-1 receptor pathway or mTOR pathway)
- Antiangiogenic agents

- Vaccines designed to elicit T-cell immunity, with specificity for tumor-specific fusion peptides
- Antibody targeting of immunotoxins to tumor cells.

SUGGESTED READINGS

Arndt CA, Crist WM. Common musculoskeletal tumors of childhood and adolescence. *N Engl J Med.* 1999;341:342–52.

Bernstein M, Kovar H, Paulussen M, et al. Ewing sarcoma family of tumors: Ewing sarcoma of bone and soft tissue and the peripheral primitive neuroectodermal tumors. In: Pizzo PA, Poplack DG, eds. *Principles and Practice of Pediatric Oncology.* Philadelphia: Lippincott–Raven; 2006:1003–32.

Carvajal R, Meyers P. Ewing's sarcoma and primitive neuroectodermal family of tumors. *Hematol Oncol Clin North Am.* 2005;19(3):501–25, vi–vii.

Ferrari S, Palmerini E. Adjuvant and neoadjuvant combination chemotherapy for osteogenic sarcoma. *Curr Opin Oncol.* 2007;19(4):341–6.

Lamoureux F, Trichet V, Chipoy C, Blanchard F, Gouin F, Redini F. Recent advances in the management of osteosarcoma and forthcoming therapeutic strategies. *Expert Rev Anticancer Ther.* 2007;7(2): 169–81.

Link PM, Gebhardt MC, Meyers PA. Osteosarcoma. In: Pizzo PA, Poplack DG, eds. *Principles and Practice of Pediatric Oncology.* Philadelphia: Lippincott–Raven; 2006:1075–115.

Marina NM, Pappo AS, Parham DM, et al. Chemotherapy dose-intensification for pediatric patients with Ewing's family of tumors and desmoplastic small round-cell tumors: a feasibility study at St. Jude Children's Research Hospital. *J Clin Oncol.* 1999;17(1):180–90.

Meyers PA. High-dose therapy with autologous stem cell rescue for pediatric sarcomas. *Curr Opin Oncol.* 2004;16(2):120–5.

NCCN. Clinical Practice Guidelines in Oncology: Bone Cancer. v.1.2008. Available at: http://www.nccn.org/professionals/physician_gls/PDF/bone.pdf

PDQR. Cancer Information Summaries: Pediatric Treatment. Available at: http://cancernet.nci.nih.gov/cancertopics/pdq/pediatrictreatment

Völker T, Denecke T, Steffen I, et al. Positron emission tomography for staging of pediatric sarcoma patients: results of a prospective multicenter trial. *J Clin Oncol.* 2007;25(34):5435–41.

Wan X, Helman LJ. The biology behind mTOR inhibition in sarcoma. *Oncologist.* 2007;12(8): 1007–18.

Wexler LH, Meyer, Helman LJ. Rhabdomyosarcoma and undifferentiated sarcomas. In: Pizzo PA, Poplack DG, eds. *Principles and Practice of Pediatric Oncology.* Philadelphia: Lippincott–Raven; 2006:972–1001.

SECTION 8

Skin Cancer

22

Skin Cancer and Melanoma

Upendra P. Hegde and Sewa S. Legha

The skin is the largest organ of the human body that is embryologically derived from the neuroecto-derm and the mesoderm. It consists of three layers: epidermis, dermis, and subcutis. Cancer of the skin arises from cell types and structures in various layers of the skin (1) (Table 22.1). The direct exposure to a wide variety of environmental carcinogens predisposes skin cells to genetic damage and increased incidence of cancer. The skin cancers are best divided into melanoma and nonmelanoma.

MELANOMA

Melanoma is a skin tumor that originates from the melanocyte, a cell derived from the neural crest that migrates during embryogenesis predominantly to the skin and less commonly to other tissues such as the meninges, the ocular choroid, the mucosa of the upper aerodigestive tract, and the lower genito-urinary tract where melanoma is rarely encountered.

Epidemiology

- Melanoma ranks as the seventh leading type of cancer in the United States.
- The estimated lifetime risk of developing melanoma in U.S. whites is about 1 in 60.
- In the United States 62,480 new cases of melanoma are expected to be diagnosed in 2008, with pro-jected deaths of 8,420 (2).
- The incidence of melanoma is 10 times greater in whites than in African Americans.
- The incidence of cutaneous melanoma in U.S. whites is 20 cases per 100,000 population although some geographic areas have higher rates.
- The rate of rise of incidence has decreased from 6% a year in the 1970s to 3% a year from the 1980s to 2000. Since the year 2000, the rate of rise of melanoma incidence has stabilized.
- Australia has the highest incidence of melanoma in the world, approximately 40 cases per 100,000 population per year.

TABLE 22.1. *Cells of epidermis, dermis, and respective tumor types*

Cells of epidermis	Tumor type incidence	Cells of dermis	Tumor type[a]
Melanocyte	Melanoma 5%–7%	Fibroblast	Benign and malignant fibrous tumor
Epidermal basal cell	Basal cell carcinoma 60%	Histiocyte	Histiocytic tumor
Keratinocyte	Squamous cell carci-noma 30%	Mast cell	Mast cell tumor
Merkel cell	Merkel cell tumor 1%–2%	Vasculature	Angioma and angiosarcoma; lymphangioma
Langerhans cell	Histiocytosis X <1%	Lymphocyte	Non-Hodgkin's lymphoma
Appendage cells	Appendageal tumors <1%	—	—

[a]Incidence of tumors in dermis <1% each type.

277

Etiology

- Sunlight exposure: Ultraviolet B rays (Fig. 22.1).
  - Intermittent intense exposure
  - Exposure at a young age
  - Individuals with propensity for sunburns and inability to tan or poor tanners
  - Individuals with fair skin, blue eyes, blonde or red hair
- Age: High incidence in young and middle-aged adults (except lentigo maligna melanoma on sun-exposed surfaces in the elderly)
- Sex: Slightly more common in male subjects than in females
- Ethnicity: Higher incidence in Northern Europeans than in Eastern and Southern Europeans
- Familial melanoma: One in 10 patients with melanoma has a family history of melanoma

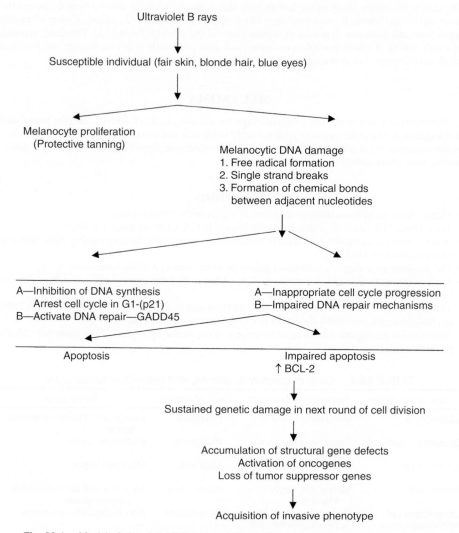

Fig. 22.1. Model of ultraviolet B light-mediated pathogenesis of cutaneous melanoma.

TABLE 22.2. *Differences between acquired melanocytic and dysplastic nevus*

Acquired melanocytic nevus	Dysplastic nevus
Develops in early childhood through fourth decade	Develops throughout life
<5 mm in diameter, sharp borders, evenly pigmented	6–8 mm in diameter, irregular borders, variegated pigment, and topographic asymmetry
Risk for melanoma development increases by 10-fold if more than 100 in number	Risk factor for melanoma development

Characteristic features of familial melanoma include:

– Multiple melanomas
– Melanoma at young age
– Melanoma often associated with dysplastic nevi
– Locus for melanoma or the dysplastic nevus resides in the distal portion of the short arm of chromosome 1
– Other genetic loci are possible, which include chromosome 9 (loss of 9p21)

Precursor lesions of melanoma include:

– Dysplastic nevi and acquired melanocytic nevi (Table 22.2)
– Congenital nevi

Risk Factors for Melanoma

• Xeroderma pigmentosum
• Familial atypical mole melanoma syndrome (FAMMS)
• Advanced age
• Immune suppression
• Sun exposure/sun-sensitive phenotype
• Melanoma in a first-degree relative
• Previous history of melanoma

Common Chromosomal Abnormalities in Melanoma

Early chromosomal abnormalities:

• Loss of 10q
• Loss of 9p

Late chromosomal abnormalities:

• Deletion of 6q
• Loss of terminal part of 1p
• Duplication of chromosome 7
• Deletion of 11q23

Mutation of chromosome 16q24 (which encodes the melanocyte-stimulating hormone receptor implicated in the pigmentation process) is a low-risk melanoma susceptibility gene that may increase risk of familial melanoma in families segregating CDKN2A gene mutation (3).

Clinicohistologic Types of Melanoma

The detection of melanoma cells (depth of invasion) in the dermis and subcutaneous fat (microstaging) has prognostic implications and was initially described by Clark et al. (4) and subsequently by Breslow (5) (Table 22.3).

TABLE 22.3. *Cutaneous melanoma microstaging
(Clark level and Breslow thickness)*

Clark level	Microscopic level of melanoma invasion	Breslow thickness	Tumor thickness (T) (AJCC) (6)
I	Melanoma limited to the epidermis (in situ melanoma)	1 mm or less	T1
II	Invasive melanoma with superficial infiltration to the papillary dermis	1.01–2 mm	T2
III	Melanoma extending to the superficial vascular plexus in the dermis	2.01–4 mm	T3
IV	Primary melanoma involving the reticular dermis	More than 4 mm	T4
V	Melanoma invading the subcutaneous fat	—	—

Source: From Ref. 6.

Clark et al. subdivided melanoma invasion of the papillary dermis into a deep group in which tumor cells accumulate at the junction of the papillary and reticular dermis and a superficial group in which tumor cells did not invade deeper layers (Fig. 22.2).

Breslow used an ocular micrometer to measure the vertical depth of penetration of tumor from the granular layer of the epidermis or from the base of the ulcerated melanoma to the deepest identifiable contiguous melanoma cell (Breslow thickness). This proved to be more accurate and reproducible than the Clark method of microstaging.

Clinical Features of Melanoma

Cutaneous melanoma can occur anywhere in the body. The most common sites are the lower extremities in women and the trunk in men. The classic signs in a pigmented skin lesion are:

- Asymmetry
- Borders that are irregular

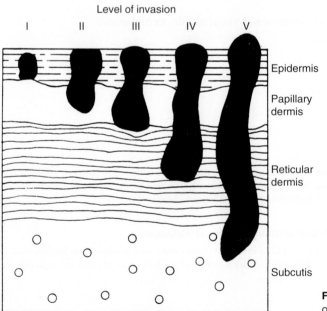

Fig. 22.2. Schematic diagram of Clark levels of invasion.

TABLE 22.4. *Immunologic markers for diagnosis of melanoma*

Antigen	Result
S-100 protein	+
Cytokeratin	−
Premelanosomal protein (HMB-45)	+
Vimentin	+
Nerve growth factor receptor	+
Tyrosinase-related protein-1 (MEL-5)	+

- Color is variegated
- Diameter of at least 6 mm; progressive change in size, nodularity, ulceration, or bleeding with or without pruritus

Less than 1% of melanoma skin lesions lack pigment. These are called amelanotic melanomas.

Diagnosis

Biopsy of a suspicious skin lesion reveals melanoma cells arising from the stratum basale of epidermis (dermoepidermal junction). The tumor cells invade the dermis, demonstrate radial and/or vertical growth phase, and stain for melanoma-specific immunologic markers (Table 22.4). A combination of clinical and histologic features provides prognostic information (Table 22.5).

Prognosis

The prognosis of patients with cutaneous melanoma is inversely proportional to the American Joint Committee for Cancer (AJCC) stage (Table 22.6 and Fig. 22.3), depth, and presence of ulceration (Fig. 22.4). Most melanomas are diagnosed early (thin melanoma, <1 mm deep) and the majority (>95%) are cured, as are about 85% of stage IIA melanoma patients. The relapse rate and mortality is considerably higher (40%–50%) in patients with stage IIB, IIC, and III melanoma. The 5-year survival is less than <5% in patients with stage IV melanoma with presently available treatment (6,7).

Cutaneous Melanoma: Prevention and Early Diagnosis

Patient education and close surveillance are key factors in the prevention and early diagnosis of cutaneous melanoma.

- General awareness about risks of developing melanoma, ways to reduce the risk with lifestyle changes that include avoidance of excessive sun exposure (midday sun between 10 AM and 4 PM) and

TABLE 22.5. *Prognostic factors of melanoma*

Good prognostic factors	Poor prognostic factors
Thin tumor (tumor ≤1 mm deep)	Thick tumor (tumor >1 mm deep)
No ulceration of tumor	Tumor ulceration present
Radial growth pattern	Vertical growth phase
Absence of foci of regression and/or tumor satellites in the reticular dermis and subcutaneous fat	Nodular histology
	Presence of foci of regression and/or tumor satellites in reticular dermis and subcutaneous fat
Absence of vascular and/or lymphatic invasion	Presence of vascular and/or lymphatic invasion
Low tumor cell mitotic rate	High tumor cell mitotic rate
Tumor involving an extremity	Tumor involving the trunk, head, and neck
Early stage (stage I and II)	Late stage at presentation (stage III and IV)

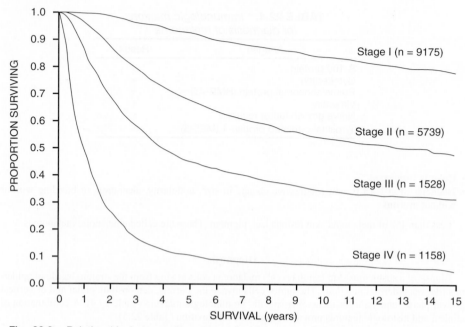

Fig. 22.3. Relationship between the stage of melanoma and survival (15-year follow-up). (Kaplan-Meier survival curves are adapted from Ref. 6)

tanning booths, sun protective measures such as effective use of sun block with protection factor (SPF) >15, and light clothing
- Performance of periodic self-examination and recognition of suspicious skin lesions
- Close skin surveillance by a dermatologist is recommended in high-risk patients.
    - Digital photography is used for tracking suspicious skin lesions over time in patients with multiple nevi or dysplastic nevus syndrome.

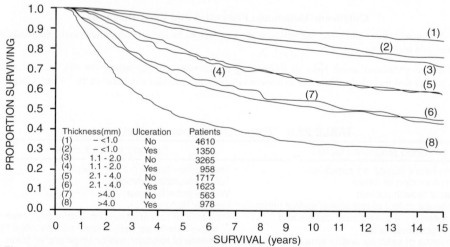

Fig. 22.4. Relationship between the Breslow depth, ulceration of melanoma, and survival. (Kaplan-Meier survival curves are adapted from Ref. 7)

TABLE 22.6. *Revised American Joint Committee for Cancer staging system for cutaneous melanoma (2001)*

T classification	Breslow's tumor thickness	Ulceration status
T1	≤1.0 mm	a: without ulceration and Clark level II/III
		b: with ulceration or Clark level IV/V
T2	1.01–2.0 mm	a: without ulceration
		b: with ulceration
T3	2.01–4.0 mm	a: without ulceration
		b: with ulceration
T4	4.0 mm or more	a without ulceration
		b: with ulceration

N classification	Number of metastatic nodes	Nodal metastatic mass
N1	1 node	a: micrometastasis
		b: macrometastasis
N2	2–3 nodes	a: micrometastasis
		b: macrometastasis
		c: in-transit met(s)/satellite(s) without metastatic nodes
N3	4 or more metastatic nodes, or matted nodes, or in-transit met(s)/satellite(s) with metastatic node(s)	

M classification	Metastatic site	Serum lactate dehydrogenase
M1a	Distant skin, subcutaneous, or nodal metastasis	Normal
M1b	Lung metastasis	Normal
M1c	Other visceral metastasis, distant metastasis	Elevated

Stage groupings for cutaneous melanoma

Clinical staging	T	N	M	Pathologic staging	T	N	M
0	Tis	N0	M0	0	Tis	N0	M0
IA	T1a	N0	M0	IA	T1a	N0	M0
IB	T1b	N0	M0		T1b	N0	M0
	T2a	N0	M0	IB	T2a	N0	M0
					T2b	N0	M0
IIA	T2b	N0	M0	IIA	T3a	N0	M0
	T3a	N0	M0		T3b	N0	M0
				IIB	T4a	N0	M0
IIB	T3b	N0	M0		T4b	N0	M0
	T4a	N0	M0	IIC			
IIC	T4b	N0	M0	IIIA	T1-4a	N1a	M0
III	Any T	N1–N3	M0		T1-4a	N2a	M0
				IIIB	T1-4b	N1a	M0
					T1-4b	N2a	M0
					T1-4a	N1b	M0
					T1-4a	N2b	M0
					T1-4a/b	N2C	M0
				IIIC	T1-4b	N1b	M0
					T1-4b	N2b	M0
					Any T	N3	M0
IV	Any T	Any N	M1	IV	Any T	Any N	pM1

Source: From Ref. 4.

— Dermoscopy (epiluminescence microscopy) performed by a trained operator, utilizes either a dermatoscope or 10× ocular scope (microscope ocular eyepiece held upside down) to visualize a variety of structures and patterns in pigmented skin lesions that are not discernible to the naked eye. The procedure has a potential to improve diagnostic sensitivity.

Melanoma Management : General Principles and Issues in Treatment

An algorithm for melanoma management is presented in Figure 22.5.

Surgical Treatment of Primary Melanoma

Principle: Complete surgical excision of the primary melanoma (Table 22.7 shows recommended margin of surgical excision), confirmed by comprehensive histologic examination of the entire excised specimen, forms the basis of surgical treatment (8).

Risk of local recurrence relates to completeness of resection of the primary tumor, but is not significantly associated with the extent of surgical margin of excision.

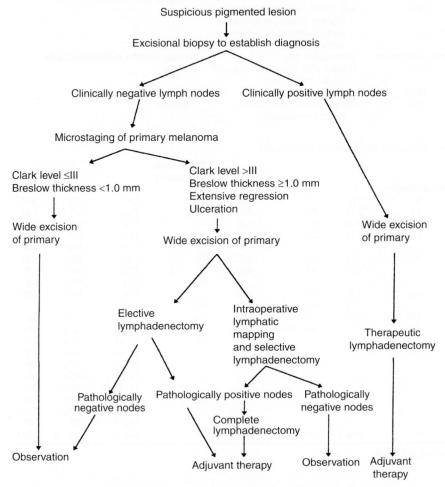

Fig. 22.5. Algorithm for melanoma management.

TABLE 22.7. *Recommended margin of surgical excision based upon pathologic stage of primary cutaneous melanoma*

Pathologic stage	Thickness	Margin of excision
ptis	Melanoma in situ	5 mm
pT1 and pT2	0–2 mm	1 cm
pT3	2–4 mm	1–2 cm
pT4	>4 mm	2–3 cm

Assessment of the Regional Lymph Node Metastasis and Lymph Node Dissection

Principle: Invasion of the dermal lymphatics by deep and invasive melanoma leads to lymph node metastasis of the respective regional lymph node basin. The tumor, uninterrupted at this site, may spread to deeper lymphatics or hematogenously to systemic organs.

Lymph node dissection can be classified as follows:

- Elective: Although clinically not palpable, the lymph nodes are dissected from the respective lymph node basin because of high suspicion of melanoma metastasis.
- Therapeutic: When the lymph nodes are clinically palpable and are suspected to be involved.
- Delayed: When initially nonpalpable lymph nodes appear to enlarge over a follow-up period.

Characteristics of a sentinel lymph node are as follows:

- First lymph node in the lymph node basin to which the primary melanoma drains
- Lymph node at the greatest risk of metastasis
- Easily accessible
- Helps to identify potential lymph node metastasis of cutaneous melanoma

SURGICAL APPROACH TO OBTAINING A SENTINEL LYMPH NODE

Preoperative lymphoscintigraphy uses vital blue dye and provides a road map of the lymph node basin. Intra operative lymphoscintigraphy uses radio colloid injection around the primary tumor, and a handheld device detects the radioactivity from the involved lymph node thereby acting as a navigator to the involved lymph node. The combination of vital blue dye and technetium-labeled sulfur colloid helps the surgeon to identify the sentinel lymph node in the respective lymph node basin in 94% of cases (9).

Surgical treatment implications of sentinel lymph node biopsy are as follows:

- Complete lymphadenectomy is recommended in patients with positive sentinel lymph node.
- Negative sentinel lymph node spares the patient morbidities of the complete lymph adenectomy.

Adjuvant Treatment of Cutaneous Melanoma in Patients at High Risk of Recurrence

INTERFERON TREATMENT

Principle: There is a high rate of relapse of cutaneous melanoma (35%–75%) among patients with stages IIB, IIC, and III disease after primary surgical treatment. Prolonged use of alpha interferon treatment (high dose, low dose, intermediate dose for variable periods of time) has been extensively studied in large prospective randomized clinical trials as an adjuvant treatment to assess reduction of recurrences and improvement of survival outcomes (10,11).

The results of these studies are summarized in Table 22.8.

- Alpha interferon treatment conferred consistent relapse and disease-free survival benefit.
- Impact upon overall survival has been variable and less consistent.
- High-dose alpha interferon is superior when compared to low-dose.
- Pegylated form of alpha interferon (slow release) given subcutaneously once weekly for 5 years conferred relapse-free survival advantage without overall survival benefit.

TABLE 22.8. *Use of adjuvant interferon treatment in stage*
IIb or III cutaneous melanoma

Study group (accrual)	Treatment regimen
ECOG E 1684 (287 patients)	High-dose interferon treatment *Induction phase:* Interferon α-2b, 20 million units/m^2/dose i.v., 5 d/wk $\times$ 4 wk (total dose/wk, 100 million units/m^2), followed by *Maintenance phase:* Interferon α-2b, 10 million units/m^2 s.c., three times/wk for 48 wk (total dose/wk, 30 million units/m^2) vs. observation
ECOG E 1690 (642 patients)	High-dose interferon treatment (as above) vs. low-dose interferon α-2b, (3 million units/m^2 s.c., three times/wk for 104 wk (total dose/wk, 9 million units/m^2) vs. observation
ECOG E 1697 (1,444 patients)	Interferon α-2b: Induction phase of high-dose interferon only of 4 wk as above vs. observation
UKCCCR Study (674 patients)	Interferon α-2a, 3 million units/m^2 s.c., three times/wk for 2 yr or until recurrence of melanoma (total dose/wk, 9 million units/m^2) vs. observation
EORTC study 18952 (1,388 patients)	Interferon α-2b, 10 million units/m^2/dose s.c. 5 d/wk for 4 wk (total dose/wk, 50 million units/m^2), followed by interferon α-2b, 10 million units/m^2 s.c., three times/wk for 1 yr (total dose/wk, 30 million units/m^2) vs. interferon α-2b, 5 million units/m^2 s.c., three times/wk for 2 yr (total dose/wk, 15 million units/m^2) vs. observation

ECOG, Eastern Cooperative Oncology Group; AJCC, American Joint Committee for Cancer; UKCCCR, The UK Coordinating Committee on Cancer Research; EORTC, European Organization for the Research and Treatment of Cancer; i.v. intravenous; s.c., subcutaneous; vs., versus.

Toxicity of high-dose interferon therapy adversely affects quality of life and may compromise the intended benefit of interferon therapy. The decision to use interferon in the adjuvant setting of melanoma treatment should be based on the perceived relative merits of disease control, quality of life, and financial cost.

RADIATION THERAPY

- Adjuvant to lymph node dissection in head and neck melanoma (12)
- Adjuvant to lymph node dissection if the involved lymph node shows extracapsular spread of melanoma
- Multiple large lymph node metastases (four or more lymph nodes)
- Local recurrence in a previously dissected lymph node basin
- Desmoplastic melanoma with neurotropism
- Brain metastasis of melanoma

Studies by Skibber et al. (13) and others have suggested that external radiation to the brain after surgical resection of the solitary brain metastasis from malignant melanoma has survival benefits.

Isolated Limb Perfusion as a Treatment of Melanoma

Principle: To deliver maximally tolerated chemotherapy doses to a regionally confined tumor area while limiting systemic toxicity. Hyperthermia and oxygenation of the circulation potentiate the tumoricidal effects of the chemotherapeutic agents that include melphalan (L-PAM), thiotepa, mechlorethamine with or without tumor necrosis factor, and gamma interferon (14). This procedure provides palliative benefit to patients with in-transit metastasis of melanoma (Table 22.9).

TABLE 22.9. *Isolated limb perfusion in melanoma*

Advantages	Disadvantages
Provide local control of the disease	Expensive and invasive procedure that is available only at selected institutions
Help resolve local symptoms such as edema, ulceration, and bleeding	Procedure provides effective palliation of local symptoms but no survival benefit
Relieves pain	Potential complications of the procedure include ischemia of the limb, peripheral neuropathy, bone marrow suppression

Management of Metastatic Melanoma

The management options for a patient with metastatic melanoma include surgical resection of an isolated metastatic site, chemotherapy, biological therapy, biochemotherapy, and experimental therapy such as immune-based treatments and targeted therapy (Table 22.10).

Single-Agent Chemotherapy

- Dacarbazine is the only FDA-approved chemotherapeutic agent for melanoma treatment that has a response rate of about 10% to 20%.
- Temozolomide is a synthetic analog of dacarbazine that is orally bioavailable, crosses the blood-brain barrier, has comparable efficacy, and a reduced toxicity profile.
- Other chemotherapeutic agents with activity as single agents include cisplatin, carboplatin, vinblastine, vinorelbine, and taxanes (paclitaxel) (Table 22.11).

Combination Chemotherapy

Commonly used combination chemotherapy regimens (Table 22.12) include:

- M.D. Anderson regimen: CVD (cisplatin, vinblastine, dacarbazine)
- Dartmouth regimen: CBDT (cisplatin, carmustine, dacarbazine, and tamoxifen)

TABLE 22.10. *Treatment options for metastatic melanoma*

Stage of melanoma	Management options

Stage IV melanoma	*Single-agent chemotherapy*
	  Dacarbazine (FDA approved) or oral temozolomide
	Combination chemotherapy
	  CVD (M.D. Anderson regimen)
	  CBDT (Dartmouth regimen)
	Biochemotherapy
	  High dose IL-2 (highly selected patients)
	  Good performance
	  Preserved organ function
	  Relative contraindication in patients with brain metastasis
	Experimental therapy
	  Anti-CTLA 4 antibody
	  Targeted therapy

Stage IV melanoma (isolated visceral metastasis or stage M1a disease)	*Surgery* Surgical excision of metastatic tumor or use of minimally invasive surgical techniques (cryoablation or radiofrequency ablation)
Brain metastasis or localized pain from metastasis	*Radiation therapy*

TABLE 22.11. *Single-agent chemotherapy for meta-static melanoma and response rates*

Chemotherapeutic agent	Response rates (%)
Dacarbazine	12–15
Temozolomide (DTIC analog)	21
Nitrosoureas (BCNU/CCNU)	10–20
Cisplatin	15–20
Carboplatin	19
Vinca alkaloids (vinblastine)	15–25
Vindesine	14–26
Paclitaxel	10–24
Docetaxel	6–17
Fotemustine	20

DTIC, dacarbazine.

– Randomized studies indicate that single-agent dacarbazine is the benchmark, but its response rates in recent trials are as low as 7% to 12% (median duration of response 3–4 months).
– Combination chemotherapy provides improved response rates (25%–30%) compared to single-agent dacarbazine, but with increased toxicity and no clear survival benefit.

A phase 3 multicenter randomized clinical trial of dacarbazine alone versus the Dartmouth regimen (i.e., cisplatin, carmustine, dacarbazine, and tamoxifen) in patients with metastatic melanoma failed to show a statistically significant survival benefit (15).

Biologic Agents Active in Melanoma

Alpha interferon was the first recombinant cytokine investigated in phase 1/2 clinical trials of patients with metastatic melanoma on the basis of its antiproliferative and immunomodulatory effects.

• The response rate in metastatic melanoma was approximately 15%.
• One-third of these responses were complete and durable.
• Responses could be observed up to 6 months after the therapy was initiated.
• Clinical benefit was pronounced in those without frequent interruptions (due to side effects).
• Patients with small-volume tumors did better than those with large-volume tumors.

TABLE 22.12. *Description of combination chemotherapy regimens in metastatic melanoma*

Chemotherapy regimens	Treatment description	Response rates (%)
CVD (M.D. Anderson Cancer Center)	Cisplatin, 20 mg/m^2/d i.v. for 4 days (2,3,4,5) (total dose/cycle, 80 mg/m^2) Vinblastine, 1.6 mg/m^2/d i.v. for 5 days (1,2,3,4,5) (total dose/cycle, 8 mg/m^2) Dacarbazine, 800 mg/m^2 i.v. on d 1 (total cycle dose 800 mg/m^2) cycle repeats every 21 days	21–48
CBDT (the Dartmouth regimen)	Cisplatin, 25 mg/m^2/d i.v. for 3 days (1,2,3) (total dose/cycle, 75 mg/m^2) Carmustine,150 mg/m^2 i.v. d 1 (every odd-numbered cycle i.e., every 43 days total dose every two cycles, 150 mg/m^2 Dacarbazine, 220 mg/m^2/d i.v. for 3 days (1,2,3) (total dose/cycle, 660 mg/m^2) Tamoxifen, 10 mg twice daily PO during the therapy Cycle repeated every 21 days	19–55

The study by Falkson et al. (16) reported treatment of patients with metastatic melanoma containing either dacarbazine alone or a combination of dacarbazine and alpha interferon 2b. The results suggested response rates of 20% and median survival of 9.6 months with dacarbazine alone versus response rates of 53% and median survival of 17.6 months in patients with dacarbazine with interferon alpha 2b. These results could not be reproduced in subsequent randomized phase 3 studies.

INTERLEUKIN-2 (IL-2)–BASED THERAPY

- IL-2 is a T-cell growth factor produced primarily by T-helper cells.
- Interacts with IL-2 receptors expressed on activated T cells and causes:
  - Increased production of other interleukins, gamma interferon, and tumor necrosis factor
  - Proliferation and differentiation of both B and T lymphocytes and cytotoxic cells
- Antitumor effects are mediated by its ability to cause proliferation of natural killer cells (NK cells), lymphokine-activated killer cells (LAKs), and cytotoxic T lymphocytes.

The U.S. Food and Drug Administration (FDA) approved dosage of IL-2 for treatment of metastatic melanoma at 600,000 IU or 720,000 IU per kg body weight administered as a bolus over 15 minutes every 8 hours for a maximum of 14 doses on days 1 to 5 and 15 to 19 (17). Imaging studies are repeated after two such courses to evaluate efficacy. In responding patients, the treatment is continued unless the patient has significant side effects or the physician decides to stop treatment for safety reasons.

- The overall response rate is about 16%, which includes a complete response rate of 6%.
- The responses are observed in all the disease sites.
- Durable responses are achieved in those who achieved complete responses.
- Good baseline performance and chemo-naive status is predictive of response.
- The toxicity profile results from capillary leak syndrome that is dependent on dose, route, and duration of administration. Common toxicity profile is as follows:
  - High fever, fluid retention
  - Gastrointestinal system side effects (i.e., nausea, vomiting, and diarrhea)
  - Cardiovascular system side effects (i.e., hypotension or arrhythmias)
  - Pulmonary side effects (i.e., hypoxemia and pleural effusions)
  - Renal side effects (i.e., azotemia, renal failure)
  - Central nervous system side effects (i.e., confusion and delirium)

Toxicity of high-dose IL-2 is accentuated in the presence of active comorbidities highlighting the importance of rigorous patient selection for safe IL-2 treatment. The treatment is also safer when administered by health care professionals who have experience treating patients with high-dose IL-2 treatment.

Lower doses of IL-2 administered either subcutaneously or as a continuous intravenous infusion at 9 to 18 million IU/m^2/day for 4 to 5 days have been studied in patients not eligible for high-dose IL-2 treatment. Although total response rates as high as 20% have been reported, complete responses appear to be lower than those with high-dose IL-2.

Biochemotherapy of Melanoma: Rationale

- Preclinical studies suggest that a combination of chemotherapeutic agents and biologic agents (biochemotherapy) confers additive or synergistic effects against melanoma tumor cells.
- Chemotherapeutic agents and biological agents differ in their mechanisms of antimelanoma effects.
- No overlapping toxicity
- No cross resistance

Biochemotherapy built upon CVD combination chemotherapy and biologic agents such as infusional IL-2 (moderate dose) and subcutaneous interferon alpha showed encouraging response rates and durable survival in selected patients (Table 22.13) (18).

The original results of biochemotherapy were not consistently reproduced by others. A recent meta-analysis of 18 clinical trials comparing biochemotherapy to chemotherapy in patients with stage IV

TABLE 22.13. *Biochemotherapy of metastatic melanoma*

Biologic and chemotherapeutic agents	Response rates
Cisplatin 20 mg/m^2 d 1,2,3,4 Vinblastine 1.6 mg/m^2 d 1,2,3,4 Dacarbazine, 800 mg/m^2 d 1 Recombinant interleukin-2, administered continuous 24 hr infusion at 9 MIU/m^2 d 1,2,3,4 Interferon alpha 2-b 5 MIU/m^2 sc d 1,2,3,4,5 Cycle repeated every 21 days with supportive care	Overall response rate of 64% Complete response rate of 21% Partial response of 43%

MIU, million international units.

melanoma confirmed high response rates (40%–50%) with biochemotherapy that did not translate into improved survival.

Immune-Based Therapy of Melanoma

Melanoma is a landmark tumor for immune strategies of treatment that include:

- Peptide vaccines consisting of melanoma-specific antigens (Table 22.14)
- Dendritic cell–based vaccines derived from peripheral blood mononuclear cells pulsed in vitro with tumor lysate or tumor-specific peptides

The immunization mechanism can be described as follows:

- The melanoma-specific peptide taken up by antigen-presenting cells (as in peptide vaccine) and mononuclear cell–derived dendritic cells pulsed with tumor antigens (as in dendritic cell–based vaccine), present the melanoma antigens to the cytotoxic T lymphocytes in the context of HLA class I molecule (adaptive arm of the immune system—the first signal).
- Cytotoxic T lymphocyte activation against tumor antigen requires engagement of costimulatory receptors on the surface of the CTLs (CD28) with costimulatory ligands expressed by the antigen-presenting cell (B7-1 and B7-2-the second signal).
- Proof of principle of therapeutic immune strategies in patients with cutaneous melanoma include demonstration of clinical responses to melanoma vaccines accompanied by generation of melanoma-specific cytotoxic T lymphocyte in peripheral blood.
- Natural brakes against melanoma-specific T cell responses are generated by regulatory T cells and CTLA-4 antigen expression by CTLs that lead to immune tolerance.

Prerequisites for a successful immune strategy of melanoma treatment include the following:

- Potent tumor-specific antigen and functional antigen presenting cell (APC)
- Generation of robust and sustained melanoma-specific cytotoxic T cell response
- Generation of facilitatory cytokines (immune microenvironment)
- Lack of immune tolerance

Heat-shock proteins isolated from cancer cells of mice and rats elicited specific immunity to the cancers from which they were derived. This observation led to the discovery that autologous tumor-derived heat-shock proteins chaperone tumor-specific peptides and present them through antigen-presenting cells to the CTLs generating T cell tumor immunity. Preliminary phase 1 and 2 studies of this strategy in humans have shown clinically relevant tumor-specific immune responses (20).

TABLE 22.14. *Melanoma-associated antigen epitopes*

Antigen	HLA restriction	Cellular location
MAGE-1	A1/Cw 1601	Cytoplasm
MAGE-3	A1/A2	Cytoplasm
MART1/Mela-A	A2	Cytoplasm
Tyrosinase	A2/A24	Melanosomal

Enhancement of immune-based treatment of cutaneous melanoma is the subject of current studies:

- Design and successful development of monoclonal antibody to CTLA-4 antigen showed promise in preclinical studies in mice. Early results of anti–CTLA-4 antibody in human subjects with metastatic melanoma have shown response rates between 10% and 15% that included occasional complete responses (21). Toxicity included severe autoimmune complications highlighting enhanced immune activity.
- Regulatory T cell blockade
- A toll-like receptor 7 agonist (imiquimod) is in clinical trials to assess its adjuvant role in potentiating the efficacy of peptide vaccine in cutaneous melanoma.

Targeted Therapy of Melanoma

Targeted therapy of melanoma is based upon a clear understanding of the functional genetic machinery that creates coordinated transduction of signals inside cells that maintain tissue homeostasis by controlling proliferation, differentiation, and cell death.

Understanding the aberrancy of cellular signaling due to gene mutations, the hallmark of cancer, provide an attractive target for intervention. At least three signal transduction pathways have been implicated in the genesis of melanoma:

- The mitogen-activated protein kinase (MAPK) pathway
- The phosphatidylinositol 3-kinase pathway (PI3K)
- The cyclic AMP (cAMP) pathway

High mutation rates (60%–70%) of intracellular molecule B-Raf, a serine/threonine kinase that occupies a central place in cell signaling inside a tumor cell, serves as an attractive target for melanoma treatment (22). Additional targets include molecules in the angiogenesis pathway such as vascular endothelial growth factor or its receptors.

The present generations of multiple tyrosine kinase inhibitors (sorafenib/sunitinib) and antiangiogenesis agent (bevacizumab) have not shown significant activity in melanoma in humans when used as single agents, suggesting cross-talk between different cellular signaling pathways.

Combined targeting of multiple molecules upstream and downstream in several signaling pathways is important in blocking relevant pathways, and provides a rationale for combining multiple targeted agents or combining targeted agents with chemotherapeutic agents. This insight into the molecular biology of melanoma has generated new ideas and optimism with regard to availability of a number of targeted agents that are currently in clinical trials. Results of such trials will be available in the near future.

Uveal Choroidal Melanoma

Uveal choroidal melanoma is the most common primary malignancy of the eye.

- Estimated incidence in the United States is six to seven cases per 1 million people.
- Depth and diameter determine the treatment indication and prognosis (Table 22.15).
- Benign choroidal nevi are up to 5 mm and 1 mm in diameter and depth, respectively.

Monosomy of chromosome 3 is a common cytogenetic abnormality and confers poor disease-free survival and high risk of death from melanoma. Other cytogenetic abnormalities involve chromosomes 1, 6, and 8.

TABLE 22.15. *Relationship of depth and diameter of uveal melanoma and 10-year survival*

Uveal choroidal melanoma (size)	Diameter (mm)	Depth (mm)	10-year survival (%)
Small	<10	<3	80
Medium	10–15	3–5	60
Large	>15	>5	34.8

Management of Uveal Choroidal Melanoma

- Local ablative treatment such as brachytherapy (iodine-125 plaque therapy), photo radiation, cryo-therapy, ultrasonic hyperthermia
- Surgical therapies include local resection, or enucleation of the eye.
- The most common site of metastasis is the liver, although in later stages the tumor can spread to other sites such as the lungs, bones, and skin.
- Systemic chemotherapy or biologic therapy is ineffective in metastatic uveal melanoma.
- Experimental therapies for liver metastasis include in situ ablative therapies such as radiofrequency ablation and hyperthermic isolated perfusion using melphalan.

Follow-up of patients with uveal choroidal melanoma after local treatment include close surveillance for liver metastasis with liver function tests and imaging studies of the liver that include sonography every 6 months in the first 5 years for early diagnosis of liver metastasis.

Indications for Enucleation of the Eye

- Tumor growing in a blind eye
- Melanoma involving more than half of the iris
- Tumor involving the anterior chamber of the eye or extraocular extension
- Failure of previous local therapy

NONMELANOMA SKIN CANCER

There are two major types of nonmelanoma skin cancers: basal cell carcinoma and squamous cell carcinoma. Together they account for nearly one million cases in the United States per year. The immune system plays an important role in the pathogenesis of nonmelanoma skin cancers, as demonstrated clinically by their increased incidence in patients with immune-suppressed states, such as the aging population and transplant recipients. Histologically, the regressing nonmelanoma skin cancers show infiltration of the tumor by activated T cells and cytokines such as interferon (IFN) alpha, TNF-beta, and IL-2.

Basal Cell Carcinoma

- Basal cell carcinoma is the most common cancer in the U.S. white population.
- It accounts for 75% of one million new cases of nonmelanoma skin cancers.
- Usual location is skin of head and neck region
- Presents as a shiny pink translucent papule with telangiectasia
- Nodular variant presents with central depression and rolled margins that may bleed from trauma.
- Pigmented basal cell carcinoma: Nodular tumor with brown to black pigment
- Sclerosing or morphea-type basal cell carcinoma: Yellowish, infiltrated, with indistinct borders, remains undiagnosed for a long time. Management includes Mohs surgery.
- Less common presentations include hyperkeratotic-type carcinoma, which usually involves head and neck area, exhibits sessile growth on the lower trunk, is multicentric on face with ulcer and scar tissues, and is of the giant exophytic type and the cystic type presenting as a blue-gray nodule on the face.

Squamous Cell Carcinoma

- Usually found in elderly white men with sun-damaged skin
- Common sites include back of the hand, forearm, face, and neck; single or multiple lesions
- Firm, indurated, expanding nodule, often at the site of actinic keratose
- The nodule may be ulcerated, and regional lymph nodes may be enlarged.

Squamous Cell Carcinoma of a Mucocutaneous Site

- Elderly men with chronic history of smoking, alcohol use, or chewing tobacco or betel nut
- Common sites include mouth and lower lip.
- Lesions usually start as erosion or a nodule that ulcerates.

Other sites of origin include sole of the foot (verrucous form) and male genitalia related with human papillomavirus in underlying condylomata of Buschke-Lowenstein tumor.

Diagnosis of Nonmelanoma Skin Cancer

Detailed clinical history should include duration of the lesion, symptoms such as pain or itching, and recent changes of the surface in addition to the following:

- Chronic sun exposure and recreational and occupational history
- Radiation and arsenic exposure, chronic ulcer/burn scar, or osteomyelitis
- Ethnic background and type of skin

A complete skin examination includes:

- Examination of scalp, ears, palms, soles, interdigital areas, and mucous membranes
- Evaluation of the extent of sun damage to skin (i.e., solar elastosis, scaling, erythema, telangiectasia, and solar lentigines)
- Assessment of the locoregional lymph nodes and distant metastases

An excisional or incisional tumor biopsy in small or large tumor, respectively, is obtained for histologic diagnosis. A shave biopsy with a scalpel may be used in noduloulcerative, cystic, or superficial type.

Treatment of Nonmelanoma Skin Cancer

Complete surgical resection with negative margins of at least 4 to 6 mm is recommended with lymph node resection if enlarged. Plastic surgery may be needed to close the defects produced by excision of the tumor.

Mohs Surgery

Mohs surgery allows excision of the tumor until the negative margins are achieved. It includes micrographic surgery that is guided by examination of a frozen section to ascertain complete resection.

Imiquimod is an FDA-approved agent for treatment of superficial basal cell carcinoma when used in cream form. The drug works via toll-like receptor agonistic activity and causes stimulation of innate and adaptive immune systems. Common side effects include local skin rashes, burning sensation, erythema, edema, induration, erosion, and pruritus.

Radiation Therapy

X-rays delivered at a total dose of 2,000 to 3,000 cGy penetrate up to 2 to 5 mm, where most of the basal cell and squamous cell carcinomas infiltrate. The total dose is divided into multiple smaller doses, usually over 3 to 4 weeks, to reduce side effects.

MERKEL CELL CARCINOMA

Merkel cell carcinoma occurs due to the neoplastic proliferation of the Merkel cells located in the basal layer of the epidermis and hair follicles. These cells, which originate from the neural crest, are a member of the amine precursor uptake and decarboxylation cell system (APUD). Merkel cells are important for tactile sensations in lower animals and function as a mechanoreceptor in humans.

Characteristics of Merkel Cell Tumor

- Occurs in the elderly population with chronically sun-damaged areas of skin
- Common sites include head and neck skin; less common sites are extremities and genitals
- Presents as 0.5 to 1 cm intracutaneous, firm, bluish-purple, nontender nodule
- Histologically, a small round cell tumor containing neurosecretory cytoplasmic granules may look similar to small cell carcinoma or melanoma, Ewing's sarcoma, and lymphoma.

- Tumor cells stain positive for neuron-specific enolase and anticytokeratin antibody CAM 5.2.
- Recent identification of polyomaviral DNA integration in merkel tumor cells indicate implication of polyomavirus in the pathegonesis of this tumor. Higher incidence of this tumor in the aging population may have clinical relevance to the aging immune system (23).
- Early spread occurs to locoregional lymph nodes and hematogenously to the distant sites.

Management of Merkel Cell Tumor

Management of Merkel cell tumor includes complete primary surgical excision with lymph node assessment by sentinel lymph node procedure and lymph node dissection if necessary, as in cutaneous melanoma. Adjuvant radiation treatment is recommended in patients at high risk of local recurrence due to incomplete resection or larger tumor size (2 cm or more).

Metastatic Merkel cell tumor is managed with systemic chemotherapy. Effective chemotherapeutic agents include cisplatin, etoposide, adriamycin, cyclophosphamide, vincristine, and irinotecan. Although the tumor is responsive to chemotherapy, high recurrence rates lead to uniformly poor outcomes.

RARE TUMORS ARISING FROM THE SKIN

Rarely, skin appendageal tumors arise in the following locations:

- Hair follicle
- Sebaceous gland
- Arrector pili muscle
- Apocrine sweat gland

Most of these tumors are benign and carcinomas are rare. The treatment principle of carcinomas includes complete surgical excision and lymph node assessment as in melanoma.

Dermatofibrosarcoma Protuberans

A rare fibrohistiocytic tumor arising in the skin and subcutaneous tissue of intermediate malignant potential demonstrating slow growth and consistent cytogenetic abnormality t(17;22) in more than 90% of patients, with the following characteristics:

- Common tumor sites include trunk and extremities
- Frequent local recurrences occur after surgical resection
- Low propensity to distant metastasis

The translocation t(17;22) between chromosome 17 and 22 places PDGFβ under the control of COL1A1, resulting in up-regulation, expression, and activation of tyrosine kinase PDGFβ (24). Recent reports suggest high response rates to imatinib mesylate. This potent and specific inhibitor of PDGFRβ is effectively used in neoadjuvant setting and in patients with recurrent disease.

REFERENCES

1. Santa Cruz DJ, Hurt MA In: Steinberg SS, ed. *Diagnostic Surgical Pathology,* 2nd ed., vol. 1. New York: Raven Press, 1999: 57–101.
2. Jemal A, Siegel R, Ward E, et al. Cancer statistics. *CA Cancer J Clin* 2008; 58: 71–96.
3. Marquette A, Bagot M, Bensussan A, Dumaz N. Recent discoveries in the genetics of melanoma and their therapeutic implications. *Arch Immunol Ther Exp* 2007; 55: 363–372.
4. Clark WH Jr, From L, Bernadino EA, et al. The histogenesis and biologic behavior of primary human malignant melanomas of skin. *Cancer Res* 1969; 29: 705.
5. Breslow A. Thickness, cross-sectional areas and depth of invasion in the prognosis of cutaneous melanoma. *Ann Surg* 1970; 172: 902.

6. Balch CM, Buzaid AC, Soong S-J, et al. Final version of the American Joint Committee on Cancer staging system for cutaneous melanoma. *J Clin Oncol* 2001; 19: 3655–3648.
7. Balch CM, Soong S-J, Gershenwald JE, et al. Prognostic factors analysis of 17,600 melanoma patients: Validation of the American Joint Committee on Cancer melanoma staging system. *J Clin Oncol* 2001; 19: 3622–3634.
8. McCarthy WH, Shaw HM. The surgical treatment of primary melanoma. *Hematol Oncol Clin North Am* 1988; 12: 797–805.
9. Morton DL. Sentinel lymphadenectomy for patients with clinical stage I melanoma. *J Surg Oncol* 1997; 66: 267–269.
10. Grobb JJ, Dreno B, Salmoniere P, et al. Randomized trial of interferon alpha-2a as adjuvant therapy in resected primary melanoma thicker than 1.5 mm without clinically detectable node metastasis. *Lancet* 1998; 351: 905–1910.
11. Kirkwood JM, Ibrahim JG, Sondak VK, et al. High- and low dose interferon alfa-2b in high-risk melanoma: First analysis of intergroup trial E1690/S9111/C9190. *J Clin Oncol* 2000; 18: 2444–2458.
12. Ang KK, Byers RM, Peters LJ, et al. Regional radiotherapy as adjuvant for head and neck malignant melanoma: preliminary results. *Arch Otolaryngol Head Neck Surg* 1990; 116: 9.
13. Skibber JM, Soong S-J, Aushin AC, et al. Cranial irradiation after surgical excision of brain metastasis in melanoma patients. *Ann Surg Oncol* 1996; 3: 118–123.
14. Ghussen F, Nage IK, Groth W, et al. Hyperthermic perfusion with chemotherapy and melanoma of the extremities. *World J Surg* 1989; 13: 598.
15. Chapman PB, Einhorn LH, Meyers ML, et al. Phase III multicenter randomized trial of the Dartmouth regimen versus dacarbazine in patients with metastatic melanoma. *J Clin Oncol* 1999; 17: 2745–2751.
16. Falkson JM. Improved results with the addition of interferon alpha-2b to dacarbazine in the treatment of patients with metastatic malignant melanoma. *J Clin Oncol* 1991; 9: 1403–1408.
17. Rosenberg SA, Yang JC, Topalian SL, et al. Treatment of 283 consecutive patients with metastatic melanoma or renal cell cancer using high-dose bolus interleukin 2. *JAMA* 1994; 271: 907–913.
18. Legha SS, Ring S, Bedikian A, et al. Treatment of metastatic melanoma with combined chemotherapy containing cisplatin, vinblastine, dacarbazine (CVD) and biotherapy using interleukin 2 and interferon alpha. *Ann Oncol* 1996; 7: 827–835.
19. Mukherji B, Chakraborty NG, Sporn JR, et al. Induction of peptide antigen reactive cytolytic T cells following immunization with MAGE-1 peptide pulsed autologous antigen presenting cells. *PNAS* 1995; 92: 8078–8082.
20. Belli F, Testori A, Rivoltini L, et al. Vaccination of metastatic melanoma patients with autologous tumor-derived heat shock protein gp96-peptide complexes: clinical and immunologic findings. *J Clin Oncol* 2002; 20: 4169–4180.
21. O'Day SJ, Hamid O, Urba WJ. Targeting cytotoxic T-Lymphocyte antigen-4 (CTLA-4): A novel strategy for the treatment of melanoma and other malignancies. *Cancer* 2007; 110: 2614–2627.
22. Davies H, Bignell GR, Cox C, et al. Mutations of the BRAF gene in human cancer. *Nature* 2002; 417: 949–954.
23. FengH, Shuda M, Chang Y, Moore PS. Clonal integration of a polyomavirus in human merkel cell carcinoma. *Science* 2008; 319: 1096–1100.
24. Takahira T, Oda Y, Tamiya S, et al. Detection of COL1A1-PDGFB fusion transcripts and PDGFB/PDGFRB mRNA expression in dermatofibrosarcoma protuberans. *Mod Pathol* 2007; 20: 68–675.

SECTION 9

Hematologic Malignancies

23

Acute Leukemia

Aaron Cumpston and Michael Craig

Acute leukemia represents a very aggressive, malignant transformation of an early hematologic precursor. The malignant clone is arrested in an immature blast form, proliferates abnormally, and no longer has the ability to undergo maturation. In contrast, the chronic leukemias are characterized by resistance to apoptosis and by accumulation of nonfunctional cells. Accumulation of the blasts within the bone marrow results in progressive hematopoietic failure, with associated infection, anemia, and thrombocytopenia. It is these complications that often prompt evaluation in newly diagnosed patients.

Acute leukemia continues to present a grave diagnosis because of its rapid clinical course. Patients require aggressive and urgent evaluation and treatment initiation. As a general rule, treatment is expected to improve quality of life and prolong survival. Unfortunately, many patients present at an advanced age and with comorbid conditions, making cytotoxic treatment difficult. Elderly or unwell patients who are given the best supportive care survive only for a few months.

The immature, clonally proliferating cells that form blasts may be derived from myeloid or lymphoid cell lines. Transformation of granulocyte, RBC, or platelet (myeloid) precursors results in acute myelogenous leukemia (AML). Acute lymphoblastic leukemia (ALL) originates from B or T lymphocytes. This general division has implications for different treatment and diagnostic approaches. It is the first step in classifying the leukemic process occurring in the patient.

EPIDEMIOLOGY

- Estimated new cases in the United States in 2007 was 13,400 for AML and 5,200 for ALL.
- AML accounts for 9,000 deaths and ALL accounts for 1,400 deaths annually in the United States.
- The risk of developing AML increases with advanced age, the median age being 60 to 69.
- Seventy-five percent of newly diagnosed patients with AML are older than 60.
- ALL is more common in children; 60% to 70% of cases are found in patients younger than 20 years.

RISK FACTORS

Most patients will have no identifiable risk for developing leukemia. Table 23.1 lists the conditions that are identified with an increased risk for developing acute leukemia. Most studies have evaluated the relationship between the risk factors and AML. The conditions that are most associated with AML are chronic benzene exposure, exposure to ionizing radiation, and previous chemotherapy.

Ionizing Radiation Exposure Explored in Atomic Bomb Survivors

- Ionizing radiations have a latency period of 5 to 20 years and a peak period of 5 to 9 years in atomic bomb survivors.
- They exhibit a 20- to 30-fold increased risk of AML and chronic myelogenous leukemia (CML).

TABLE 23.1. *Risk factors for acute leukemia*

Exposure
Ionizing radiation, benzene, cytotoxic drugs, alkylating agents, cigarette smoking, ethanol use by the mother
Acquired disorders
Myelodysplastic syndrome, paroxysmal nocturnal hemoglobinuria, polycythemia vera, chronic myelogenous leukemia, myeloproliferative disorders, idiopathic myelofibrosis, aplastic anemia, eosinophilic fasciitis, myeloma, primary mediastinal germ cell tumor (residual teratoma elements evolve into myeloid progenitors that evolve into AML years later)
Genetic predisposition
Down syndrome, Fanconi anemia, Diamond-Blackfan anemia, Kostmann syndrome, Klinefelter syndrome, Chromosome 21q disorder, Wiskott-Aldrich syndrome, ataxia-telangiectasia, dyskeratosis congenita, combined immunodeficiency syndrome, von Recklinghausen disease, neurofibromatosis 1, Shwachman syndrome
Familial
Nonidentical sibling (1:800), monozygotic twin (1:5), first-degree relative (three times increased risk)
Infection
Human T cell leukemia virus and T cell ALL

AML, acute myelogenous leukemia; ALL, acute lymphoblastic leukemia.

Chemotherapy

- Therapy-related AML may account for 10% to 20% of new cases.
- Leukemia associated with alkylating agents may be associated with cytogenetic changes of chromosomes 5, 7, and 13. Often there is a multiyear latent-phase myelodysplastic syndrome preceding the development of AML.
- Topoisomerase II agents, often with an abnormal chromosome 11q23 in the blasts, can rapidly evolve after initial therapy. Usually, these are preceded by only a brief myelodysplastic state rapidly evolving to AML.
- Previous high-dose therapy with autologous transplant leads to a cumulative risk of 2.6% by 5 years, especially with total body irradiation (TBI)–containing regimens.

CLINICAL SIGNS AND SYMPTOMS

1. Ineffective hematopoiesis—results from marrow infiltration by the malignant cells
   - Anemia: pallor, fatigue, and shortness of breath
   - Thrombocytopenia: epistaxis, petechiae, and easy bruising
   - Neutropenia: fever and pyogenic infection.
2. Infiltration of other organs
   - Skin: leukemia cutis in 10%
   - Gum hypertrophy: especially in monocytic leukemia (AML M5)
   - Granulocytic sarcoma: localized tumor composed of blast cells; it imparts poorer prognosis; these sarcomas are occasionally extramedullary leukemia masses associated with 8;21 translocation
   - Liver, spleen, and lymph nodes: common in ALL, occasionally in monocytic leukemia (AML M5)
   - Thymic mass: present in 15% of ALL in adults
   - Testicular infiltration: also a site of relapse for ALL
   - Retinal involvement: may occur in ALL
3. Central nervous system (CNS) and meningeal involvement
   - 5%–10% of cases at diagnosis, mainly ALL, inv(16) [French-American-British (FAB) M4Eo], and high blast count
   - Analysis and prophylaxis are given in ALL to decrease CNS relapse
   - Symptoms: headache and cranial nerve palsy, but mostly asymptomatic

4. Disseminated intravascular coagulation (DIC) and bleeding
   - Very common with acute promyelocytic leukemia (APL); mechanism is related to tissue factor release by granules and fibrinolysis; generally improves with all-trans retinoic acid (ATRA) of which early initiation is imperative
   - Can be present in AML inv(16) or monocytic leukemia or can be related to sepsis
5. Leukostasis
   - Occurs with elevated blast count; 25% of patients with ALL present with white blood cell (WBC) count >50,000
   - Symptoms result from capillary plugging by leukemic cells; it is associated with large nondeformable blasts in AML and ALL, and is rarely seen in CLL
   - Common signs: dyspnea, headache, confusion, and hypoxia
   - Initial treatment includes leukapheresis, aggressive hydration, and chemotherapy to rapidly lower the circulating blast percentage with drugs (e.g., oral hydroxyurea or intravenous cyclophosphamide)
   - Transfusions should be avoided because these may increase viscosity
   - Leukapheresis is repeated daily in conjunction with chemotherapy until the blast count is <50,000

DIAGNOSTIC EVALUATION

- History and physical examination are an essential part of diagnosis of acute leukemia.
- Complete blood count (CBC) and differential, manual examination of peripheral smear, and peripheral blood flow cytometry are considered when circulating blasts are sufficiently abundant to establish a diagnosis.
- Coagulation tests include prothrombin time (PT), partial thromboplastin time (PTT), D-dimer, and fibrinogen.
- Electrolytes with calcium, magnesium, phosphorus, and uric acid. Low glucose, potassium, and PO_2 (partial pressure of oxygen) can occur with delay in analysis of high blast count.
- Bone marrow biopsy and aspirate (with analysis for morphology), cytogenetics, flow cytometry, and cytochemical stains (Sudan black, myeloperoxidase, acid phosphatase, and specific and nonspecific esterase) are used for diagnosis.
- Human leukocyte antigen (HLA) testing of patients who are transplant candidates—the test is performed before the patient becomes cytopenic. Specimen requirements are minimal when DNA-based HLA typing is performed.
- Hepatitis B and C, cytomegalovirus, herpes simplex virus, human T-cell leukemia virus, and human immunodeficiency virus antibody titers are obtained.
- Pregnancy test (β-human chorionic gonadotropin).
- Electrocardiogram (ECG) and analysis of cardiac ejection fraction should be done prior to treatment with anthracyclines.
- Lumbar puncture—performed when signs and symptoms of neurologic involvement are present. Low platelets should be corrected. The procedure may be performed after reduction of peripheral blast count to avoid inoculation of blasts into uninvolved cerebrospinal fluid (CSF). Obtain cell count, opening pressure, protein level, and submit cytocentrifuge specimen for cytology.
- Central venous access should be obtained. An implanted port-type catheter is not recommended. Coagulation abnormalities should be corrected if present. It is often possible to initiate induction therapy with normal peripheral veins and await subsidence of coagulopathy to reduce risk of procedural complications.
- Supplemental testing of fluorescent in situ hybridization (FISH) assay for 15;17 translocation is performed when APL is suspected; and BCR-ABL test is performed when CML in blast phase or ALL is suspected.
- Cytogenetic analysis of blasts will contribute dramatically to subsequent preferred management and prognosis.

INITIAL MANAGEMENT

The initial management of acute leukemia involves the following:

- Hydration with IV fluids (2–3 L/m^2 per day)
- Tumor lysis prophylaxis should be started.
- Blood product support suggestions for prophylactic transfusions are hemoglobin level <8 and platelet level <10,000. Platelet trigger threshold can be higher in the context of fever or bleeding (<20,000 suggested), cryoprecipitate can be used if fibrinogen level is <100, and fresh frozen plasma (FFP) can be used to correct significantly elevated levels of PT and PTT. The minimum "safe" platelet level required to prevent spontaneous hemorrhage is not known. Additional platelet optimization strategies include avoidance of nonsteroidal anti-inflammatory drugs (NSAIDs), aspirin, and clopidogrel-like agents.
- Blood products should be irradiated and a WBC filter (if CMV-negative blood inventory is not available) should be used in those patients who are future allogeneic transplant candidates.
- Fever and neutropenia require blood and urine cultures, followed by treatment with appropriate antibiotics (see Chapter 36), and imaging.
- Therapeutic anticoagulation should be given with extreme caution in patients during periods of extreme thrombocytopenia. Adjustment of prophylactic platelet transfusion thresholds or anticoagulants is required.
- Suppression of menses: medroxyprogesterone (Provera) 10 mg daily or twice daily.

Tumor Lysis Syndrome

- Tumor lysis syndrome can be spontaneous or can be induced by chemotherapy.
- Risk factors include elevated uric acid, high WBC count, elevated lactate dehydrogenase (LDH), and high tumor burden.
- Laboratory tests indicate elevated potassium, phosphorus, and uric acid; with a resulting decrease in calcium.
- The patients should be initiated on allopurinol 300 mg twice daily for 3 days, followed by once daily until risk is resolved.
- For hydration, alkalinizing fluids (0.5NS with 50 mEq sodium bicarbonate) could be considered to increase solubility of uric acid, minimizing intratubular precipitation. Caution should be taken since alkanizing the urine also promotes calcium-phosphate complex deposition.
- Rasburicase (Elitek) should be used if the patient has hyperuricemia and an elevated creatinine on presentation or has hyperuricemia uncontrolled with allopurinol.
- Hemodialysis may be required in refractory cases or urgently in the setting of life-threatening hyperkalemia, or volume overload if oliguric (see Chapter 38).

CLASSIFICATION OF ACUTE MYELOGENOUS LEUKEMIA

There are two current systems to classify AML. The most commonly used criteria is from the World Health Organization (WHO) and incorporates recurrent cytogenetic abnormalities and prognostic groups (Table 23.2). Marrow blasts should make up 20% of the nucleated cells within the aspirate unless t(8;21) or inv(16) is present. The French-American-British (FAB) classification is also used and classifies AML into eight subtypes. The blasts may be characterized as myeloid lineage by the presence of Auer rods; a positive myeloperoxidase, Sudan black, or nonspecific esterase stain; and the immunophenotype shown by flow cytometry. Cell surface markers associated with myeloid cell lines include CD13, CD33, CD34, c-kit, and HLA-DR. Monocytic markers include CD64, CD11b, and CD14. CD41 (platelet glycophorin) is associated with megakaryocytic leukemia, and glycophorin A is present on erythroblasts. HLA-DR–negative blast phenotype is commonly seen in APL and serves as a rapidly available test in confirming the suspicion of this subtype requiring a specific induction therapy.

TABLE 23.2. *The World Health Organization (WHO) and French-American-British (FAB) classification of acute myeloid leukemia*

AML with recurrent genetic abnormalities
AML with t(8;21) (usually FAB M2)
AML with abnormal bone marrow eosinophils and inv(16) or t(16;16) (usually FAB M4Eo)
Acute promyelocytic leukemia with t(15;17) (FAB M3)
AML with 11q23 abnormalities
AML with multilineage dysplasia
Following MDS or myeloproliferative disorder
Without prior MDS but with dysplasia in 50% cells in two cell lines
AML and MDS, therapy-related
Alkylating agent or radiation related
Topoisomerase II related
Others
AML not otherwise categorized
AML minimally differentiated (FAB M0)
AML without maturation (FAB M1)
AML with maturation (FAB M2)
Acute myelomonocytic leukemia (FAB M4)
Acute monocytic leukemia (FAB M5)
Acute erythroid leukemia (FAB M6)
Acute megakaryocytic leukemia (FAB M7)
Acute basophilic leukemia
Acute panmyelosis with myelofibrosis
Myeloid sarcoma

AML, acute myelogenous leukemia; MDS, myelodysplasia.

CLASSIFICATION OF ACUTE LYMPHOBLASTIC LEUKEMIA

The WHO classification of ALL divides the disease into precursor B cell, precursor T cell, and Burkitt cell leukemia. Immunophenotyping of B-lineage ALL reveals lymphoid markers (CD19, CD20, CD10, TdT, and immunoglobulin). T cell markers include TdT, CD2, CD3, CD4, CD5, and CD7. Burkitt cell leukemia is characterized by a translocation between chromosome 8 (the *c-myc* gene) and chromosome 14 (immunoglobulin heavy chain), or chromosome 2 or 22 (light chain) regions.

PROGNOSTIC GROUPS IN ACUTE MYELOGENOUS LEUKEMIA

Those patients who are older (>60 years) and those with an elevated blast count at diagnosis (>20,000) have a worse prognosis. Chemotherapy-related AML and prior history of myelodysplasia (MDS) imparts a lower chance of obtaining complete remission (CR) and long-term survival. Table 23.3 illustrates the prognostic groups according to cytogenetics.

PROGNOSTIC GROUPS IN ACUTE LYMPHOBLASTIC LEUKEMIA

As in AML, patients with ALL have a worse prognosis when presenting with advanced age or elevated WBC count. Burkitt cell (mature B-cell) leukemia or lymphoma has an improved prognosis with intensive chemotherapy and CNS treatment; it usually has a translocation involving chromosome 8q24. Table 23.4 lists the prognostic groups according to cytogenetic analysis. The presence of t(9;22) (Philadelphia chromosome) is the most common abnormality in adults. It is present in 20% to 30% of patients with ALL and in up to 50% of patients in the B cell lineage. Long-term survival is dismal in this group if treated by chemotherapy alone, and patients are recommended to undergo allogeneic transplantation if they are a suitable candidate in first CR.

TABLE 23.3. *Cytogenetic risk groups in treated adult acute myelogenous leukemia cases*

Favorable risk (5-yr survival with therapy approximately 55%)
t(15;17)
inv(16), del(16q), t(16;16)
t(8;21) with or without complex karyotype and del(9q)
Standard risk (5-yr survival with therapy approximately 25%)
no cytogenetic abnormality identified (i.e., normal)
all other cytogenetic abnormalities not associated with a specific prognosis
Poor risk (5-yr survival with therapy approximately 5%)
−5, −7
inv(3) or t(3;3)
t(9;22)
11q23 (MLL) abnormalities, excluding t(9;11)
three or more abnormalities
t(6;9)

TABLE 23.4. *Prognostic groups in adult acute lymphoblastic leukemia*

Poor risk	Good risk
t(9;22)	8q24 translocations
t(4;11)	t(12;21)
Hypodiploid	t(10;14)
t(1;19)	t(7;10)

TREATMENT INDUCTION IN ACUTE MYELOGENOUS LEUKEMIA [NON–t(15;17) ACUTE PROMYELOCYTIC LEUKEMIA]

The goal of induction chemotherapy is to obtain CR, which has been shown to correlate with improved survival. CR is the elimination of the malignant clone (marrow blasts <5%) and recovery of hematopoiesis [absolute neutrophil count (ANC) >1,000 and platelet count >100,000]. Patients typically have a leukemia cell burden of approximately 10×10^{12} that is reduced to approximately 10×10^9 by induction. This residual disease is essentially undetectable but will lead to relapse in weeks to months if more therapy is not administered. Additional intensive "consolidation" cycles of chemotherapy are given to further reduce the residual burden in the hope that host immune mechanisms can suppress the residual leukemia population, thereby leading to sustained CR. The general approach to induction chemotherapy for adults is shown in Table 23.5. Patients should be considered for clinical trials if available.

In general:
• Addition of high-dose cytarabine (HDAC) or etoposide has been evaluated in published regimens for induction that may benefit some patients younger than 60. These additions have not been demonstrated to be conclusively superior to 3 days of anthracycline and 7 days of cytarabine alone.

TABLE 23.5. *Standard induction for acute myelogenous leukemia*

"7 + 3," 7 d of cytarabine and 3 d of anthracycline
Cytarabine 100–200 mg/m² daily as continuous infusion × 7 d with
  Idarubicin 12 mg/m² daily bolus for 3 d
          OR
  Daunorubicin 45–60 mg/m² daily bolus for 3 d

TABLE 23.6. *Consolidation of acute myelogenous leukemia*

Age <60
Cytarabine 3 gm/m^2 infused over 3 h, q12h on d 1, 3, and 5 (six doses)
Creatinine 1.5–1.9 mg/dL: Decrease cytarabine 1.5 g/m^2 per dose
Age >60
"5 + 2:" Cytarabine 100 mg/m^2 daily as continuous infusion for 5 d and anthracycline agent
(idarubicin 12 mg/m^2 or daunorubicin 45–60 mg/m^2) bolus daily for 2 d
OR
Intermediate-dose cytarabine: [(1–1.5 gm/m^2 q12h on d 1, 3, 5]) OR [(1–1.5 gm/m^2 daily x ×
4–5 days])

- Bone marrow aspiration should be repeated at approximately day 14. If significant residual blasts are present, induction chemotherapy should be repeated (consider "5 + 2" in Table 23.6). If significant disease is present (<50% reduction in disease volume), induction should be repeated or a change in the regimen to age-appropriate HDAC should be considered.
- Older (>65) patients may benefit from treatment. HDAC should be avoided because of excess CNS toxicity and commonly observed poor survival prospects regardless of therapy selection.

SUPPORTIVE CARE

- Infection is a major cause of morbidity and mortality. Prophylactic antibiotics and antifungals are often used during prolonged neutropenia with uncertain benefit. Broad-spectrum antimicrobials are used for neutropenic fever (see Chapter 35).
- Growth factors such as granulocyte colony-stimulating factor (G-CSF) are associated with shortened length of neutropenia and are of demonstrated value in patients older than 55 years. Growth factors are not routinely recommended in younger patients but can be safely added if necessary. Initiation of G-CSF is delayed until after day 14, when bone marrow shows a satisfactory induction pattern. Growth factors may have the most benefit in those patients with infectious complications.
- Steroid eye drops are required during HDAC infusions to reduce risk of exfoliative keratitis.

TREATMENT : ACUTE MYELOGENOUS LEUKEMIA CONSOLIDATION, NON–T(15;17)

The consolidation options for those patients who enter CR are shown in Table 23.6. HDAC especially may benefit those patients with good-risk disease [t(8;21) or inv(16)]. Consolidation usually consists of four cycles (the minimum effective dose and number of cycles is not clear). Older patients do not seem to benefit from more than one to two consolidation cycles. Patients with preceding MDS or poor-risk cytogenetics should be considered for allogeneic transplantation. Lumbar puncture should be done at first remission for patients with monocytic histologies or a WBC >100,000 at diagnosis.

TREATMENT FOR ACUTE PROMYELOCYTIC LEUKEMIA, T(15;17)

The t(15;17) brings together the retinoic acid receptor-α and the promyelocytic leukemia genes, allowing for transduction of a novel protein (PML/RARα). The protein plays a role in blocking differentiation of the promyelocyte, thereby allowing abnormal accumulation within the marrow space. Because the characteristic translocation occurs in this subgroup of AML, therapy incorporates ATRA, which acts as a differentiating agent. Table 23.7 shows a treatment summary in APL.

TABLE 23.7. *Treatment of acute promyelocytic leukemia*

Induction
ATRA 45 mg/m²/d PO divided into two doses, daily until CR and
Anthracycline: Idarubicin 12 mg/m² alternate days for four doses (d 2, 4, 6, 8[a])
Consolidation stratified by low risk and high risk
Low risk (WBC <10,000 and platelet count >40 at diagnosis)
  Alternating anthracycline/anthracenedione: Idarubicin 5 mg/m² daily for 4 d (first consolidation),
    then mitoxantrone 10 mg/m² daily for 5 d (second consolidation), followed by idarubicin
    12 mg/m² times one dose (third consolidation)
High risk (WBC ≥10,000 or platelet count ≤40 at diagnosis)
  Alternating anthracycline/anthracenedione: Idarubicin 7 mg/m² daily for 4 d (first consolidation),
    then mitoxantrone 10 mg/m² daily for 5 d (second consolidation), followed by idarubicin
    12 mg/m² daily for 2 d (third consolidation)
                        PLUS
ATRA 45 mg/m²/d PO divided into two doses, daily for 15 d (days 1–15 of each consolidation
  cycle)
Maintenance (2 yr)
  ATRA 45 mg/m² daily for 15 d q3mo
  Mercaptopurine 50 mg/m² daily
  MTX 15 mg/m² weekly

ATRA, all-trans retinoic acid; 6-MP, 6-mercaptopurine; MTX, methotrexate.
[a]Consider omitting day 8 idarubicin in patients older than 70 years.

- Therapy with ATRA should be started immediately upon suspicion of APL; therapy can be tailored pending genetic confirmation.
- Time to attain remission may be more than 30 days and a bone marrow biopsy is not performed on day 14.
- PCR should be followed for PML-RAR: reinduction therapy should be considered if PCR is still positive post-consolidation; also, levels should be followed during the maintenance phase. A return of the transcript to positive heralds relapse.
- ATRA syndrome (retinoic acid syndrome) consists of capillary leak and cytokine release resulting in fever, leukocytosis, respiratory compromise (dyspnea and infiltrates), weight gain, effusions (pleural and pericardial), renal failure, and hypotension. This syndrome occurs in 25% of patients during induction, often around day 7, and is associated with a rapidly rising neutrophil count. Treat with dexamethasone 10 mg IV BID × 3 days, then taper over 2 weeks. Discontinuation of ATRA or use of leukocyte apheresis should be considered in severe cases. ATRA may still be safely employed in maintenance-phase therapy because the ATRA syndrome is limited to the induction-period neutrophilia.
- A similar differentiation syndrome, not involving ATRA, is seen with the use of arsenic trioxide.
- Prognosis with APL is very good, with 90% of patients attaining a CR and 70% long-term disease-free survival.
- Those patients with WBC counts >10,000 and platelets <40,000 at diagnosis may have increased risk of relapse. An intensified consolidation regimen has been shown to benefit these patients.
- ATRA + arsenic trioxide is an alternative option for untreated patients unable to tolerate anthralcines.

Relapsed Disease

1. Arsenic trioxide 0.15 mg/kg/day until second CR
   - Median of 57 days to remission
   - Baseline electrolytes (Ca, K, Mg), creatinine, and ECG (for prolonged QT interval)
   - Monitoring: At least weekly electrolytes and ECG. Keep K>4.0 and Mg>2.0 and reassess if QTc interval >500
   - Patients commonly develop APL differentiation syndrome similar to ATRA
   - Eighty-five percent of patients achieve CR
   - Arsenic trioxide may be given as consolidation at a dose of 0.15 mg/kg/day, 5 days per week (Monday through Friday) for 25 doses.

2. Gemtuzumab ozogamicin (Mylotarg)—if the patient has recently been treated with arsenic
3. Patients achieving CR (PCR-negative) should receive consolidation with an autologous transplant, if eligible. Patients with persistent positive PCR results should be considered for an allogeneic transplant.

TREATMENT OF RELAPSED OR REFRACTORY ACUTE MYELOGENOUS LEUKEMIA

Relapse of AML after initial CR is very common (60–80% of all cases). Relapse occurring within 6 months of induction or a patient never attaining remission with induction (refractory disease) complicates many induction attempts. The prognosis for long-term survival in this subset of patients is very poor with chemotherapy alone, and all patients who are able to tolerate the treatment should be evaluated for allogeneic transplantation. Some treatment approaches are described below.

1. Gemtuzumab ozogamicin (Mylotarg)
   - Gemtuzumab ozogamicin is an anti-CD33 monoclonal antibody conjugated with calicheamicin.
   - The dosage is 9 mg/m^2 as 2-hour infusion on days 1 and 15.
   - Thirty percent of patients achieved CR (13% without complete platelet recovery).
   - Side effects include infusion reactions (may be seen up to 24 hours after infusion), myelosuppression, and increased liver enzymes.
   - WBC count should be reduced to <30,000 before treatment.
   - Gemtuzumab ozogamicin in combination with allogeneic transplantation may result in increased risk of veno-occlusive disease (VOD).
   - Overall treatment-related morbidity can be considered similar to that of conventional chemotherapy induction.
2. Reinduction with "7 + 3" or high-dose cytarabine
   - Reinduction may be an option for those patients who relapse more than 6 to 12 months after induction.
   - Subsequent remissions are usually of shorter duration (<50% of the duration of the preceding remission).
3. Etoposide, mitoxantrone, ± cytarabine (EM or MEC)
4. FLAG: fludarabine, cytarabine, and G-CSF (can be combined with idarubicin or mitoxantrone)
5. Liposomal daunorubicin and cytarabine combination at high doses
6. In cases of isolated CNS relapse, it should be considered that systemic relapse almost always follows soon and that a systemic therapy is also required.

TREATMENT OF ACUTE LYMPHOCYTIC LEUKEMIA

General scheme: induction, consolidation, maintenance, and CNS treatment

Several strategies exist for the treatment of adult ALL. Table 23.8 illustrates the Hyper-CVAD (cyclophosphamide, vincristine, doxorubicin, and dexamethasone) regimen employed in many North American centers. The Larson regimen reported by Cancer and Leukemia Group B (CALGB) Study 9111, shown in Table 23.9, is also commonly employed. Other options based on the Hoelzer and Linker regimen are also available. Burkitt-cell leukemia (mature-B ALL, L3) is not included because of high resistance to typical induction chemotherapy. It can be treated with hyper-CVAD without maintenance therapy but requires aggressive CNS treatment to prevent relapse.

SUPPORTIVE CARE

The regimens described previously incorporate growth factors to reduce neutropenia and allow more scheduled chemotherapy to proceed. All patients will require blood product support at some point during the treatment. Those patients treated with hyper-CVAD receive prophylactic antimicrobials (i.e., levofloxacin 500 mg daily, fluconazole 200 mg daily, and valacyclovir 500 mg daily).

TABLE 23.8. *The hyper-CVAD and MTX/HIDAC regimen*

Cycle 1, 3, 5, 7
Cyclophosphamide 300 mg/m^2 i.v. over 3 h q12h d 1–3 (six doses)
Mesna 600 mg/m^2/d i.v. as continuous infusion d 1–3
Vincristine 2 mg i.v. d 4, 11
Doxorubicin 50 mg/m^2 i.v. d 4
Dexamethasone 40 mg PO daily d 1–4 and 11–14
G-CSF 10 μg/kg/d SQ starting after chemotherapy
Cycle 2, 4, 6, 8
Methotrexate 200 mg/m^2 i.v. over 2 h on d 1, followed by
Methotrexate 800 mg/m^2 i.v. over 22 h on d 1
Leucovorin 50 mg starting 12 h after methotrexate completed, followed by leucovorin 15 mg every 6 h × eight doses, dose adjusted on the basis of methotrexate levels.
Cytarabine 3 g/m^2 i.v. over 2 h every 12 h on d 2 and 3 (four doses)
Methylprednisolone 50 mg i.v. twice daily d 1–3
G-CSF 10 μg/kg/d SQ starting after chemotherapy
CNS prophylaxis[a]
Methotrexate 12 mg intrathecal (IT) on d 2
Cytarabine 100 mg IT on d 8
Maintenance therapy[b] **(POMP)** × **2 years**
Mercaptopurine 50 mg PO three times daily
Methotrexate 20 mg/m^2 PO, weekly
Vincristine 2 mg i.v. monthly
Prednisone 200 mg/d for 5 d each month
Dosage adjustments
Vincristine reduced to 1 mg if bilirubin 2–3 mg/dL (omitted if bilirubin >3 mg/dL)
Doxorubicin decreased to 50% for bilirubin 2–3 mg/dL, decreased to 25% if bilirubin 3–5 mg/dL, and omitted if bilirubin >5 mg/dL
Methotrexate reduced to 50% if creatinine clearance 10–50 mL/min, and a decrease to 50–75% for delayed excretion, nephrotoxicity, or grade ≥3 mucositis with prior courses
High-dose cytarabine decreased to 1 g/m^2 if patient ≥60 yr, creatinine ≥1.5 mg/dL, or MTX level >20 μmol/L at the completion of the MTX infusion

G-CSF, granulocyte colony-stimulating factor; CNS, central nervous system; MTX, methotrexate.
[a]Dosing interval based on risk stratification (see text).
[b]Maintenance therapy is not given in Burkitt-cell leukemia/lymphoma.

THERAPY FOR CENTRAL NERVOUS SYSTEM DISEASE

- CNS is a sanctuary site.
- CNS disease is diagnosed by the presence of neurologic deficits at diagnosis *or* by five or more blasts per microliter of CSF.
- Therapy for CNS disease is intrathecal (IT) methotrexate (MTX) or cytarabine (Ara-C), often alternating. These will be given twice weekly until disease clears, then weekly for 4 weeks, and then resume prophylaxis schedule. Radiation (fractionated to 2,400–3,000 cGy) can also be considered, being aware of potential late-term cognitive toxicities.
- Prophylaxis decreases CNS relapse from 30% to <5%. The prophylactic radiation and chemotherapy schedule intensity are dependent on the relapse risk.
- In the hyper-CVAD regimen, patients with high-risk disease (i.e., LDH level >2.3 times upper limit of normal or elevated proliferative index) should receive eight prophylactic IT treatments, and those with low-risk disease (no factors) receive six prophylactic IT treatments. Patients with mature B-cell disease or a history of documented CNS involvement will require 16 IT therapies. No prophylactic cranial irradiation is given.

TREATMENT OF RELAPSED ACUTE LYMPHOBLASTIC LEUKEMIA

Marrow is the most common site of relapse, but relapse can occur in testes, eye, and CNS. Patients with late relapse (more than 1 year from induction) may respond to reinduction with the original regi-

TABLE 23.9. *The Larson regimen*

Course I: Induction (4 wk)
Cyclophosphamide 1,200 mg/m^2 i.v. d 1[a]
Daunorubicin 45 mg/m^2 i. v. d 1–3[a]
Vincristine 2 mg i.v. d 1, 8, 15, 22
Prednisone 60 mg/m^2/d PO d 1–21[a]
L-Asparaginase (*Escherichia coli*) 6,000 IU/m^2 SQ/IM d 5, 8, 11, 15, 18, 22
G-CSF 5 μg/kg/d SQ starting d 4
Course IIA (4 wk; repeat once for Course IIB)
Methotrexate 15 mg intrathecal (IT) d 1
Cyclophosphamide 1,000 mg/m^2 i.v. d 1
6-Mercaptopurine 60 mg/m^2/d PO d 1–14
Cytarabine 75 mg/m^2/d SQ d 1–4 and 8–11
Vincristine 2 mg i.v. d 15 and 22 (two doses)
L-Asparaginase (*E. coli*) 6,000 IU/m^2 SQ/IM d 15, 18, 22, 25 (four doses)
G-CSF 5 μg/kg/d SQ starting d 2
Course III: CNS prophylaxis and interim maintenance (12 wk)
IT Methotrexate 15 mg d 1, 8, 15, 22, 29
Cranial irradiation 2,400 cGy (fractionated) d 1–12
6-Mercaptopurine 60 mg/m^2/d PO d 1–70
Methotrexate 20 mg/m^2 PO d 36, 43, 50, 57, 64
Course iv: Late intensification (8 wk)
Doxorubicin 30 mg/m^2 i.v. d 1, 8, 15
Vincristine 2 mg i.v. d 1, 8, 15
Dexamethasone 10 mg/m^2/d PO d 1–14
Cyclophosphamide 1,000 mg/m^2 i.v. d 29
6-Thioguanine 60 mg/m^2/d PO d 29–42
Cytarabine 75 mg/m^2/d SQ d 29–32 and 36–39
Course V: Prolonged maintenance (continue until 24 months after diagnosis)
Vincristine 2 mg i.v. d 1 of every 4 wk
Prednisone 60 mg/m^2/d PO d 1–5 of every 4 wk
6-Mercaptopurine 60 mg/m^2/d PO d 1–28
Methotrexate 20 mg/m^2 PO d 1, 8, 15, 22

CNS, central nervous system.
[a]Dosage reductions for age >60 yr: cyclophosphamide 800 mg/m^2 d 1, daunorubicin 30 mg/m^2 d 1–3, and prednisone 60 mg/m^2 d 1–7.

men. Early relapse or refractory disease will require transplantation or changing treatment plan. Several options are available, including:

- High-dose cytarabine with idarubicin, mitoxantrone, or fludarabine
- Methotrexate, vincristine, asparaginase, steroids (MOAD)
- Imatinib, dasatinib, or nilotinib (if Ph-positive)
- Hyper-CVAD, if not given initially
- Vinorelbine with mitoxantrone, fludarabine, steroids, or rituximab
- Nelarabine
- Clofarabine

USE OF TARGETED THERAPIES IN ACUTE LYMPHOBLASTIC LEUKEMIA

1. Rituximab (Rituxan)
   – Anti-CD20 chimeric murine–human monoclonal antibody
   – Given in addition to the previously noted regimens in front-line treatment, if CD20+
2. Alemtuzumab (Campath)
   – Anti-CD52 chimeric monoclonal antibody employed in CLL
   – Limited experience in relapsed and refractory ALL, but may have a role

3. Imatinib (Gleevec), dasatinib (Sprycel), and nilotinib (Tasigna)
   - Tyrosine kinase inhibitors targeting the Philadelphia chromosome [t(9;22)]
   - Imatinib should be considered in addition to previously noted regimens in front-line treatment, if Ph-positive
   - Role in maintenance therapy is unknown at this time, but could be considered
   - May be used as treatment or palliation in patients unable to tolerate aggressive chemotherapy

TRANSPLANTATION

Autologous Transplant

- Autologous transplant appears to have minimal benefit in acute leukemia in CR1
- Autologous transplant could be considered for patients achieving CR2, without availability of an allogeneic donor
- It may be performed in older patients (age >60).

Allogeneic Transplant

- Allogeneic transplant has the added benefit of "graft versus leukemia" effect.
- In the setting of unrelated donor searches, the prolonged time needed to identify a donor needs to be considered at the time of diagnosis. Referral to a transplant center is preferred as early as possible in the treatment plan.
- It is considered for all patients with relapsed or refractory disease, as it is the option that may yield long-term survival.
- It is performed in the first CR or early in the course for those patients with poor-risk cytogenetics or MDS, especially with a matched-related donor.
- Patients with intermediate-risk cytogenetics may be offered allogeneic transplant if they have a sibling donor.
- Gene mutations may be able to help stratify intermediate-risk patients as poorer or more favorable outcome; assisting in the decision of the usefulness of transplantation in CR1. NPM1 mutations (without FLT3/ITD) and possibly CEBPA mutations may have a good prognosis and may not benefit from transplant in CR1. FLT3 mutations appear to be a negative predictor of outcome.
- When transplanted in CR1, overall survival is 60%; it decreases to <40% when performed for patients in CR2, and is <10% for patients with refractory disease.
- Nonmyeloablative transplantation is reasonable for those patients unable to proceed with ablative treatment secondary to age or comorbidities.

PROGNOSIS AND SURVIVAL

Adults with acute leukemia remain at high risk for disease-related and treatment-related complications. In AML, the prognostic characteristics of the disease are associated with survival. Good-risk AML is associated with 80% to 90% CR rate, and long-term disease-free survival is 60% to 70% in younger patients treated with HDAC. Poor-risk features are associated with only a 50% to 60% chance of obtaining a CR, and a high risk of relapse is observed in those patients who enter CR.

CR and long-term outcome have improved for adult patients with ALL who were receiving intensive courses of chemotherapy. With the Larson regimen, 85% obtained CR (39% older than 60 years). The hyper-CVAD course yielded a CR of 91% (79% for patients older than 60 years). Median duration of CR was 30 months with Larson regimen and was 33 months with hyper-CVAD. Five-year survival was approximately 40%.

SUGGESTED READINGS

Bloomfield C, Lawrence D, Byrd J, et al. Frequency of prolonged remission duration after high-dose cytarabine in acute myeloid leukemia varies by cytogenetic subtype. *Cancer Res* 1998;58:4173–4179.

Byrd J, Mrozek K, Dodge R, et al. Pretreatment cytogenetic abnormalities are predictive of induction success, cumulative incidence of relapse, and overall survival in adult patients with de novo acute myeloid leukemia: results from Cancer and Leukemia Group B (CALGB 8461). *Blood* 2002; 100:4325–4336.

Cortes J, Estey E, O'Brien S, et al. High-dose liposomal daunorubicin and high-dose cytarabine combination in patients with refractory or relapsed acute myelogenous leukemia. *Cancer* 2001;92:7–14.

Davies S, Rowe J, Appelbaum F. Indications for hematopoietic cell transplantation in acute leukemia. *Biol Blood Marrow Transplant* 2008;14:154–164.

Estey E, Garcia-Manero G, Ferrajoli A, et al. Use of all-trans retinoic acid plus arsenic trioxide as an alternative to chemotherapy in untreated acute promyelocytic leukemia. *Blood* 2006;107:3469–3473.

Estey E. How I treat older patients with AML. *Blood* 2000;96:1670–1673.

Estey E. Therapeutic options for acute myelogenous leukemia. *Cancer* 2001;92:1059–1073.

Farag S, Ruppert A, Mrozek K, et al. Outcome of induction and postremission therapy in younger adults with acute myeloid leukemia with normal karyotype: a CALGB study. *J Clin Oncol* 2005;23: 482–493.

Ferrando A, Look AT. Clinical implications of recurring chromosomal and associated molecular abnormalities in acute lymphoblastic leukemia. *Semin Hematol* 2000;37:381–395.

Garcia-Manero G, Kantarjian HM. The hyper-CVAD regimen in adult acute lymphocytic leukemia. *Hematol Oncol Clin North Am* 2000;14:1381–1396.

Garcia-Manero G, Thomas D. Salvage therapy for refractory or relapsed acute lymphocytic leukemia. *Hematol Oncol Clin North Am* 2001;15:163–205.

Grimwade D, Walker H, Harrison G, et al. The predictive value of hierarchical cytogenetic classification in older adults with acute myeloid leukemia (AML): analysis of 1065 patients entered into the United Kingdom Medical Research Council AML11 trial. *Blood* 2001;98:1312–1320.

Harris N, Jaffe E, Diebold J, et al. World Health Organization classification of neoplastic diseases of the hematopoietic and lymphoid tissues: report of the Clinical Advisory Committee metting-Airlie House, Virginia, November 1997. *J Clin Oncol* 1999;17:3835–3849.

Hoelzer D, Gokbuget N, Digel W, et al. Outcome of adult patients with T-lymphoblastic lymphoma treated according to protocols for acute lymphoblastic leukemia. *Blood* 2002;99:4379–4385.

Kantarjian H, Thomas D, O'Brien S, et al. Long-term follow-up results of hyperfractionated cyclophosphamide, vincristine, doxorubicin, and dexamethasone (Hyper-CVAD), a dose intensive regimen, in adult acute lymphocytic leukemia. *Cancer* 2004;101:2788–2801.

Larson RA, Dodge RK, Linker CA, et al. A randomized controlled trial of filgrastim during remission induction and consolidation chemotherapy for adults with acute lymphoblastic leukemia: CALGB Study 9111. *Blood* 1998;92:1556–1564.

Larson RA. Recent clinical trials in acute lymphoblastic leukemia by the Cancer and Leukemia Group B. *Hematol Oncol Clin North Am* 2000;14:1367–1379.

Leone G, Voso MT, Sica S, et al. Therapy related leukemias: susceptibility, prevention, and treatment. *Leuk Lymphoma* 2001;41:255–276.

Marcucci G, Radmacher M, Maharry K, et al. MicroRNA expression in cytogenetically normal acute myeloid leukemia. *N Engl J Med* 2008;358:1919–1928.

Maris M, Niederwieser D, Sandmaier B, et al. HLA-matched unrelated donor hematopoietic cell transplantation after nonmyeloablative conditioning for patients with hematologic malignancies. *Blood* 2003;102:2021–2030.

Mrozek K, Heerema N, Bloomfield C. Cytogenetics in acute leukemia. *Blood Rev* 2004;18:115–136.

Oliansky D, Appelbaum F, Cassileth P, et al. The role of cytotoxic therapy with hematopoietic stem cell transplantation in the therapy of acute myelogenous leukemia in adults: an evidence-based review. *Biol Blood Marrow Transplant* 2008;14:137–180.

Pui C, Evans W. Treatment of acute lymphoblastic leukemia. *N Engl J Med* 2006;354:166–178.

Sanz M, Martin G, Gonzalez M, et al. Risk-adapted treatment of acute promyelocytic leukemia with all-trans-retinoic acid and anthracycline monochemotherapy: a multicenter study by the PETHEMA group. *Blood* 2004;103:1237–1243.

Sanz M, Tallman M, Lo-Coco F. Tricks of the trade for the appropriate management of newly diagnosed acute promyelocytic leukemia. *Blood* 2005;105:3019–3025.

Schlenk R, Dohner K, Drauter J, et al. Mutations and treatment outcome in cytogenetically normal acute myeloid leukemia. *N Engl J Med* 2008;358:1909–1918.

Sievers EL, Larson RA, Stadmauer EA, et al. Efficacy and safety of gemtuzumab ozogamicin in patients with CD33-positive acute myeloid leukemia in first relapse. *J Clin Oncol* 2001;19:3244–3254.

Soignet SL, Frankel SR, Douer D, et al. United States multicenter trial of arsenic trioxide in relapsed acute promyelocytic leukemia. *J Clin Oncol* 2001;19:3852–3860.

Tallman M, Nabhan C, Feusner J, et al. Acute promyelocytic leukemia: evolving therapeutic strategies. *Blood* 2002;99:759–767.

Thomas D, Faderl S, Cortes J, et al. Treatment of Philadelphia chromosome-positive acute lymphocytic leukemia with hyper-CVAD and imatinib mesylate. *Blood* 2004;103:4396–4407.

Thomas D, Faderl S, O'Brien S, et al. Chemoimmunotherapy with Hyper-CVAD plus rituximab for the treatment of adult Burkitt and Burkitt-type lymphoma or acute lymphoblastic leukemia. *Cancer* 2006;106:1569–1580.

Weick J, Kopecky K, Appelbaum F, et al. A randomized investigation of high-dose versus standard-dose cytosine arabinoside with daunorubicin in patients with previously untreated acute myeloid leukemia: a Southwest Oncology Group Study. *Blood* 1996;88:2841–2851.

24

Chronic Lymphoid Leukemias

Saad Jamshed and Bruce D. Cheson

Chronic lymphocytic leukemia (CLL) is the most common leukemia in the United States, with 15,000 new cases diagnosed annually. It tends to be a disease of the elderly diagnosed with a median age at presentation of 65 years. Major advances have been made in the management of patients with CLL. These include improved ability to accurately make the diagnosis, better prognostic studies, better supportive care and improved treatments. Additional chronic lymphoid leukemias discussed in this chapter are prolymphocytic leukemia (PLL) and hairy cell leukemia (HCL).

PRESENTATION AND DIAGNOSIS

CLL is usually suspected on routine laboratory testing with an increased absolute lymphocyte count. Although patients may be asymptomatic at presentation, symptoms usually associated with CLL include fatigue, weight loss, fever, night sweats, increased frequency of infections, autoimmune anemia, or thrombocytopenia. On examination, lymphadenopathy and/or splenomegaly may be noted.

According to guidelines published by the National Cancer Institute–sponsored Working Group (NCI-WG), the diagnosis of CLL requires the following three criteria:

- Absolute lymphocytosis ($\geq 5 \times 10^3$ per μL), with cells having a morphologically mature appearance
- Monoclonal B cell phenotype [CD19, CD20 (dim), CD23] coexpressing CD5 with a low level of surface immunoglobulin (Ig)
- Whereas a bone marrow is not needed to make the diagnosis, if done the threshold should be $\geq 30\%$ lymphocytes. A bone marrow can be helpful in ascertaining the cause of cytopenias and should be done prior to treatment and to evaluate response to treatment.

STAGING AND PROGNOSIS

The most commonly used staging methods include the Rai, modified Rai, and the Binet staging systems. Prognosis based on modified Rai staging system is outlined in Table 24.1.

TABLE 24.1. *Staging and prognosis of chronic lymphocytic leukemia*

Rai	Modified Rai	Criteria	Median survival
0	Low risk	Lymphocytosis only ($\geq 15 \times 10^3/\mu$L in peripheral blood)	>10 yr
1	Intermediate risk	Lymphocytosis with enlarged nodes	7 yr
2	Intermediate risk	Lymphocytosis with increased splenic or hepatic size	
3	High risk	Lymphocytosis with anemia (Hb ≤ 11 g/dL)	5 yr
4	High risk	Lymphocytosis with thrombocytopenia ($\leq 100 \times 10^3/\mu$L)	

Hb, hemoglobin.
Note: Survival as reported in the orginal publication.

Newly identified prognostic factors that predict an inferior outcome include the cytogenetic abnormalities 11q-, 17p- and complex karyotypes; an elevated serum β-2-microglobulin level, unmutated immunoglobulin variable region heavy chain genes (IgVH), Zeta-associated protein 70 (ZAP-70) over expression and elevated CD38 expression. On the other hand, trisomy 12 and normal cytogenetics are associated with an intermediate outcome, while 13q- is associated with a favorable outcome. The utility of these factors lies in prognosis and at this time should not be used in deciding when or how to treat patients.

Computerized tomography (CT) is not required at diagnosis or for staging but it may be useful to evaluate the presence of enlarged lymph nodes potentially causing complications. Positron emission tomography (PET) scanning is generally of no value, although it might be helpful when transformation into a more aggressive lymphoma is suspected.

COMPLICATIONS

Patients with CLL may develop cytopenias, infections, aggressive transformation, and secondary malignancies. These complications can occur as a consequence of the disease or its therapy.

Frequent infections, often sinopulmonary, are often related to hypogammagobulinemia, an inadequate humoral response, and impaired complement activation. Thrombocytopenia and anemia can be autoimmune, secondary to marrow infiltration, or chemotherapy effect. Pure red cell aplasia, although rare, is possibly caused by suppressor T cells. Cyclosporine may be effective with a reticulocyte response within a few weeks.

Transformation to Richter syndrome (large B cell lymphoma), PLL, acute lymphocytic leukemia (ALL), and multiple myeloma occurs in 10% to 15% of cases. Patients are also at increased risk of developing secondary malignancies of the gastrointestinal tract, lung, skin, and other common sites. Therefore, appropriate screening is recommended.

TREATMENT

CLL can exhibit an indolent course, often not requiring treatment at diagnosis. Treatment is indicated in the presence of the following:

- Significant and persistent fatigue
- Weight loss
- Fever without infection
- Recurrent infections
- Night sweats
- Significant anemia
- Thrombocytopenia
- Disfiguring or bulky lymphadenopathy and/or significant splenomegaly

The degree of lymphocytosis is not an indication for treatment, although a rapid lymphocyte doubling time may support the decision to treat.

Historically, the most common initial systemic therapy has been chlorambucil or fludarabine. Incorporation of monoclonal antibodies with fludarabine has improved response rates to 90% to 95%, and appears to improve survival. Therefore rituximab and fludarabine (FR) and fludarabine, cyclophosphamide, and rituximab (FCR) are the current standards. Bendamustine and alemtuzumab have shown a response rate of 68% and 83%, respectively, and are also approved for initial therapy as well as in the relapsed setting.

CLL is incurable and patients develop recurrent disease requiring additional treatment. Selection of the optimal salvage treatment depends on age, performance status, prior treatment, adverse effects and duration of remission to prior therapy, and extent of disease. Options include purine nucleoside analogs, alkylating agents, monoclonal antibodies, stem cell transplantation, combination chemotherapy, and investigational treatments (Table 24.2).

TABLE 24.2. *Therapy for chronic lymphocytic leukemia*

Therapy	Comments
Chlorambucil	Dose: Either daily 4–8 mg/d, or pulse schedule of 40–80 mg PO over 1–3 d Q2–4 wk; toxicity: myelosuppression
Fludarabine	Dose: 25 mg/m^2 i.v. d1–5 q4wk for 6 mo; toxicity: myelosuppression and prolonged immunosuppression
Bendamustine	Dose: 100 mg/m^2 i.v. d1–2 q4wk; toxicity: myelosuppression
Alemtuzumab	Dose: Escalated from 3, 10–30 mg s.c. or i.v. three times a week for 12 wk; toxicity: infections and myelosuppression; prophylaxis for PCP and CMV
Rituximab	Dose: 375 mg/m^2 i.v. qwk for 4 wk; toxicity: infusion reaction
Combination therapy	Fludarabine 25 mg/m^2 i.v. d1–5 + rituximab 375 mg/m^2 i.v. d1 q4wk (FR) for 6 mo; fludarabine 25 mg/m^2 + cyclophosphamide 250 mg/m^2, both d2–4 of cycle1 and d1–3 of cycles 2–6 + rituximab on d1 at 375 mg/m^2 for cycle 1 and 500 mg/m^2 of cycles 2–6 (FCR); bendamustine 70 mg/m^2 on d1 at 375 mg/m^2 for cycle 1 and 500 mg/m^2 of cycles 2–6 (BR); other regimens: pentostatin + cyclophosphamide + rituximab (PCR); cyclophosphamide + adriamycin + vincristine + prednisone (CHOP)
Stem cell transplantation	Patients with multiple relapses; allogeneic transplantation with nonmyeloablative approaches allow older patients and patients with comorbidities to undergo transplant; toxicities: opportunistic infections and graft-versus-host disease
Investigational	Flavopiridol; lenalidomide; pro-apoptotic antibodies (oblimersen, obatoclax, ABT-263); combination of bendamustine with other agents

CLL, chronic lymphocytic leukemia; PCP, pneumocystis jiveruci; CMV, cytomegalovirus; i.v., intravenously.

While receiving therapy patients with white blood cell counts >50.000/μL and/or bulky lymph nodes should receive tumor lysis prophylaxis. Patients should receive appropriate anti-infective agents against pneumocystis jiveruci, varicella zoster, and/or fungi.

OTHER CHRONIC LYMPHOID LEUKEMIAS

Other rare lymphoproliferative disorders include PLL (Table 24.3) and hairy cell leukemia (HCL) (Table 24.4).

TABLE 24.3. *Prolymphocytic leukemia*

Clinical findings	Hepatosplenomegaly; very high lymphocyte count; patients with T-PLL may have pleural effusion and skin lesions
Clinical course	B-PLL: variable course; indolent in some, while others with anemia, thrombocytopenia, and a high lymphocyte count have a shorter survival T-PLL: more aggressive than B-PLL or CLL
Morphology	Large cells with abundant cytoplasm and prominent nucleolus within a convoluted nucleus with immature chromatin
Phenotypic features	B-PLL: surface expression of CD19, CD20, CD22, CD24, IgM and IgD; usually negative for CD5, CD23 T-PLL: surface expression of CD2, CD3, CD4, CD5, CD7, CD45RO, occasionally CD8; rearrangement of the T-cell–receptor gene
Treatment	B-PLL: anecdotal reports of treatment with nucleoside analogues and monoclonal antibodies T-PLL: High response rates with short duration of remission with alemtuzumab and allogeneic stem cell transplantation

CLL, chronic lymphocytic leukemia; B-PLL, B-cell prolymphocytic leukemia; T-PLL, T-cell prolymphocytic leukemia; Ig, surface immunoglobulin.

TABLE 24.4. *Hairy cell leukemia*

Clinical findings	Male predominance, pancytopenia, splenomegaly, infections; less often lymphadenopathy, necrotizing vasculitis, lytic bone abnormalities
Morphology	Lymphocytes with cytoplasmic projections, TRAP-stain positive
Bone marrow	Aspiration frequently unsuccessful, "dry tap" secondary to fibrosis; marrow biopsy reveals "hairy" cells and classic "fried-egg" appearance
Immunology	High-intensity sIg, CD19, 20, 21, 22, 11c, 25, 103, PCA-1 and Bly7, and light and heavy chain Ig rearrangements
Treatment indications	Life-threatening infections, vasculitis, bony involvement, symptomatic splenomegaly, leukocytosis, neutropenia ($<$0.5–1.0 × 10^9/mL), anemia (Hb, $<$8–10 g/dL), thrombocytopenia ($<$50–100 × 10^9/mL)
Treatment	*First-line* Cladribine; RR: 80–95%, dose: 0.1 mg/kg/d by CI over 7 d; pentostatin; RR: 75–80%, dose: 4 mg/m^2 i.v. every other week for 3–6 mo *Relapsed/recurrent disease* Retreatment with nucleoside analogs; interferon-α; RR: $>$70%, dose: 2 million units/m^2 s.c. three times/wk; splenectomy is reserved for those with bleeding and thrombocytopenia or for those whom systemic chemotherapy has failed; rituximab RR: 24–80%, dose: 375 mg/m^2 i.v. qwk for four doses *Promising* BL22, anti-CD22 monoclonal antibody linked to pseudomonas exotoxin A, RR: 70% CR in cladribine-refractory patients.

TRAP, tartrate-resistant acid phosphatase; sIg, surface immunoglobulin; Hb, hemoglobin; CI, continuous infusion; RR, response rate; CR, complete response.

SUGGESTED READINGS

Byrd JC, Peterson BL, Morrison VA, et al. Randomized phase 2 study of fludarabine with concurrent versus sequential treatment with rituximab in symptomatic, untreated patients with B-cell chronic lymphocytic leukemia: Results from Cancer and Leukemia Group B 9712 (CALGB 9712). *Blood* 2003;101:6–14.

Chanan-Khan A, Miller KC, Musial L, et al. Clinical efficacy of lenalidomide in patients with relapsed or refractory chronic lymphocytic leukemia: results of a phase II study. *J Clin Oncol* 2006;24: 5343–5349.

Cheson BD, Bennett JM, Grever M, et al. National Cancer Institute-sponsored Working Group guidelines for chronic lymphocytic leukemia: revised guidelines for diagnosis and treatment. *Blood* 1996;87:4990–4997.

Cheson BD, Sorensen JM, Vena DA, et al. Treatment of hairy cell leukemia with 2-chlorodeoxyadenosine via the Group C protocol mechanism of the National Cancer Institute: a report of 979 patients. *J Clin Oncol* 1998;16:3007–3015.

Clark FJ, Radia D, Rassam SM, et al. High remission rate in T-cell prolymphocytic leukemia with Campath-1H. *Blood* 2001;98:1721–1726.

Cortes J, O'Brien S, Loscertales J, et al. Cyclsporin A for the treatment of cytopenia associated with chronic lymphocytic leukemia. *Cancer* 2001;92:2016–2022.

Döhner H, Stilgenbauer S, Benner A, et al. Genomic aberrations and survival in chronic lymphocytic leukemia. *N Engl J Med* 2000;343:1910–1916.

Flinn IW, Neuberg DS, Grever MR, et al. Phase III trial of fludarabine plus cyclophosphamide compared with fludarabine for patients with previously untreated chronic lymphocytic leukemia: US Intergroup Trial E2997. *J Clin Oncol* 2007;25:793–798.

Grever M, Kopecky K, Foucar MK, et al. Randomized comparison of pentostatin versus interferon alfa-2a in previously untreated patients with hairy cell leukemia: an intergroup study. *J Clin Oncol* 1995;13:974–982.

Hainsworth JD, Litchy S, Barton JH, et al. Single-agent rituximab as first-line and maintenance treatment for patients with chronic lymphocytic leukemia or small lymphocytic lymphoma: a phase II trial of the Minnie Pearl Cancer Res Network. *J Clin Oncol* 2003;21:1746–1751.

Hamblin TJ, Davis Z, Gardiner A, et al. Unmutated Ig V(H) genes are associated with a more aggressive form of chronic lymphocytic leukemia. *Blood* 1999;94:1848–1854.

Hillmen P, Skotnicki AB, Robak T, et al. Alemtuzumab compared with chlorambucil as first-line therapy for chronic lymphocytic leukemia. *J Clin Oncol* 2007;25:5616–5623.

Kay NE,Geyer SM, Call TG, et al. Combination chemoimmunotherapy with pentostatin, cyclophospha-mide, and rituximab shows significant clinical activity with low accompanying toxicity in previously untreated B chronic lymphocytic leukemia. *Blood* 2007;109:405–411.

Keating MJ, Flinn I, Jain V, et al. Therapeutic role of alemtuzumab (Campath-1H) in patients who have failed fludarabine: results of a large international study. *Blood* 2002;99:3554–3556.

Keating MJ, O'Brien S, Albitar M, et al. Early results of a chemoimmunotherapy regimen of fludara-bine, cyclophosphamide, and rituximab as initial therapy for chronic lymphocytic leukemia. *J Clin Oncol* 2005;23:4079–4088.

Kreitman RJ, Squires DR, Stetler-Stevenson M, et al. Phase I trial of recombinant immunotoxin RFB4(dsFy)-PE38 (BL22) in patients with B-cell malignancies. *J Clin Oncol* 2005;23:6719–6729.

Maloisel F, Benboubker L, Gardembas M, et al. Long-term outcome with pentostatin treatment in hairy cell leukemia patients. A French retrospective study of 238 patients. *Leukemia* 2003;12:45–41.

Piro LD, Carrera CJ, Carson DA, et al. Lasting remissions in hairy-cell leukemia induced by a single infusion of 2-chlorodeoxyadenosine. *N Engl J Med* 1990;322:1117–1121.

Rai KR, Peterson BL, Appelbaum FR, et al. Fludarabine compared with chlorambucil as primary therapy for chronic lymphocytic leukemia. *N Engl J Med* 2000;343:1750–1757.

Rai KR, Sawitsky A, Cronkite EP, et al. Clinical staging of chronic lymphocytic leukemia. *Blood* 1975; 46:219–234.

Tsimberidou AM, Keating MJ. Richter syndrome: biology, incidence and therapeutic strategies. *Cancer* 2005;103:216–228.

25

Chronic Myeloid Leukemia

Ebru Koca and Muzaffar H. Qazilbash

EPIDEMIOLOGY

The annual incidence of chronic myeloid leukemia (CML) is one to two cases per 100,000 of general population, accounting for 15% to 20% of all leukemia in adults. The median age at diagnosis is 45 to 55 years but the disease can be seen in all age groups including children. Approximately 30% of the patients are over 60 years of age. There is male predominance and women appear to have a survival advantage (1).

PATHOPHYSIOLOGY

CML is a disease of hematopoietic stem cells. The hallmark of CML is the Philadelphia chromosome (Ph-chromosome), a reciprocal translocation between the long arms of chromosomes 9 and 22 [t(9;22)]. The translocation results in the transfer of the Ableson (ABL) gene on chromosome 9 to an area of chromosome 22 termed the breakpoint cluster region, resulting in the BCR-ABL fusion gene. This fusion gene encodes a chimeric protein with dysregulated tyrosine kinase activity that plays a role in the pathogeneis of CML.

The fusion protein varies in size depending on the site of chromosomal break. More than 90% of CML patients express the 210-kDa oncoprotein, while less than 10% express either a 185-kDa or 230-kDa oncoprotein. The latter was found to be associated with a lower white cell count and slower progression to blastic crisis. The blast phase is characterized by multiple additional chromosomal and molecular abnormalities, such as duplicate Ph-chromosome or trisomy 8 (1–3).

DIAGNOSIS AND CLINICAL FEATURES

Symptoms

- Patients in the early chronic phase may be asymptomatic
- Fatigue
- Anorexia
- Weight loss
- Sweats and low-grade fever
- Left upper quadrant discomfort/early satiety
- Dyspnea on exertion

Signs

The most common finding is splenomegaly, which is present in up to 50% of the patients. In about 10% of patients the spleen is not enlarged even on splenic scan.

Laboratory Features

CML is characterized with the following laboratory features:

- Increased white blood cell count (usually $>25 \times 10^9$/L) with "left shift"
- Thrombocytosis in approximately 50% of cases
- Mild anemia
- Myeloid cells at all stages of maturation and basophilia with or without eosinophilia in peripheral smear
- Marked myeloid hyperplasia in bone marrow
- Increased megakaryocytes
- Mild to moderate myelofibrosis
- Leukocyte alkaline phosphatase (LAP) is nearly always low

Diagnosis is confirmed by identification of Ph-chromosome on cytogenetic analysis or the detection of BCR-ABL fusion transcript by polymerase chain reaction (PCR) in peripheral blood or bone marrow. About 5% to 10% of cases are negative for Ph-chromosome on standard karyotypic analysis. In these patients, diagnosis is established by finding the BCR-ABL transcript by fluorescence in situ hybridization (FISH) or by PCR (1).

Differential Diagnosis

- Leukoerythroblastic reaction in response to infection, inflammation, or malignancy
- Chronic myelomonocytic leukemia
- Atypical CML
- Idiopathic myelofibrosis
- Essential thrombocytosis
- Polycythemia vera

STAGING AND PROGNOSTIC FACTORS

CML typically progresses over time. The chronic phase is almost always followed by an accelerated or blast phase, where it acquires the characteristics of acute leukemia (Table 25.1) (4).

A sudden transition to blast phase is called *blast crisis*. Features of a blast crisis include fever, malaise, progressive and painful splenomegaly and/or hepatomegaly, bone pain, worsening anemia, thrombocytopenia, and thrombotic or bleeding complications.

TABLE 25.1. *WHO criteria for chronic myeloid leukemia stages*

Stage	Features
Chronic phase	Blast cells in blood or marrow <10%
	Basophils in blood <20%
	Platelets $>100 \times 10^9$/L
Accelerated phase	Blast cells in blood or marrow 10%–19%
	Basophils in blood 20% or more
	Persistent thrombocytopenia unrelated to therapy
	Thrombocytosis unresponsive to therapy
	Progressive splenomegaly and increasing WBC count unresponsive to therapy
	Cytogenetic evidence of clonal evolution
Blastic phase	Blast cells in blood or bone marrow ≥20%
	Extramedullary blast proliferation
	Large foci or clusters of blasts in the bone marrow biopsy

Source: From Ref. 4.

TABLE 25.2. *Sokal and Hasford risk indexes*

Risk category	Risk index	Median survival
Sokal		
Low	<0.8	5 yr
Intermediate	0.8–1.2	3.5 yr
High	>1.2	2.5 yr
Hasford		
Low	≤780	98 mo
Intermediate	781–1,480	65 mo
High	>1,480	42 mo

Sokal risk index was defined based on patients treated with conventional chemotherapy. Hasford risk index was defined based on patients treated with rIFNα-based regimens.

Sokal score: EXP [0,0116 × (age −43.4) + 0.0345 × (spleen size [cm below costal marigin]−7.51) + 0.188 × [(platelet count/700)^2 − 0.563] + 0.0887 × (myeloblasts − 2.1)].

Hasford score: [0.666 when age ≥50 yr + 0.042 × (spleen size [cm below costal marigin]) + 1.0956 (when platelet count ≥ 1500 × 10^9 /L) + 0.0584 × myeloblasts + 0.2039 (when basophils ≥3%) + 0.0413 × eosinophils (%)] × 1000.

Source: From Refs. 5 and 6.

It is important to recognize the prognostic factors prior to and during therapy. Phase of the disease at the time of diagnosis predicts the response, duration of response, and survival. Sokal and Hasford risk scores are derived from patients treated with conventional chemotherapy or recombinant Interferon alfa (rIFNa), and use clinical and laboratory features at diagnosis such as age, spleen size, platelet count, and blast percentage in peripheral blood (Table 25.2) (5,6). They are also useful in the imatinib era. According to the 5-year data from the IRIS trial (International Randomized Study of Interferon vs. STI571), overall survival at 54 months were 94%, 88%, and 81% for low, intermediate, and high Sokal risk patients, respectively ($P < 0.01$) (7,8). Appearance of additional chromosomal abnormalities during treatment, such as Ph duplication or deletions of derivatives of chromosome 9, seems to predict a worse prognosis. Time to and the magnitude of hematological, cytogenetic, and molecular responses also provide important prognostic information (Table 25.3) (1,9,10).

TREATMENT

The treatment options for CML include conventional cytotoxic chemotherapy with hydroxyurea and busulfan, rIFNα, allogeneic hematopoietic stem cell transplantation, and most recently imatinib and newer tyrosine kinase inhibitors.

Hydroxyurea

Hydroxyurea is a cytotoxic antiproliferative agent that is administered orally and is well tolerated. It allows rapid control of blood counts and induces hematologic responses in 50% to 80% of patients. However, it does not prevent or delay the progression to blast phase. It is currently used for initial cytoreduction as an adjunct to more definitive therapies (11).

TABLE 25.3. *Prognostic factors*

Disease phase at diagnosis
Prognostic scores in early disease phase (Hasford and Sokal risk indexes)
Cytogenetic changes during disease course
Degree and timing of hematological, cytogenetic, and molecular response to treatment

Interferon

rIFNα-based regimens were the standard therapy for chronic-phase CML before the discovery of imatinib. Follow-up for large studies of rIFNα showed 9- or 10-year overall survival between 27% and 53%. Adverse events are not life-threatening, but it impairs quality of life in many patients (12,13).

Tyrosine Kinase Inhibitors

Imatinib Mesylate

Imatinib not only revolutionized the treatment and prognosis of CML but also challenged general ideas about cancer treatment. Imatinib is a phenylaminopyrimidine derivative that inhibits the BCR-ABL tyrosine kinase by competitive binding at the ATP-binding site (14). Although active in all phases of CML, the most durable responses are seen in newly diagnosed patients in chronic phase. Results of the IRIS trial showed a hematological remission rate of 98%, a major cytogenic response rate of 92%, and a complete cytogenetic remission rate of 87% at 5 years in patients with chronic-phase CML receiving imatinib as initial treatment (7). An estimated 7% of patients progressed to accelerated-phase CML or blast crisis. As a result, imatinib 400 mg daily has been established as standard of care for patients with newly diagnosed chronic-phase CML. The main adverse events seen with imatinib are skin rash, muscle cramps, myelosuppression, diarrhea, and liver function test abnormalities.

The high rate of complete cytogenetic response with imatinib has shifted the goal of therapy to achieving molecular responses measured by PCR. Response criteria are summarized in Table 25.4 (15). Duration of remission and survival are related to the depth of clinical response achieved. This makes molecular monitoring an essential component of CML management. A suggested monitoring schema is summarized in Table 25.5 (1).

Second-Generation Tyrosine Kinase Inhibitors

Second-generation tyrosine kinase inhibitors include dasatinib, nilotinib, and bosutinib that are more potent than imatinib. Dasatinib is approved by the U.S. Food and Drug Administration at a dose of 70 mg twice daily for patients resistant to or intolerant of imatinib. Common side effects of dasatinib are cytopenia and pleural effusion. There are several third-generation tyrosine kinase inhibitors undergoing clinical trials. These agents have activity against BCR-ABL/T315I mutation that is mainly responsible for resistance to imatinib and second-generation tyrosine kinase inhibitors (16).

Treatment options for patients with imatinib resistance include allogeneic stem cell transplantation; interferon with or without chemotherapy; and dose escalation of imatinib, dasatinib, or investigational agents.

Allogeneic Stem Cell Transplantation

Allogeneic stem cell transplantation is a potentially curative treatment for CML. It is associated with a relatively high treatment-related mortality due to graft-versus-host disease and infectious complications.

TABLE 25.4. *Response criteria*

Definitions for response criteria	
Hematological response	*Complete:* Platelet count <450 × 10⁹/L, WBC <10 × 10⁹/L, no immature granulocytes, basophils <10% in blood, and no palpable spleen
Cytogenetic response	*Minimum:* Proportion of cells with Ph chromosome 66–95% *Minor:* Proportion of cells with Ph chromosome 36–65% *Partial:* Proportion of cells with Ph chromosome 1–35% *Complete:* Proportion of cells with Ph chromosome 0%
Molecular response	*Major:* BCR-ABL/control gene ratio <0.1 *Complete:* Transcripts nondetectable and nonquantifiable

Source: From Ref. 15.

TABLE 25.5.   *Monitoring suggestions for chronic-phase*
CML patients treated with imatinib

Hematological response	Monitor every 2 wk until complete hematologic response achieved, then at 3 mo intervals.
Cytogenetic response (by bone marrow aspiration)	Monitor every 6 mo until complete cytogenetic response confirmed, then at 1 yr intervals.
Molecular response	Monitor at 3 mo intervals, perform mutational analysis if response is suboptimum, treatment failure occurs, or transcript concentrations rise.

Source: From Ref. 1.

According to European Group for Blood and Marrow Transplantation (EBMT) data, patients undergoing allogeneic transplantation in first chronic phase had a 20-year overall survival of about 40% (17). Improvements in HLA typing, management of infections, supportive care, conditioning regimens, and immunosuppressions have contributed to a significant improvement in transplant outcomes. Donor lymphocyte infusion can induce durable remissions in selected patients with relapsed disease. Reduced-intensity regimens have been safely used in older patients and patients with comorbidities (18).

Allogeneic stem cell transplantation is recommended as second-line treatment after imatinib failure in low-risk patients. For patients with advanced-phase CML, it remains an effective treatment strategy regardless of response to imatinib therapy. Patient's preference and economic reasons should also be considered in making a decision.

TREATMENT SUMMARY

Fig. 25.1 is a management algorithm for CML. Imatinib 400 mg daily is the standard treatment for newly diagnosed chronic-phase CML. If imatinib fails or response is poor, dose escalation of imatinib,

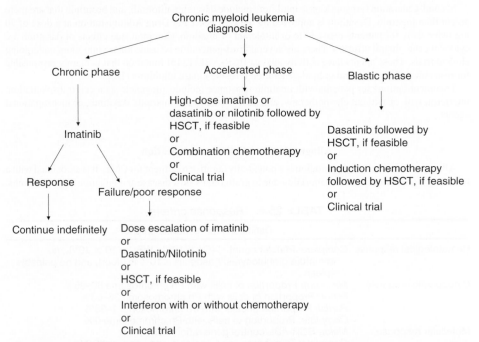

Fig. 25.1.   Management algorithm for newly diagnosed CML (From Refs. 1,15,16,19). (HSCT, hematopoietic stem cell transplantation.)

second-generation tyrosine kinase inhibitors, allogeneic stem cell transplantation, or a clinical trial with investigational agents are alternatives. For patients who present with accelerated-phase CML, starting treatment with higher doses of imatinib or other tyrosine kinase inhibitors followed by allogeneic stem cell transplantation, combination chemotherapy, or clinical trials can be considered. Allogeneic stem cell transplantation after second-generation tyrosine kinase inhibitors or induction chemotherapy and clinical trials can be considered for patients diagnosed in blastic phase (1,15, 16,19).

REFERENCES

1. Hehlmann R, Hochhaus A, Baccarani M, European LeukemiaNet. Chronic myeloid leukaemia. *Lancet* 2007;370:342–350.
2. Rowley JD. A new consistent chromosomal abnormality in chronic myelogenous leukaemia identified by quinacrine fluorescence and Giemsa staining. *Nature* 1973;243:290–293.
3. Sawyers CL. Chronic myeloid leukemia. *N Engl J Med* 1999;340:1330–1340.
4. Vardiman JW, Harris NL, Brunning RD. The World Health Organization (WHO) classification of the myeloid neoplasms. *Blood* 2002;100:2292–2302.
5. Sokal JE. Prognosis in chronic myeloid leukaemia: biology of the disease vs. treatment. *Baillieres Clin Haematol* 1987;1:907–929.
6. Hasford J, Pfirrmann M, Hehlmann R, et al. A new prognostic score for survival of patients with chronic myeloid leukemia treated with interferon alfa. Writing Committee for the Collaborative CML Prognostic Factors Project Group. *J Natl Cancer Inst* 1998;90:850–858.
7. O'Brien SG, Guilhot F, Larson RA, et al. Imatinib mesylate compared with interferon and low-dose cytarabine for newly diagnosed chronic-phase chronic myeloid leukemia. *N Engl J Med* 2003;348:994–1004.
8. Druker BJ, Guilhot F, O'Brien SG, et al. Five-year follow-up of patients receiving imatinib mesylate for chronic myeloid leukemia. *N Engl J Med* 2006;355:2408–2417.
9. Hasford J, Pfirrmann M, Shepherd P, et al. The impact of the combination of baseline risk group and cytogenetic response on the survival of patients with chronic myeloid leukemia treated with interferon alpha. *Haematologica* 2005;90:335–340.
10. Branford S. Chronic myeloid leukemia: molecular monitoring in clinical practice. *Hematology Am Soc Hematol Educ Program* 2007;2007:376–383.
11. Hehlmann R, Berger U, Pfirrmann M, et al. Randomized comparison of interferon alpha and hydroxyurea with hydroxyurea monotherapy in chronic myeloid leukemia (CML-study II): prolongation of survival by the combination of interferon alpha and hydroxyurea. *Leukemia* 2003;17:1529–1537.
12. Silver RT, Woolf SH, Hehlmann R, et al. An evidence-based analysis of the effect of busulfan, hydroxyurea, interferon, and allogeneic bone marrow transplantation in treating the chronic phase of chronic myeloid leukemia: developed for the American Society of Hematology. *Blood* 1999;94:1517–1536.
13. Baccarani M, Russo D, Rosti G, Martinelli G. Interferon-alfa for chronic myeloid leukemia. *Semin Hemato* 2003;40:22–33.
14. Druker BJ, Talpaz M, Resta DJ, et al. Efficacy and safety of a specific inhibitor of the BCR-ABL tyrosine kinase in chronic myeloid leukemia. *N Engl J Med* 2001;344:1031–1037.
15. Baccarani M, Saglio G, Goldman J, et al. Evolving concepts in the management of chronic myeloid leukemia: recommendations from an expert panel on behalf of the European LeukemiaNet. *Blood* 2006;108:1809–1820.
16. Shah NP. Medical management of CML. *Hematology Am Soc Hematol Educ Program* 2007;2007:371–375.
17. Gratwohl A, Brand R, Apperley J, et al. Allogeneic hematopoietic stem cell transplantation for chronic myeloid leukemia in Europe 2006: transplant activity, long-term data and current results. An analysis by the Chronic Leukemia Working Party of the European Group for Blood and Marrow Transplantation (EBMT). *Haematologica* 2006;91:513–521.

18. Kebriaei P, Detry MA, Giralt S, et al. Long-term follow-up of allogeneic hematopoietic stem-cell transplantation with reduced-intensity conditioning for patients with chronic myeloid leukemia. *Blood* 2007;110:3456–3462.

19. National Comprehensive Cancer Network® (NCCN) Clinical Practice Guidelines in Oncology. Chronic Myelogenous Leukemia. http://www.nccn.org/professionals/physician_gls/PDF/cml.pdf. Accessed June 10, 2008.

26

Chronic Myeloproliferative Diseases

Manish Monga and Marcel P. Devetten

Myeloproliferative disorders include several clonal hematological diseases that arise in a hematopoietic stem cell. The World Health Organization (WHO) revised the classification in 2008: the terms *disease* or *disorder* for both myeloproliferative disorders (MPDs) and MDS/MPD, are replaced by *neoplasm*, that is, myeloproliferative neoplasm (MPN). In addition, a new category of myeloid neoplasms associated with eosinophilia and abnormalities of PDGFRA, PDGFRB, or FGFR1 was introduced. Although not discussed in this chapter, these newly recognized disorders are of clinical significance because of their unique sensitivity to treatment with the tyrosine kinase inhibitor imatinib mesylate.

The 2008 WHO classification scheme for myeloid neoplasms (Table 26.1) designates seven conditions as MPNs:

1. BCR-ABL–positive chronic myeloid leukemia (CML)
2. Chronic neutrophilic leukemia
3. Chronic eosinophilic leukemia/hypereosinophilic syndrome
4. Primary myelofibrosis (MF, also known as agnogenic myeloid metaplasia)
5. Polycythemia vera (PV)
6. Essential thrombocythemia (ET)
7. Mast cell disease

In addition, a category of *MPNs unclassifiable* is recognized. CML is also discussed in Chapter 25 because of its specific association with the Philadelphia chromosome translocation (*bcr-abl* tyrosine

TABLE 26.1. *The 2008 World Health Organization Classification Scheme for myeloid neoplasms*

1. Acute myeloid leukemia
2. Myelodysplastic syndrome (MDS)
3. Myeloproliferative neoplasms (MPN)
   - 3.1 Chronic myeloid leukemia
   - 3.2 Polycythemia vera
   - 3.3 Essential thrombocythemia
   - 3.4 Primary myelofibrosis
   - 3.5 Chronic neutrophilic leukemia
   - 3.6 Chronic eosinophilic leukemia
   - 3.7 Mast cell disease
   - 3.8 MPNs, unclassifiable
4. MDS/MPN
   - 4.1 Chronic myelomonocytic leukemia
   - 4.2 Juvenile myelomonocytic leukemia
   - 4.3 Atypical chronic myeloid leukemia, BCR-ABL negative
   - 4.4 MDS/MPN unclassifiable
5. Myeloid neoplasms associated with eosinophilia and abnormalities of PDGFRA, PDGFRB, or FGFR1
   - 5.1 Myeloid neoplasms associated with PDGFRA rearrangement
   - 5.2 Myeloid neoplasms associated with PDGFRB rearrangement
   - 5.3 Myeloid neoplasms associated with FGFR1 rearrangement (8p11 myeloproliferative syndrome)

kinase), and because of its unique treatment paradigm. This chapter is limited to a discussion of the three "classical" clinical entities: PV, ET, and MF. These three disorders share characteristics, including marrow hypercellularity, a propensity to thrombosis and hemorrhage, and a risk of leukemic transformation. Treatment for PV, ET, and MF is generally directed toward minimizing morbidity and prolonging survival by preventing complications such as hemorrhage and thrombosis, in the case of PV and ET, and alleviating anemia and symptoms associated with splenomegaly in the case of MF. Bone marrow transplantation is a potentially curative option that should be considered for MF.

PATHOPHYSIOLOGY AND DIAGNOSIS

Molecular Mechanism and Diagnostic Criteria

Janus Kinase 2 (JAK-2), a cytoplasmic tyrosine kinase, is critical for instigating intracellular signaling by the receptors for erythropoietin, thrombopoietin, interleukin-3, granulocyte colony-stimulating factor (G-CSF), and granulocyte macrophage colony-stimulating factor (GM-CSF). A mutation in JAK-2 substituting phenylalanine for a valine at position 617 of the JAK-2 protein (V617F) causes cytokine-independent (constitutive) activation of downstream messengers through the JAK-STAT, PI3K, and AKT pathways. JAK-2 mutations in the MPDs are not found in the germline but are acquired. Ninety-five percent of patients with PV and 50% to 60% with ET or idiopathic myelofibrosis have the characteristic JAK-2 V617F mutation. Additional genetic mutations, such as the mutation in the transmembrane domain of the thrombopoietin receptor (cMPL) known as cMPLW515L/K and alternative mutations in exon 12 of JAK-2 have recently been described. JAK-2 V617F mutation is also found in a small minority of patients with hypereosinphilic syndrome, chronic myelomonocytic leukemia, chronic neutrophilic leukemia, myelodysplasia, or acute myeloid leukemia but not in patients with lymphoid or other malignancies or other hematological disorders. JAK-2 mutation is found in more than 50% of patients with Budd-Chiari syndrome suggestive of a masked myeloproliferative disorder. The 2008 WHO revised criteria for diagnosis of PV, ET, and MF recognize the importance of JAK2 mutations by incorporating JAK-2 V617F as a major diagnostic criterium (Table 26.2). Testing for the JAK-2 V617F mutation detection by different techniques (PCR, restriction enzyme digestive pyrosequencing) is sensitive and specific, and readily available as a diagnostic tool.

Even with a positive JAK-2 mutation and low erythropoietin level, bone marrow biopsy is recommended in cases of PV. In JAK-2 mutation-negative thrombocytosis or bone marrow fibrosis, CML should be ruled out by performing a fluorescence in situ hybridization (FISH) analysis for BCR-ABL.

PROGNOSIS

Median Survivals

- Patients with PV have a median survival of 1.5 to 13 years. In a recent multicountry prospective study of 1,638 patients with PV, the 5-year event-free survival was 82%, with a relatively low risk of death from cardiovascular disease and a high risk of death from noncardiovascular causes (mainly hematologic transformations).
- The median survival is more than 10 years for patients with ET.
- For patients with MF, the median survival is 3 to 5 years.

Rate of Transformation to Acute Leukemia

- The estimated incidence of acute leukemia in 1,638 patients with PV prospectively followed in the ECLAP study was 1.3%, with an estimated annual incidence of 0.5 per 100.000 per year. Older age and exposure to P32, busulfan, or pipobroman were independent risk factors.
- The cumulative rate of transformation for patients with ET is 2% to 4% respectively at 10 and 20 years since diagnosis.
- The cumulative rate of transformation for patients with MF is 10% at 10 years.

TABLE 26.2. *WHO diagnostic criteria for polycythemia vera, essential thrombocythemia, and primary myelofibrosis*

	Polycythemia vera	Essential thrombocythemia	Primary myelofibrosis
Major criteria	Hgb >18.5 g/dL (men) >16.5 g/dL (women) or Hgb or Hct >99th percentile of reference range for age, sex or altitude of residence or Hgb >17 g/dL (men) or >15 g/dL (women) if associated with a sustained increase of >2 g/dL from baseline that cannot be attributed to correction of iron deficiency or elevated red cell mass >25% above mean predicted value. Presence of JAK-2 mutation	Platelet count ≥450 × 10⁹/L Megakaryocyte proliferation with large and mature morphology; no granulocyte or erythroid proliferation. Not meeting WHO criteria for CML, PV, PMF, MDS, or other myeloid neoplasms. Presence of JAK-2 mutation or no evidence of reactive thrombocytosis	Megakaryocyte proliferation and atypia accompanied by either reticulin and/or collagen fibrosis, or in the absence of reticulin fibrosis, the megakaryocyte changes must be accompanied by increased marrow cellularity, granulocytic proliferation, and often-decreased erythropoiesis. Not meeting WHO criteria for CML, PV, PMF, MDS, or other myeloid neoplasms. Presence of JAK-2 mutation or no evidence of reactive marrow fibrosis
Minor criteria	BM trilineage myeloproliferation Subnormal serum Epo level Endogenous erythroid colony growth		Leukoerythroblastosis Increased serum LDH Anemia Palpable splenomegaly

Note: Diagnosis of PV requires meeting either both major criteria and one minor criterion or the first major criterion and two minor criteria. Diagnosis of ET requires meeting all four major criteria. Diagnosis of MF requires meeting all three major criteria and two minor criteria.

Spent Phase

Both PV and ET may progress to post-PV MF or post-ET MF, previously referred to as the spent phase, which clinically resembles primary MF and is characterized by progressive cytopenias, splenomegaly, and marrow fibrosis. The cumulative rate of transformation is 5% and 10% at 10 years to 20 years respectively for ET and 10% to 20% for the same time line for PV.

Risk Factors for Thrombosis

In two prospective studies, the ECLAP study and the MRC-PT1, the cumulative rate of cardiovascular events in patients with PV ranged from 2.5% to 5% per patient-year and from 1.9% to 3% per patient-year for patients with ET. Arterial thrombosis accounts for 60% to 70% of the events, and is the major cause of death.

- In PV, older age (>60), a hematocrit equal to or >45%, and a previous history of thrombosis are risk factors. Surgery should be avoided in patients until a hematocrit <45% has been maintained for more than 2 months.
- In ET, age over 60 years and the presence of other cardiovascular risk factors (e.g., smoking and previous thrombosis) increase the risk for thrombosis.

TABLE 26.3. *Distinguishing features of the myeloproliferative neoplasms*

	CML	PV	ET	MF
Hematocrit	N or ↓	↑↑	N	↓
WBC count	↑↑↑	↑	N	↑ or ↓
Platelet count	↑ or ↓	↑	↑↑↑	↑ or
Splenomegaly	+++	+	+	+++
Cytogenetic abnormality	Ph chromosome	±	−	±
LAP score[a]	↓	↑↑	N or ↑	N or ↑
Marrow fibrosis	±	± or ↓	±	+++ (Dry tap)
Marrow cellularity	↑↑↑ myeloid	↑↑	↑↑ megakaryocytes	N or ↓
Basophils ≥2%	+	±	±	Usually +

CML, chronic myeloid leukemia; PV, polycythemia vera; ET, essential thrombocytopenia; MF, myelofibrosis; N, normal; WBC, white blood cell; LAP, leukocyte alkaline phosphatase; MPN, myeloproliferative neoplasm.
[a]See Chapter 25.

In ET, an association between platelet count and thrombosis has not been established, but platelet cytoreduction on treatment with hydoxiurea (HU) has been associated with a *reduced* risk.

Risk Factors for Hemorrhage

• In ET, a platelet count >2 × 10⁶ per μL is a risk factor for hemorrhage.

Distinguishing Between the Myeloproliferative Disorders

All the MPDs can present because of incidentally noted abnormal blood counts. Table 26.3 illustrates differences between the various MPNs. Otherwise, PV can demonstrate symptoms of increased red blood cell (RBC) mass, such as headaches, vertigo, tinnitus, and blurred vision. A distinctive symptom in PV is pruritus aggravated by hot water. Cerebrovascular ischemia, digital ischemia, erythromelalgia, and spontaneous abortions resulting from arterial thrombosis are more commonly seen in patients with ET. Patients with MF may have symptoms related to anemia or may experience abdominal fullness or early satiety because of splenomegaly. Hypermetabolic symptoms such as weight loss and sweating can be seen in all types of MPDs. ET is diagnosed after excluding PV; MF is diagnosed after excluding PV and ET because marrow fibrosis can be a sequela of the other MPDs. The thrombotic episodes seen in all the MPDs can occur in unusual locations such as the hepatic vein (Budd-Chiari syndrome) and portal vein. Platelet function tests or bleeding times are of little use in diagnosing or in guiding the management of MPNs.

TREATMENT

Current drug therapies do not alter the natural history of PV, ET, and MF. Recent discovery of JAK-2 and MPL mutations in MPNs have given prospects of targeted therapy in these disorders. Present strategies are aimed at reducing risks of complications related to thrombosis, anemia, splenomegaly, and others. Current management and risk stratification in PV, ET, and MF are shown in Table 26.4.

Polycythemia Vera

A reasonable treatment strategy for PV is based on risk stratification:

• Low risk: Patients younger than 60 years, with no personal history of vascular events and no additional risk factors for cardiovascular disease are at low risk. Phlebotomy alone with or without low-dose aspirin should be recommended.
• Intermediate risk: Patients younger than 60 years, with no personal history of vascular events who do have additional cardiovascular risk factors are at intermediate risk. Phlebotomy alone is adequate therapy; use of low-dose aspirin is encouraged.

TABLE 26.4. *Current management and risk stratification for PV, ET, and MF*

Risk category	PV	ET	MF age <50	MF age >50
Low	Low-dose aspirin + phlebotomy	Low-dose aspirin	Observation or experimental drug therapy	Observation or experimental drug therapy
Intermediate	Low-dose aspirin + phlebotomy	Low-dose aspirin	Experimental drug therapy or Allotransplant	Experimental drug therapy or conventional drug therapy
High	Low-dose aspirin + phlebotomy + hydroxyurea	Low-dose aspirin + hydroxyurea	Allotransplant or experimental drug therapy	Allotransplant or experimental drug therapy

PV, polycythemia vera; ET, essential thrombocytopenia; MF, myelofibrosis.

- High risk: Patients who are 60 years or older or with a positive history of thrombosis are at high risk. HU (with or without concommittant phlebotomy) and low-dose aspirin are recommended therapies.

Maintaining a hematocrit <45% dramatically decreases the incidence of thrombotic complications (in PV, 35% of initial thrombotic events are fatal). This is preferably achieved through phlebotomy; alternatives are myelosuppressive oral chemotherapy or IFN-α. Selection among these options is guided by data from the ECLAP study. A randomized study of 518 patients with PV has shown that treatment with low-dose aspirin (100 mg/day) lowers the risk of cardiovascular death, nonfatal myocardial infarction, and nonfatal stroke.

- Spent phase: Options to alleviate cytopenia associated with massive splenomegaly include HU, IFN-α, and EPO. Analgesia may be required for splenic infarct pain. It is difficult to treat cytopenia associated with marrow fibrosis and massive splenomegaly. Splenectomy can be followed by progressive hepatomegaly and can eventually transform to acute leukemia. In selected patients, allogeneic transplantation can be curative.
- Pruritus: Intractable pruritus responds to IFN-α in up to 81% of patients. In low-risk patients in whom IFN-α is not indicated, paroxetine, a selective serotonin reuptake inhibitor, can alleviate symptoms in most cases.
- Hyperuricemia: Allopurinol should be started before chemotherapy to decrease the risk of urate nephropathy (300 mg/day given orally; dose reduction needed in renal insufficiency).

Essential Thrombocythemia

Treatment in ET must be provided on the basis of the fact that life expectancy in this condition is nearly normal and that platelet reduction with HU may be associated with an increased risk for transformation to leukemia. Treatment is directed at preventing thrombosis and hemorrhage in those patients deemed to be at risk for these complications. These patients have a history of thrombosis, with associated cardiovascular risk factors such as smoking and age older than 60 years, and have a platelet count $>1.5 \times 10^6$ per μL. Increased WBC might be an additional risk factor for thrombosis.

- A randomized trial of HU versus placebo in 114 high-risk patients showed a significant reduction of thrombotic events in the treatment arm (3.6% vs. 24%). The HU dose was adjusted to achieve a platelet count of $<600 \times 10^3$ per μL. Anagrelide is a nonmutagenic orally active agent that produces selective platelet cytoreduction by interfering with megakaryocyte maturation. In a randomized study of 809 patients with high-risk ET, hydroxyurea plus low-dose aspirin was superior to anagrelide plus low-dose aspirin. IFN-α can also effectively cause platelet cytoreduction. The therapeutic target platelet count for reduction of thrombosis is below $400,000 \times 10^3$ per μL. Plateletpheresis is used as an emergency therapy when ongoing thrombosis cannot be adequately managed with chemotherapy and antithrombotic agents.
- Clinically significant acquired von Willebrand syndrome (ristocetin cofactor activity <30%) should be excluded before the use of aspirin in patients with platelet count of more than $1,000 \times 10^9$/L.

Myelofibrosis

- Risk stratification of MF according to the Mayo Prognostic Scoring System: one point each for hemoglobin <10 g/dL, leukocyte count 4 or >30 × 10⁹/L, platelet count <100 × 10⁹/L, or monocyte count ≥1 × 10⁹/L; low-risk: score 0; intermediate-risk: score 1; high-risk: score ≤2, median survival 93 months for low-risk patients, 26 months for intermediate-risk patients, and 13 months for high-risk patients
- Palliative therapy for MF is directed toward alleviating anemia and painful splenomegaly. For anemia, androgens, thalidomide, and prednisone has been tried with mixed results. Transfusion support (with iron chelation when indicated) may be necessary. Splenectomy, as performed in experienced centers, is associated with an operative mortality of <10%, and in addition to alleviating pain, discomfort, and early satiety, it can improve anemia. Increasing white blood cell counts and platelet counts after splenectomy may necessitate HU therapy. IFN-α is an experimental therapy for MF. Revlimid can be used for 5q-cytogenetic abnormality MF in approximately 3% of all MF patients. A small study with low-dose thalidomide (up to 200 mg daily) showed improvement in cytopenias in some patients.
- Curative therapy: Allogeneic transplantation should be considered for patients younger than 55 years who have MF; 5-year survivals with a related or an unrelated matched transplant are 54% and 48%, respectively, as determined by the European Group for Blood and Marrow Transplantation (EBMT). A recommendation for transplantation is not clear-cut in asymptomatic patients without cytogenetic abnormalities and no cytopenia because the median survival in this group is >14 years with palliative therapy alone. Although the outcome with transplantation also is adversely affected by these features, poor prognostic features such as hemoglobin level <10 g/dL; white blood cell count <4 × 10³ per μL or >30 × 10³ per μL; more than 10% of circulating blasts, promyelocytes, or myelocytes; or abnormal cytogenetics should prompt consideration for transplantation. Pretransplantation splenectomy, although not necessary in every patient, is associated with faster engraftment and can be considered in those with massive splenomegaly. Marrow fibrosis is reversible with transplantation.

SUGGESTED READINGS

Berk PD, Goldberg JD, Donovoun PB, et al. Therapeutic recommendations in polycythemia vera based on Polycythemia Vera Study Group protocols. *Semin Hematol* 1986;23:132–143.

Cortelazzo S, Finazzi G, Ruggeri M, et al. Hydroxyurea for patients with essential thrombocythemia and a high risk for thrombosis. *N Engl J Med* 1995;332:1132–1136.

Fruchtman SM, Mack K, Kaplan ME, et al. From efficacy to safety: a polycythemia vera study group report on hydroxyurea in patient with polycythemia vera. *Semin Hematol* 1997;34:17–23.

Guardiola P, Anderson JE, Bandini G, et al. Allogeneic stem cell transplantation for agnogenic myeloid metaplasia: a European Group for Blood and Marrow Transplantation, Societe Francaise de Greffe de Moelle, Gruppo Italiano per il Trapianto del Midollo Osseo, and Fred Hutchinson Cancer Research Center collaborative study. *Blood* 1999;93:2831–2838.

Harris NL, Jaffe ES, Diebold J, et al. World Health Organization classification of neoplastic diseases of the hematopoietic and lymphoid tissues: report of the Clinical Advisory Committee meeting, Airlie House, Virginia, November 1997. *J Clin Oncol* 1999;17:3835–3849.

Harrison CN, Campbell PJ, Buck G, et al. Hydroxyurea compared with anagrelide in high-risk essential thrombocythemia. *N Engl J Med* 2005;353:33–45.

Hoffman R, Mesa RA, Vannucchi AM. Myeloproliferative Disorders. In *Hematology 2007* (American Society of Hematology Education Program Book), American Society of Hematology, 2007.

Kaplan ME, Mack K, Goldberg JD, et al. Long term management of polycythemia vera with hydroxyurea: a progress report. *Semin Hematol* 1986;23:167–171.

Landolfi R, Marchioli R, Kutti J, et al. Efficacy and safety of low-dose aspirin in polycythemia vera (ECLAP study). *N Engl J Med* 2004;350:114–124.

Silver RT. Interferon-alpha: effects of long-term treatment for polycythemia vera. *Semin Hematol* 1997; 34:40–50.

Spivak J. Polycythemia vera: myths, mechanisms, and management. *Blood* 2002;100:4272–4290.

Tefferi A, Thiele J, Orazi A, et al. Proposals and rationale for revision of the World Health Organization diagnostic criteria for polycythemia vera, essential thrombocythemia, and primary myelofibrosis: recommendations from an ad hoc international expert panel. *Blood.* 2007;110(4):1092–1097.

27

Multiple Myeloma

Sattva S. Neelapu and Cynthia E. Dunbar

EPIDEMIOLOGY

- In 2009, 20,580 new cases and 10,580 deaths from multiple myeloma (MM) are estimated in the United States.
- The incidence rate of myeloma is five to seven new cases per 100,000 population per year in the United States. Incidence among African Americans is twice that in whites and three times that in Asians and Pacific Islanders.
- The median age at diagnosis is 70 years.
- An increased incidence of myeloma in atomic bomb survivors implicates excessive radiation as a risk factor, but there is little evidence to implicate other environmental causes. Familial clustering has been reported in some cases.

PATHOPHYSIOLOGY

MM is characterized by the proliferation and accumulation of clonal plasma cells. The involvement of B cells is somewhat controversial, but the extent of somatic mutation in the complementarity-determining regions (the antigen-binding portions) of the variable gene segment suggests that the proliferation of the clone is antigen driven at some point, although the identity of the antigen or antigens is unknown (Fig. 27.1). Five recurrent translocations involving the heavy chain locus on chromosome 14 have been identified and are present in approximately 40% of all myeloma tumors. Deletion of chromosome 13q is also common and portends a very poor prognosis. The clinical features of MM are a result of bone marrow infiltration by the malignant clone; damage from high levels of immunoglobulins or free light chains in the circulation or glomeruli; the secretion of osteoclast-activating factors such as RANKL (receptor activator of NF-κB ligand) and MIP-1 (macrophage inflammatory protein-1) with resultant bone damage; decreased production of the natural RANKL inhibitor OPG (osteoprotegerin); and impaired immunity, both cell-mediated and humoral.

CLINICAL FEATURES

- Bone pain is present in 80% of patients with MM, and 70% of the patients develop pathologic fractures during the course of their disease. Any patient with spontaneous fractures, severe persistent bone pain, or unexplained severe osteoporosis should be evaluated for myeloma.
- Other common clinical features include fatigue, normocytic normochromic anemia (70%), and hypercalcemia (20%).
- Renal insufficiency is seen in at least 25% of patients at diagnosis and may be caused by hypercalcemia and related dehydration, light chain deposition in the tubules or glomeruli, or amyloid deposition. In some patients, amyloidosis can cause a nephrotic syndrome (<5%). Acquired Fanconi syndrome with glycosuria, phosphaturia, and aminoaciduria can occur.
- Infections are an important cause of morbidity and mortality in patients with MM.
- Hyperviscosity symptoms are rare except with immunoglobulin (Ig)A and IgG3 subtypes.

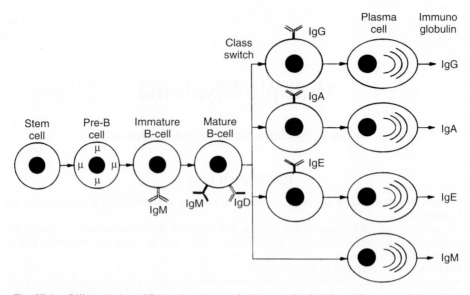

Fig. 27.1. Differentiation of B lymphocytes and plasma cells. A pleiotropic stem cell gives rise to the pre–B cell that has acquired the capacity to synthesize heavy chains (μ). The immature B cell can synthesize light chains so that a complete immunoglobulin M (IgM) molecule is formed and expressed on the cell surface. Mature B cells express both IgM and IgD on their surfaces. These cells can either mature into IgM-secreting plasmacytoid lymphocytes or undergo a class switch to express IgG, IgA, or IgE on their surfaces. The latter cells can undergo terminal differentiation into IgG- or IgE-secreting plasma cells. (Used with permission from Stamatovannopoulos G, Nienhuis AW, Leder P, et al., eds. *The molecular basis of blood diseases.* Philadelphia: WB Saunders, 1987.)

DIAGNOSIS

- The criteria for the diagnosis of monoclonal gammopathies proposed by the International Myeloma Working Group are shown in Table 27.1 (1).
- The diagnostic and staging workup of MM should include a history and physical examination, complete blood count with differential; levels of serum electrolytes, blood urea nitrogen, serum creatinine, calcium, phosphate, magnesium, uric acid, β_2-microglobulin, and lactate dehydrogenase; serum protein electrophoresis (SPEP) and immunofixation; serum free light chains; 24-hour urine protein electrophoresis (UPEP) and immunofixation; quantitative immunoglobulins; 24-hour urine for Bence Jones reaction; at least a unilateral bone marrow aspirate and biopsy; and a radiographic skeletal survey. A nuclear medicine bone scan is not indicated because lytic lesions are not visualized on bone scans. Any patient with significant back pain should undergo a magnetic resonance imaging (MRI) of the spine to evaluate cord compression.
- An SPEP and/or serum immunofixation is inadequate because some myeloma clones secrete only light chains, which are rapidly cleared from the plasma to the urine (Fig. 27.2). Serum free light chains, UPEP, and/or urine immunofixation are useful in such patients.
- The circulating monoclonal protein is IgG in 50% of cases, IgA in 20%, light chain only (Bence Jones proteinemia) in 20%, IgD in 2%, and biclonal in 1%.
- Because bone marrow involvement may be focal rather than diffuse, repeated bone marrow sampling may be needed before diagnostic infiltrates of more than 10% plasma cells are identified.
- Radiologic changes include punched-out lytic lesions, osteoporosis, and fractures.

TABLE 27.1. *International Myeloma Working Group criteria for diagnosis of monoclonal gammopathies*

Disorder	Clonal plasma cells	Monoclonal (M) protein	End organ damage due to plasma cell proliferative process[a]
Monoclonal gammopathy of undetermined significance (MGUS)	<10% in bone marrow	<3 g/dL in serum	None
Asymptomatic (smoldering) multiple myeloma[b]	≥10% in bone marrow	≥3 g/dL in serum	None
Symptomatic multiple myeloma	Present in bone marrow (any amount)	Present in serum and/or urine (any amount)	Present
Nonsecretory multiple myeloma	≥10% in bone marrow	None	Present
Solitary or multiple plasma-cytomas	Present at site of bony or extramedullary tumor Normal bone marrow	May or may not be present	None other than localized bone lesion(s)

[a]End organ damage may include one or more of the following: hypercalcemia, renal insufficiency, anemia, lytic bone lesions, hyperviscosity, amyloidosis, or recurrent bacterial infections.
[b]A diagnosis of asymptomatic multiple myeloma would require presence of ≥10% clonal plasma cells in bone marrow and/or M-protein in serum of ≥3 g/dL.
Source: Adapted from Ref. 1.

STAGING

The new International Staging System (ISS) (2) that replaced the previously used Durie-Salmon staging system (3) for MM is shown in Table 27.2.

PROGNOSIS

- The ISS provides useful prognostic grouping in patients aged greater versus less than 65 years and in those who received conventional or high-dose transplantation therapy.
- Other laboratory parameters such as hemoglobin concentration, creatinine, calcium, lactate dehydrogenase, immunoglobulin subtype, plasmablastic morphology, circulating plasma cells, and C-reactive protein have also been shown to be independent risk factors for survival in myeloma.
- A high plasma-cell–labeling index also strongly predicts poor prognosis, but this test is not commonly available.
- Deletion of chromosome 13 is one of the best characterized cytogenetic abnormalities associated with poor outcome. Other common cytogenetic abnormalities associated with poor adverse outcome include t(4;14), t(14;16), and deletion of 17p.
- Recent analysis of the Surveillance, Epidemiology, and End Results (SEER) database suggests that the 5-year relative survival of patients with myeloma improved from 28.8% to 34.7%, and 10-year relative survival increased from 11.1% to 17.4% between 1990 to 1992 and 2002 to 2004. The improvement in survival was most significant for patients under the age of 60 years (4). In another study from the Mayo Clinic, an improved outcome was observed in patients with myeloma with the use of novel therapies, both in the relapsed setting as well as at diagnosis (5).

TREATMENT

- Monoclonal gammopathy of undetermined significance (MGUS): Patients with MGUS are monitored indefinitely without treatment because 20% to 25% of them will eventually progress to myeloma at

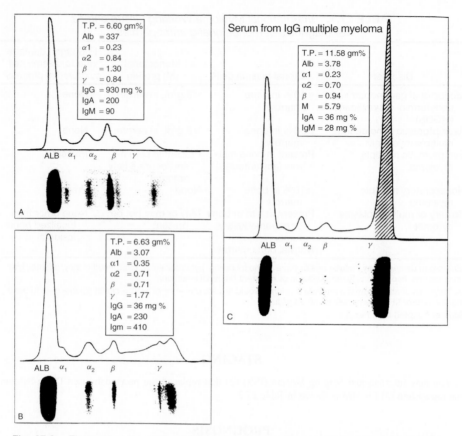

Fig. 27.2. Electrophoretic pattern of (A) normal human serum, (B) hypergammaglobulinemia, and (C) immunoglobulin G (IgG) multiple myeloma. (Used with permission from Lee GR,
Bithell TC, Foerster J, et al., eds. *Wintrobe's clinical hematology.* Philadelphia: Lea & Febiger,
1993.)

a rate of approximately 1% per year. Checking SPEP or UPEP every 6 months along with watchful
waiting for other symptoms is appropriate. Early intervention studies to date have shown no benefit
for thalidomide or steroids.

- Asymptomatic (smoldering) MM: These patients can also be observed closely without therapy. Treatment is indicated when there is evidence of disease progression to symptomatic disease. The median
time from diagnosis to symptomatic progression is 2 to 3 years.

TABLE 27.2. *International Staging System for multiple myeloma (2)*

Stage	Criteria	% of patients	Median survival (months)
I	Serum β_2-microglobulin <3.5 mg/L Serum albumin ≥3.5 g/dL	28	62
II	Not fitting stage I or III Serum β_2-microglobulin 3.5–5.4 mg/L Serum albumin <3.5 g/dL	33	44
III	Serum β_2-microglobulin ≥5.5 mg/L	39	29

Source: Adapted from Ref. 2.

- Solitary plasmacytoma: These patients are treated with radiation therapy (solitary bone) and/or surgical removal (extraosseous plasmacytomas) of the affected area, followed by close monitoring of M protein because of the risk of overt MM.
- Multiple myeloma: To date, there is no clear curative therapy available for most MM patients. However, in the past decade, the availability of novel highly active drugs such as thalidomide, bortezomib, and lenalidomide has significantly improved the outcome of patients with MM. The goal of standard therapy is to improve quality of life, delay disease progression, and prolong survival. The treatment choice for symptomatic myeloma depends on eligibility for transplantation and risk factors (Fig. 27.3). Eligible patients should always be considered for enrollment in clinical trials that evaluate novel treatment strategies. The proposed criteria by the International Myeloma Working Group (IMWG) for evaluating disease response and progression in myeloma patients are outlined in Table 27.3 (6).

Initial Therapies

Induction Treatment for Patients Eligible for Transplantation

- Infusional therapy with vincristine, doxorubicin, and dexamethasone (VAD) was commonly used for many years as an induction regimen prior to autologous stem cell transplantation. However, VAD is no longer used as initial therapy since several novel drug combinations using thalidomide, bortezomib or lenalidomide have been shown to be superior to VAD.

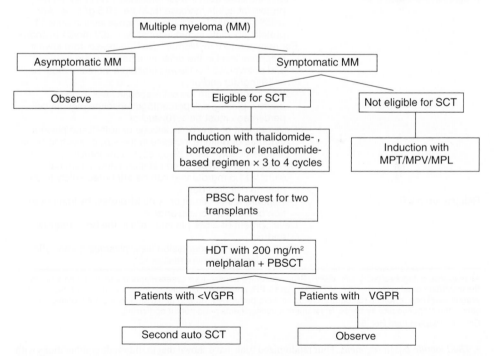

Fig. 27.3. A suggested treatment algorithm for newly diagnosed myeloma patients. All patients should receive supportive care and must be considered for bisphosphonate treatment and clinical trials. (SCT, stem cell transplantation; MPT, melphalan, prednisone, and thalidomide; MPV, melphalan, prednisone, and bortezomib; MPL, melphalan, prednisone, and lenalidomide; HDT, high-dose therapy; PBSCT, peripheral blood stem cell transplantation; VGPR, very good partial response.)

TABLE 27.3. *International Myeloma Working Group uniform response criteria*

Response subcategory	Response criteria
Stringent complete response (sCR)	CR as defined below *plus* Normal free-light-chain (FLC) assay ratio *plus* Absence of clonal cells in bone marrow by immunohisto-chemistry or immunofluorescence
Complete response (CR)	Negative immunofixation on the serum and urine *and* disappearance of any soft-tissue plasmacytomas *and* <5% plasma cells in bone marrow
Very good partial response (VGPR)	Serum and urine M-protein detectable by immunofixation but not on electrophoresis or ≥90% reduction in serum M-protein plus urine M-protein level <100 mg/24 h
Partial response (PR)	≥50% reduction in serum M-protein and reduction in 24-h urine M-protein by ≥90% or to <200 mg/24 h For nonsecretory myeloma, ≥50% decrease in the difference between involved and uninvolved FLC levels If serum and urine M-protein and serum free-light-chain assay are unmeasurable, ≥50% reduction in plasma cells in the bone marrow provided baseline percentage was ≥30% If present at baseline, ≥50% reduction in the size of soft-tissue plasmacytomas
Stable disease (SD)	Not meeting criteria for CR, VGPR, PR, or PD
Progressive disease (PD)	≥25% increase from lowest response level in serum M-protein (absolute increase must be ≥0.5 g/dL) *and/or* ≥25% increase from lowest response level in urine M-protein (absolute increase must be ≥200 mg/24 h) *and/or* For nonsecretory myeloma, ≥25% increase from lowest response level in the difference between the involved and uninvolved FLC levels (absolute increase must be > 10 mg/dL) *and/or* ≥25% increase from lowest response level in bone marrow plasma cell percentage (absolute plasma cell percentage must be ≥10) *and/or* Development of new bone lesions or soft-tissue plasma-cytomas or definite increase in the size of existing bone lesions or soft-tissue plasmacytomas *and/or* Development of hypercalcemia (corrected serum calcium >11.5 mg/dL) that can be attributed solely to the plasma cell disorder
Relapse from CR	Reappearance of serum or urine M-protein by immunofixation or electrophoresis *and/or* Development of ≥5% plasma cells in the bone marrow and/or Any other sign of progression (new plasmacytoma, lytic bone lesions, or hypercalcemia)

All response categories (sCR, CR, VGPR, PR) require two consecutive assessments made at any time before the institution of any new therapy. sCR, CR, VGPR, PR, and SD also require no known evidence of new or progressive bone lesions if radiographic studies were performed. Radiographic studies are not required to satisfy the response requirements. Bone marrow assessments need not be confirmed.
Source: Adapted from Ref. 6.

- *Thalidomide-based regimens.* Four randomized trials have shown that thalidomide combinations with dexamethasone (TD) or doxorubicin and dexamethasone (TAD), or VAD (Thal+VAD) were superior to high-dose dexamethasone alone and/or VAD (7–10) (Tables 27.4 and 27.8).
- *Bortezomib-based regimens.* Randomized trials have shown bortezomib in combination with dexamethasone is superior to VAD and bortezomib in combination with thalidomide and dexamethasone (VTD) is superior to TD alone (11,12) (see Tables 27.4 and 27.8).

TABLE 27.4. *Responses to induction therapy for transplant-eligible myeloma patients*

Regimen	OR (CR + PR)	CR + VGPR	Reference(s)
TD vs. dex	63% vs. 46%	44% vs. 16%	7,8
TAD vs. VAD	72% vs. 54%	33% vs. 15%	9
Thal + VAD-doxil vs. VAD-doxil	81% vs. 63%	54% vs. 31%	10
Bortezomib + dex vs. VAD	89% vs. 71%	50% vs. 24%	11
Bortezomib + TD vs. TD	93% vs. 80%	60% vs. 25%	12
Lenalidomide + high-dose dex vs. high-dose dex	85% vs. 51%	79% vs. 26%	13
Lenalidomide + low-dose dex vs. lenalidomide + high-dose dex	70% vs. 82%	42% vs. 52%	14

OR, overall response; CR, complete response; PR, partial response; VGPR, very good partial response; dex, dexamethasone; Thal, thalidomide; TD, thalidomide and dexamethasone; TAD, thalidomide, doxorubicin, and dexamethasone; VAD, vincristine, doxorubicin, and dexamethasone.

- *Lenalidomide-based regimens.* Similar to thalidomide and bortezomib combinations, lenalidomide plus high-dose dexamethasone was shown to be superior to high-dose dexamethasone alone in terms of overall response rates and progression-free survival (13). Interim results of an Eastern Cooperative Oncology Group randomized trial of lenalidomide plus high-dose dexamethasone versus lenalidomide plus low-dose dexamethasone show significantly better overall survival and safety with lenalidomide plus low-dose dexamethasone (14) (see Tables 27.4 and 27.8).

In summary, the preferred novel combinations for induction therapy in patients eligible for transplantation are TAD, Thal+VAD, bortezomib + dexamethasone, VTD, and lenalidomide plus low-dose dexamethasone. Although thalidomide combinations are the most commonly used induction regimens, bortezomib or lenalidomide-based regimens are preferable in specific clinical scenarios. For patients at risk of DVT and in patients with renal insufficiency, bortezomib + dexamethasone is preferred; for patients with history of peripheral neuropathy, lenalidomide plus low-dose dexamethasone would be a better choice; and for patients with diabetes mellitus, lenalidomide plus low-dose dexamethsone or bortezomib in combination with liposomal doxorubicin (15) would be good choices.

Autologous Stem Cell Transplantation

- Two large randomized trials, the InterGroupe Francophone du Myelome 90 (IFM 90) trial and the Medical Research Council Myeloma VII Trial, demonstrated that high-dose therapy (HDT) followed by autologous stem cell transplantation (SCT) significantly improves response rate and survival compared to conventional chemotherapy in myeloma patients younger than 65 years with good performance status (Table 27.5) (16, 17). The IFM 95 randomized trial demonstrated that 200 mg/m^2 of melphalan is less toxic and at least as effective a conditioning regimen as total body irradiation of 8 Gy with 140 mg/m^2 melphalan before autologous SCT (18). Although SCT is commonly performed following three to four cycles of induction chemotherapy, a randomized trial comparing early versus

TABLE 27.5. *Results for conventional chemotherapy (CC) versus high-dose therapy (HDT) followed by autologous stem cell transplantation (SCT)*

Treatment	OR (CR + PR)	CR	Median EFS/PFS	Median OS	Reference
CC vs. HDT (IFM 90)	57% vs. 81%	5% vs. 22%	18 vs. 28 mo	44 vs. 57 mo	16
CC vs. HDT (MRC7)	48% vs. 86%	8% vs. 44%	20 vs. 32 mo	42 vs. 54 mo	17

OR, overall response; CR, complete response; PR, partial response; IFM, InterGroupe Francophone du Myelome; CC, conventional chemotherapy; HDT, high-dose therapy; EFS, event-free survival; PFS, progression-free survival; OS, overall survival; MRC, Medical Research Council.

TABLE 27.6. *Results for single versus double autologous stem cell transplantation (SCT)*

Treatment	OR (CR + PR)	CR + VGPR/nCR	Median EFS	Median OS	TRM	Reference
Single vs. Double SCT (IFM 94)	84% vs. 88%	42% vs. 50%	25 vs. 30 mo	48 vs. 58 mo	4% vs. 6%	21
Single vs. Double SCT (Bologna 96)	n/a	33% vs. 47%	23 vs. 35 mo	65 vs. 71 mo	3% vs. 4%	22

OR, overall response; CR, complete response; PR, partial response; VGPR, very good partial response; nCR, near complete response; SCT, stem cell transplantation; EFS, event-free survival; OS, overall survival; TRM, treatment-related mortality.

late transplantation demonstrated that SCT can be delayed until relapse without compromising survival provided that the stem cells are harvested and cryopreserved early in the disease course (19). Moreover, a Spanish randomized trial suggested that patients responding to induction therapy had similar overall and progression-free survival with either autologous SCT or eight additional courses of chemotherapy (20). Therefore, the timing of SCT is based on patient preference and other clinical conditions.

- Although the benefit of autologous SCT in terms of event-free and overall survival is yet to be proven after induction therapy with novel agents, it is generally recommended as it has been shown to improve the complete remission rate (11,12).
- The IFM 94 trial (21) and the Bologna 96 Clinical study from Italy (22) established that *double transplantation* is superior to single autologous transplantation and should be considered as a treatment option, especially for patients younger than 60 years who do not have a very good partial response (defined as >90% reduction in serum M-protein level) after single transplantation (Table 27.6).

Induction Treatment for Patients Not Eligible for Transplantation

- *Melphalan and prednisone (MP) combinations.* MP has been the standard treatment regimen for MM for more than 40 years. However, randomized trials have now shown that in patients ≥65 years of age combination of MP with any of the new agents (thalidomide, bortezomib, and lenalidomide) is significantly superior to MP in terms of response rate, event-free survival, and overall survival, although increased toxicity with the newer regimens needs to be considered when choosing therapy (Tables 27.7 and 27.8) (23–26). These new combinations of MPT, MPV, and MPL are now considered standard of care for elderly patients. The duration of therapy is usually six cycles with the newer combinations.

TABLE 27.7. *Results with induction therapy in newly diagnosed elderly myeloma patients*

Regimen	OR (CR + PR)	CR + VGPR	EFS/PFS/TTP	OS	Reference
MPT vs. MP	76% vs. 48%	28% vs. 7%	54% vs. 27% at 24 mo	80% vs. 64% at 36 mo	23
MPT vs. MP	76% vs. 35%	47% vs. 7%	28 vs. 18 mo	52 vs. 33 mo median OS	24
Bortezomib + MP (MPV) vs. MP	82% vs. 50%	45% vs. 10%	24 vs. 17 mo	83% vs. 70% at 24 mo	25
Lenalidomide + MP (MPL)	81%	48%	92% at 12 mo	100% at 12 mo	26

OR, overall response; CR, complete response; PR, partial response; VGPR, very good partial response; EFS, event-free survival; PFS, progression-free survival; TTP, time to progression; OS, overall survival; MP, melphalan and prednisone; MPT, melphalan, prednisone, and thalidomide.

TABLE 27.8. *Chemotherapy regimens in multiple myeloma*

Regimen	Treatment description	Cycle duration	Response rate	Reference(s)
TD	Dexamethasone 40 mg/d PO d 1–4, 9–12, and 17–20 Thalidomide 200 mg/d PO daily at bedtime	28 d	63% in untreated patients	7,8
TAD	Thalidomide 200–400 mg/d PO daily at bedtime Doxorubicin 9 mg/m²/d i.v. rapid infusion d 1–4 (total dose/cycle = 36 mg/m²) Dexamethasone 40 mg/d PO d 1–4, 9–12, and 17–20 (total dose/cycle = 480 mg)	28 d	72% in untreated patients	9
Thal + VAD-doxil	Thalidomide 200 mg/d PO daily at bedtime Vincristine 2 mg i.v. bolus on d 1 Pegylated liposomal doxorubicin 40 mg/m² i.v. 60 min infusion d 1 Dexamethasone 40 mg/d PO d 1–4, 9–12, and 17–20 for cycle 1 and on days 1–4 for cycles 2–4	28 d	81% in untreated patients	10
MPT	Melphalan 4 mg/m²/d PO d 1–7 Prednisone 40 mg/m²/d PO d 1–7 Thalidomide 100 mg/d PO daily at bedtime	28 d	76% in untreated patients	23,24
Bortezomib + dexamethasone	Bortezomib 1.3 mg/m²/d i.v. on d 1, 4, 8, and 11 (total dose/cycle = 5.2 mg/m²) Dexamethasone 40 mg/d PO on d 1–4 and 9–12 during cycles 1 and 2; and d 1–4 only during cycles 3 and 4	21 d	80% in untreated patients	11
Bortezomib + TD (VTD)	Bortezomib 1.3 mg/m²/d i.v. on d 1, 4, 8, and 11 Thalidomide 200 mg/d PO daily at bedtime Dexamethasone 40 mg/d PO on d 1, 2, 4, 5, 8, 9, 11, and 12	21 d	93% in untreated patients	12
Bortezomib + Pegylated liposomal doxorubicin	Bortezomib 1.3 mg/m²/d i.v. on d 1, 4, 8, and 11 Pegylated liposomal doxorubicin 30 mg/m² i.v. 60 min infusion on d 4	21 d	44% in relapsed or refractory patients	15
MPV	Melphalan 9 mg/m²/d PO d 1–4 Prednisone 60 mg/m²/d PO d 1–4 Bortezomib 1.3 mg/m²/d i.v. on d 1, 4, 8, 11, 22, 25, 29, and 32 for four cycles and on d 1, 8, 22, and 29 for five cycles	42 d	88% in untreated patients	25

(Continued)

TABLE 27.8.   *(Continued)*

Regimen	Treatment description	Cycle duration	Response rate	Reference(s)
Lenalidomide + high-dose dexamethasone	Lenalidomide 25 mg/d PO on d 1–21 Dexamethasone 40 mg/d PO on d 1–4, 9–12, and 17–20	28 d	82% in untreated patients	13,14
Lenalidomide + low-dose dexamethasone	Lenalidomide 25 mg/d PO on d 1–21 Dexamethasone 40 mg/d PO on d 1, 8, 15, and 22	28 d	70% in untreated patients	14
MPL	Melphalan 0.18 mg/kg/d PO on d 1–4 Prednisone 2 mg/kg/d PO on d 1–4 Lenalidomide 10 mg/d PO on d 1–21	28 d	81% in untreated patients	26
MP	Melphalan 10 mg/m^2/d PO d 1–4 (total dose/cycle = 40 mg/m^2) Prednisone 60 mg/m^2/d PO d 1–4 (total dose/cycle = 240 mg/m^2)	4–6 wk	53% in untreated patients	43
Pulse dexamethasone	Dexamethasone 40 mg/d PO d 1–4, 9–12, and 17–20 for odd cycles and d 1–4 for even cycles (total dose/cycle = 480 mg for odd cycles and 160 mg for even cycles)	28 d	43% in untreated patients	36
VAD	Vincristine 0.4 mg/m^2/d continuous i.v. infusion d 1–4 (total dose/cycle = 1.6 mg/m^2) Doxorubicin 9 mg/m^2/d continuous i.v. infusion d 1–4 (total dose/cycle = 36 mg/m^2) Dexamethasone 40 mg/d PO d 1–4, 9–12, and 17–20 for odd cycles and d 1–4 for even cycles	21 d	55%–84% in untreated patients	37
CVAD	Cyclophosphamide 225 mg/m^2/dose i.v. every 12 h on d 1–4 (total dose/cycle = 1,800 mg/m^2) Vincristine 0.4 mg/m^2/d continuous i.v. infusion d 1–4 (total dose/cycle = 1.6 mg/m^2) Doxorubicin 9 mg/m^2/d continuous i.v. infusion d 1–4 (total dose/cycle = 36 mg/m^2) Dexamethasone 40 mg/d PO d 1–4, 9–12, and 17–20 for odd cycles and d 1–4 for even cycles	21 d	40% in relapsed or refractory patients	38

(Continued)

TABLE 27.8. *(Continued)*

Regimen	Treatment description	Cycle duration	Response rate	Reference(s)
DCEP	Dexamethasone 40 mg/d PO d 1–4 (total dose/cycle = 160 mg) Cyclophosphamide 400 mg/m²/d continuous i.v. infusion d 1–4 (total dose/cycle = 1,600 mg/m²) Etoposide 40 mg/m²/d continuous i.v. infusion d 1–4 (total dose/cycle = 160 mg/m²) Cisplatin 10 mg/m²/d continuous i.v. infusion d 1–4 (total dose/cycle = 40 mg/m²)	4–6 wk	41% in refractory patients	39,40
DTPACE	Dexamethasone 40 mg/d PO d 1–4 Thalidomide 400 mg/d PO daily at bedtime (continuous) Cisplatin 10 mg/m²/d continuous i.v. infusion d 1–4 (total dose/cycle = 40 mg/m²) Doxorubicin 10 mg/m²/d continuous i.v. infusion d 1–4 (total dose/cycle = 40 mg/m²) Cyclophosphamide 400 mg/m²/d continuous i.v. infusion d 1–4 (total dose/cycle = 1,600 mg/m²) Etoposide 40 mg/m²/d continuous i.v. infusion d 1–4 (total dose/cycle = 160 mg/m²)	4–6 wk	40% in refractory patients	41
Thalidomide	Thalidomide start at 200 mg/d PO daily at bedtime for 2 wk; increase dose by 200 mg every 2 wk to a maximum of 800 mg/d	Continuous	32% in refractory patients	35
HDT + AutoSCT	Conditioning regimen: Melphalan 200 mg/m² i.v. infusion over 30 min on d 2 (total dose/cycle = 200 mg/m²) PBSC transplantation on d 0	N/A	>80% in untreated patients	16,17
Pamidronate	Pamidronate 90 mg i.v. infusion over 2 h (total dose/cycle = 90 mg)	Monthly	N/A	27
Zoledronic acid	Zoledronic acid 4 mg i.v. infusion over 15 min (total dose/cycle = 4 mg)	Monthly	N/A	28,29

SCT, stem cell transplantation; HDT, high-dose therapy.

The preference for one regimen over the other may depend on the patient's comorbid conditions and other social factors. For patients at risk of DVT and in patients with renal insufficiency, MPV is preferred; for patients with history of peripheral neuropathy, MPL should be the choice; if costs are a concern, MPT is least expensive; if oral therapy is desired, MPT or MPL would be good choices.

Maintenance Treatment

- Maintenance therapy with interferon or corticosteroids has shown little benefit and is no longer recommended.
- The role of maintenance therapy with thalidomide, lenalidomide, and bortezomib is not definitively established and should be performed only in the context of a clinical trial.

SUPPORTIVE MEASURES

- Bisphosphonates should be considered for all patients with evidence of lytic bone lesions and/or osteopenia. Intravenous pamidronate given monthly reduced bone pain and the incidence of pathologic fractures and the need for surgery or irradiation to the bone in patients with advanced myeloma (27). A randomized trial demonstrated that zoledronic acid is as effective as pamidronate in reducing skeletal complications, in addition to having the advantage of a shorter administration time (28,29). However, pamidronate may be preferred due to the greater risk of development of osteonecrosis of the jaw with zoledronic acid.
- Other supportive measures in myeloma include adequate analgesia and/or local irradiation for bone pain, radiation or surgery for spinal cord compression, surgery for impending pathologic fractures, erythropoietin for anemia, treatment and prevention of hypercalcemia, avoidance of dehydration by a high fluid intake of approximately 3 L/day to maintain renal function, and dialysis if necessary. Intravenous immunoglobulin therapy may be beneficial for patients with recurrent life-threatening infections.
- Prophylactic anticoagulation to decrease the risk of thrombotic complications is recommended for myeloma patients receiving thalidomide or lenalidomide-based therapies. The IMWG recommends a prophylaxis strategy according to a risk-assessment model (30). Risk factors to be considered include obesity, history of venous thromboembolism, central venous catheter, infections, diabetes, cardiac disease, chronic renal disease, immobilization, surgery, inherited thrombophilia, eythropoietin usage, myeloma diagnosis per se, hyperviscosity, and therapy with high-dose dexamethasone, doxorubicin or multiagent chemotherapy in combination with thalidomide or lenalidomide. Patients with more than one risk factor may receive prophylaxis with aspirin (81–325 mg once daily). Low molecular weight heparin (equivalent to a dose of enoxaparin 40 mg/day) is recommended for patients with ≥ 2 risk factors. Warfarin targeting a therapeutic INR of 2 to 3 is an alternative to low molecular weight heparin.

REFRACTORY OR RELAPSED DISEASE

- Patients relapsing more than 6 months after primary induction therapy may be retreated with the same regimen or other novel agent combinations. Patients who have had only one autologous SCT, may be considered for a second autologous SCT following second remission.
- Patients relapsing within 6 months after primary induction therapy or patients with primary refractory disease need to be treated with combination salvage therapies using conventional chemotherapeutic agents and/or novel agents.
- Novel agents that are FDA-approved based on phase 3 trials for use in relapsed and/or refractory MM include single-agent bortezomib (31,32), bortezomib in combination with pegylated liposomal doxorubicin (15), and lenalidomide in combination with dexamethasone (33,34) (see Table 27.8).
- Other salvage regimens that have shown efficacy include thalidomide with or without dexamethasone (35), bortezomib in combination with dexamethasone, single-agent lenalidomide, high-dose pulse dexamethasone (36), VAD (37), cyclophosphamide-VAD (38), high-dose cyclophosphamide, DCEP (39,40), and DTPACE (41) (see Table 27.8).
- Allogeneic transplantation may potentially benefit a small percentage of patients because of a powerful graft-versus-myeloma effect. However, myeloablative allotransplants were associated with high treatment-related mortality (TRM) of up to 50% because of severe graft-versus-host disease, opportunistic infections, and complications resulting from a second aggressive conditioning regimen in patients already surviving and relapsing following autologous transplantation.
- The recent experience with nonmyeloablative allogeneic transplantation suggests that the TRM could be reduced to <10% to 20%, but this strategy should currently be considered investigational (42). Nevertheless, up to 50% of patients relapse following allogeneic transplantation; therefore, at present, this option is far from ideal for most patients.

REFERENCES

1. International Myeloma Working Group. Criteria for the classification of monoclonal gammopathies, multiple myeloma and related disorders: a report of the International Myeloma Working Group. *Br J Haematol.* 2003 Jun;121(5):749–57.

2. Greipp PR, San Miguel J, Durie BG, et al. International staging system for multiple myeloma. *J Clin Oncol.* 2005 May 20;23(15):3412–20. Epub 2005 Apr 4. Erratum in: *J Clin Oncol.* 2005 Sep 1;23(25):6281. Harousseau, Jean-Luc (corrected to Avet-Loiseau, Herve).

3. Durie BG, Salmon SE. A clinical staging system for multiple myeloma. Correlation of measured myeloma cell mass with presenting clinical features, response to treatment, and survival. *Cancer.* 1975 Sep;36(3):842–54.

4. Brenner H, Gondos A, Pulte D. Recent major improvement in long-term survival of younger patients with multiple myeloma. *Blood.* 2008 Mar 1;111(5):2521–6. Epub 2007 Sep 27.

5. Kumar SK, Rajkumar SV, Dispenzieri A, et al. Improved survival in multiple myeloma and the impact of novel therapies. *Blood.* 2008 Mar 1;111(5):2516–20. Epub 2007 Nov 1.

6. Durie BG, Harousseau JL, Miguel JS, et al. International Myeloma Working Group. International uniform response criteria for multiple myeloma. *Leukemia.* 2006 Sep;20(9):1467–73. Epub 2006 Jul 20. Erratum in: *Leukemia.* 2006 Dec;20(12):2220; *Leukemia.* 2007 May;21(5):1134.

7. Rajkumar SV, Blood E, Vesole D, Fonseca R, Greipp PR; Eastern Cooperative Oncology Group. Phase III clinical trial of thalidomide plus dexamethasone compared with dexamethasone alone in newly diagnosed multiple myeloma: a clinical trial coordinated by the Eastern Cooperative Oncology Group. *J Clin Oncol.* 2006 Jan 20;24(3):431–6. Epub 2005 Dec 19.

8. Rajkumar SV, Rosiñol L, Hussein M, et al. Multicenter, randomized, double-blind, placebo-controlled study of thalidomide plus dexamethasone compared with dexamethasone as initial therapy for newly diagnosed multiple myeloma. *J Clin Oncol.* 2008 May 1;26(13):2171–7. Epub 2008 Mar 24.

9. Lokhorst HM, Schmidt-Wolf I, Sonneveld P, et al. Dutch-Belgian HOVON; German GMMG. Thalidomide in induction treatment increases the very good partial response rate before and after high-dose therapy in previously untreated multiple myeloma. *Haematologica.* 2008 Jan;93(1):124–7.

10. Zervas K, Mihou D, Katodritou E, et al. Greek Myeloma Study Group. VAD-doxil versus VAD-doxil plus thalidomide as initial treatment for multiple myeloma: results of a multicenter randomized trial of the Greek Myeloma Study Group. *Ann Oncol.* 2007 Aug;18(8):1369–75.

11. Harousseau JL, Mathiot C, Attal M, et al. VELCADE/Dexamethasone (Vel/D) versus VAD as induction treatment prior to autologous stem cell transplantion (ASCT) in newly diagnosed multiple myeloma (MM): Updated results of the IFM 2005/01 trial. *Blood.* 2007 Nov;110:450.

12. Cavo M, Patriarca F, Tacchetti P, et al. Bortezomib (Velcade®)-Thalidomide-Dexamethasone (VTD) vs Thalidomide-Dexamethasone (TD) in preparation for autologous stem-cell (SC) transplantation (ASCT) in newly diagnosed multiple myeloma (MM). *Blood.* 2007 Nov;110:73.

13. Zonder JA, Crowley J, Hussein MA, et al. Superiority of lenalidomide (Len) plus high-dose dexamethasone (HD) compared to HD alone as treatment of newly-diagnosed multiple myeloma (NDMM): results of the randomized, double-blinded, placebo-controlled SWOG trial S0232. *Blood.* 2007 Nov;110:77.

14. Rajkumar SV, Jacobus S, Callander N, et al. A randomized trial of lenalidomide plus high-dose dexamethasone (RD) versus lenalidomide plus low-dose dexamethasone (RD) in newly diagnosed multiple myeloma (E4A03): a trial coordinated by the Eastern Cooperative Oncology Group. *Blood.* 2007 Nov;110:74.

15. Orlowski RZ, Nagler A, Sonneveld P, et al. Randomized phase III study of pegylated liposomal doxorubicin plus bortezomib compared with bortezomib alone in relapsed or refractory multiple myeloma: combination therapy improves time to progression. *J Clin Oncol.* 2007 Sep 1;25(25):3892–901. Epub 2007 Aug 6.

16. Attal M, Harousseau JL, Stoppa AM, et al. A prospective, randomized trial of autologous bone marrow transplantation and chemotherapy in multiple myeloma. Intergroupe Français du Myélome. *N Engl J Med.* 1996 Jul 11;335(2):91–7.

17. Child JA, Morgan GJ, Davies FE, et al. Medical research council adult leukaemia working party. High-dose chemotherapy with hematopoietic stem-cell rescue for multiple myeloma. *N Engl J Med.* 2003 May 8;348(19):1875–83.

18. Moreau P, Facon T, Attal M, et al. Intergroupe Francophone du Myélome. Comparison of 200 mg/m(2) melphalan and 8 Gy total body irradiation plus 140 mg/m(2) melphalan as conditioning regimens for peripheral blood stem cell transplantation in patients with newly diagnosed multiple myeloma: final analysis of the Intergroupe Francophone du Myélome 9502 randomized trial. *Blood.* 2002 Feb 1;99(3):731–5.

19. Fermand JP, Ravaud P, Chevret S, et al. High-dose therapy and autologous peripheral blood stem cell transplantation in multiple myeloma: up-front or rescue treatment? Results of a multicenter sequential randomized clinical trial. *Blood.* 1998 Nov 1;92(9):3131–6.

20. Bladé J, Rosiñol L, Sureda A, et al. Programa para el Estudio de la Terapéutica en Hemopatía Maligna (PETHEMA). High-dose therapy intensification compared with continued standard chemotherapy in multiple myeloma patients responding to the initial chemotherapy: long-term results from a prospective randomized trial from the Spanish cooperative group PETHEMA. *Blood.* 2005 Dec 1;106(12):3755–9. Epub 2005 Aug 16.

21. Attal M, Harousseau JL, Facon T, et al. InterGroupe Francophone du Myélome. Single versus double autologous stem-cell transplantation for multiple myeloma. *N Engl J Med.* 2003 Dec 25;349(26):2495–502. Erratum in: *N Engl J Med.* 2004 Jun 17;350(25):2628.

22. Cavo M, Tosi P, Zamagni E, et al. Prospective, randomized study of single compared with double autologous stem-cell transplantation for multiple myeloma: Bologna 96 clinical study. *J Clin Oncol.* 2007 Jun 10;25(17):2434–41. Epub 2007 May 7.

23. Palumbo A, Bringhen S, Caravita T, et al. Italian Multiple Myeloma Network, GIMEMA. Oral melphalan and prednisone chemotherapy plus thalidomide compared with melphalan and prednisone alone in elderly patients with multiple myeloma: randomised controlled trial. *Lancet.* 2006 Mar 11;367(9513):825–31.

24. Facon T, Mary JY, Hulin C, et al. Intergroupe Francophone du Myélome. Melphalan and prednisone plus thalidomide versus melphalan and prednisone alone or reduced-intensity autologous stem cell transplantation in elderly patients with multiple myeloma (IFM 99-06): a randomised trial. *Lancet.* 2007 Oct 6;370(9594):1209–18.

25. San Miguel JF, Schlag R, Khuageva N, et al. MMY-3002: a phase 3 study comparing bortezomib-melphalan-prednisone (VMP) with melphalan-prednisone (MP) in newly diagnosed multiple myeloma. *Blood.* 2007 Nov;110:76.

26. Palumbo A, Falco P, Corradini P, et al. GIMEMA—Italian Multiple Myeloma Network. Melphalan, prednisone, and lenalidomide treatment for newly diagnosed myeloma: a report from the GIMEMA—Italian Multiple Myeloma Network. *J Clin Oncol.* 2007 Oct 1;25(28):4459–65. Epub 2007 Sep 4.

27. Berenson JR, Lichtenstein A, Porter L, et al. Efficacy of pamidronate in reducing skeletal events in patients with advanced multiple myeloma. Myeloma Aredia Study Group. *N Engl J Med.* 1996 Feb 22;334(8):488–93.

28. Rosen LS, Gordon D, Kaminski M, et al. Zoledronic acid versus pamidronate in the treatment of skeletal metastases in patients with breast cancer or osteolytic lesions of multiple myeloma: a phase III, double-blind, comparative trial. *Cancer J.* 2001 Sep-Oct;7(5):377–87.

29. Rosen LS, Gordon D, Kaminski M, et al. Long-term efficacy and safety of zoledronic acid compared with pamidronate disodium in the treatment of skeletal complications in patients with advanced multiple myeloma or breast carcinoma: a randomized, double-blind, multicenter, comparative trial. *Cancer.* 2003 Oct 15;98(8):1735–44.

30. Palumbo A, Rajkumar SV, Dimopoulos MA, et al. International Myeloma Working Group. Prevention of thalidomide- and lenalidomide-associated thrombosis in myeloma. *Leukemia.* 2008 Feb;22(2):414–23. Epub 2007 Dec 20.

31. Richardson PG, Barlogie B, Berenson J, et al. A phase 2 study of bortezomib in relapsed, refractory myeloma. *N Engl J Med.* 2003 Jun 26;348(26):2609–17.

32. Richardson PG, Barlogie B, Berenson J, et al. Extended follow-up of a phase II trial in relapsed, refractory multiple myeloma: final time-to-event results from the SUMMIT trial. *Cancer.* 2006 Mar 15;106(6):1316–9.

33. Dimopoulos M, Spencer A, Attal M, et al. Multiple Myeloma (010) Study Investigators. Lenalidomide plus dexamethasone for relapsed or refractory multiple myeloma. *N Engl J Med.* 2007 Nov 22;357(21):2123–32.

34. Weber DM, Chen C, Niesvizky R, et al. Multiple Myeloma (009) Study Investigators. Lenalidomide plus dexamethasone for relapsed multiple myeloma in North America. *N Engl J Med.* 2007 Nov 22;357(21):2133–42.

35. Singhal S, Mehta J, Desikan R, et al. Antitumor activity of thalidomide in refractory multiple myeloma. *N Engl J Med.* 1999 Nov 18;341(21):1565–71. Erratum in: *N Engl J Med.* 2000 Feb 3;342(5):364.
36. Alexanian R, Barlogie B, Dixon D. High-dose glucocorticoid treatment of resistant myeloma. *Ann Intern Med.* 1986 Jul;105(1):8–11.
37. Barlogie B, Smith L, Alexanian R. Effective treatment of advanced multiple myeloma refractory to alkylating agents. *N Engl J Med.* 1984 May 24;310(21):1353–6.
38. Dimopoulos MA, Weber D, Kantarjian H, Delasalle KB, Alexanian R. HyperCVAD for VAD-resistant multiple myeloma. *Am J Hematol.* 1996 Jun;52(2):77–81.
39. Munshi NC, Desikan KR, Jagannath S, et al. Dexamethasone, cyclophosphamide, etoposide and cis-platinum (DCEP), an effective regimen for relapse after high-dose chemotherapy and autologous transplantation. *Blood* 1996;88(Suppl. 1):2331a.
40. Lazzarino M, Corso A, Barbarano L, et al. DCEP (dexamethasone, cyclophosphamide, etoposide, and cisplatin) is an effective regimen for peripheral blood stem cell collection in multiple myeloma. *Bone Marrow Transplant.* 2001 Nov;28(9):835–9.
41. Lee CK, Barlogie B, Munshi N, et al. DTPACE: an effective, novel combination chemotherapy with thalidomide for previously treated patients with myeloma. *J Clin Oncol.* 2003 Jul 15;21(14):2732–9.
42. Maloney DG, Molina AJ, Sahebi F, et al. Allografting with nonmyeloablative conditioning following cytoreductive autografts for the treatment of patients with multiple myeloma. *Blood.* 2003 Nov 1;102(9):3447–54.
43. Myeloma Trialists' Collaborative Group. Combination chemotherapy versus melphalan plus prednisone as treatment for multiple myeloma: an overview of 6,633 patients from 27 randomized trials. *J Clin Oncol.* 1998:3832–3842.

28

Non-Hodgkin Lymphoma

Kevin K. Tay, Wyndham H. Wilson, and Kieron Dunleavy

Non-Hodgkin lymphoma (NHL) represents a group of diverse diseases that vary in clinical behavior and morphologic appearance. The various types of NHL can be correlated to neoplastic lymphoid cells that are arrested at different stages of normal differentiation.

EPIDEMIOLOGY

NHL is the fifth most common malignancy in adult males and females in the United States (1). Over the last 20 years, the incidence of NHL has been steadily increasing at approximately 2% to 3% per year; 66,120 new cases were expected to be diagnosed in 2008 (1). The increasing incidence of NHL can be attributed to many factors, including an increase in the population at risk of AIDS-related lymphoma and an increase in the reporting and detection of lymphoma. While the median age at diagnosis for NHL is in the sixth and seventh decades, certain subtypes such as primary mediastinal B cell lymphoma (PMBL) and Burkitt lymphoma (BL) occur in much younger populations. NHL is more common in Western countries and different subtypes have particular geographic predilections.

PATHOGENESIS AND MOLECULAR CHARACTERIZATION

For different NHL subtypes, cytogenetics, gene rearrangement, and molecular markers are closely associated with histogenesis, and mechanisms of lymphomagenesis. Tumor clonality may be assessed by immunoglobulin (Ig) gene rearrangement in B cells and by T cell–receptor (TCR) rearrangement in T cells. Cytogenetics and/or oncogene rearrangement by polymerase chain reaction (PCR) may also be useful to assess clonality. However, the absence of clonality does not exclude a malignant lymphoid process, whereas the presence of clonality does not always confirm it.

Several chromosomal translocations are strongly associated with different subtypes of NHL (Tables 28.1 and 28.2). The main cytogenetic abnormality that occurs in follicular lymphoma is the t(14;18) translocation with rearrangement and overexpression of the antiapoptotic gene bcl-2, which is present in over 85% of follicular lymphomas (2). Diffuse large B cell lymphoma (DLBCL) is characterized by various molecular abnormalities that include the overexpression of bcl-2 and the transcription factor bcl-6 (3). Virtually all cases of mantle cell lymphomas (MCL) contain the t(11;14) with cyclin D1 overexpression, which promotes progression from G_1 to S phase of the cell cycle (3). The commonly associated translocations seen in BL are the t(8;14), t(2;8), and t(8;22), which places the c-myc gene under the immunoglobulin heavy chain promoter (see Table 28.1) (3).

Immunodeficiency or immune dysregulation is a major risk factor for the development of NHL. Examples of this include HIV infection, iatrogenic immune suppression (post organ transplant), congenital immune deficiencies, and chronic autoimmune diseases (rheumatoid arthritis, Sjogren's syndrome, and Hashimoto's thyroiditis). Infectious agents have also been implicated as risk factors; Epstein-Barr virus (EBV) is associated with many lymphomas including endemic BL, angioimmunoblastic T cell lymphoma (AILT), extranodal NK/T cell lymphoma, and AIDS-related lymphomas (ARLs); Kaposi sarcoma–associated herpesvirus (KSHV, also known as human herpesvirus-8 or HHV-8) is etiologically linked to primary effusion lymphomas and multicentric Castleman disease; and human retrovi-

TABLE 28.1. *Molecular characteristics of B cell lymphomas*

Histology	Cytogenetics	Oncogene/ protein	Ig gene rearrangements
			Heavy κγ
Chronic lymphocytic leukemia/small lymphocytic lymphoma	Trisomy 12[a]; deletions of 13q14 and 11q22–23	—	+ +
Lymphoplasmacytoid lymphoma/Waldenström macroglobulinemia	t(9;14)	PAX-5 gene	+ +
Follicular[b]	t(14;18)	BCL-2	+ / −
Marginal zone[c]	Trisomy 3, t(11;18)	—	+ / −
Mantle cell lymphoma	t(11;14)	BCL–1/cyclin D1	+ / −
Diffuse large B cell[d]	t(14;18), 3q27, 17p	BCL-2, BCL-6, P53	+ +
Primary mediastinal B cell lymphoma	Gains 9p	REL gene, MAL gene overexpression	+ +
Lymphoblastic lymphoma/ leukemia	t(9;22), t(12;21), t(1;19)	BCR/ABL, TEL/ AML1, PBX/E2A	+ ±
Burkitt lymphoma	t(8;14)(q24;q32), t(2;8)(11p; q24), t(8;22)(q24;q11)	C-MYC	+ +

[a]Trisomy 12 is seen in 30% of cases and abnormalities in 13q are present in 25% of patients.
[b]t(14;18) is present in 75% to 95% of FL.
[c]Cytogenetic abnormalities have been seen in extranodal MZ NHL.
[d]Bcl-2 rearrangements in up to 30% and Bcl-6 in up to 45% of cases of DLBCL.

ruses such as human T cell lymphoma virus 1 (HTLV-1) is linked to adult T cell leukemia/lymphoma. Infectious agents have also been implicated in lymphomagenesis through stimulating B cell clones: examples include hepatitis C virus and splenic marginal zone lymphomas, *Helicobacter pylori* and gastric mucosa-associated lymphoid tissue (MALT) lymphoma, as well as chlamydia psittaci and ocular MALT lymphomas. Environmental and occupational exposures, especially organic compounds (organophosphate insecticides), have also been etiologically linked to the development of lymphoma.

TABLE 28.2. *Molecular characteristics of T cell lymphomas*

Histology	Cytogenetics	Oncoprotein	TCR gene rearrangements
T-CLL/T-PLL	Inv14(q11;q32), Trisomy 8q	Bcl-3	+
Mycosis fungoides			+
Peripheral T cell lymphoma unspecified	Loss of 9p,5q, 12q, Zap70		+
Angioimmunoblastic T cell lymphoma[a]	Trisomy 3 or 5, EBV+		+
ATL	HTLV-1 integration+		+
Enteropathy T cell	EBV+		β+
Hepatosplenic γ/Δ			δγ+
Systemic ALCL[b,c]	t(2;5)	Alk+	+
Precursor T-lymphoblastic lymphoma/leukemia	Variable t(7;9)	Tcl-4	Variable

TCR, T cell–receptor; CLL, chronic lymphocytic leukemia; PLL, prolymphocytic leukemia; ATL, adult T cell lymphoma/leukemia; EBV, Epstein-Barr virus; ALCL, anaplastic large cell lymphoma.
[a]TCR gene rearrangement is present in 75% and IgH in 10%.
[b]TCR gene rearrangement in 60%+.
[c]Alk: ALK gene.

CLASSIFICATION OF NON-HODGKIN LYMPHOMAS

Lymphomas are classified according to the World Health Organization (WHO) classification system (3). This classification evolved from an international collaboration of pathologists and clinicians and is based on various insights into the molecular pathogenesis of lymphoma, including the identification of hallmark genetic abnormalities. NHLs are broadly classified as B cell lymphomas or T cell lymphomas depending on the lymphocyte lineage giving rise to the tumor. Within each lineage or category of cell of origin, malignancies are described and defined by morphologic features, immunophenotype, genotype, and clinical behavior.

Staging for Non-Hodgkin Lymphoma

- Staging evaluation of NHL should include a complete history and physical examination and clinical laboratory assessment of organ function. In addition, viral serology for HIV, HTLV-1, and hepatitis B and C viruses needs to be considered if indicated by risk or by lymphoma subtype.
- Routine blood tests, including lactate dehydrogenase (LDH), should be performed.
- T cell subset analysis (e.g., CD4 cell count) should be done if the patient is HIV-positive.
- Radiologic evaluation should include chest x-ray and computerized tomographic scans of chest, abdomen, and pelvis. FDG positron emission tomography (PET) scans are useful in certain scenarios as discussed later.

Staging procedures

- Bone marrow (BM) aspirate and biopsy
- Lumbar puncture with cytology and flow cytometry in patients deemed at increased risk for central nervous system (CNS) disease—this includes all patients with BL or ARL and DLBCLs with several or specific extranodal sites of disease such as bone marrow or testis.
- The Ann Arbor staging system, originally designed for Hodgkin lymphoma, is widely used in the staging of NHL. However due to the tremendous heterogeneity of NHL and the lack of contiguous orderly spread from one lymph node region to another in these diseases, this staging system is of limited prognostic value (Table 28.3).

Diagnostic Confirmation by Tissue Biopsy

The single most useful diagnostic test for a patient with suspected lymphoma is a properly evaluated, technically adequate excisional lymph node biopsy and optimal pathologic evaluation usually requires an entire lymph node. Needle biopsies may yield inadequate tissue for diagnosis and should be avoided. Important studies for diagnostic confirmation often include assessment of clonality, immunophenotyping, cytogenetic analysis, and molecular studies. Oncogene rearrangement and/or overexpression of oncoproteins can also be diagnostically useful:

- t(8;14) or c-myc in Burkitt lymphoma
- t(14;18) or bcl-2 in follicular lymphoma
- t(2;5) or anaplastic lymphoma kinase (ALK) in anaplastic large-cell lymphoma
- t(11;14) or bcl-1/cyclin D1 in MCL
- Trisomy 3 or trisomy 18 (marginal zone lymphoma)
- Some tumors (e.g., T cell–rich B cell lymphoma or lymphomatoid granulomatosis) have an excess of reactive T cells that may obscure the minority of diagnostic malignant B cells if inadequate tissue is obtained.

Restaging for Response Evaluation

- On completion of therapy, staging studies should be repeated (CT scanning and bone marrow biopsy if positive previously). FDG-PET scanning is useful for the evaluation of residual masses at the completion of therapy. It may also be useful at initial staging and when performed during therapy to predict therapeutic outcome.

TABLE 28.3. *Staging classification of lymphoma*

Stage	Ann Arbor classification	Cotswold modification
I	Involvement of a single lymph node region (I) or of a single extralymphatic organ or site (I_E)	Involvement of a single lymph node region or lymphoid structure
II	Involvement of two or more lymph node regions on the same side of the diaphragm alone (II) or with involvement of limited, contiguous extralymphatic organ or tissue (II_E)	Involvement of two or more lymph node regions on the same side of the diaphragm (the mediastinum is considered a single site, whereas the hilar lymph nodes are considered bilaterally); the number of anatomic sites should be indicated by a subscript (e.g., II_3)
III	Involvement of lymph node regions on both sides of the diaphragm (III), which may include the spleen (III_S); a limited contiguous extralymphatic organ or site (III_E); or both (III_{ES})	Involvement of lymph node regions on both sides of the diaphragm: III_1 (with or without involvement of splenic hilar, celiac, or portal nodes) and III_2 (with involvement of para-aortic, iliac, and mesenteric nodes)
IV	Multiple or disseminated foci of involvement of one or more extralymphatic organs or tissues, with or without lymphatic involvement	Involvement of one or more extranodal sites in addition to a site for which the designation E has been used

Note: All cases are subclassified to indicate the absence (A) or presence (B) of the systemic symptoms of significant fever [>38.0°C (100.4°F)], night sweats, and unexplained weight loss exceeding 10% of normal body weight within the previous 6 months. The clinical stage (CS) denotes the stage as determined by all diagnostic examinations and a single diagnostic biopsy only. In the Ann Arbor classification, the term pathologic stage (PS) is used if a second biopsy of any kind has been obtained, whether negative or positive. In the Cotswold modification, the PS is determined by laparotomy; X designates bulky disease (widening of the mediastinum by more than one-third or the presence of a nodal mass >10 cm), and E designates involvement of a single extranodal site that is contiguous or proximal to the known nodal site.

Prognostic Features

- Prognostic assessment and modeling: The International Prognostic Index (IPI) has been applied to untreated aggressive lymphoma (Table 28.4). It is based on an international project that correlated clinical variables and outcome in 2,031 patients with untreated aggressive lymphoma.
- There are five clinical factors that make up the IPI and 1 point is assigned for each feature. The 5-year survivals were 73%, 51%, 43%, and 26% for scores of 0 to 1, 2, 3, and 4 to 5 respectively. The factors are:
  - Age >60 years
  - Eastern Cooperative Oncology Group (ECOG) performance status 2 or higher
  - LDH level greater than normal
  - Two or more extranodal sites
  - Ann Arbor stage III or IV disease

TABLE 28.4. *International Prognostic Index for aggressive non-Hodgkin lymphoma*

Risk category	IPI score	CR rate (%)	5-year disease-free survival (%)	5-year survival (%)
Low	0 or 1	87	70	73
Low-intermediate	2	67	50	51
High-intermediate	3	55	49	43
High	4 or 5	44	40	26

CR, complete response; ECOG, Eastern Cooperative Oncology Group; IPI, International Prognostic Index; LDH, lactate dehydrogenase.

One point is given for the presence of each of the following characteristics: age >60 years, elevated serum LDH level, ECOG performance status ≥2, Ann Arbor stage III or IV, and more than two extranodal sites.

TABLE 28.5. *Follicular Lymphoma International Prognostic Index*

Risk category	FLIPI score[a]	5-year survival (%)	10-year survival (%)
Low	0 or 1	91	71
Intermediate	2	78	51
High	3 or more	52	36

[a]One point is given for the presence of each of the following characteristics: age >60 years, elevated serum LDH level, hemoglobin level <12.0 g/dL, Ann Arbor stage III or IV, and number of involved nodal areas >4.

A validated clinical prognostic index has also been applied to patients with untreated follicular lymphoma. The Follicular Lymphoma International Prognostic Index (FLIPI) is based on patient age, disease stage, serum LDH level, hemoglobin value, and the number of nodal areas, and it has been found to reliably predict survival (Table 28.5).

- Gene expression profiling is emerging as an important prognostic tool in NHL. In DLBCL the gene expression of morphologically similar tumors can show marked heterogeneity and can be classified into gene signatures that correspond to the cellular origin of the lymphoma. Based on these signatures, DLBCL can be divided into at least three different subtypes: germinal center B cell (GCB), activated B cell (ABC), and PMBL (4). The overall survival (OS) is different in each group—patients with the GCB gene expression patterns have a better prognosis compared to the ABC type (5). Immunohistochemistry may be used to predict GCB and non-GCB subtypes of DLBCL but these techniques require further refinement and validation in prospective clinical trials.
- The gene expression profile of BL has been elucidated recently and has demonstrated that molecular profiling identifies cases of BL that have been histologically classified as DLBCL (6). Given the difference in treatment strategies for BL and DLBCL, techniques that enhance the accuracy of diagnostic distinction between BL and DLBCL are important in ensuring optimal therapy of these diseases. Gene expression profiling has also generated survival predictors in MCL, chronic lymphocytic leukemia, and T cell lymphomas (7–9). Although molecular profiling at this time is largely an experimental technique that is not widely available, it promises to improve pathologic diagnostic accuracy and predict outcome with greater precision. In addition, it can elucidate lymphomagenesis pathways, thus identifying pertinent cellular targets and therefore paving the way for more individualized therapy.

Management of Indolent Lymphomas

B Cell

Follicular lymphoma: After DLBCL, this is the second most prevalent subtype of NHL and constitutes 35% of NHL in adults in the United States (3). Patients are typically older and have disseminated disease at diagnosis. During the course of the illness, transformation from follicular to large-cell lymphoma occurs in 35% of patients and overall median survival is approximately 10 years (3).

Follicular lymphoma is graded (1–3) according to the number of centroblasts per high power field. Histologic grade has been correlated with prognosis but is poorly reproducible. Clinical approaches to grades 1 to 3A are similar, whereas grade 3B is considered a variant of DLBCL for the purposes of treatment and is curable with treatment.

Patients with early-stage FL may achieve prolonged remissions (and possibly cure?) with radiation treatment alone, either utilizing involved field or extended field irradiation. In early-stage FL, radiation treatment has an OS of over 60% at 10 years, and there is no clear evidence that extended field irradiation improves OS. In addition, late onset radiation-induced toxicities and second primary cancers remain a concern and are increased with more extensive radiation fields (10). However, in a recent report from the Stanford group on patients with early-stage disease, there was no difference in survival when "watching and waiting" or deferring therapy was compared to early intervention (11).

As grades 1 to 3A follicular lymphoma are considered incurable, several different therapeutic approaches are reasonable. For selected patients, deferred therapy is reasonable. There are many effective systemic therapies for follicular lymphoma ranging from single-agent chemotherapy (fludarabine, cyclophosphamide) to a variety of combination chemotherapy regimens. Rituximab, the monoclonal antibody against CD20 is very effective in follicular lymphoma with response rates of up to 73% in untreated patients and 43% in patients with relapsed or refractory disease (12,13). For patients who previously responded to rituximab, the response rate with retreatment is 40% (14). Chemotherapy regimens with rituximab are very effective and can produce durable responses. In a randomized study of CHOP with or without rituximab for the treatment of newly diagnosed advanced-stage follicular lymphoma, the addition of rituximab was associated with a significant higher response rate and survival benefit (15). Rituximab also has a potential role in maintenance therapy where it may improve progression-free survival (16).

Radioimmunotherapy has been investigated in and is approved for use in relapsed or refractory follicular lymphoma. It involves the delivery of targeted radiotherapy to tumor tissue by conjugating an anti-CD20 antibody to either yttrium-90 (ibritumomab tiuxetan) or iodine-131 (tositumomab). In a randomized trial of relapsed or refractory follicular or transformed lymphoma, the overall response rate was better with ibritumomab tiuxetan than with rituximab (80% vs. 56%) (17). Radioimmunotherapy is also being investigated in combination with systemic chemotherapy.

B-chronic lymphocytic leukemia/small lymphocytic lymphoma (SLL): SLL represents the nonleukemic equivalent of CLL and both diseases are biologically related. Most patients are elderly. Whereas all patients with CLL have peripheral blood and marrow involvement at diagnosis, SLL can be diagnosed in the absence of marrow or peripheral blood disease. The treatment of these diseases is similar to that of follicular lymphoma with fludarabine and rituximab having important therapeutic roles.

Lymphoplasmacytoid lymphoma/Waldenström macroglobulinemia: This is an indolent lymphoma composed of mature plasmacytoid lymphocytes that produce monoclonal IgM. It primarily affects older patients and sites of involvement include bone marrow and spleen. Paraproteinemia with IgM and hyperviscosity symptoms may occur. Treatment is usually initiated when patients become symptomatic and the therapeutic approach is similar to that of other indolent B cell lymphomas with purine analogs and rituximab having important therapeutic roles.

Marginal zone lymphoma: Extranodal marginal zone B cell lymphomas of mucosa-associated lymphoid tissue (MALT lymphoma) make up 7% to 8% of all B cell lymphomas and many of these are primary gastric lymphomas (3). They occur in the gastrointestinal tract, salivary glands, thyroid gland, lungs, ocular adnexae, breast, and other extranodal sites and most patients present with early-stage disease. A past history of a chronic inflammatory disorder like *Helicobacter*-associated chronic gastritis or Sjögren syndrome is common. In a small minority of patients with gastric MALT lymphomas who have superficial, node-negative disease, sustained remissions have been observed after *Helicobacter* eradication with antibiotic therapy (18). Otherwise, these tumors are sensitive to chemotherapy, rituximab, or radiotherapy, alone or in combination; treatment of early-stage disease can result in long remissions. MALT lymphomas tend to run an indolent course, remaining localized for long periods of time. Nodal marginal zone lymphoma is a rare, indolent primary nodal B cell neoplasm and is considered the nodal counterpart of MALT lymphoma.

Finally, splenic marginal zone lymphoma, considered a separate entity in the WHO classification, involves the spleen, splenic hilar lymph nodes, marrow, and peripheral blood. Characterized by an indolent course, it is classically often treated with splenectomy; however, rituximab may ultimately replace this approach.

T Cell

Cutaneous T cell lymphomas: These include mycosis fungoides (MF), Sézary syndrome, primary cutaneous ALCL, and lymphomatoid papulosis. MF is a cutaneous T cell lymphoma characterized by multiple cutaneous plaques, nodules, and/or generalized erythroderma. Nodal involvement and leukemic phases (Sézary syndrome) are late occurrences.

The disease may be relatively indolent over prolonged periods of time, but in older patients with advanced-stage disease, the prognosis is poor and survival short. In MF, a variety of active treatments are available for good-prognosis disease, but the extent to which outcomes are related to therapy or to the natural history of the disease is often not well documented. Reported treatments include low-dose oral methotrexate, topical bexarotene gel, topical gel formulation combining methotrexate and laurocapram, and topical nitrogen mustard. Combined-modality therapy, including subcutaneous interferon-α and oral isotretinoin followed by total-skin electron beam therapy and long-term maintenance therapy with topical nitrogen mustard and interferon-α, has been reported as being useful.

Extracorporeal photopheresis with or without other modalities has been reported. Patients with progressive disease and those with systemic dissemination may be treated with methotrexate and corticosteroids, although responses are usually poor and transient. Novel agents for this disease include the synthetic retinoid X receptor–selective retinoid bexarotene, the fusion toxin denileukin diftitox; and histone deacetlyase inhibitors.

Primary cutaneous ALCL affects the skin; this disease is distinct from systemic ALCL. In cases of localized skin involvement, skin-directed therapies can be used; extracutaneous disease requires more aggressive therapies. Lymphomatoid papulosis usually runs a benign course and sometimes requires therapies such as low-dose methotrexate.

Aggressive Non-Hodgkin Lymphomas

B Cell Lymphoma

Diffuse large B cell lymphoma: DLBCL represents the most prevalent histologic subtype of NHL and compromises 30% to 40% of these diseases (3). Though the median age at diagnosis is in the seventh decade, DLBCL affects children and adults of all ages. Several morphological variants have been identified which include centroblastic, immunoblastic, T cell–rich/histiocyte-rich, and anaplastic. There are several clinical and pathologic variants of DLBCL and extranodal involvement is seen in 40% of cases. Certain subtypes are associated with specific clinical patterns of presentation and natural histories. For example, PMBL is usually seen in young women with disease typically localized to the mediastinum. It is important to recognize that DLBCL can arise de novo or as a result of histologic transformation from an indolent lymphoma. Though this differentiation may not affect treatment choice initially, it does affect prognosis and should be recognized at diagnosis.

Radiation therapy alone is inadequate treatment for DLBCL and is associated with high rates of recurrence, locally and distally. Hence, all stages of disease require at least systemic chemotherapy. For early-stage disease, the benefit of adding radiation therapy to chemotherapy is controversial. Combined-modality therapy became standard following a randomized study that showed a survival advantage of limited-course CHOP plus involved field radiation over full-course CHOP in early-stage (I/II) aggressive lymphoma (19). However, this standard was questioned when longer follow-up showed a convergence of the OS curves because of increased late systemic relapses in the combined-modality arm. A prospective Group d'Etade des Lymphomas l'Adulte study of 576 patients with early-stage aggressive lymphoma, randomized to receive CHOP alone (four cycles) or CHOP plus radiation, demonstrated that combined-modality therapy was not superior to chemotherapy alone. In view of these results as well as the improved outcome of rituximab with CHOP (R-CHOP), radiation therapy should not be routinely recommended for early-stage disease (20).

One exception to this recommendation may be in the treatment of patients with PMBL following chemotherapy, where there may be some role for radiation therapy depending on the chemotherapy regimen used: however, recent results using dose-adjusted EPOCH with rituximab suggest that radiation may not be required for most patients who receive this regimen, thus eliminating the risk of long-term toxicities (21).

Advanced-stage DLBCL is treated with systemic chemotherapy. The CHOP regimen was developed over 30 years ago and a randomized trial established it as the standard, based on it demonstrating equivalent efficacy to other more toxic regimens. Since then, different regimens have been developed in an attempt to improve the outcome of this disease and define a new standard for the treatment of DLBCL. The study that has had the most significant impact on practice was performed by the GELA, which found that patients with DLBCL over 60 years of age were randomized to receive CHOP or R-CHOP and the results demonstrated that patients who received R-CHOP had a higher 5-year event-free survival (47% vs. 29%) (22,23). The benefit of adding rituximab to CHOP was further validated in the U.S. Intergroup study, performed in a similar patient population and the MabThera International Trial (MINT) study, which randomized good-prognosis patients under 60 years of age to receive CHOP or a CHOP-like regimen with or without rituximab (24). Dose-adjusted EPOCH-R is another regimen that has shown promising results in phase 2 studies and is currently being compared to R-CHOP in a randomized CALGB study (25). More recently, dose-dense CHOP (given every 2 weeks) versus CHOP given every 3 weeks, with or without the addition of etoposide (CHOEP vs. CHOP), was evaluated in young as well as older patients (26,27). Young patients with good-prognosis aggressive lymphomas had better survival with the addition of etoposide. In elderly patients, better results were seen with dose-dense CHOP, but not with CHOEP (Table 28.6).

There is no proven role for high-dose chemotherapy and autologous stem cell transplantation (SCT) in the initial treatment of DLBCL. High-dose chemotherapy is also associated with late toxicities such as leukemia and secondary myelodysplasia.

Primary central nervous system lymphoma (PCNSL): PCNSL is a rare, highly aggressive lymphoma confined to the CNS that is usually of DLBCL histology. It may occur de novo or in the setting of immunosuppression, as with HIV infection. It usually presents with multifocal intracranial disease in patients who are HIV infected and with solitary disease in HIV-negative patients. The treatment of this entity is different from that of systemic DLBCL as many of the chemotherapy agents used in systemic disease do not cross the blood-brain barrier and therefore may not be very effective except where there is disruption of the barrier by lymphoma. High-dose methotrexate (HD-MTX) remains the cornerstone of most chemotherapy regimens in PCNSL, but when used alone, it produces a progression-free survival of just over 12 months (28). Radiation therapy itself is also effective in achieving tumor response, but responses tend to be short-lived and almost all patients ultimately relapse. The combination of these two modalites (HD-MTX followed by whole brain radiotherapy, WBRT) is associated with a CR rate of up to 88% and median progression-free survival rates of approximately 3 years (29). However, chemotherapy followed by radiation is associated with severe long-term neurotoxicity and for this reason there has been much interest in developing regimens that may obviate or defer the need for radiation until relapse (30).

Burkitt lymphoma: BL is the most aggressive lymphoma and constitutes 3% to 5% of all lymphomas. It is characterized by a very high tumor proliferation rate and spontaneous cell death, clinically presenting with an acute onset and rapid progression of symptoms. Phenotypically, BL cells are CD20-positive, CD10-positive, and TdT-negative, consistent with a germinal center origin, which has been confirmed by gene expression profiling. This disease was initially identified in equatorial Africa, where it was found to be associated with EBV and translocation of the c-myc oncogene, now regarded as endemic BL. This subtype typically affects young children and often presents with jaw and facial bone disease. BL occurs in the sporadic form in Western countries, predominantly affecting children and young adults. It usually presents with bulky abdominal disease, extranodal involvement of the GI tract, particularly ileocecal disease, and is associated with EBV in 30% to 50% of cases. Immunodeficiency-associated BL usually

TABLE 28.6. *Regimens for initial treatment of DLBCL*

Therapy	Patient group	Survival	Reference
R-CHOP (GELA)	Age ≥60 yr; all IPI	EFS: 47% at 5 yr OS: 58% at 5 yr	23
R-CHOP (U.S. Inter-group)	Age ≥60 yr; all IPI	FFS: 53% at 3 yr	24
R-CHOP–like (MINT)	Age ≤60 yr; low IPI	EFS: 79% at 3 yr OS: 93% at 3 yr	53
ACVBP	Age ≥60 yr; at least 1 IPI factor	EFS: 39% at 5 yr	54
		OS: 46% at 5 yr	54
DA-EPOCH-R	Age ≥18 yr; all IPI	PFS: 82% at 43 mo OS: 79% at 43 mo	25
CHOEP-21	Age 18–60 yr; good-prognosis disease	EFS: 69.2% at 5 yr	26
CHOP-14	Age 61–75 yr; all IPI	EFS: 43.8% at 5 yr OS: 53% at 5 yr	27
R-CHOP-14	Age ≥60 yr; all IPI	EFS: 66% at 3 yr OS: 78% at 3 yr	55

occurs in HIV-positive populations, is associated with nodal disease, and is variably associated with EBV. CNS involvement is not uncommon, particularly when there is bulky or disseminated disease.

Therapy for BL must be instituted rapidly due to the very high tumor proliferation rate of BL, which led to the development of dose-intense regimens with a short cycle time, theoretically to minimize tumor regrowth between cycles. Examples of these regimens include the French LMB and German Berlin-Frankfurt-Munster (BFM) protocols and the National Cancer Institute CODOX-M/IVAC regimen (31–33). With the goal of improving the therapeutic index of BL and minimizing treatment-related toxicity, regimens such as DA-EPOCH-R are being investigated and results thus far are promising (34).

Mantle cell lymphoma: MCL is a distinct subtype of B cell lymphoma that occurs at a median age of 60 years and has a male preponderance. MCL has attributes of both indolent and aggressive lymphomas, namely the lack of curability and a relatively aggressive clinical course with a historical median survival of 3 years or less. This is, however, improving in parallel with the development of more effective upfront therapies. Most patients present with advanced-stage disease, frequently involving the spleen, bone marrow, peripheral blood, and gastrointestinal tract. The blastic variant of MCL is associated with more aggressive disease and a shorter survival. The t(11;14) translocation occurs in almost all cases with overexpression of the cyclin-D1 (bcl-1) gene product (3). Although the overall response rate in MCL is 89% with CHOP, the median OS is merely 37 months (35). Recently, the M.D. Anderson group published their experience with hyper-CVAD and rituximab alternating with high-dose methotrexate and cytarabine in patients with untreated MCL (36). The complete response rate was 87% and a 3-year failure-free survival of 64%. Though this regimen was very effective, it was also associated with considerable toxicity, especially in older patients, leading the authors to not recommend it in patients over 65 years of age.

The role of high-dose chemotherapy and autologous SCT in MCL has been investigated in several phase 2 studies (37). At this time, autologous transplantation has not proven to be a curative strategy and has not demonstrated a significant survival advantage over conventional therapy. Nonmyeloablative allogeneic SCT has also been investigated in MCL and certainly may have a role in patients with recurrent disease (37).

With regard to novel agents, the proteasome inhibitor bortezomib, has shown promising results in patients with relapsed or refractory MCL. In a multicenter study the overall response rate was 33% (38). The mTOR inhibitor temsirolimus has also shown activity in relapsed MCL with a response rate of 38% (39). Other promising strategies include combining rituximab with thalidomide and the use of lenalidomide (40,41).

EBV-associated lymphoproliferative disorders: Several lymphoproliferative disorders are associated EBV infection. Post-transplant lymphoproliferative disorder (PTLD) encompasses a broad spectrum of diseases with varying degrees of clinical aggressiveness and usually occurs following solid organ transplantation. It can be treated by the withdrawal of immunosuppression but rituximab or chemotherapy may be necessary in cases that are resistant to withdrawal of immunosuppression.

HIV-associated lymphomas are typically monoclonal B cell aggressive subtypes, either DLBCL or BL. The incidence of DLBCL is up to 100 times more common and BL up to 1,000 times more common in the setting of HIV infection. Many cases are associated with EBV. Most patients have advanced disease on presentation and often have extranodal sites of involvement. Therapy for HIV-associated lymphomas is dependent on the specific lymphoma subtype, but since highly antiretroviral therapy has become more available, the outcome for these diseases has improved significantly and many subtypes are highly curable. The infusional regimen EPOCH, with HAART suspension, produced a 74% complete response rate and 72% OS at a median-time follow-up of 53 months (42). The role of rituximab is controversial in HIV-associated lymphomas as it has been associated with increased infections (43).

Chronic immunosuppressive drugs such as methotrexate are also associated with an increased incidence of EBV-associated lymphoproliferative disorders. Lymphomatoid granulomatosis is a rare EBV-associated lymphoproliferative disorder that mostly involves extranodal sites. Lymphoproliferative disorders associated with primary immune deficiencies are most commonly seen in the pediatric population. B cell lymphoma is the most common subtype seen although T cell lymphomas are more common in ataxic telangiectasia. These malignancies generally respond poorly to standard therapy.

T Cell Lymphomas

Lymphomas that are derived from T and NK cells are relatively uncommon and only account for approximately 10% to 15% of all NHLs (3). Their incidence varies significantly by geographic location, with an increased frequency in Asia. The natural history of mature T cell and NK cell lymphomas ranges from indolent to aggressive. Unlike aggressive B cell lymphomas, the majority of aggressive T/NK cell lymphomas are incurable. Important exceptions include anaplastic large cell lymphoma (ALCL), which is highly curable when it expresses the ALK fusion protein and early-stage, extranodal, T/NK cell, nasal-type lymphoma (44). The Non-Hodgkin Lymphoma Classification Project examined all newly diagnosed cases of lymphoma over a 2-year period from several different international centers (45). A survival analysis of these cases demonstrated a very poor outcome of PTL compared to DLBCL and ALCL. Slightly more than a quarter of patients with low IPI scores were still alive without disease at 5 years. This contrasted significantly with cases of ALCL where 80% of patients were alive at 5 years, irrespective of the IPI score.

Anaplastic large cell lymphoma: Systemic ALCL (cutaneous ALCL is discussed in an earlier section) is typically a disease of children and young adults and comprises approximately 3% of all lymphomas in adults. ALCL may involve both nodal and extranodal sites, including skin, bone, or soft tissues. Fifty percent of the patients may have constitutional symptoms and advanced stages at presentation. ALCL is associated with the t(2;5)(p23;q35) translocation, resulting in the expression of the nucleophosmin ALK. This is important to consider when discussing treatment as ALK positivity, present in two-thirds of cases, is associated with a better prognosis than ALK-negative disease (44). ALCL responds very well to CHOP-based therapies and has an excellent prognosis with a cure rate of approximately 70%, even in advanced cases.

Extranodal NK/T cell lymphoma, nasal type: This is a very rare, predominantly extranodal lymphoma that is characterized by a broad morphological spectrum. It is prevalent in Asia and Central and South America and is almost always associated with EBV. It has a predilection for the nasal cavity, nasopharynx, palate, skin, gastrointestinal tract, and testis. Disease outside the nasal cavity is usually highly aggressive and associated with a very poor prognosis. Optimal therapy has not been defined due to the rarity of this disease and lack of prospective clinical trials, but the use of involved-field external-beam radiation with or without chemotherapy for early-stage disease confined to the nasal cavity has shown promising results.

Angioimmunoblastic T cell lymphoma: AILT is another rare type of T cell lymphoma that is associated with scattered EBV-positive B cells in biopsy specimens. It occurs in older patients and is characterized by fever, rash, diffuse lymphadenopathy, organomegaly, hemolytic anemia, and polyclonal hypergammaglobulinemia (46). Patients are usually susceptible to opportunistic infections and may develop secondary EBV lymphomas. Most patients actually succumb to these complications rather than die from the disease itself. No optimal therapy has been defined for AILT and it has a low curative potential with conventional-dose chemotherapy. Nonetheless, anthracycline-based regimens and purine analogs are often used, but novel approaches such as the use of cyclosporine have shown some promising activity (47).

Hepatosplenic T cell lymphoma: This is a very rare type of T cell lymphoma that is characterized by a proliferation of clonal cells expressing the γ/δ isotype, isochromosome 7q translocation. It usually presents with marked hepatosplenomegaly and bone marrow involvement. There is typically an absence of peripheral lymphadenopathy and a prior history of immunosuppressive therapy for organ transplant is relatively common. The prognosis of this disease is extremely poor and although patients usually respond to chemotherapy, these responses are short-lived and survival rates are low. Although experimental, patients should be considered for allogeneic transplant in first remission.

Peripheral T cell lymphoma, unspecified (PTL-nos): This is a group of diseases that are not included in other T cell lymphoma categories in the WHO classification. This group of lymphomas is very diverse both morphologically and clinically. Patients usually have a poor outcome with conventional chemotherapy. The poor outcome of PTL-nos has led to the investigation of novel approaches to treat these diseases. Purine analogs are associated with good response rates but unfortunately are rarely curative. Alemtuzumab, a monoclonal antibody that binds to the CD52 antigen, which is expressed on many PTL-nos, has shown activity with a 36% response rate in one series of heavily pretreated patients. At this time several combination studies of alemtuzumab with doxorubicin-based chemotherapy are ongoing (48). Several studies have looked at the role of autologous SCT but the outcome has been poor. Alogeneic transplantation as a therapeutic strategy is also being investigated.

Precursor B and T cell lymphoma: Precursor B-lymphoblastic and T-lymphoblastic lymphomas (LBL) are highly aggressive diseases that are cytologically identical to acute lymphoblastic leukemia. They are usually T cell lymphomas and are more common in adolescent boys or young men. Patients often present with leucocytosis and a large mediastinal mass. Treatment is with regimens that are used for acute leukemia and include CNS prophylaxis.

Salvage Treatment of Relapsed Aggressive Lymphoma

Treatment options for relapsed aggressive DLBCL include salvage chemotherapy and high-dose chemotherapy with autologous or allogeneic SCT. The choice of treatment modality should be individualized and it is important to consider several factors before instituting treatment, such as the timing of relapse in relation to initial therapy, the type of therapy previously used, performance status of patients, and projected tolerance of different therapies.

ICE, ESHAP, and EPOCH are some examples of active salvage chemotherapy regimens used in patients with relapsed or refractory DLBCL, yielding CR rates ranging from 27% to 37% (49–51). The addition of rituximab appears to have enhanced the activity of several salvage regimens. There is a commonly held belief that salvage regimens should include agents that are different from previous therapies to avoid the development of drug resistance. However, recent evidence questions this notion and indicates that drug-specific mechanisms are less important than other determinants of sensitivity to apoptosis as a cause of drug resistance. Therefore, salvage regimens developed around the most active upfront agents should have high activity in relapsed patients.

Patients with chemotherapy-sensitive disease have the best outcome with autologous SCT. This strategy has become standard in many settings at initial relapse and has yielded overall and event-free survivals of 40% to 50% and 30% to 40% respectively (52). As with salvage chemotherapy, the incorporation of rituximab and radioimmunoconjugate therapy into conditioning regimens may be improving outcomes. However, in projecting the outcome of autologous transplantation at relapse, one must consider that improvements in upfront therapy over the past few years, such as the use of more effective regimens and the addition of rituximab, may diminish the relative benefit of autologous SCT in the future. Patients with chemotherapy-resistant disease have a poor outcome with autologous SCT and should be considered for experimental treatments, such as allogeneic SCT. Although most patients relapse with disseminated disease, some relapses may be localized and salvageable with radiation treatment. Two diseases to which this principle may apply are PMBL, which can remain localized even at relapse, and PTLDs, which may sometimes have an isolated resistant EBV clone following chemotherapy.

The salvage therapy of MCL and BL is much less successful and these diseases are rarely curable when at relapse. The outcome for relapsed aggressive T cell lymphomas also tends to be poor with the exception of ALCL that can be successfully salvaged with chemotherapy and/or transplantation.

REFERENCES

1. Jemal A, Siegel R, Ward E, et al. Cancer statistics, 2008. *CA Cancer J Clin.* 2008;58:71–96.
2. Weiss LM, Warnke RA, Sklar J, Cleary ML. Molecular analysis of the t(14;18) chromosomal translocation in malignant lymphomas. *N Engl J Med.* 1987;317:1185–1189.
3. Jaffe ES, Harris NL, Stein H, Vardiman JW. *World Health Organization Classification of Tumours. Pathology and Genetics of Tumours of Hematopoietic and Lymphoid Tissues.* IARC Press: Lyon, 2001.
4. Alizadeh AA, Eisen MB, Davis RE, et al. Distinct types of diffuse large B-cell lymphoma identified by gene expression profiling. *Nature.* 2000;403:503–511.
5. Rosenwald A, Wright G, Chan WC, et al. The use of molecular profiling to predict survival after chemotherapy for diffuse large-B-cell lymphoma. *N Engl J Med.* 2002;346:1937–1947.
6. Dave SS, Fu K, Wright GW, et al. Molecular diagnosis of Burkitt's lymphoma. *N Engl J Med.* 2006;354:2431–2442.

7. Rosenwald A, Alizadeh AA, Widhopf G, et al. Relation of gene expression phenotype to immunoglobulin mutation genotype in B cell chronic lymphocytic leukemia. *J Exp Med.* 2001;194: 1639–1647.

8. Rosenwald A, Wright G, Wiestner A, et al. The proliferation gene expression signature is a quantitative integrator of oncogenic events that predicts survival in mantle cell lymphoma. *Cancer Cell.* 2003;3:185–197.

9. Lamant L, de Reynies A, Duplantier MM, et al. Gene-expression profiling of systemic anaplastic large-cell lymphoma reveals differences based on ALK status and two distinct morphologic ALK+ subtypes. *Blood.* 2007;109:2156–2164.

10. Mac Manus MP, Hoppe RT. Is radiotherapy curative for stage I and II low-grade follicular lymphoma? Results of a long-term follow-up study of patients treated at Stanford University. *J Clin Oncol.* 1996 Apr;14(4):1282–1290.

11. Advani R, Rosenberg SA, Horning SJ. Stage I and II follicular non-Hodgkin's lymphoma: long-term follow-up of no initial therapy. *J Clin Oncol.* 2004;22:1454–1459.

12. Davis TA, White CA, Grillo-Lopez AJ, et al. Single-agent monoclonal antibody efficacy in bulky non-Hodgkin's lymphoma: results of a phase II trial of rituximab. *J Clin Oncol.* 1999;17: 1851–1857.

13. Colombat P, Salles G, Brousse N, et al. Rituximab (anti-CD20 monoclonal antibody) as single first-line therapy for patients with follicular lymphoma with a low tumor burden: clinical and molecular evaluation. *Blood.* 2001;97:101–106.

14. Davis TA, Grillo-Lopez AJ, White CA, et al. Rituximab anti-CD20 monoclonal antibody therapy in non-Hodgkin's lymphoma: safety and efficacy of re-treatment. *J Clin Oncol.* 2000;18:3135–3143.

15. Hiddemann W, Kneba M, Dreyling M, et al. Front-line therapy with rituximab added to the combination of cyclophosphamide, doxorubicin, vincristine and prednisone (CHOP) significantly improves the outcome of patients with advanced stage follicular lymphomas as compared to CHOP alone—results of a prospective randomized study of the german low grade lymphoma study group (GLSG). *Blood.* 2005.

16. Hainsworth JD. Prolonging remission with rituximab maintenance therapy. *Semin Oncol.* 2004; 31:17–21.

17. Witzig TE, Gordon LI, Cabanillas F, et al. Randomized controlled trial of yttrium-90-labeled ibritumomab tiuxetan radioimmunotherapy versus rituximab immunotherapy for patients with relapsed or refractory low-grade, follicular, or transformed B-cell non-Hodgkin's lymphoma. *J Clin Oncol.* 2002 May 15;20(10):2453–2463.

18. Wotherspoon AC, Doglioni C, Diss TC, et al. Regression of primary low-grade B-cell gastric lymphoma of mucosa-associated lymphoid tissue type after eradication of *Helicobacter pylori*. *Lancet.* 1993;342:575–577.

19. Miller TP, Dahlberg S, Cassady JR, et al. Chemotherapy alone compared with chemotherapy plus radiotherapy for localized intermediate- and high-grade non-Hodgkin's lymphoma. *N Engl J Med.* 1998;339:21–26.

20. Bonnet C, Fillet G, Mounier N, et al. CHOP alone compared with CHOP plus radiotherapy for localized aggressive lymphoma in elderly patients: a study by the Groupe d'Etude des Lymphomes de l'Adulte. *J Clin Oncol.* 2007;25:787–792.

21. Dunleavy K, Pittaluga S, Janik J, et al. Primary mediastinal large b-cell lymphoma (PMBL) may be significantly improved by the addition of rituximab to dose-adjusted EPOCH and obviates the need for radiation: results from a prospective study of 44 patients. *Blood* (ASH Annual Meeting Abstracts). 2006;108.

22. Coiffier B, Lepage E, Briere J, et al. CHOP chemotherapy plus rituximab compared with CHOP alone in elderly patients with diffuse large-B-cell lymphoma. *N Engl J Med.* 2002;346:235–242.

23. Feugier P, Van Hoof A, Sebban C, et al. Long-term results of the R-CHOP study in the treatment of elderly patients with diffuse large B-cell lymphoma: a study by the Groupe d'Etude des Lymphomes de l'Adulte. *J Clin Oncol.* 2005;23:4117–4126.

24. Habermann TM, Weller EA, Morrison VA, et al. Rituximab-CHOP versus CHOP alone or with maintenance rituximab in older patients with diffuse large B-cell lymphoma. *J Clin Oncol.* 2006;24:3121–3127.

25. Wilson WH, Dunleavy K, Pittaluga S, et al. Phase II study of dose-adjusted EPOCH and rituximab in untreated diffuse large B-cell lymphoma with analysis of germinal center and post-germinal center biomarkers. *J Clin Oncol.* 2008;26:2717–2724.

26. Pfreundschuh M, Trumper L, Kloess M, et al. Two-weekly or 3-weekly CHOP chemotherapy with or without etoposide for the treatment of young patients with good-prognosis (normal LDH) aggressive lymphomas: results of the NHL-B1 trial of the DSHNHL. *Blood.* 2004;104:626–633.

27. Pfreundschuh M, Trumper L, Kloess M, et al. Two-weekly or 3-weekly CHOP chemotherapy with or without etoposide for the treatment of elderly patients with aggressive lymphomas: results of the NHL-B2 trial of the DSHNHL. *Blood.* 2004;104:634–641.

28. Batchelor T, Carson K, O'Neill A, et al. Treatment of primary CNS lymphoma with methotrexate and deferred radiotherapy: a report of NABTT 96-07. *J Clin Oncol.* 2003;21:1044–1049.

29. Gavrilovic IT, Hormigo A, Yahalom J, DeAngelis LM, Abrey LE. Long-term follow-up of high-dose methotrexate-based therapy with and without whole brain irradiation for newly diagnosed primary CNS lymphoma. *J Clin Oncol.* 2006;24:4570–4574.

30. Pels H, Schmidt-Wolf IG, Glasmacher A, et al. Primary central nervous system lymphoma: results of a pilot and phase II study of systemic and intraventricular chemotherapy with deferred radio-therapy. *J Clin Oncol.* 2003;21:4489–4495.

31. Divine M, Casassus P, Koscielny S, et al. Burkitt lymphoma in adults: a prospective study of 72 patients treated with an adapted pediatric LMB protocol. *Ann Oncol.* 2005;16:1928–1935.

32. Reiter A, Schrappe M, Parwaresch R, et al. Non-Hodgkin's lymphomas of childhood and ado-lescence: results of a treatment stratified for biologic subtypes and stage—a report of the Berlin-Frankfurt-Munster Group. *J Clin Oncol.* 1995;13:359–372.

33. Magrath I, Adde M, Shad A, et al. Adults and children with small non-cleaved-cell lymphoma have a similar excellent outcome when treated with the same chemotherapy regimen. *J Clin Oncol.* 1996;14:925–934.

34. Dunleavy K, Healey Bird BR, Pittaluga S, et al. Efficacy and toxicity of dose-adjusted EPOCH-rituximab in adults with newly diagnosed Burkitt lymphoma. *Journal of Clinical Oncology.* 2007;25.

35. Meusers P, Engelhard M, Bartels H, et al. Multicentre randomized therapeutic trial for advanced centrocytic lymphoma: anthracycline does not improve the prognosis. *Hematol Oncol.* 1989;7:365–380.

36. Romaguera JE, Fayad L, Rodriguez MA, et al. High rate of durable remissions after treatment of newly diagnosed aggressive mantle-cell lymphoma with rituximab plus hyper-CVAD alternating with rituximab plus high-dose methotrexate and cytarabine. *J Clin Oncol.* 2005;23:7013–7023.

37. Jacobsen E, Freedman A. An update on the role of high-dose therapy with autologous or allogeneic stem cell transplantation in mantle cell lymphoma. *Curr Opin Oncol.* 2004;16:106–113.

38. Fisher RI, Bernstein SH, Kahl BS, et al. Multicenter phase II study of bortezomib in patients with relapsed or refractory mantle cell lymphoma. *J Clin Oncol.* 2006;24:4867–4874.

39. Witzig TE, Geyer SM, Ghobrial I, et al. Phase II trial of single-agent temsirolimus (CCI-779) for relapsed mantle cell lymphoma. *J Clin Oncol.* 2005;23:5347–5356.

40. Kaufmann H, Raderer M, Wohrer S, et al. Antitumor activity of rituximab plus thalidomide in pa-tients with relapsed/refractory mantle cell lymphoma. *Blood.* 2004;104:2269–2271.

41. Wiernik PH, Lossos IS, Tuscano JM, et al. Lenalidomide monotherapy in relapsed or refractory aggressive non-Hodgkin's lymphoma. *J Clin Oncol.* 2008;26:4952–4957.

42. Little RF, Pittaluga S, Grant N, et al. Highly effective treatment of acquired immunodeficiency syndrome-related lymphoma with dose-adjusted EPOCH: impact of antiretroviral therapy suspen-sion and tumor biology. *Blood.* 2003;101:4653–4659.

43. Kaplan LD, Lee JY, Ambinder RF, et al. Rituximab does not improve clinical outcome in a randomized phase 3 trial of CHOP with or without rituximab in patients with HIV-associated non-Hodgkin lymphoma: AIDS-Malignancies Consortium Trial 010. *Blood.* 2005;106:1538–1543.

44. Gascoyne RD, Aoun P, Wu D, et al. Prognostic significance of anaplastic lymphoma kinase (ALK) protein expression in adults with anaplastic large cell lymphoma. *Blood.* 1999;93:3913–3921.

45. A clinical evaluation of the International Lymphoma Study Group classification of non-Hodgkin's lymphoma. The Non-Hodgkin's Lymphoma Classification Project. *Blood.* 1997;89:3909–3918.

46. Dunleavy K, Wilson WH, Jaffe ES. Angioimmunoblastic T cell lymphoma: pathobiological insights and clinical implications. *Curr Opin Hematol.* 2007;14:348–353.
47. Advani R, Horwitz S, Zelenetz A, Horning SJ. Angioimmunoblastic T cell lymphoma: treatment experience with cyclosporine. *Leuk Lymphoma.* 2007;48:521–525.
48. Enblad G, Hagberg H, Erlanson M, et al. A pilot study of alemtuzumab (anti-CD52 monoclonal antibody) therapy for patients with relapsed or chemotherapy-refractory peripheral T-cell lymphomas. *Blood.* 2004;103:2920–2924.
49. Moskowitz CH, Bertino JR, Glassman JR, et al. Ifosfamide, carboplatin, and etoposide: a highly effective cytoreduction and peripheral-blood progenitor-cell mobilization regimen for transplant-eligible patients with non-Hodgkin's lymphoma. *J Clin Oncol.* 1999;17:3776–3785.
50. Velasquez WS, McLaughlin P, Tucker S, et al. ESHAP—an effective chemotherapy regimen in refractory and relapsing lymphoma: a 4-year follow-up study. *J Clin Oncol.* 1994;12:1169–1176.
51. Gutierrez M, Chabner BA, Pearson D, et al. Role of a doxorubicin-containing regimen in relapsed and resistant lymphomas: an 8-year follow-up study of EPOCH. *J Clin Oncol.* 2000;18:3633–3642.
52. Shipp MA, Abeloff MD, Antman KH, et al. International consensus conference on high-dose therapy with hematopoietic stem cell transplantation in aggressive non-Hodgkin's lymphomas: report of the jury. *J Clin Oncol.* 1999;17:423–429.
53. Pfreundschuh M, Trimper L, Osterborg A, et al. CHOP-like chemotherapy plus rituximab versus CHOP-like chemotherapy alone in young patients with good-prognosis diffuse large B cell lymphoma: A randomized controlled trial by the MabThera International Trial group. *Lancet Oncol.* 2006;7:379–391.
54. Tilly H, Lepage E, Coiffer B, et al. Intensive conventional chemotherapy (ACVBP regimen) compared with standard CHOP for proor-prognosis aggressive non-Hodgkin lymphoma. *Blood.* 2003;102:4284–4289.
55. Pfreundschuh M, Schubert J, Ziepert M, et al. Six versus eight cycles of bi-weekly CHOIP-14 with or without rituximab in elderly patients with aggressive CD201 B cell lymphomas: A randomized controlled trial (RICOVER-60). *Lancet Oncol.* 2008;9:105–116.

29

Hodgkin Lymphoma

Ayman Saad, Michael Craig, and Wyndham H. Wilson

EPIDEMIOLOGY

Hodgkin lymphoma (HL) is a common lymphoid malignancy of young adults. It represents about 11% of all lymphomas. The annual incidence of HL is 3.2 per 100,000 individuals. Unlike non-Hodgkin lymphoma, HL incidence has not increased over the past decades. It affects males only slightly more often than females (1.3:1 ratio). In the United States, it affects people of European descent more than those of African descent. It has a bimodal age distribution with the first peak in third decade (earlier age in developing countries) and a second peak after the age of 50 years.

ETIOLOGY AND RISK FACTORS

The etiology of HL is unclear.

- Epstein-Barr virus (EBV) infection increases the risk of classical HL (particularly mixed cellularity type) by twofold to threefold. Tumor cells of HL are positive for EBV in about 50% of patients in Western countries and in up to 90% of patients in developing countries.
- HIV infection increases risk of classical HL by 5- to 10-fold.
- Family history of classical HL increases risk to develop disease by threefold to ninefold. No heritable genetic abnormality has been identified.

PATHOLOGY

HL is a neoplastic disease of B-cell origin. It is characterized by the presence of multinucleated giant cells, Reed-Sternberg (RS) cells, amidst an inflammatory background that is composed of lymphocytes, eosinophils, monocytes, and histiocytes.

RS cells are derived from the germinal B cell center and they constitute ≤1% of the affected tissues. They often exhibit two mirror-image nuclei (owl's eyes appearance) (Fig. 29.1).

Pathological Classification

The World Health Organization (WHO) classified HL based on histopathological and immunophenotypic features (Table 29.1) into:

- Classical HL
- Nodular lymphocyte predominant HL (NLPHL)

Table 29.2 summarizes the clinical pathological features of the disease subtypes.

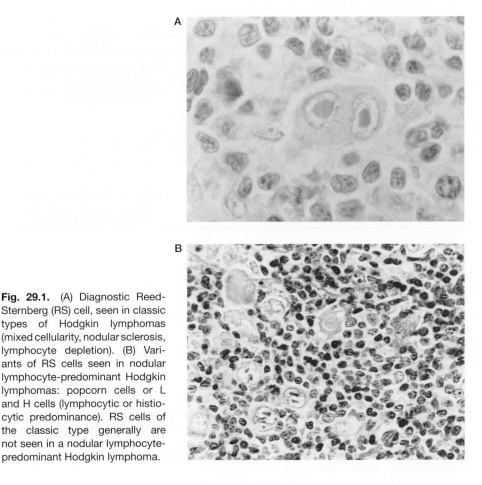

Fig. 29.1. (A) Diagnostic Reed-Sternberg (RS) cell, seen in classic types of Hodgkin lymphomas (mixed cellularity, nodular sclerosis, lymphocyte depletion). (B) Variants of RS cells seen in nodular lymphocyte-predominant Hodgkin lymphomas: popcorn cells or L and H cells (lymphocytic or histiocytic predominance). RS cells of the classic type generally are not seen in a nodular lymphocyte-predominant Hodgkin lymphoma.

CLINICAL FEATURES

- Lymphadenopathy: commonly cervical, axillary, or mediastinal. Enlarged nodes are not tender with a characteristic firm rubbery consistency. Lymph node pain may occasionally be precipitated by alcohol intake.
- B symptoms
  - Unexplained weight loss (>10% body weight over 6 months before diagnosis)
  - Fever of >38°C, intermittent with 1- to 2-week cycles

TABLE 29.1. *Immunophenotypic features of Hodgkin lymphoma*

	Classical type	Nodular lymphocyte predominant
CD45	Negative	Positive
CD30	Positive	Variable (weak)
CD15	Positive (80% of cases)	Negative
CD20	Variable	Positive

TABLE 29.2. *WHO classification of Hodgkin disease*

Pathologic type	Pathologic features	Clinical features
Nodular sclerosing	Nodular growth pattern with broad bands of fibrosis	Most common type; frequent mediastinal involvement
Mixed cellularity	Numerous RS cells in a rich inflammatory background and fine reticular fibrosis; most often positive for Epstein-Barr virus	Second most common type; can be HIV-associated
Lymphocyte rich	More lymphocytes with paucity of RS cells	Common in elderly; has good prognosis
Lymphocyte depleted	More frequent RS cells with depletion of normal lymphocytes	Rare, commonly seen in elderly; can be HIV-associated; has poor prognosis
Nodular lymphocyte predominant	No RS cells, but characterized by "popcorn" cells (lobulated nucleus)	More common in adult males; early stage with good prognosis, but frequent relapses

- Drenching night sweats
- Pruritis and fatigue are *not* considered "B" symptoms.

Staging

The modified Ann Arbor staging of lymphoma is used to clinically stage HL (Table 29.3).

Diagnostic Evaluation

Excisional biopsy of enlarged lymph node is recommended for initial diagnosis. A core biopsy may be appropriate if adequate to avoid major surgery. A fine-needle aspiration is *not* recommended for initial diagnosis.

Staging laparotomy with splenectomy is no longer performed because chemotherapy is now employed in early disease stages.

TABLE 29.3. *Cotswolds modified Ann Arbor staging of lymphoma*

Stage I	Single lymph node region, lymphoid structure (e.g., spleen, thymus, or Waldeyer ring), or single extralymphatic site (IE)
Stage II	Two or more lymph node regions on the same side of the diaphragm, or localized extranodal extension (contagious to a nodal site) plus one or more nodal regions (IIE).
Stage III	The number of anatomic sites should be indicated by numeric subscript (e.g II_3). Lymph node regions on both sides of the diaphragm. This may be accompanied by localized extranodal site (IIIE), or splenic involvement (IIIS), or both (IIIE+S).
Stage IV	Dissemination to one or more extranodal sites (beyond those designated E) with or without associated nodal involvement.
	Each stage is designated A or B, where B means presence and A means absence of B symptom.
	X: A mass >10 cm or a mediastinal mass larger than one-third of the thoracic diameter.
	E: Extranodal site contiguous or proximal to a known nodal site.

Laboratory Tests

- Complete blood count (CBC): thrombocytosis may be seen.
- Erythrocyte sedimentation rate (ESR): adverse prognostic biomarker, if elevated
- Lactate dehydrogenase (LDH): adverse prognostic biomarker, if elevated
- Liver function tests: If abnormal, may be associated with liver involvement.
- Alkaline phosphatase: May be nonspecifically high or associated with bone involvement.
- Renal function test, electrolytes, and uric acid

Radiologic Studies

- Chest radiograph
- Computerized tomography (CT) scan of the chest, abdomen, and pelvis are required for staging. CT scan of the neck may sometimes be needed.
- Positron emission tomography (PET) scan is useful to evaluate equivocal disease seen in the CT scan and occult disease, including normal size nodes and bone. PET scan is more sensitive than CT scan, but can be falsely positive. The effect of stage migration due to upstaging by PET scan must be considered when discussing prognosis with the patient.

Bone Marrow Biopsy and Aspiration

Required in clinical stage IB, IIB, III, or IV.

Evaluation for Specific Treatments

- Left ventricular ejection fraction using multigated acquisition scan (MUGA scan) or echocardiography before anthracycline treatment should be performed as medically indicated.
- Pulmonary function tests are recommended prior to bleomycin treatment.

Additional Workup/Procedures

- Pregnancy test for female in childbearing age
- HIV test for patients at risk for infection
- Semen cryopreservation: considered for males before chemotherapy or pelvic irradiation
- Oophoropexy for premenopausal females before pelvic irradiation
- Vaccination (pneumococcal, hemophilus influenzae, and meningococcal) prior to splenic irradiation is recommended.

MANAGEMENT

- National statistics have shown significant improvement of the 5-year survival rates of HL over the past four decades. HL is a potentially curable disease, particularly in early stages. Thus, long-term toxicity is a major consideration of treatment.
- Early-stage disease may be treated with radiation alone (in best-prognosis patients); combined-modality chemotherapy and radiation treatment (RT), or chemotherapy alone.
- Advanced-stage disease is usually treated with chemotherapy alone.
- Radiation consolidation may be appropriate to limited sites that are PET positive following a full course of chemotherapy but should be omitted in patients with PET-negative residual masses. Based on pre-PET studies, only routine radiation consolidation in patients with massive (>10 cm or one-third the diameter of the chest on CXR) mediastinal disease appears to impact overall survival; however, radiation consolidation may not be necessary in PET-negative mediastinal masses.

TABLE 29.4. *CALGB study comparing different regimens in Hodgkin lymphoma*

Regimen	Complete response rate (%)	5-year overall survival rate (%)
MOPP	67	66
ABVD	82	73
Alternating MOPP/ABVD	83	75

Principles of Chemotherapy

- The gold standard regimen for HL in the United States is ABVD since it superseded MOPP regimen in the large randomized trial of the Cancer and Leukemia Group B (CALGB) in 1992 (Table 29.4). ABVD regimen was associated with less risk of leukemia and infertility compared to MOPP regimen.
- The German Hodgkin's Lymphoma Study Group (GHLSG) developed the BEACOPP regimen and showed it to be superior to COPP-ABVD in advanced HL. Furthermore, they showed that an increased dose was superior to standard dose BEACOPP but was also more toxic.
- Stanford V is a dose-intense regimen combined with radiation consolidation and may be a less desirable alternative in advanced disease where the survival benefit of radiation is uncertain. Stanford V is given for three cycles in all stages except for stage IA, IIA nonbulky for which only two cycles are used. The cumulative dose of doxorubicin and bleomycin in Stanford V is less than those in ABVD, with potentially less risk for cardiac and pulmonary toxicity.

Chemotherapy regimens are described in Table 29.5.

TABLE 29.5. *Commonly used chemotherapy regimens for Hodgkin lymphoma*

ABVD (every 28 days)	Doxorubicin 25 mg/m²/dose i. v. on day 1 and 15 Bleomycin 10 units/m²/dose i. v. on day 1 and 15 Vinblastine 6 mg/m²/dose i. v. on day 1 and 15 Dacarbazine (DTIC) 375 mg/m²/dose i. v. on day 1 and 15
Standard BEACOPP (every 3 weeks)	Bleomycin 10 IU/m² i. v. on day 8 Etoposide (VP-16) 100 mg/m² i. v. on day 1–3 Doxorubicin (Adriamycin) 25 mg/m² on day 1 Cyclophosphamide (Cytoxan) 650 mg/m² on day 1 Vincristine 1.4 mg/m² (max 2 mg) on day 8 Procarbazine 100 mg/m² PO on day 1–7 Prednisone 40 mg/m² PO on day 1–14
Increased-dose BEACOPP (every 3 weeks)	Bleomycin 10 IU/m² i. v. on day 8 Etoposide (VP-16) 200 mg/m² i. v. on day 1–3 Doxorubicin (Adriamycin) 35 mg/m² on day 1 Cyclophosphamide (Cytoxan) 1,200 mg/m² on day 1 Vincristine 1.4 mg/m² (max 2 mg) on day 8 Procarbazine 100 mg/m² PO on day 1–7 Prednisone 40 mg/m² PO on day 1–14 Filgrastim (G-CSF) support is needed
Stanford V (every 4 weeks) × three cycles (12 weeks)	Nitrogen mustard 6 mg/m² i. v. day 1 Doxorubicin (Adriamycin) 25 mg/m² i. v. day1 and 15 Vinblastine 6 mg/m² i. v. day 1 and 15 Vincristine 1.4 mg/m² i. v. day 8 and 22 (maximum dose is 2 mg/dose). Bleomycin 5 U/m² i. v. day 8 and 22 Etoposide (VP-16) 60 mg/m² i. v. day 15 and 16 Prednisone 40 mg po qod × 10 weeks, then taper by 10 mg every other day between weeks 10 and 12 For patients older than 50, reduce vinblastine to 4 mg/m² and vincristine to 1 mg/m² in cycle 3

Principles of Radiotherapy

- Radiation therapy for HL targets sites with either clinical disease (involved field) or involved *plus* adjacent areas (extended field). Extended fields are either "mantle field" for the cervical, axillary and mediastinal regions or "inverted Y field" for para-aortic and pelvic regions (Fig. 29.2). One or both extended fields were popularly used as RT monotherapy based on the principle that HL spreads to contagious lymph nodes.

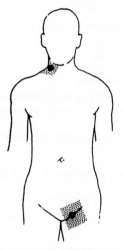

A Involved field irradiation

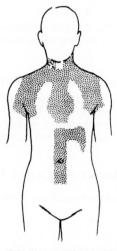

B Subtotal nodal irradiation including mantle and spade fields

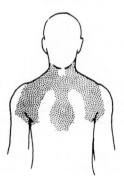

C Mantle field irradiation

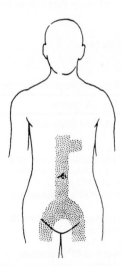

D Inverted-Y field irradiation

Fig. 29.2. Radiation therapy fields used in treating Hodgkin disease (A, B, C, and D). When the fields shown in C and D are combined, this is commonly called total nodal irradiation (TNI). (Used with permission from Haskell CM. *Cancer Treatment.* 4th ed. Philadelphia: WB Saunders, 1995:965.)

TABLE 29.6. *Radiation therapy dose used in treatment of Hodgkin lymphoma*

RT alone (less common)	Up to 30–44 Gy to involved regions
	Up to 30–36 Gy to involved sites
Bulky stage I–IV (after chemotherapy)	Up to 20–36 Gy
Nonbulky stage I–IV (after chemotherapy)	Up to 20–30 Gy

Note: Lower doses are used for nodular lymphocyte–predominant Hodgkin lymphoma.

- Dose of RT depends on the extent of the disease (Table 29.6). In combined modality therapy, RT is initiated within 4 weeks of finishing chemotherapy.

Treatment Response Evaluation

All patients (early and late stages) should receive interim restaging during treatment to evaluate the response to treatment. Restaging should be repeated 3 months after the end of treatment if complete remission was not achieved in the interim assessment.

Revised response criteria for lymphoma, including PET scan are now widely used (Table 29.7).

TREATMENT OF EARLY DISEASE (STAGES I AND II)

Early classical HL should be treated with intent to cure. Poor risk factors have been identified in this subset of patients.

Unfavorable Prognostic Features for Early Stages (I and II)

- B symptoms (fevers and/or weight loss)
- Bulky disease: a mass >10 cm in diameter or high mediastinal mass ratio (> one-third of intrathoracic diameter)
- ESR >50
- More than three sites of disease

TABLE 29.7. *Revised response criteria for lymphoma (including PET scan)*

Response	Lymph nodes	Spleen and liver	Bone marrow
CR	If PET +ve HL: any mass size if PET –ve If PET –ve HL: no mass	Not palpable	Negative for HL (if done)
PR	If PET +ve HL: persistence of one or more +ve sites with ≥50% reduction of SPD If PET –ve HL: ≥50% reduction of SPD	≥50% reduction of SPD of nodules	Irrelevant if +ve initially
SD	No change of disease or failure to attain a response or PD		
PD	New lesion >1.5 cm ≥50% increase of SPD of more than one node ≥50% increase of the longest diameter of one node that was initially at least 1 cm in the short axis	>50% increase of SPD from nadir	New involvement

CR, complete response; PR, partial response; SD, stable disease; PD, progressive disease; SPD, sum of the product of the diameters.

Treatment paradigm will account only for the first two risk factors (B symptoms and bulky disease):

- Favorable early disease (nonbulky stages IA–IIA): These patients are treated with either ABVD × 6 cycles or ABVD × 4 cycles followed by involved field RT. The cure rate of these patients is >90%.
- Unfavorable early disease (stages I and II with either B symptoms or bulky disease): These patients are also treated with ABVD × 6 to 8 cycles alone or ABVD four to six cycles with involved field radiation. The use of RT is more compelling with bulky disease. The use of at least 6 cycles of ABVD is compelling with B symptoms. PET scans should be used to determine if RT is necessary for residual abnormalities.

TREATMENT OF ADVANCED DISEASE (STAGES III AND IV)

Aggressive histology (e.g., mixed cellularity or lymphocyte depletion) is more common among patients with advanced classical HL. However, other prognostic factors have been identified in this subset of patients.

Unfavorable Prognostic Features for Advanced Stages (III and IV)

International prognostic score (IPS) factors are as follows:

- Disseminated disease (stage IV)
- Age >45 years
- Male gender
- Leukocytosis with WBC $\geq$15,000/mm$_3$
- Lymphopenia (<600/mm^3 or <8% of total WBC)
- Hemoglobin <10.5 gm/dL
- Albumin level <4 gm/dL

The 5-year progression-free survival decreases with higher IPS score as follows: 0 factors (84%), 1 factor (77%), 2 factors (67%), 3 factors (60%), 4 factors (51%), and 5 or more factors (42%).

The goal of treatment of advanced classical HL should be curative. The primary treatment of advanced disease is chemotherapy. ABVD is the gold standard in the United States. The recommended initial treatment is 6 to 8 cycles of ABVD including 2 cycles to be administered after complete resolution of the disease by imaging studies. BEACOPP is an effective alternative, particularly in patients with unfavorable disease (e.g., $\geq$4 unfavorable factors). The recommended initial treatment is 8 cycles of BEACOPP. Following ABVD or BEACOPP, involved field RT for PET-positive bulky disease sites should be administered. Patients with PET-negative residual masses do not appear to benefit from RT; however, this has not been adequately studied in patients with massive mediastinal Hodgkin lymphoma. If Stanford V (three cycles) is used, RT is an integral part of this regimen, which will be dependent on the treatment center and may impact efficacy.

TREATMENT OF NODULAR LYMPHOCYTE–PREDOMINANT HODGKIN LYMPHOMA

This subtype represents 5% of HL. Unlike classical Hodgkin lymphoma, NLPHL is strongly CD20 positive and typically behaves like an indolent non-Hodgkin lymphoma. While conventional Hodgkin lymphoma approaches continue to be applied to NLPHL, as outlined below, there are compelling biologic and clinical arguments for a different therapeutic approach.

Conventional Treatment Approaches

- Stage IA can be treated with RT alone (involved or extended fields) or observed in some cases.
- Stage IIA can be treated with RT alone or ABVD ± RT or observed in some cases.
- Stages IB, IIB, III, and IV are treated with ABVD ± involved field RT in early-stage disease.

Alternative Treatment Approaches

In the absence of a curative outcome with initial treatment, side effects of treatment become a significant cause of morbidity and mortality. Hence, due to the usually indolent nature of this disease, side effects must be weighed against benefit. In early-stage disease, observation and/or surgical resection may be appropriate. The high efficacy of rituximab strongly suggests it should be part of all systemic treatment approaches, including as a single agent or with chemotherapy. The optimal chemotherapy regimen remains unknown. While ABVD is the "historical" standard, regimens designed for non-Hodgkin lymphomas such as CHOP or dose-escalated EPOCH with rituximab are also appropriate. It is important to recognize the "aggressive" presentations of NLPHL such as those with disseminated disease, including the bones and bone marrow and aggressive histologic features. Such cases should be treated as aggressive B cell lymphomas.

Follow-up After Completion of Treatment

The purpose of follow-up is detection of disease relapse and late treatment-related complications.

- Clinical evaluation with CBC, ESR, chemistry panel every 3 months for 2 years, then every 6 months for 5 years
- CT of chest, abdomen, and pelvis every 3 to 6 months for 3 years, then annually for up to 5 years. Surveillance PET scan is controversial because of high false-positive results. Pathologic confirmation is always recommended for abnormal scans.
- Annual influenza vaccine is considered in patients who received bleomycin or chest RT.
- TSH annually if neck RT was given (risk of hypothyroidism).
- Annual mammogram screening should start 8 years after or at age of 40 years, whichever is earlier, for patients who received RT above the diaphragm. Breast MRI is also recommended by the American Cancer Society in addition to mammogram in younger patients. Breast self-exam should be encouraged.

LATE TREATMENT–RELATED COMPLICATIONS

- Hypothyroidism can occur after neck RT.
- Breast cancer can occur in females after chest or axillary RT. The risk is higher in patients who receive RT at younger age. It occurs after an average of 15 years after finishing treatment.
- Lung cancer: high risk is evident patients who received RT to chest and smoke cigarettes.
- Infertility risk is significantly higher with MOPP regimen compared to ABVD.
- Leukemia and myelodysplastic syndromes (more with MOPP regimen).
- Pulmonary toxicity after bleomycin treatment. Risk may be increased when G-CSF is used during treatment.
- Cardiac toxicity secondary to anthracycline is uncommon (total cumulative anthracycline dose is not high). The risk for coronary artery disease is also increased after mediastinal RT.
- Lhermitte sign: it is an infrequent complication that can occur 6 to 12 weeks after neck RT and resolves spontaneously. Patients feel electric-like shock sensation radiating down the back and extremities when neck is flexed. This sign is attributed to transient spinal cord demyelinization.
- Capsulated organism infection (pneumococcal, meningococcal, and hemophilus) can occur in patients not vaccinated after splenic RT or splenectomy (rarely used now).

TREATMENT OF RELAPSED HODGKIN LYMPHOMA

- Relapsed disease always requires pathologic confirmation.
- Classical HL:
  - If RT was the primary treatment, conventional chemotherapy (ABVD) with or without involved RT can be very effective treatment.

TABLE 29.8. *Salvage chemotherapy regimen for Hodgkin lymphoma*

ESHAP (etoposide, methylprednisolone, high-dose cytarabine and cisplatin)
ICE (ifosfamide, carboplatin, and etoposide)
DHAP (dexamethasone, high-dose cytarabine, and cisplatin)
EIP (etoposide, ifosfamide, and cisplatin)

- If conventional chemotherapy (with or without RT) was the primary treatment, salvage chemotherapy such as ICE, DHAP, ESHAP (Table 29.8) followed by autologous progenitor (stem) cell therapy is the treatment of choice.
- Gemcitabine combinations also have activity in advanced disease.
- NLPHL: Relapsed disease is best approached as an indolent lymphoma and includes observation, rituximab alone or with chemotherapy and/or RT.

Palliative Treatment

1. Sequential single-agent chemotherapy such as gemcitabine or vinblastine
2. Radiation treatment can be used to relieve pain or pressure symptoms of bulky masses.
3. Investigational treatment is encouraged through enrollment in clinical trials.

SUGGESTED READINGS

Aisenberg AC. Problems in Hodgkin's disease management. *Blood.* 1999;93:761–779.

Byrne BJ, Gockerman JP. Salvage therapy in Hodgkin's lymphoma. *Oncologist.* 2007;12:156–167.

Canellos GP, Anderson JR, Propert KJ, et al. Chemotherapy of advanced Hodgkin's disease with MOPP, ABVD, or MOPP alternating with ABVD. *N Engl J Med.* 1992;327:1478–1484.

Connors JM, Klimo P, Adams G, et al. Treatment of advanced Hodgkin's disease with chemotherapy—comparison of MOPP/ABV hybrid regimen with alternating courses of MOPP and ABVD: a report from the National Cancer Institute of Canada clinical trials group. *J Clin Oncol.* 1997;15:1638–1645.

Diehl V, Engert A, Re D. New strategies for the treatment of advanced-stage Hodgkin's lymphoma. *Hematol Oncol Clin North Am.* 2007;21:897–914.

Duggan DB, Petroni GR, Johnson JL, et al. Randomized comparison of ABVD and MOPP/ABV hybrid for the treatment of advanced Hodgkin's disease: report of an Intergroup trial. *J Clin Oncol.* 2003;21:607–614.

Fabian CJ, Mansfield CM, Dahlberg S, et al. Low-dose involved field radiation after chemotherapy in advanced Hodgkin disease. A Southwest Oncology Group randomized study. *Ann Intern Med.* 1994;120:903–912.

Federico M, Bellei M, Brice P, et al. High-dose therapy and autologous stem-cell transplantation versus conventional therapy for patients with advanced Hodgkin's lymphoma responding to front-line therapy. *J Clin Oncol.* 2003;21:2320–2325.

Ferme C, Eghbali H, Meerwaldt JH, et al. Chemotherapy plus involved-field radiation in early-stage Hodgkin's disease. *N Engl J Med.* 2007;357:1916–1927.

Harris NL. Hodgkin's disease: classification and differential diagnosis. *Mod Pathol.* 1999;12:159–175.

Horning SJ, Hoppe RT, Breslin S, Bartlett NL, Brown BW, Rosenberg SA. Stanford V and radiotherapy for locally extensive and advanced Hodgkin's disease: mature results of a prospective clinical trial. *J Clin Oncol.* 2002;20:630–637.

Lister TA, Crowther D, Sutcliffe SB, et al. Report of a committee convened to discuss the evaluation and staging of patients with Hodgkin's disease: Cotswolds meeting. *J Clin Oncol.* 1989;7:1630–1636.

Macdonald DA, Connors JM. New strategies for the treatment of early stages of Hodgkin's lymphoma. *Hematol Oncol Clin North Am.* 2007;21:871–880.

Schmitz N, Pfistner B, Sextro M, et al. Aggressive conventional chemotherapy compared with high-dose chemotherapy with autologous haemopoietic stem-cell transplantation for relapsed chemosensitive Hodgkin's disease: a randomised trial. *Lancet.* 2002;359:2065–2071.

Specht L, Gray RG, Clarke MJ, Peto R. Influence of more extensive radiotherapy and adjuvant chemotherapy on long-term outcome of early-stage Hodgkin's disease: a meta-analysis of 23 randomized trials involving 3,888 patients. International Hodgkin's Disease Collaborative Group. *J Clin Oncol.* 1998;16:830–843.

van Leeuwen FE, Klokman WJ, Hagenbeek A, et al. Second cancer risk following Hodgkin's disease: a 20-year follow-up study. *J Clin Oncol.* 1994;12:312–325.

30

Hematopoietic Stem Cell Transplantation

Akm Hossain, Michael Craig, Jame Abraham, and Richard W. Childs

Hematopoietic stem cell transplantation (HSCT) remains an effective treatment option for many patients with a wide range of malignant and nonmalignant conditions. In addition to autologous and matched related donor myeloablative allogeneic transplantations, many patients may be offered unrelated donor, nonmyeloablative, haploidentical, or cord blood transplantation. An estimated more than 60,000 transplantations were performed worldwide in 2005. Although transplantation may be associated with significant morbidity and mortality, recent advances in supportive care, human leukocyte antigen (HLA) typing, treatments for graft versus host disease (GVHD), better management of complications, and improved understanding of new drugs have led to improved outcomes for patients undergoing the procedure. An overview of autologous and allogeneic transplantation is provided in this chapter, along with a discussion of the complications and their management.

HEMATOPOIETIC STEM CELLS

Hematopoietic stem cells (HSCs) are immature precursor cells residing within the marrow space that are capable of giving rise to most of the cellular elements within the blood, including lymphoid, erythroid, and myeloid cell lines. These cells are defined by their ability to rescue lethally irradiated animals from marrow aplasia. In humans, most HSCs express the CD34 antigen and lack lineage-specific markers, although a population of CD34$^-$ stem cells has also been described. The number of CD34$^+$ cells that are present in the graft has an impact on transplant outcome; in the allogeneic setting, fewer CD34$^+$ cells are associated with a higher risk of transplant-related mortality and delays in the time to hematopoietic recovery in contrast to more CD34$^+$ cells where transplant-related mortality, hematological recovery, and the risk of disease relapse is decreased. HSCs can be obtained from peripheral blood following mobilization or directly from the bone marrow, or umbilical cord blood (discussed in subsequent text).

Peripheral Blood Stem Cell Collection

- Growth factors [granulocyte colony-stimulating factor (G-CSF) or granulocyte-macrophage colony-stimulating factor (GM-CSF)] are used to "mobilize" or increase the number of HSCs and progenitor cells in the peripheral blood.
- Cells are collected by apheresis procedure on day 5 or 6.
- In the autologous transplant setting, chemotherapy may be given (providing an additional antineoplastic effect) before growth factors, with apheresis being performed during hematopoietic recovery.
- Fewer complications and morbidity are experienced by the donor.
- Peripheral blood stem cell (PBSC) grafts result in more rapid engraftment than marrow grafts.
- The minimum goal of PBSC collection is 2×10^6 CD34$^+$ cells per kg of the recipient (range 2.0–8.0).
- Recently, the CXCR4 antagonist plerixafor was shown to enhance G-CSF mobilization of CD34+ cells in patients with non-Hodgkin lymphoma and myeloma being mobilized for autologous transplantation

Umbilical Cord Blood Transplantation

- HSCs can be collected from umbilical cord blood of placenta after delivery and frozen and stored viably.
- Enriched source of stem cells in a relative small volume of blood in comparison to bone marrow or PBSC
- Rapidly available and reduced requirement of HLA matching
- Higher total nucleated cell doses and better degrees of HLA match are associated with improved transplant outcome.
- Hematologic engraftment is typically delayed, and graft rejection occurs more commonly compared to transplants utilizing other stem cell sources.
- Dual cord blood transplantation from two different cord blood donors can be used to increase the dose of transplanted cells resulting in improve engraftment.

Bone Marrow Harvest

- Traditional source of HSCs; used less often than peripheral blood grafts.
- Bone marrow is harvested from posterior iliac crests under general anesthesia.
- A harvest of 15 mL/kg of aspirated marrow is generally considered safe to the donor.
- The goal cell dose is 2.0×10^8 mononuclear cells per kg of recipient weight.
- Complications to the donor may include pain, infection, neuropathy, and anemia.
- Severe complications occur in $<0.5\%$ of procedures.

CURRENT INDICATIONS FOR TRANSPLANTATION

Many malignant and nonmalignant disorders have been treated successfully with HSCT; the National Marrow Donor Program (NMDP) currently lists more than 70 diseases. Most transplants are performed for malignant conditions, including acute myeloid and lymphocytic leukemias, chronic myelogenous leukemia (CML), multiple myeloma, non-Hodgkin and Hodgkin lymphoma, and chronic lymphocytic leukemia (CLL). Stem cell disorders (e.g., aplastic anemia and paroxysmal nocturnal hemoglobinuria), inherited immune system defects (e.g., severe combined immunodeficiency and Wiskott-Aldrich syndrome), erythrocyte disorders (e.g., sickle cell anemia and β-thalassemia), and congenital metabolic diseases may be cured by allogeneic HSCT.

PRETRANSPLANTATION EVALUATION

Prior to treatment, a thorough discussion highlighting the transplantation procedure as well as risks and benefits associated with the procedure should take place between the physician and the patient.

1. Human leukocyte antigen testing (HLA typing) of the patient and a search for an HLA-matched donor (beginning with siblings) is required if an allogeneic transplant is being considered.
2. Medical history and evaluation
   - Review of original diagnosis and previous treatments, including radiation
   - Concomitant medical problems
   - Current medications, important past medications, and allergies
   - Determination of current disease status (i.e., in remission, relapse, minimal residual disease, etc.)
   - Restaging and confirmation of metastatic spread
   - Transfusion history and complications, as well as ABO typing
   - Psychosocial evaluation and delineation of a caregiver
3. Physical examination
   - Thorough physical examination
   - Evaluation of oral cavity and dentition
   - Neurologic evaluation if disease could involve the central nervous system
   - Karnofsky performance status (preferred value $>70\%$)

4. Organ function analysis
   - Renal function: creatinine clearance >60 mL per minute
   - Hepatic function: alanine aminotransferase (AST) and aspartate aminotransferase (ALT) less than twice the upper level of normal and bilirubin <2.00 µg/dL
   - Cardiac evaluation (electrocardiogram [ECG] and echocardiography [ECHO] or multiple-gated acquisition imaging [MUGA] with ejection fraction >40%)
   - Chest x-ray and pulmonary function testing, including diffusing capacity of lung for carbon monoxide (DLCO) and forced vital capacity (FVC).
5. Infectious disease evaluation
   - Serology for cytomegalovirus (CMV), human immunodeficiency virus (HIV), and hepatitis
   - Serology for herpes simplex virus (HSV), Epstein-Barr virus (EBV), and varicella
   - Assess for prior history of invasive fungal (aspergillus) infection.
6. Consideration of referral to reproductive center for sperm banking or in vitro fertilization

AUTOLOGOUS STEM CELL TRANSPLANTATION

High-dose chemotherapy (HDCT) without stem cell rescue may result in prolonged cytopenias. Autologous stem cells are collected and then reinfused into the patient after the completion of HDCT to reconstitute the hematopoietic system.

- Autologous transplantation is most effective in chemotherapy-sensitive tumors or as a consolidation therapy for patients in remission.
- HDCT may also overcome intrinsic tumor resistance to chemotherapy.
- Most grafts use PBSCs collected by apheresis.
- The product is frozen viably in dimethyl sulfoxide (DMSO) and thawed just prior to infusion.
- Reactions during transfusion are rare and may include bronchospasm, flushing, hypertension, or hypotension secondary to DMSO.
- Pancytopenia typically persists for 10 to 20 days and can be shortened using PBSC transplants and growth factors.
- Antimicrobials (antibacterial, antifungal, and antiviral) and blood products are typically given to support the patient in the first few weeks following transplantation.
- Infectious complications may occur as a consequence of the patient being profoundly immunosuppressed.
- New protocols are currently exploring tandem autologous transplants (two stem cell rescues after HDCT) and autologous followed by nonmyeloablative allogeneic transplantation.
- Late toxicities include the development of myelodysplasia, especially in regimens with total body irradiation (TBI) and frequent infections.

ALLOGENEIC STEM CELL TRANSPLANTATION

Introduction

Allogeneic stem cell transplantation has progressed from a treatment of last resort to first-line therapy for some patients. Extensive planning and coordination of care is required for all transplantation candidates, usually involving a network of physicians and support staff. The NMDP is an invaluable resource for physicians and their patients for the purpose of unrelated transplantation. The NMDP Web site is www.marrow.org. All physicians may perform a free initial search for an HLA-matched unrelated donor in the NMDP, which maintains a registry of more than 5 million potential donors.

Graft Versus Malignancy

The main therapeutic benefit of allogeneic transplant depends on the potential of the donor's immune system to recognize and eradicate the malignant or abnormal stem cell clone [the so-called graft-versus-leukemia (GVL) or graft-versus-tumor (GVT) effect]. This immune effect is evidenced by the lower relapse rate of hematological malignancies in patients who undergo allogeneic transplantation than in those who undergo autologous transplantation, as well as by an increased relapse rate in patients receiving a transplant from a syngeneic (identical twin) donor or an allograft that has undergone T-cell depletion. In addition, patients who develop GVHD have a lower risk of relapse than those who do not, and those who relapse after transplantation may be induced into a second remission with a donor lymphocyte infusion (DLI). CML, low-grade lymphoma, and acute myelogenous leukemia (AML) are most susceptible to the GVT effect, whereas acute lymphoblastic leukemia and high-grade lymphomas are relatively resistant to GVT. GVL is predominantly mediated by donor-derived T cells, although new evidence supports a potential contribution from nonspecific cytokines (both host and/or donor derived) and donor-derived natural killer (NK) cells in some settings.

Sources of Donor Hematopoietic Progenitor Cells

Matched Related Donor

- The probability of HLA identity between siblings is 25%.
- In the United States, approximately 30% of patients will have an HLA-matched sibling.
- The risk of GVHD increases as the HLA disparity between the patient and donor increases; therefore, most transplant centers prefer a 6/6 or 5/6 HLA match.

Syngeneic Donor

- Rarely, an identical twin can serve as the donor.
- Because GVHD does not occur (although reported in rare cases), post-transplantation immunosuppression is not required (although the risk of disease relapse is higher in this setting).

Matched Unrelated Donor

- Search through the NMDP for appropriate HLA match.
- Time from identifying a preliminary donor to collecting the allograft is typically 4 months.
- Seventy percent of whites will have an HLA-matched donor.
- It is more difficult to find matched donors for certain minority groups.
- Thirty percent of searches through the NMDP result in a transplant.
- The risk of GVHD and graft failure increases with increasing HLA mismatches. Recent data suggest high-resolution matched unrelated transplants have outcome similar to matched sibling transplants.

Umbilical Cord Transplantation

- Umbilical cords are obtained from umbilical vessels at delivery and are cryopreserved; a registry records the HLA type of the donor.
- Lymphocytes from cord grafts are immunologically immature, which appears to decrease the risk of acute GVHD that is associated with using an HLA-mismatched graft.
- Low stem cell numbers in the graft lead to increased risk of graft failure and a prolonged interval to hematopoietical recovery.

Haploidentical Donor

- Parent or sibling may serve as donor, with HLA match restricted to partial matching.
- Large numbers of CD34$^+$ cells increase the chances of engraftment.
- T cell depletion of the allograft is required to reduce the risk of lethal GVHD.
- The process results in prolonged immune recovery, increasing infection risks.

Donor Evaluation

Careful donor selection and evaluation is an integral part of the pretransplantation workup. The donor must be healthy and able to withstand the apheresis procedure or a bone marrow harvest.

1. Donor HLA typing
2. ABO typing
3. History-relevant information of the donor
   - Any previous malignancy within 5 years, except nonmelanoma skin cancer (absolute exclusion criteria)
   - Cardiac or coronary artery disease
   - Complications to anesthesia
   - History of lung disease
   - Back or spine disorders
   - Medications
4. Infection exposure
   - HIV, human T-lymphotropic virus (HTLV), hepatitis, CMV, HSV, and EBV
5. Pregnancy

Human Leukocyte Antigen Typing

The HLA system is a series of cell surface proteins, which play an important role in immune function. The system is intimately involved in cell-to-cell interactions and recognition. The genes encoding the HLA system are located on chromosome 6 and are codominantly expressed. A striking feature of the HLA system is its enormous diversity. HLA class I molecules include HLA-A, HLA-B, and HLA-C loci. HLA class II molecules are made up of more than 15 antigens, with HLA-DR having the greatest impact on transplantation outcome. Further complexity of the HLA system was revealed with the advent of molecular-based HLA typing, showing that HLA antigens previously identified by serologic testing were actually diverse when classified by DNA analysis. Current recommendations include matching of the donor and recipient at the allele level for HLA-A, HLA-B, HLA-C, HLA-DRB1, and HLA-DQB1 loci.

Stages of Transplant

Conditioning ("The Preparative Regimen")

- The goals of the conditioning regimen include immunosuppression of the recipient to prevent graft rejection and to eradicate residual disease or abnormal cell populations.
- Conditioning strategies can be categorized as myeloablative (conventional conditioning) or reduced intensity (aka nonmyeloablative) strategies (see section on nonmyeloablative transplants). Several myeloablative conditioning regimens are currently being used, with the most common regimens incorporating high-dose cyclophosphamide combined with either TBI or busulfan. The choice of a particular conditioning regimen is guided by factors such as the sensitivity of the malignancy to drugs in the regimen, the toxicities inherent to individual conditioning agents, and the age and performance status of the patient.
- Initial side effects of the transplantation procedure that are related to the preparative regimen include mucositis, nausea, diarrhea, alopecia, pancytopenia, and seizures (with busulfan).
- Late effects of transplant conditioning include lung toxicity, hypothyroidism, growth retardation, and second malignancy (e.g., breast cancer, lung cancer).

Transplantation Phase

- The transplantation phase usually starts 24 hours after completing the preparative regimen.
- Infusion of donor product is usually well tolerated by the recipient with pre- and post-transplant aggressive hydration.
- The day of transplantation is traditionally referred to as "day 0."

ENGRAFTMENT

- Engraftment is defined as time to develop a sustained absolute granulocyte count of >500 cells per µL.

- Platelet recovery usually lags behind granulocyte recovery.
- Duration of conditioning-induced cytopenias depends on the number of CD34$^+$ cells transplanted with the graft, use of growth factors, and agents used for GVHD prophylaxis.

Supportive Care Phase

- Hematological support is provided with blood products.
- Infection prophylaxis and treatment form a part of this phase.
- GVHD and other transplantation-related complications occur in this phase.

Infections

Infection remains a major cause of morbidity for patients undergoing HSC transplantation. Fig. 30.1 displays an overview of potential pathogens. Indwelling catheters are a common source of infections, and sepsis may occur during the neutropenia phase of the transplantation. Current approaches to minimize the risk of life-threatening infections include the use of prophylactic antimicrobial, antifungal, and antiviral agents, as well as aggressive screening for common transplantation-associated infections.

Neutropenic Fever

See Chapter 35 for overview of management of neutropenic fever.

Cytomegalovirus Infection

- CMV infection is a major cause of morbidity and mortality, especially pneumonia and colitis.
- In addition to pneumonia, symptoms may include fever, hepatitis, enteritis, and marrow suppression.
- CMV infection most commonly occurs as a result of the reactivation of a prior infection in the patient or because of the transfer of an infection from the donor (rare). New infection with CMV can also occur.
- The infection usually occurs after engraftment and may coincide with GVHD or with the use of immunosuppressive agents used to treat GVHD. The window of risk for viral reactivation is greatest from the day of engraftment to 100 days after transplantation.
- Screening for viral reactivation is performed weekly after transplantation by measuring the CMV antigen levels or by polymerase chain reaction (PCR).
- Initial treatment is with intravenous ganciclovir $\pm$ intravenous immunoglobulin treatment.
- Foscarnet is an alternative treatment (especially in patients with cytopenias).

Invasive Fungal Infection

- Invasive fungal infection is another cause of significant morbidity, with presentation of pneumonia, sinusitis, cellulitis, or blood infection.
- Common agents are *Aspergillus*, *Fusarium*, and *Zygomycetes*, as well as *Candida* species.
- Expanded selection of antifungal agents may improve outcome.
- *Candida* fungal prophylaxis with fluconazole is used by many centers.

Hematologic Support

- Hematologic support is provided by replacement of blood and platelet products as needed.
- All blood products should be irradiated prior to infusion.
- Leukocyte reduction filters are indicated to reduce CMV transmission and to reduce febrile reactions.

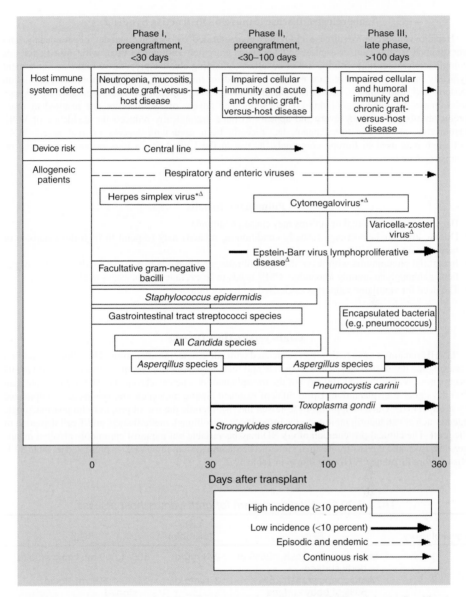

Fig. 30.1. Phases of opportunistic infections among allogenic HSCT recipients. (*, without standard prophylaxis; Δ, primarily among persons who are seropositive before transplant). (Used with permission from Centers for Disease Control and Prevention. Guidelines for preventing opportunistic infections among hematopoietic stem cell transplant recipients: recommendations of CDC, the Infectious Disease Society of America, and the American Society of Blood and Marrow Transplantation. *MMWR Morb Mortal Wkly Rep* 2000;49(No. RR-10): 1–60.)

CHAPTER 30

Venoocclusive Disease (Sinusoid Obstructive Syndrome)

Hepatic venoocclusive disease (VOD) is characterized by jaundice, tender hepatomegaly, and unexplained weight gain or ascites. VOD remains extremely difficult to treat, with the risk for this complication increasing with the use of busulfan-containing ablative preparative regimens. Treatment typically involves supportive care measures focused on maintaining renal function, the coagulation system, and fluid balance. Monitoring busulfan drug levels with appropriate dose adjusting appears to decrease the incidence of this complication. The advent of IV busulfan has resulted in more predictable busulfan drug levels and appears to have dramatically reduced the incidence of VOD. Defibrotide, an investigational agent, has recently been used with success to treat severe VOD. Although it is used in Europe commonly, its use in the United States is occasional and based on compassionate use.

Pulmonary Toxicity

- Bacterial, viral, or fungal organisms may cause pneumonia.
- Diffuse alveolar hemorrhage (usually conditioning related) may respond to high-dose steroids or recombinant factor VIIa.
- Interstitial pneumonitis with fever, diffuse infiltrates, and hypoxia may occur in 10% to 20% of patients; although commonly idiopathic, CMV needs to be excluded as the cause in all the cases.
- The need for ventilator support is associated with poor outcome.

Graft-Versus-Host Disease

GVHD remains a main toxic effect associated with allogeneic transplantation. This clinical condition results when donor-derived T cells recognize and react against normal recipient tissues. Acute GVHD occurs most within the first 100 days of the transplantation, whereas chronic GVHD occurs more than 100 days after transplantation. Up to 50% of matched sibling allogeneic transplants are complicated by acute GVHD. Current approaches to lessen the risk include the use of prophylactic pharmacologic agents such as calcineurin inhibitors (cyclosporine or tacrolimus), methotrexate, and T cell depletion of the graft. The clinical presentation of GVHD may be variable but the most commonly affected organs are skin, liver, and the gastrointestinal system. The staging system for GVHD is presented in Table 30.1. Risk factors for acute GVHD are shown in Table 30.2.

TABLE 30.1. *Staging system for graft-versus-host disease*

Level of injury	Skin	Liver (bilirubin)	Gut
1	Maculopapular rash <25% of body surface	2–3 mg/dL	500–1,000 mL liquid stool/d
2	Maculopapular rash 25%–50% of body surface	3–6 mg/dL	1,000–1,500 mL liquid stool/d
3	Generalized erythroderma	6–16 mg/dL	>1,500 mL liquid stool/d
4	Generalized erythroderma with bullae or desquamation	>15 mg/dL	Severe abdominal pain with or without ileus
Clinical grade	Skin	Liver	GI tract
I	1 or 2	None	None
II	1–3	1	1
III	2 or 3	2 or 3	2 or 3
IV	2–4	2–4	2–4

GI, gastrointestinal.

TABLE 30.2. *Risk factors for acute graft-versus-host disease*

Level of HLA mismatch
Infection (e.g., CMV, varicella, etc.)
Use of unrelated donors
Older patients
Donor with a prior history of pregnancy
Sex-mismatched transplant (female allografts into male recipients)
Intensive conditioning regimens

HLA, human leukocyte antigen; CMV, cytomegalovirus.

Prevention of Acute Graft-Versus-Host Disease

- T cell depletion of the allograft or combinations of cyclosporine, methotrexate, tacrolimus, prednisone, or mycophenolate mofetil may prevent acute GVHD.
- A common regimen for sibling donor transplants is cyclosporine, PO or i.v., and methotrexate i.v. on days 1, 3, 6, and 11.
- Cyclosporine dose 5 mg/kg/day, divided in two doses; the goal is to maintain therapeutic blood levels, which may range from 150 to 400 ng/mL.
- Tacrolimus dose 0.05 to 0.1 mg/kg/day, divided in two doses; the goal is to maintain levels at 5 to 15 ng/mL.
- Many medications may interact with immunosuppressant drugs.
- Donor T cell depletion prior to transplant decreases risk of GVHD but may increase the risk of relapse.
- T cell depletion may be accomplished by various methods, such as $CD34^+$ selection of the graft or the use of monoclonal antibodies directed against T cell antigens.

Treatment of Acute Graft-Versus-Host Disease

- Initially, methylprednisolone should be given at a dose of 1 to 2 mg/kg/day.
- For those patients who do not respond or for those who have a partial response, additional agents can be added with variable success (Table 30.3); clinical trials should be considered.

Prophylactic antifungal therapy against aspergillus should be considered in patients who develop GVHD requiring high dose or prolonged corticosteroid treatment.

Chronic Graft-Versus-Host Disease

- Chronic GVHD typically occurs after 100 days from transplantation.
- Prior history of acute GVHD and the use of PBSC allografts are risk factors.
- Chronic GVHD presents with variable organ involvement (skin, liver, and GI tract) and symptoms, including clinical presentations that may resemble autoimmune disorders (i.e., lichenoid skin changes, sicca syndrome, scleroderma-like skin changes, chronic hepatitis, and bronchiolitis obliterans).

TABLE 30.3. *Treatments that may be useful for acute graft-versus-host disease*

Methylprednisolone
Cyclosporine/tacrolimus
Azathioprine
Daclizumab
Infliximab
Muromonab-CD3 (OKT3)
Photopheresis
Antithymocyte globulin

- Chronic GVHD is often accompanied by cytopenias and immunodeficiency.
- Treatment involves prolonged courses of steroids and other immunosuppressive agents as well as prophylactic antibiotics (e.g., penicillin). Some trials have shown a benefit from thalidomide, mycophenolate mofetil, pentostatin, photopheresis, and Psoralen-UV-A (PUVA) (for chronic skin GVHD).

Relapse After Transplant

Relapse of malignant disease after allogeneic transplant is an ominous event, especially for aggressive malignancies such as AML and ALL. Most relapses occur within 2 years of transplantation. Relapse within 6 months of transplantation is associated with worse survival compared to patients relapsing more than 6 months post transplant. Immunosuppression is typically withdrawn to enhance a GVT effect, and in some cases, a DLI is given (lymphocytes from the original stem cell donor). This frequently results in GVHD, which may also be associated with a GVT response. The most favorable responses to DLI have been seen in patients with CML, especially those in the molecular or chronic phase of relapse. Second transplant for relapsed disease rarely results in long-term disease free survival

Reduced-Intensity Transplantation (Nonmyeloablative Transplantation)

Reduced-intensity transplantation or nonmyeloablative transplantation (NST) relies principally on the graft-versus-malignancy effect. Instead of intense myeloablative preparative regimens, this technique incorporates immunosuppression to allow for engraftment of donor cells. The most common preparative regimen consists of fludarabine combined with low-dose TBI or alkylating agent such as cyclophosphamide or busulfan. Nonmyeloablative transplants may be performed in older adults (i.e., older than 60 years) because regimen-related toxicities are less in this case. A mixture of donor and recipient hematopoietic cells is present just after transplant (called mixed chimerism). As immune suppression is removed, the surviving recipient cells are gradually eradicated by the donor immune system, ultimately resulting in full donor engraftment. GVT effects have been observed to occur in CML, AML, CLL, lymphoma, multiple myeloma, as well as in select metastatic solid tumors. Clinical trials investigating GVT effects in renal cell carcinoma and a variety of other metastatic solid tumors are ongoing.

CONCLUSION

HSC transplantation has dramatically improved over the last several decades into an effective therapeutic treatment for a variety of malignant and nonmalignant conditions. The improved safety profile of the procedure and the increasing availability of unrelated donors has led to an increase in the number of transplants performed each year. There have been improvements in survival, less acute complications, and improved treatment of chronic complications. The number of patients who benefit from this procedure will likely increase as future transplantation strategies continue to evolve that limit complications and expand the stem cell source, while maximizing beneficial donor immune-mediated graft-versus-malignancy effects.

SUGGESTED READINGS

American Society of Blood and Marrow Transplantation. Web site *www.asbmt.org*

Bensinger WI, Storb R. Allogeneic peripheral blood stem cell transplantation. *Rev Clin Exp Hematol.* 2001 Jun;5(2):67–86.

Centers for Disease Control and Prevention. Guidelines for preventing opportunistic infections among hematopoietic stem cell transplant recipients: recommendations of the CDC, the Infectious Disease Society of America, and the American Society of Blood and Marrow Transplantation. *MMWR Morb Mortal Wkly Rep.* 2000;49(No. RR-10):1–125.

Childs R, Chernoff A, Contentin N, et al. Regression of metastatic renal-cell carcinoma after nonmyeloablative allogeneic peripheral-blood stem-cell transplantation. *N Engl J Med* 2000;343:750–758.

Greb A, Bohlius J, Schiefer D, Schwarzer G, Schulz H, Engert A. High-dose chemotherapy with autologous stem cell transplantation in the first line treatment of aggressive non-Hodgkin lymphoma (NHL) in adults. *Cochrane Database Syst Rev.* 2008 Jan 23;(1):CD004024.

Hurley C, Lowe L, Logan B, et al. National Marrow Donor Program HLA-matching guidelines for unrelated marrow transplants. *Biol Blood Marrow Transplant* 2003;9:610–615.

International Bone Marrow Transplant Registry. Web site *www.ibmtr.org*

Lickliter JD, McGlave PB, DeFor TE, et al. Matched-pair analysis of peripheral blood stem cells compared to marrow for allogeneic transplantation. *Bone Marrow Transplant.* 2000 Oct;26(7):723–728.

Messina C, Faraci M, de Fazio V, et al. Prevention and treatment of acute GvHD. *Bone Marrow Transplant.* 2008 Jun;41(Suppl 2):S65–70.

National Marrow Donor Program. Web site *www.marrow.org*

The American Society of Hematology education program book. Washington, DC: American Society of Hematology, 2007. Web site *www.hematology.org*

SECTION 10

Other Malignancies

31

Carcinoma of Unknown Primary

Hung T. Khong

DEFINITION

Carcinoma of unknown primary (CUP) is defined as the detection of one or more metastatic tumors for which standardized evaluation, including history and physical examination, routine blood work, urinalysis, chest x-ray, computed tomography (CT) scan, and histologic evaluation, fails to identify the primary site.

EPIDEMIOLOGY

- Incidence: 2% to 7% of all diagnosed oncologic cases in the United States are CUP.
- Gender: male-to-female ratio is approximately 1:1.
- Age: highest incidence is in the sixth decade of life.

CLINICAL FEATURES AND PROGNOSIS

Clinical Features

- At presentation, most patients (97%) complain of symptoms at metastatic site(s). Common presenting sites and common metastatic sites are listed in Tables 31.1 and 31.2.
- Nonspecific constitutional symptoms also are common, such as anorexia, weight loss, and fatigue.
- At diagnosis, more than 50% of patients have multiple sites (more than two) of metastatic involvement.

Prognosis

- In general, the median survival time of patients with CUP is 3 to 4 months; however, some recent studies have reported a median survival duration of 5 to 12 months.
- Less than 20% of patients survive at 1 year and less than 10% at 5 years (Fig. 31.1).

TABLE 31.1. *Common presenting sites*

Site	%	Range (%)
Lymph node	26	14–37
Lung	17	16–19
Bone	15	13–30
Liver	11	4–19
Brain	8	7–10
Pleura	7	2–12
Skin	5	0–22
Peritoneum	4	1–6

In each patient, the metastatic site that was apparent or symptomatic first was the only one counted. Data were collected from three series involving a total of 611 patients.

Sources: From Refs. 15–17, with permission.

TABLE 31.2. *Common metastatic sites*

Site	%	Range (%)
Lymph nodes	41	20–42
Liver	34	33–43
Bone	29	29
Lung	27	26–31
Pleura	11	11–12
Peritoneum	9	
Brain	6	6
Adrenal gland	6	4–6
Skin	4	
Bone marrow	3	

All principal metastatic sites in each patient were counted. Data were collected from two series involving a total of 1,051 patients. Data reported from subspecialty practices were excluded.

Sources: From Refs 18 and 19, with permission.

Poor prognostic factors include the following:

- Male gender
- Adenocarcinoma histology
- Increasing number of involved organ sites
- Hepatic or adrenal involvement
- Supraclavicular lymphadenopathy

Advantageous prognostic factors include the following:

- Nonsupraclavicular lymphadenopathy
- Neuroendocrine histology
- A study of 1,000 patients (from the M.D. Anderson Cancer Center) revealed several prognostic subgroups. Some of these are shown in Table 31.3.

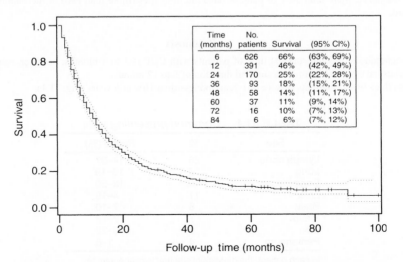

Time (months)	No. patients	Survival	(95% CI%)
6	626	66%	(63%, 69%)
12	391	46%	(42%, 49%)
24	170	25%	(22%, 28%)
36	93	18%	(15%, 21%)
48	58	14%	(11%, 17%)
60	37	11%	(9%, 14%)
72	16	10%	(7%, 13%)
84	6	6%	(7%, 12%)

Fig. 31.1. Kaplan–Meier survival curve of 1,000 consecutive patients with cancer of unknown primary (CUP). Median survival is 11 months (95% confidence interval [CI], 10–12 months).

TABLE 31.3. *Median survival in some prognostic subgroups*

Median survival time (mo)			
40	24	5	5
1 or 2 metastatic organ sites, nonadenocarcinoma, and no involvement of liver, bone, adrenal, or pleura	Liver mets and neuroendocrine histology	Liver mets, not neuroendocrine histology, and age >61.5 yr	Adrenal mets

Mets, metastasis.

The median survival for all patients in this study was 11 months.

DIAGNOSIS

- The recommended initial evaluation is listed in Table 31.4.
- Generous tissue samples should be obtained at the first biopsy.
- Accurate pathologic evaluation is critical.
- Light microscopic examination: Four major histologic subtypes can be identified by the initial light microscopic examination (Fig. 31.2).
- Immunoperoxidase staining (IPS) should be performed in all CUP cases of poorly differentiated carcinomas (PDCs). Table 31.5 lists some immunoperoxidase stains that are most useful.
- Electron microscopy should be considered if the tumor cannot be identified by IPS.
- Most common primary sites are listed in Table 31.6.
- Recently, gene and protein microarray technologies have emerged as valuable tools in the diagnosis of CUP. One assay that is commercially available in the United States is the CancerTYPE ID, a 92-gene RT-qPCR that provides a molecular classification of 39 tumor types in metastatic cancer with 87% accuracy.

WELL-DIFFERENTIATED OR MODERATELY DIFFERENTIATED ADENOCARCINOMA OF UNKNOWN PRIMARY

Clinical Features

- Accounts for about 60% of CUP cases; typically affecting elderly patients
- Metastatic tumors at multiple sites
- Poor performance status (PS) at diagnosis
- Common metastatic sites: lymph nodes, liver, lung, and bone
- Most common primary sites identified: the lung and pancreas (45%) (see Table 31.6)

TABLE 31.4. *Initial evaluation*

Complete H & P (attention to breast and pelvic examination in women; prostate and testicular examination in men; and head/neck and rectal examination in all patients)
CBC
Chemistry profiles
Urinalysis
Stool testing for occult blood
CXR
Symptom directed endoscopy
Consider PET scan in the initial conventional workup.

H & P, history and physical examination; CBC, complete blood count; CXR, chest x-ray.

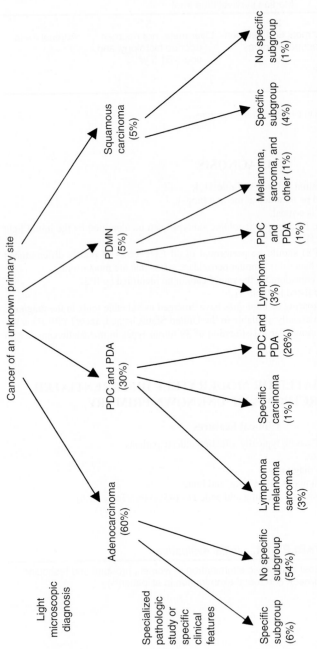

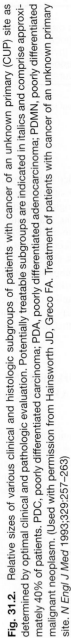

Fig. 31.2. Relative sizes of various clinical and histologic subgroups of patients with cancer of an unknown primary (CUP) site as determined by optimal clinical and pathologic evaluation. Potentially treatable subgroups are indicated in italics and comprise approximately 40% of patients. PDC, poorly differentiated carcinoma; PDA, poorly differentiated adenocarcinoma; PDMN, poorly differentiated malignant neoplasm. (Used with permission from Hainsworth JD, Greco FA. Treatment of patients with cancer of an unknown primary site. *N Engl J Med* 1993;329:257–263)

TABLE 31.5. *Immunoperoxidase staining in the differential diagnosis of carcinoma of unknown primary site*

Tumor type	Cytokeratin	Leukocyte common antigen	S100 protein, HMB 45	Neuron-specific enolase, chromogranin	Vimentin desmin
			Immunoperoxidase stains		
Carcinoma	+	−	−	±	−
Lymphoma	−	+	−	−	−
Melanoma	−	−	+	±	−
Sarcoma	−	−	−	−	+
Neuroendocrine	+	−	−	+	−

HMB, β-hydroxy β-methylbutyrate monohydrate.

- Poor prognosis (median survival of 3–4 months)
- Primary site is rarely found (<15% before death); an exhaustive search is not indicated.

Further Workup

Additional studies that should be performed include prostate-specific antigen (PSA) serum level and/or IPS for men, and mammography, serum CA 15-3, serum CA 125, and estrogen receptor/

TABLE 31.6. *Primary sites (diagnosed during life or at autopsy)*

Primary sites	%
Lung	23.7
Pancreas	21.1
Ovary	6.4
Kidney	5.5
Colorectal	5.3
Gastric	4.6
Liver	4.3
Prostate	4.1
Breast	3.4
Adrenal	2.2
Thyroid	2.2
Urinary tract/bladder	1.9
Esophagus	1.5
Lymphoma	1.5
Gall bladder/biliary tree	1.2
Testicular germ cell	1
Mesothelioma	0.5
Uterus	0.3
Others	9.3
Total	100

Data were collected from nine series involving a total of 1,453 patients with CUP. A diagnosis was made either during life or at autopsy in 582 patients. Head/neck primary and data from subspecialty practices have been excluded in the calculation (to avoid artifactual representation of certain cancers such as the high rates of pancreatic primary reported by clinics specializing in gastrointestinal malignancy).

progesterone receptor (ER/PR) (IPS) for women. CT scan of the abdomen can identify a primary site in approximately 30% of cases. In patients with CUP who have metastatic adenocarcinoma to the axillary lymph nodes and a negative mammogram, breast magnetic resonance imaging (MRI) detected a primary breast cancer in 9 (75%) of 12 patients in one study and in 19 (86%) of 22 patients in another study.

Treatment

- Most cases (90%) of well-differentiated or moderately differentiated adenocarcinoma of unknown primary show low response rates (RRs) and few complete responses with systemic chemotherapy.
- Patients in this group have a poor prognosis.
- The empiric chemotherapy for CUP is discussed in Table 31.7.
- The various subsets of patients with different types of CUP is who can be treated are discussed in the following sections.

TABLE 31.7. *Empiric chemotherapy for carcinoma of unknown primary*

Regimen (Ref.)	Treatment description	Cycle
Adenocarcinoma		
Paclitaxel, carboplatin (1)	200 mg/m^2/3 h i.v. d 1	21 d
	AUC 6 d 1	
Paclitaxel, carboplatin, etoposide (2)	200 mg/m^2/1 h i.v. d 1	21 d
	AUC 6 d 1	
	50 mg/d PO alternating with 100 mg/d PO d 1–10	
Docetaxel, carboplatin (3)	65 mg/m^2 i.v. d 1	21 d
	AUC 6 d 1	
Gemcitabine, cisplatin (4)	1,250 mg/m^2 i.v. d 1 and 8 100 mg/m^2 i.v. d 1	21 d
Gemcitabine, docetaxel (5)	1,000 mg/m^2 i.v. d 1 and 8 75 mg/m^2 i.v. d 8	21 d
Squamous cell carcinoma		
Paclitaxel, cisplatin, 5-FU (6)	175 mg/m^2/3 h i.v. d 1	21 d
	100 mg/m^2 i.v. d 2	
	500 mg/m^2/d continuous infusion over 120 h	
Docetaxel, cisplatin, 5-FU (7)	75 mg/m^2 i.v. d 1	21 d
	75 mg/m^2 i.v. d 1	
	750 mg/m^2/d continous infusion d 1–5	
Neuroendocrine tumor		
Paclitaxel, carboplatin, etoposide (8)	200 mg/m^2/1 h i.v. d 1	21 d
	AUC 6 d 1	
	50 mg/d PO alternating with 100 mg/d PO d 1–10	
Cisplatin, etoposide (9)	45 mg/m^2 i.v. d 2 and 3	28 d
	100 mg/m^2 i.v. d 1 and 3	
Cisplatin, etoposide (10,11)	60–80 mg/m^2 i.v. d 1	21–28 d
	100–120 mg/m^2 i.v. d 1 and 3	
Carboplatin, etoposide (12)	AUC 5 d 1	28 d
	100 mg/m^2 i.v. d 1, 2 and 3	
Temozolomide (13)	100–200 mg/m^2 PO d 1–5	28 d
Temozolomide, thalidomide (14)	150 mg/m^2 PO d 1–7 and d 15–21	28 d
	50–400 mg PO daily	

i.v., intravenous; AUC, area under the curve; PO, by mouth.
Source: Adapted from the National Comprehensive Cancer Network *Practice Guidelines in Oncology*, vol.1, 2008.

Peritoneal Carcinomatosis in Women

- Typical of ovarian cancer
- Occasionally associated with cancers from the gastrointestinal (GI) tract or breast
- Serum CA125 level is often elevated.
- Treatment is the same as for stage III ovarian cancer (laparotomy with surgical cytoreduction, followed by platinum-based combination chemotherapy) (see Chapter 17). It should be noted that about 20% of patients have complete remission and 16% have prolonged disease-free survival.

Women With Axillary Lymph Node Metastases

- Suggests breast cancer
- ER/PR and Her-2/neu should be checked.
- Occult breast primary is found in 55% to 75% of cases.
- Axillary node metastases in women should be treated in the same manner as stage II or III breast cancer.
- Modified radical mastectomy has been recommended.
- Alternatively, radiation therapy (XRT) to the breast can be performed after axillary node dissection.
- Adjuvant systemic chemotherapy should also be considered (see Chapter 17).
- Patients with metastatic sites in addition to axillary nodes should be treated for metastatic breast cancer (see Chapter 12).

Men With Elevated Prostate-Specific Antigen or Osteoblastic Bone Metastasis

- If the PSA serum level or tumor staining is positive, a regimen of hormonal therapy similar to that used for metastatic prostate cancer (Chapter 14) should be started.
- If osteoblastic bone metastases are present, empiric hormonal therapy should be started regardless of the PSA levels.

Patients With a Single Metastatic Site

- Surgical excision and/or XRT should be performed.

POORLY DIFFERENTIATED CARCINOMA/ ADENOCARCINOMA OF UNKNOWN PRIMARY

- Poorly differentiated carcinoma (PDC) and poorly differentiated adenocarcinoma (PDA) account for 30% of CUP (PDC accounts for two-thirds of cases and PDA accounts for one-third).
- Patients with PDC and PDA show poor response to fluorouracil-based chemotherapy and exhibit a short survival.
- Some patients have neoplasms that are highly responsive to platinating agent–based combination chemotherapeutic treatments. Some long-term survivors and cures have been described for both PDC and PDA.

Clinical Features

- Younger median age (about 40 years)
- Rapid progression of symptoms
- Evidence of rapid tumor growth
- Most common sites of metastatic involvement (50% of cases): lymph nodes, mediastinum, and retroperitoneum.

Pathologic Evaluation

- IPS is useful in the pathologic evaluation of PDC and PDA.
- Electron microscopic evaluation should be performed if tumor cannot be identified by IPS.

- Genetic analysis may be useful [e.g., i(12p), del(12p), or multiple copies of (12p) are diagnostic of germ cell tumor].

Further Workup

- Additional workup should include CT scan of chest and abdomen, and serum β-human chorionic gonadotropin (β-HCG) and α-fetoprotein (AFP).

Treatment

1. Extragonadal germ cell cancer syndrome
   - This syndrome is commonly found in young men.
   - These are predominantly midline tumors (mediastinum or retroperitoneum).
   - The syndrome is characterized by elevated levels of β-HCG, AFP, or both.
   - Genetic analysis may be diagnostic (e.g., abnormalities in chromosome 12).
   - This syndrome should be treated in the same manner as a germ cell tumor (Chapter 16).
2. Poorly differentiated neuroendocrine carcinoma
   - These carcinomas are high-grade tumors.
   - It is characterized by multiple metastatic sites.
   - The carcinomas are highly responsive to cisplatin-based chemotherapy.
   - The overall RR for combination chemotherapy was 71% (33 of 46 patients), with a complete response in 28% (13 of 46 patients); 17% of patients (8 of 46 patients) showed durable disease-free survival.
   - Patients in this group should be treated with a regimen of combination chemotherapy including a platinating agent and etoposide (see Table 31.7). It should be noted that other patients with PDC or PDA should receive an empiric therapy of platinating agent–based chemotherapy (see Table 31.7). (In a prospective study of 220 patients, the overall RR was 62%, with a complete RR of 26%. Thirteen percent of patients were considered cured.)

POORLY DIFFERENTIATED MALIGNANT NEOPLASMS OF UNKNOWN PRIMARY

- Found in 5% of all patients with CUP
- Specialized pathologic study found 35% to 65% of the malignant neoplasms to be lymphomas; carcinomas accounted for most of the remaining cases. Less than 15% of the neoplasms are melanoma and sarcoma.

SQUAMOUS CELL CARCINOMA OF UNKNOWN PRIMARY

- Account for 5% of all patients with CUP.

Cervical Node Involvement

High Cervical Node(s)

- Workup and treatment of squamous cell CUP in the high cervical nodes is the same as that for primary head and neck cancer (see Chapter 1). PET scan may help identify the primary site in this setting.
- High long-term survival rates (30–70%) have been reported after local treatment.
- The role of chemotherapy is undetermined. However, concurrent chemoradiation is an option in patients with extracapsular spread or N2 or N3 disease.

Low Cervical or Supraclavicular Node(s)

- Histology can be squamous, adenocarcinoma, or poorly differentiated tumors.
- Poorer prognosis (particularly for adenocarcinoma histology) is because lung and GI tract are frequent primary sites.

- If no other sites of disease are found, a few patients (10–15%) will have a long-term disease-free survival with aggressive local therapy (surgery and/or XRT).
- The role of chemotherapy is undetermined.

Inguinal Lymph Node(s)

- A primary site in the genital or anorectal areas is often identified in most patients.
- Curative therapy is available for some of these patients.
- If no primary is found, surgical node dissection (with or without XRT) can offer long-term survival.

SUGGESTED READINGS

Abbruzzese JL, Abbruzzese MC, Hess KR, et al. Unknown primary carcinoma: natural history and prognostic factors in 657 consecutive patients. *J Clin Oncol.* 1994;12:1272–80.

Briasoulis E, Kalofonos H, Bafaloukos D, et al. Carboplatin plus paclitaxel in unknown primary carcinoma: a phase II Hellenic Cooperative Oncology Group Study. *J Clin Oncol.* 2000;18:3101–7.

Bugat R, Bataillard A, Lesimple T, et al. Summary of the standards, options and recommendations for the management of patients with carcinoma of unknown primary site (2002). *Br J Cancer.* 2003;89(Suppl 1):S59–66.

Calais G, Pointreau Y, Alfonsi M, et al. Randomized phase III trial comparing induction chemotherapy using cisplatin (P), fluorouracil (F) with or without docetaxel (T) for organ preservation in hypopharynx and larynx cancer. Preliminary results of GORTEC 2000-01. *J Clin Oncol.* 2006 ASCO Annual Meeting Proceedings Part I. Vol 24, No. 18S 2006:5506.

Chorost MI, Lee MC, Yeoh CB, et al. Unknown primary. *J Surg Oncol.* 2004;87:191–203.

Culine S, Lortholary A, Voigt J, et al. Cisplatin in combination with either gemcitabine or irinotecan in carcinomas of unknown primary site: results of a randomized phase II study—trial for the French Study Group on Carcinomas of Unknown Primary (GEFCAPI 01). *J Clin Oncol.* 2003; 21:3479–82.

Ekeblad S, Sundin A, Janson ET, et al. Temozolomide as monotherapy is effective in treatment of advanced malignant neuroendocrine tumors. *Clin Cancer Res.* 2007;13:2986–91.

Fjallskog ML, Granberg D, Welin S, et al. Treatment with cisplatin and etoposide in patients with neuroendocrine tumors. *Cancer.* 2001;92:1101–7.

Fletcher JW, Djulbegovic B, Soares HP, et al. Recommendations on the use of 18F-FDG PET in oncology. *J Nucl Med.* 2008;49:480–508.

Greco F, Burris H, Erland J, et al. Carcinoma of unknown primary site. *Cancer.* 2000;89:2655–60.

Greco F, Erland J, Morrissey H, et al. Carcinoma of unknown primary site: phase II trials with docetaxel plus cisplatin or carboplatin. *Ann Oncol.* 2000;11:211–5.

Greco FA, Hainsworth JD. Cancer of unknown primary site. In: DeVita VT Jr, Hellman S, Rosenberg SA, eds. *Cancer: Principles and Practice of Oncology*, 5th ed. Philadelphia, PA: Lippincott–Raven Publishers, 2005:2213–34.

Hainsworth JD, Johnson DH, Greco FA. Cisplatin-based combination chemotherapy in the treatment of poorly differentiated carcinoma and poorly differentiated adenocarcinoma of unknown primary site: results of a 12-year experience. *J Clin Oncol.* 1992;10:912–22.

Hainsworth J, Spigel D, Litchy S, et al. Phase II trial of paclitaxel, carboplatin, and etoposide in advanced poorly differentiated neuroendocrine carcinoma: a Minnie Pearl Cancer Research Network Study. *J Clin Oncol.* 2006;24:3548–54.

HealthProfessional, 2007. http://www.nci.nih.gov/cancer/topics/pdq/treatment/unknownprimary/

Hess KR, Abbruzzese MC. Lenzi R, Raber MN, Abbruzzese JL. Classification and regression tree analysis of 1000 consecutive patients with unknown primary carcinoma. *Clin Cancer Res* 1999;5(11): 3403–10.

Hitt R, Lopez-Pousa A, Martinez-Trufero J, et al. Phase III study comparing cisplatin plus fluorouracil to paclitaxel, cisplatin, and fluorouracil induction chemotherapy followed by chemoradiotherapy in locally advanced head and neck cancer. *J Clin Oncol.* 2005;23:8636–45.

Kirsten F, Chi CH, Leary JA, Ng AB, Hedley DW, Tattersall MH. Metastatic adeno or undifferentiated carcinoma from an unknown primary site-natural history and guidelines for identification of treatable subsets. *Q J Med* 1987;62(238):143–161.

Kulke MH, Stuart K, Enzinger PC, et al. Phase II study of temozolomide and thalidomide in patients with metastatic neuroendocrine tumors. *J Clin Oncol.* 2006; 24:401–6.

Le Chevalier T, Cvitkovic E, Caille P, et al. Early metastatic cancer of unknown primary origin at presentation. A clinical study of 302 consecutive autopsied patients. *Arch Intern Med* 1988;148(9): 2035–39.

Lyman GH, Preisler HD. Carcinoma of unknown primary: natural history and response to therapy. *J Med* 1978;9(6):445–459.

Morris EA, Schwartz LH, Dershaw DD, et al. MR imaging of the breast in patients with occult primary breast carcinoma. *Radiology.* 1997;205(2):437–440.

Niell H, Herndon J, Miller A, et al. Randomized phase III intergroup trial of etoposide and cisplatin with or without paclitaxel and granulocyte colony-stimulating factor in patients with extensive-stage small-cell lung cancer: Cancer and Leukemia Group B Trial 9732. *J Clin Oncol.* 2005;23:3752–9.

Okamoto H, Watanabe K, Nishiwaki Y, et al. Phase II study of area under the plasma-concentration-versus-time curve-based carboplatin plus standard-dose intravenous etoposide in elderly patients with small-cell lung cancer. *J Clin Oncol.* 1999;17:3540–45.

Pavlidis N, Briasoulis E, Hainsworth J, et al. Diagnostic and therapeutic management of cancer of an unknown primary. *Eur J Cancer.* 2003;39:1990–05.

Pouessel D, Culine S, Becht C, et al. Gemcitabine and docetaxel as front-line chemotherapy in patients with carcinoma of an unknown primary site. *Cancer.* 2004;100:1257–61.

Schiller J, Adak S, Cella D, et al. Topotecan versus observation after cisplatin plus etoposide in extensive-stage small-cell lung cancer: E7593—a phase III trial of the Eastern Cooperative Oncology Group. *J Clin Oncol.* 2001;19:2114–22.

Shildt RA, Kennedy PS, Chen TT, Athens JW, O'Bryan RM, Balcerzak SP. Management of patients with metastatic adenocarcinoma of unknown origin: a Southwest Oncology Group study. *Cancer Treat Rep* 1983;67(1):77–79.

32

Central Nervous System Tumors

Scott Miller and Patrick J. Mansky

Primary and secondary brain tumors comprise a diverse spectrum of diseases whose intracranial location poses a unique problem for the practitioner. While brain tumors are only the tenth most common cause of death from cancer, they are the second most common neurologic cause of death (after stroke) and a major cause of mortality from cancer in young adults and children. Most adult brain tumors occur in the cerebral hemispheres, but two-thirds of all pediatric brain tumors are infratentorial.

Metastatic brain tumors are found at autopsy in 25% to 40% of patients with systemic cancer. Advances in computed tomography (CT) and magnetic resonance imaging (MRI) have resulted in earlier detection and more accurate diagnosis of brain tumors, but despite these improvements, the prognosis for most patients is extremely poor. The mainstays of treatment are surgery and radiation; chemotherapy is beneficial only in a select group of tumors.

PRIMARY BRAIN TUMORS

Epidemiology

- Primary brain tumors comprise 1.3% of all cancers.
- The American Cancer Society estimates that 22,070 primary central nervous system (CNS) tumors will be diagnosed in 2009.
- According to the Surveillance, Epidemiology, and End Results registry for 2000–2005, the incidence of primary malignancies of the brain and CNS is 2.1 to 22.6 cases per 100,000 persons per year, depending on age at diagnosis (Table 32.1). Incidence initially peaks at ages 1 to 4 (4.0/100,000) and gradually increases from a low at ages 15 to 19 (2.1/100,000) to a second peak at ages 75 to 79 (22.6/100,000). Median age at diagnosis is 55.
- Primary brain tumors account for about 2.2% of all cancer deaths, with an estimated 13,000 deaths from primary brain tumors per year. CNS tumors are the most prevalent solid tumors in childhood.

TABLE 32.1. *Brain tumor frequency (%) by type and age of patient*

Histology	Age (yr)						
	0–9	10–19	20–29	30–39	40–49	50–59	60–74
Astrocytoma	60%	59%	76%	81%	86%	87%	91%
Low-grade	10%	7%	5%	5%	3%	2%	2%
Anaplastic	47%	43%	51%	55%	48%	39%	40%
GBM	1%	7%	14%	18%	33%	44%	51%
Mixed glioma	3%	4%	5%	6%	6%	4%	2%
Oligodendroglioma	1%	4%	5%	6%	6%	4%	2%
Ependymoma	9%	3%	4%	2%	1%	1%	1%
Medulloblastoma	21%	10%	6%	2%	1%	0%	0%
Embryonal/teratoid	1%	1%	0%	0%	0%	0%	0%
Meningioma	0%	0%	1%	2%	1%	2%	2%

Source: From DeVita VT Jr, Hellman S, Rosenberg SA, eds. *Cancer: Principles and Practice of Oncology.* 7th ed. Philadelphia: Lippincott–Raven; 2005, with permission.

Brain tumors are the most frequent cancer-related cause of death in children <15 years, and the third leading cause of cancer-related deaths among patients 15 to 59 years. The majority (80%) of all primary brain tumor–related deaths occur in patients >59 years.
- The most common CNS tumors are derived from glial precursors.
- There is an increased risk of brain tumors in type 1 neurofibromatosis.

Clinical Diagnosis

The most common signs in order of decreasing frequency are:

- Hemiparesis
- Cranial nerve palsies
- Papilledema
- Cognitive dysfunction
- Sensory deficits
- Hemianesthesia
- Hemianopia
- Dysphasia

The most common symptoms in order of decreasing frequency are:

- Headache
- Seizure
- Cognitive/personality changes
- Focal weakness
- Nausea/vomiting
- Speech abnormalities
- Altered consciousness

Tumors of the cerebrum may be differentiated by location according to age at onset of symptoms (Table 32.2 and Fig. 32.1).

TABLE 32.2. *Differential diagnosis of brain tumors*

Location	Tumor type	Adult	Child
Supratentorial	Glioblastoma	X	X
	Astrocytoma	X	X
	Oligodendroglioma	X	X
	Mixed glioma	X	X
	Metastatic disease	X	
	Meningioma	X	
	Sarcoma		X
	Neuroblastoma		X
Infratentorial	Astrocytoma	X	X
	Ependymoma	X	X
	Brainstem glioma	X	X
	Metastatic disease	X	
	Glioblastoma	X	
	Medulloblastoma		X
Sellar/parasellar	Pituitary tumor	X	
	Meningioma	X	
	Craniopharyngioma		X
	Optic glioma		X
	Epidermoid		X
Base of skull	Neurinoma	X	
	Meningioma	X	
	Chordoma	X	
	Carcinoma	X	
	Dermoid/epidermoid	X	

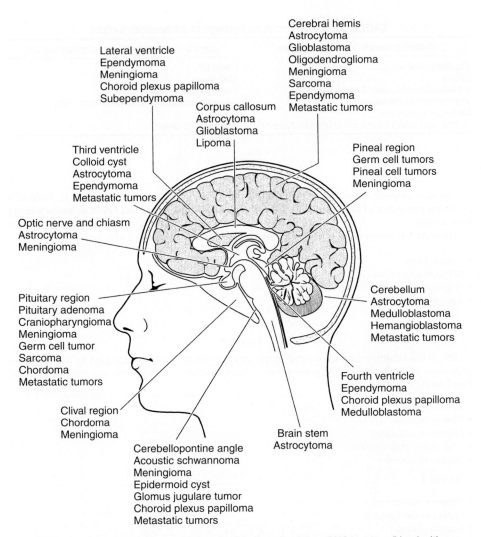

Fig. 32.1. Topologic distribution and preferred sites of primary CNS tumors. (Used with permission from Burger PC, Scheithauer BW, Vogel FS. *Surgical Pathology of the Nervous System and Its Coverings*. 3rd ed. New York: Churchill Livingstone; 1991.)

Acute Complications

Because the skull's rigidity does not allow for intracranial expansion, brain lesions routinely result in structural displacement and life-threatening consequences. Following the path of least resistance, tentorial or foramen magnum herniation may ensue (Table 32.3).

Types of Primary Brain Tumors

Broadly speaking, primary CNS tumors may be classified as gliomas and nongliomas.

TABLE 32.3. *Neurologic findings in intracranial tumors*

Tentorial/temporal lobe herniation	Cerebellar/foramen magnum herniation
Pupillary dilation	Head tilt
Ptosis	Stiff neck
Ipsilateral/contralateral hemiplegia	Neck paresthesias
Homonymous hemianopia	Tonic tensor spasms of limbs and body
Midbrain syndrome	Coma
Coma with rising blood pressure/bradycardia	Respiratory arrest

Gliomas

Gliomas comprise 45% of all intracranial tumors, with peak age in the seventh decade. Table 32.4 shows the prevalence of the pathologic subtypes of gliomas in relation to other more common primary brain tumors.

There are four major types of gliomas, based on their presumed glial cell of origin:

- Astrocytoma
- Oligodendrocytoma
- Oligoastrocytoma (mixed glioma)
- Ependymoma

GRADING

The World Health Organization's pathologic grading system, generally accepted by neuropathologists since 1993, determines the grade (level of aggressiveness) of each histologic subtype of tumor based on the following features:

- Cellular atypia
- Mitotic activity
- Degree of cellularity
- Endothelial proliferation
- Degree of necrosis

Grade 1

- Pilocytic astrocytoma
- Giant cell astrocytoma
- Ganglioglioma
- Dysembryoplastic neuroepithelial tumors

TABLE 32.4. *Prevalence of gliomas by pathologic subtype*

Subtype of glioma	Prevalence (%)
Glioblastoma	55
Astrocytoma	20.5
Ependymoma	6
Medulloblastoma	6
Oligodendroglioma	5
Choroid plexus papilloma	2
Colloid cyst	2

Grade 2

- Well-differentiated low-grade astrocytomas
- Oligodendrogliomas
- Ependymomas

Grade 3

- Anaplastic astrocytomas
- Anaplastic oligodendrogliomas
- Anaplastic ependymal tumors

Grade 4

- GBM (glioblastoma multiforme)
- Embryonal tumors

MOLECULAR GENETICS

Genetic alterations may form a continuum of progression from astrocytoma to anaplastic astrocytoma to GBM (Table 32.5). Whereas secondary or progressive gliomas often demonstrate mutations of p53 and overexpression of platelet-derived growth factor receptor (PDGFR), they seldom show amplification of epidermal growth factor receptor (EGFR). By contrast, primary (de novo) GBM usually lack p53 mutations and contain an amplified EGFR.

Glioblastoma Multiforme

- The most common adult primary brain tumor, accounting for at least 80% of malignant gliomas and 10% to 15% of all intracranial tumors.
- Categorized as grade 4
- Peak incidence is at 45 to 55 years; overall incidence is 2 to 3/100,000; male-to-female ratio is 3:2; median survival is 6 months.
- Localized equally throughout the brain; proportional to the volume of brain tissue in a particular location.
- More likely to be bihemispheric than other types of brain tumors.

TABLE 32.5. *Molecular genetics of gliomas*

Glioma	Genetic alteration
Secondary GBM (10%)	
Grade 2 astrocytoma	(+) mutant p53; PDGF-A and PDGFR overexpression
Grade 3 anaplastic astrocytoma	RB loss
	CDK4 amplification (12q13)
	LOH: 6, 9p, 19q, 11p
Grade 4 high-grade GBM	PTEN mutation
	LOH: 10q
Primary (de novo) GBM (90%)	Wild type p53
	EGFR amplification rearrangements (7p12)
	MDM2 amplification/overexpression
	RB mutation (13q13)
	CDKN2A deletion
	P16 deletion
	PTEN mutation (10q24)
	LOH: 10p and 10q

EGFR, epidermal growth factor receptor; GBM, glioblastoma multiforme; LOH, loss of heterozygosity; PDGFR, platelet-derived growth factor receptor; RB, retinoblastoma.

- Development is de novo (primary ~90%) or a progression from a lower-grade precursor lesion (secondary ~10%).

IMAGING CHARACTERISTICS

- Heterogeneous hypointense or isointense mass on CT or Tesla 1 (T1, relaxation time 1) MRI
- Heterogeneously contrast-enhancing mass
- Hypervascular appearance
- Rare calcifications

DIFFERENTIAL DIAGNOSIS

- Brain metastasis
- Cerebral abscess
- Demyelinating/inflammatory process (i.e., multiple sclerosis)
- Radiation necrosis
- Single photon emission computed tomography (SPECT) and MR cerebral perfusion imaging may distinguish radiation necrosis (hypovascular) from tumor recurrence (hypervascular).
- MR spectroscopy is increasingly used to distinguish tumor from other processes visualized on MRI.
- Gliosarcoma, a variant, has a mesenchymal component and a greater tendency for dural invasion.
- GBMs are characteristically infiltrative within brain parenchyma but rarely show extracerebral metastasis.

TREATMENT

- Current treatment recommendations for malignant gliomas (i.e., high-grade astrocytomas and GBM) include surgical resection, adjuvant radiotherapy, and, in select patients, the addition of chemotherapy. The infiltrative growth of malignant gliomas makes them likely to recur even after total primary resection.
- Radiation therapy has demonstrated a clear survival benefit in several randomized clinical trials, increasing median survival from 20 to 36 weeks. Radiation usually includes the contrast-enhanced tumor volume or peritumoral edema with a margin of 2 to 3 cm. A total dose of 60 Gy is delivered in 30 to 33 fractions over 6 weeks. Palliative treatment provides radiation to 30 Gy in 10 fractions over 2 weeks.
- The role of chemotherapy in the treatment of malignant gliomas was established by the Brain Tumor Study Group in several phase 3 trials of nitrosoureas. BCNU (carmustine) at a dose of 80 mg/m^2 daily for 3 days, repeated every 6 weeks, increased median survival from 38 to 51 weeks in patients with GBM. Because there is no solid rationale for administering BCNU over 3 days, it is now commonly given as a single intravenous infusion of 200 mg/m^2 every 6 weeks.
- Data from a randomized European Organization for Research and Treatment of Cancer (EORTC) trial in 2005 established the current standard of care for patients with newly diagnosed GBM. In that trial, 75 mg/m^2 of temozolomide was given every day concurrent with 6 weeks of standard external-beam radiotherapy (60 Gy in 30 fractions). Temozolomide was then administered postradiotherapy at a dose of 200 mg/m^2/day for 5 days every 28 days for six cycles. Patients on this regimen had a statistically significant increase in median survival (approximately 2.5 months) compared to patients who received radiotherapy alone; 2-year survival increased from 9% with radiation alone to 28% with combined treatment. A subsequent study of these patients showed a notable survival advantage in tumors that had a methylated (less active) promoter of the DNA repair enzyme promoter MGMT (methyl guanine methyl DNA transferase). Median survival was 21.7 months for patients with a methylated MGMT promoter versus 15.3 months for those without.
- Gliadel wafers, containing 3.8% carmustine, are FDA-approved for local therapy in conjunction with surgery and radiotherapy for newly diagnosed GBM, with an increased survival of 2.1 months compared to radiotherapy alone. This approach is appropriate only for a subset of patients due to the possibility of CNS leakage, increased infections, and increased need for use of steroids to treat swelling.

TABLE 32.6. *Median survival in malignant glioma*

Tumor type	Patient status	Median survival (mo)
Anaplastic astrocytoma	<50 yr, normal mental status	40–60
	>50 yr, KPS >70, symptoms >3 mo	40–60
	<50 yr, abnormal mental status	11–18
	>50 yr, symptoms <3 mo	11–18
Glioblastoma	>50 yr	11–18
	<50 yr, KPS >70	11–18
	>50 yr, KPS <70 or abnormal mental status	11–18

KPS, Karnofsky performance status.

- There is no proven approach superior to palliative care for recurrent GBM. An individualized approach that includes a possible second surgery, localized radiation, or systemic therapy is experimental. Whenever possible, patients should be enrolled in a clinical study.

PROGNOSIS

- Survival categories according to patient characteristics (Table 32.6) are based on an analysis of several Radiation Therapy Oncology Group trials.
- Given the generally poor prognosis for patients with high-grade gliomas, new treatment strategies are needed. Bevacizumab (an antiangiogenic agent) with irinotecan showed some activity in phase 2 studies for recurrent GBM, but cannot be considered standard of care until further studies are completed.
- Other promising strategies using inhibitors of the EGFR, PDGFR, ras, and mTOR (mammalian target of rapamycin) signal transduction pathways are being studied. Additional treatment strategies currently under investigation include therapeutic gene transfer and immunotherapeutic approaches.

Astrocytoma and Anaplastic Astrocytoma

Astrocytomas comprise 25% to 30% of all hemispheric gliomas.

LOW-GRADE DIFFUSE ASTROCYTOMA

Low-grade diffuse astrocytomas are categorized as grade 2 and account for approximately 5% of primary brain tumors. They occur mostly in the cerebral hemispheres, but may also occur in the brain stem. Mean age at diagnosis is 34 years.

Imaging characteristics on MRI are as follows:

- Little edema/mass effect
- Difficult to distinguish from nonmalignant infarct/cerebritis/demyelination
- Rare calcifications
- Large area of white/gray matter changes
- Differential diagnosis: infarct or cerebritis

TREATMENT

- Radiation therapy has been the standard treatment, but the timing and dose of radiation therapy have come under question. Recent EORTC studies of several hundred patients with low-grade gliomas have demonstrated no survival benefit for 60 Gy of radiation compared to 54 Gy. Thus, 54 Gy of radiation is currently considered standard. In another EORTC trial, patients with low-grade gliomas were randomized to immediate radiation at time of diagnosis versus radiation delayed until radiographic and/or clinical progression. Although median time to tumor progression was longer for the immediate radiotherapy group, there was no difference in overall survival. Recent data have shown that temozolomide can induce significant (albeit slow) preradiation tumor regression in low-grade astrocytomas. However, it does not appear that such responses are prolonged, and responses are <40% with upfront therapy.

- Pediatric low-grade supratentorial astrocytomas respond for prolonged periods to carboplatin and vincristine, although pilocytic astrocytomas tend to be more responsive than diffuse astrocytomas.
- Pilocytic astrocytomas, a subset of low-grade astrocytomas, are the most common pediatric astrocytic tumor and virtually the only type curable with complete surgical resection.
- Prolonged stabilization and tumor regression are possible with both radiotherapy and chemotherapy. The most commonly used chemotherapy regimen is carboplatin and vincristine.

PROGNOSIS

Median survival after surgery alone:

- 5 years: 19% to 32%
- 10 years: 10%

Median survival after surgery and postoperative radiation:

- 5 years: 36% to 55%
- 10 years: 26% to 43%

HIGH-GRADE DIFFUSE (ANAPLASTIC) ASTROCYTOMA

High-grade diffuse astrocytomas are categorized as grade 3 and account for approximately 5% of primary brain tumors. Mean age at diagnosis is 45 years. They are distinguished from low-grade diffuse astrocytomas by increased mitoses. They have a high propensity for transforming into GBM. Survival is 2 to 5 years.

TREATMENT

- In early trials, postoperative radiation therapy (approximately 60 Gy) increased median survival from 14 to 36 weeks. The introduction of postoperative nitrosourea-based chemotherapy regimens such as procarbazine, CCNU, and vincristine (PCV) (Table 32.7) significantly increased survival, particularly in anaplastic astrocytoma, with 50% of patients alive at 157 weeks.
- Two large retrospective studies, however, suggest that outcomes for patients treated with postradiation single-agent nitrosourea, such as BCNU and CCNU (lomustine), are just as good as outcomes for those treated with PCV.
- Retrospective data from 109 patients with anaplastic astrocytoma showed adjuvant temozolomide after resection and radiation was as effective as, and less toxic than, PCV and is preferred in the elderly. There are currently prospective trials looking at adjuvant temozolomide, and it is reasonable to extrapolate that temozolomide will prove to be active in the postradiation setting for anaplastic gliomas.

TABLE 32.7. *PCV chemotherapy regimen*

Agent	Dose	Route	Day(s)	Total dose/cycle[a]
Procarbazine	60 mg/m^2	p.o.	8–21	840 mg/m^2
CCNU (lomustine)	110 mg/m^2	p.o.	1	110 mg/m^2
Vincristine	1.4 mg/m^2	i.v.	8 and 29	2.8 mg/m^2

[a]Cycle = 6 weeks; may be extended to 8 weeks for hematologic recovery.

Source: From Levin VA, Silver P, Hannigan J, et al. Superiority of postradiotherapy adjuvant chemotherapy with CCNU, procarbazine, and vincristine (PCV) over BCNU for anaplastic astrocytoma: NCOG 6G61 final report. *Int J Radiat Oncol Biol Phys.* 1990;18:321–4, with permission.

Brainstem Gliomas

Brain stem gliomas occur predominantly in children as a group of diffuse astrocytomas of all grades. The clinical course is often malignant, regardless of grade, with typical presentation of cranial nerve VI and VII palsies.

TREATMENT

- Brain stem gliomas are rarely resectable unless there is a very large exophytic component. Even then, the intrinsic component is never completely resectable. Infiltrating pontine gliomas may be the only brain tumors for which treatment based purely on radiographic criteria, without tissue diagnosis, is considered appropriate.
- 60 Gy of radiation is delivered in standard fractionation. Earlier data pointing to an advantage for hyperfractionation have not held up.
- Chemotherapy regimens including CCNU, PCV, 5-fluorouracil, and hydroxyurea have been tested with no clear survival benefits.

Oligodendroglioma and Oligoastrocytoma (Mixed Glioma)

These diffuse cerebral tumors often appear with prominent areas of calcification on CT scan. They account for 5% to 10% of all gliomas and may have a better prognosis than astrocytomas. Like astrocytomas, low-grade gliomas may progress to a higher grade.

TREATMENT

- Low-grade oligodendrogliomas are best treated by surgical resection if most of the radiographically visible tumor can be safely removed.
- Radiation therapy has been the treatment of choice for low-grade progressive and anaplastic oligodendrogliomas. However, chemotherapy with PCV or temozolomide is increasingly being used either in the postradiation adjuvant setting or as neoadjuvant therapy to delay the potential long-term neurotoxicity of radiation therapy, particularly with large diffuse tumors that require large-field radiation.

EPENDYMOMA

Ependymomas comprise a spectrum of tumors ranging from aggressive childhood intraventricular tumors to low-grade adult spinal cord lesions. Typical locations are on the ventricular surface and the filum terminale.

Epidemiology

- Ependymomas account for 2% to 7.8% of all CNS neoplasms.
- 75% of ependymomas are low-grade.
- 50% occur before the age of 5 years.
- Intracranial tumors are 60% infratentorial, 40% supratentorial, with 50% intraventricular.
- Overall incidence of spinal seeding is approximately 7% to 15.7% for high-grade infratentorial lesions and increases with uncontrolled primary lesions.

Imaging

CT and MRI are highly suggestive of the presence of ependymoma (i.e., calcified mass on the fourth ventricle) but are not diagnostic.

Treatment

Surgery

Survival benefit only for complete resection confirmed by neuroimaging.

Radiotherapy

- When complete surgical resection is achieved, no adjuvant radiation therapy is recommended for low-grade ependymomas.
- Radiation therapy is usually warranted for low-grade ependymomas that show radiographic signs of tumor progression and for which complete surgical resection is no longer possible. Radiation is also warranted for anaplastic ependymomas.
- The entire posterior fossa is treated in infratentorial ependymomas, whereas local fields are treated in supratentorial ependymomas.
- Craniospinal irradiation is warranted for evidence of seeding by cerebrospinal fluid (CSF), cytologic or radiographic studies, or for anaplastic ependymomas.

Chemotherapy

The role of chemotherapy in ependymomas remains investigational. Multiple chemotherapeutic regimens have been tested in recurrent and anaplastic ependymomas, but response rates have been generally low, and few responses have been maintained.

Prognosis

- 5-year survival
- Low-grade tumors: 60% to 80%
- Anaplastic ependymoma: 10% to 47%
- Long-term survival
  - Surgery alone: 17% to 27%
  - Surgery plus radiation: 40% to 87%
  - Age is a dominant prognostic factor. Infants do poorly.

CHOROID PLEXUS TUMORS (NONGLIOMAS)

Choroid plexus tumors occur mostly in ventricles; in adults, occurrence is predominantly in the fourth ventricle. Tumors range from aggressive supratentorial childhood tumors to benign cerebellopontine angle tumors of adulthood. An association with Li-Fraumeni syndrome and von Hippel-Lindau syndrome has been described.

Diagnosis

- Signs of increased intracranial pressure (ICP)
- Focal findings of the fourth ventricle (ataxia and nystagmus)
- Anaplastic histologic changes warrant CSF examination for increased risk of disseminated disease.

Treatment

Surgery

- Complete resection is the goal of surgery.

Radiation Therapy/Chemotherapy

Given the rarity of these tumors, there are few prospective studies to evaluate a uniform approach. Radiation therapy, in conjunction with chemotherapy, has shown some benefit. Combinations of doxorubicin, cyclophosphamide, vincristine, and nitrosoureas have been used, as well as intraventricular methotrexate and cytarabine, but there have been no studies to evaluate these approaches.

MEDULLOBLASTOMA

Medulloblastoma is a malignant, small, blue, round cell tumor of the CNS.

Epidemiology

- Medulloblastoma, a malignant, small, blue, round cell tumor of the CNS, comprises 25% of all pediatric tumors.
- Found predominantly in the posterior fossa in children; uncommon in adults.
- 30% to 50% of medulloblastomas have isochromosome 17q.
- Associated with Gorlin syndrome and Turcot syndrome.

Clinical Presentation

- The most common presenting symptoms are signs of increased ICP and cerebellar and bulbar signs.
- At diagnosis, 5% to 25% of patients have CSF dissemination.
- <10% of patients exhibit systemic metastasis, commonly to bone.
- 40% of patients have brain stem infiltration.

Risk Stratification

- Average risk: localized disease at diagnosis; total or near-total resection
- High risk: disseminated disease at diagnosis and/or partial resection

Imaging

Typically, CT or MRI reveals contrast-enhancing posterior fossa midline lesion, most frequently arising from the cerebellar vermis.

Staging

- A modified Chang staging system is used (Table 32.8).
- Tumors are evaluated according to size, local extension, and presence of metastasis.
- CSF and spinal axis should be evaluated for metastasis with lumbar puncture and contrast-enhanced MRI.

Treatment

- Surgical resection
- Radiation therapy involves postoperative 35 Gy radiation to whole brain, with 15- to 20-Gy boost to posterior fossa. Average-risk patients may be cured with radiation alone.
- Ongoing studies are investigating the possibility of further reducing craniospinal radiation to 18 Gy in combination with local irradiation and adjuvant chemotherapy.
- Children with localized disease have shown an overall survival of >81% when treated with 23.4 Gy irradiation to the craniospinal axis, supplemented by 32.4 Gy local irradiation, followed by eight cycles of the following adjuvant chemotherapy regimen:
  - Vincristine 1.5 mg/m^2 i.v. weekly *plus*
  - CCNU 75 mg/m^2 p.o. on day 0 *plus*
  - Cisplatin 75 mg/m^2 i.v. on day 1

TABLE 32.8. *Chang staging system for medulloblastoma*

Stage	Description
T1	Tumor <3 cm in diameter, limited to midline position in the vermis, the roof of the fourth ventricle, and less frequently to the cerebellar hemisphere.
T2	Tumor >3 cm, further invading one adjacent structure or partially filling the fourth ventricle.
T3a	Tumor invading two adjacent structures or completely filling the fourth ventricle, with extension into aqueduct of Sylvius, foramen of Magendie, or foramen of Luschka, producing marked hydrocephalus.
T3b	Tumor arising from the floor of the fourth ventricle or brain stem and filling the fourth ventricle.
T4	Tumor further spreading through the aqueduct of Sylvius to involve the third ventricle or midbrain, or extending to the upper spinal cord.
M0	No evidence of gross subarachnoid or hematogenous metastasis.
M1	Microscopic tumor cells found in cerebrospinal fluid.
M2	Gross nodule seedings demonstrated in cerebellar–cerebral subarachnoid space or in the third or lateral ventricles.
M3	Gross nodule seedings in the spinal subarachnoid space.
M4	Extraneuraxial metastasis.

Results of this combination therapy were equivalent to:
- Cisplatin 75 mg m^2 i.v. on day 0 *plus*
- Vincristine 1.5 mg/m^2 i.v. weekly *plus*
- Cyclophosphamide 1,000 mg/m^2 i.v. over 60 minutes on days 21 and 22
- Small nonrandomized trials with select patients suggest that a small percentage (<20%) of patients who relapse after primary treatment can be successfully retreated and remain disease-free for >5 years with high-dose chemotherapy and stem cell support.

Prognosis

Disseminated disease is the most important prognostic factor. Other important factors are age (worse in children <3 years) and extent of resection (controversial).

Progression-free survival after chemotherapy and radiation are as follows:

- High-risk patients: 40% to 60%
- Average-risk patients: 65% to 91%

MENINGIOMAS

Meningiomas comprise up to 39% of primary CNS tumors. They are usually benign.

Genetics

- Monosomy 22, with frequent mutation of *NF2* gene on 22q
- Malignant meningiomas frequently show loss of 1p, 10, and 14q.
- Female sex, ionizing irradiation, *NF2*, and breast carcinoma are predisposing factors.

Clinical Presentation

Meningiomas commonly present in the parasagittal region, cerebral convexity, and sphenoidal ridge. Signs and symptoms include seizures, hemiparesis, visual field loss, and other focal findings.

Treatment

Surgery

- Treatment goal is complete resection.
- Recurrence after complete resection is 7% at 5 years and 20% at 10 years (higher for incompletely resected tumors).

Radiotherapy

- Adjuvant radiation: consider only for incompletely resected meningiomas as it probably reduces recurrence.
- Benign meningiomas: 54 Gy in 1.8 to 2.0 Gy fractions
- Malignant meningiomas: Increase dose to 60 Gy. Consider in postoperative adjuvant setting even after complete surgical resection, as it probably increases survival.

Chemotherapy

There is no effective drug treatment for meningiomas. Despite having estrogen and/or progesterone receptors, meningiomas are generally nonresponsive to hormonal therapy with agents such as tamoxifen. Although a small phase 2 trial suggested that the antiprogestin RU-486 had antimeningioma activity, a subsequent large randomized trial of RU-486 versus placebo for locally unresectable meningiomas showed no benefit for the drug compared to placebo.

PRIMARY BRAIN LYMPHOMA

- Intracerebral lymphoma most frequently presents as parenchymal lymphoma, but may be found in other anatomic sites such as the eye, meninges, or ependymal nodules.
- Primary CNS lymphoma accounts for <2% of all primary brain tumors, but up to one-quarter of HIV-associated lymphomas. Its prevalence in AIDS patients has declined with improved retroviral therapy.
- For unknown reasons, there has been a 10-fold increase in the last few decades in incidence of this tumor in immunocompetent patients, from 0.3/100,000 to 3/100,000. This increase has leveled off since 1995.

Risk Factors

- AIDS
- Immunosuppression for organ transplantation
- Autoimmune disease
- Congenital immunodeficiencies such as Wiscott-Aldrich syndrome
- Epstein-Barr virus (EBV) infection

Clinical Presentation

- Symptoms of intracranial mass (headaches and signs of increased ICP)
- Frontal lobe is most commonly involved, often with multiple lesions. Personality changes and decreased alertness are common.
- Multifocal disease: 42% leptomeningeal seeding at diagnosis

Diagnosis and Staging

Tissue diagnosis is paramount, except when EBV DNA is evident in the CSF of an AIDS patient, combined with hypermetabolic lesion on PET or SPECT imaging. Staging studies should include the following:

- MRI of brain with gadolinium
- Lumbar puncture
- Ophthalmologic evaluation
- Complete physical and blood work (including liver function tests)
- Chest x-ray
- Abdominal CT scan (optional if no other signs of systemic disease)

Treatment

Approximately 40% to 70% of tumors are highly steroid-sensitive. Steroids should thus be withheld, if possible, until tissue diagnosis is confirmed. A ring-enhancing lesion that "disappears" after starting steroids is strongly suggestive of CNS lymphoma, although other infectious diseases (i.e., toxoplasmosis) and inflammatory/demyelinating diseases (i.e., multiple sclerosis) must be considered.

Surgery

Surgery has no role in therapy, but is used to confirm diagnosis.

Radiotherapy

Radiotherapy yields 80% to 90% radiographic complete response. Common dosage is 40 to 60 Gy to the entire brain and meninges (C2 radiation). Median survival is 12 to 18 months.

Chemotherapy

- Methotrexate is the most active agent in CNS lymphoma. Studies suggest that preradiation chemotherapy with high-dose methotrexate significantly increases median survival and the number of long-term survivors.
- The role of radiotherapy for patients who have complete response to chemotherapy is unknown.
- The potential for long-term treatment-induced neurocognitive toxicity is considerably greater for patients receiving combined-modality treatment.
- Treatment is poorly tolerated in patients ≥60 years old. Single-agent methotrexate should be the treatment of choice for these patients unless contraindicated.
- The two most widely utilized treatment regimens for primary CNS lymphoma are the New Approaches to Brain Tumor Therapy (NABTT) regimen and the Memorial Sloan-Kettering Cancer Center (MSKCC) regimen, as outlined in Table 32.9.

GERM CELL TUMORS

Epidemiology

- Germ cell tumors (GCTs) of the CNS are typically located in the pineal region.
- The most common histologic type is germinoma, comprising 30% to 50% of all pineal tumors.
- Overall, GCTs are a rare subgroup of <1% of all intracranial tumors.

Clinical Presentation

Because the pineal region is close to the center of the brain, symptoms are generally related to increased ICP and ocular pathway cranial nerve palsies:

- Obstructive hydrocephalus (headache, nausea, vomiting, lethargy)
- Cranial nerve palsies (diplopia, upward-gaze paralysis)
- Elevated levels of serum tumor markers α-fetoprotein, β-human chorionic gonadotropin, and placental alkaline phosphatase

TABLE 32.9. *Two chemotherapy regimens for primary brain lymphoma*

	Treatment	Results
NABTT regimen[a]	High-dose methotrexate 8 g/m² every 2 wk, with leucovorin rescue to maximal response; delayed radiotherapy until tumor progression.	22 patients treated; overall response rate 74%; median progression-free survival 12.8 mo; median overall survival 22.8+ mo; no reported delayed severe neurologic toxicity
MSKCC regimen[b]	Five cycles of methotrexate 2.5 g/m², vincristine 1.4 mg/m² with maximum dose at 2.8 mg (2 m²), procarbazine 100 mg/m²/day for 7 days (cycle 1, 3, 5), and intraventricular methotrexate 12 mg followed by whole-brain radiotherapy to 45 Gy	102 patients treated; 94% response to preradiation chemotherapy; median progression-free survival 24 mo; overall survival 3.9 mo; 15% of patients experienced severe delayed neurologic toxicity

[a]New Approaches to Brain Tumor Therapy.
[b]Memorial Sloan-Kettering Cancer Center.
Source: From DeAngelis LM, Seiferheld W, Schold SC, et al. Combination chemotherapy and radiotherapy for primary central nervous system lymphoma: Radiation Therapy Oncology Group Study 93–10. *J Clin Oncol.* 2002;20(24):4643–8.

Treatment

Surgery

- Microsurgical infratentorial supracerebellar or supratentorial approach under the occipital lobe is used to establish diagnosis and to attempt resection in radioresistant tumors.
- Teratoma: Treatment is primarily surgical, possibly with radiation.

Radiation Therapy

Germinomas are exquisitely radiosensitive.

- Localized germinomas: 24 Gy to ventricular system; 26 Gy to tumor
- Disseminated germinomas: 20 to 35 Gy to craniospinal axis in addition to systemic chemotherapy

Nongerminomatous GCTs are irradiated after chemotherapy.

- Localized tumors: 24 Gy to ventricular system; 54 to 60 Gy boost to tumor
- Disseminated tumors: 54 to 60 Gy to tumor; 45 Gy to ventricles; 35 Gy to spinal cord

Chemotherapy

- Overall role of chemotherapy remains unclear; primarily used for nonseminomatous GCTs.
- Commonly used regimens include cisplatin/etoposide/bleomycin and carboplatin/etoposide/vinblastine in doses used for extragonadal GCTs.

Prognosis

- Germinomas: 5-year survival >80% with radiation only
- High survival is seen in mature teratomas.
- Prognosis is significantly poorer for nonseminomatous mixed GCTs.

TABLE 32.10. *Frequency of brain metastases*

Primary tumor	Frequency of brain metastases (%)
Lung cancer	50
Breast cancer	15–20
Unknown primary	15–19
Melanoma	10
Renal cell cancer	8–10
Colon cancer	5
Site of metastases	
Brain hemispheres	80
Cerebellum	15
Brain stem	5

METASTATIC BRAIN TUMORS

Epidemiology

- Brain metastases are the most prevalent intracranial malignancy (Table 32.10). Estimated incidence in the United States is 80,000 to 170,000 cases per year, compared to approximately 21,000 newly diagnosed primary brain tumors, highlighting the importance of proper diagnosis and management of this disease.
- An estimated 25% of adults and 6% to 10% of children with systemic cancer will develop symptomatic brain metastases.
- Lung and breast cancers are the most common primary cancers in adult metastatic brain disease.
- Sarcomas, neuroblastomas, and GCTs are the most common primary cancers in pediatric metastatic brain disease.

Clinical Presentation

Clinical signs and symptoms of brain metastasis are listed in Table 32.11.

Differential Diagnosis

- Primary brain tumors
- Abscess

TABLE 32.11. *Clinical signs and symptoms of brain metastases*

Signs	Frequency (%)
Hemiparesis	44
Change in mental status	35
Gait ataxia	13
Hemisensory loss	9
Papilledema	9
Symptoms	
Headache	42
Mental changes	31
Focal deficit	27
Seizure	20
Gait ataxia	17
Speech disturbance	10
Sensory problems	6

- Demyelination
- Cerebral infarction
- Cerebral hemorrhage
- Progressive multifocal leukoencephalopathy
- Radiation necrosis

The false-positive rate for single brain metastasis may be as high as 30%. Nonmetastatic brain lesions are equally divided between primary brain tumors and infections. Meningioma must be considered in patients with primary breast cancer with a dural-based brain lesion because the prevalence of this primary brain tumor increases in breast cancer.

Imaging

Contrast-enhanced MRI is the diagnostic imaging modality of choice. Features that favor MRI diagnosis of brain metastasis include the following:

- Multiple lesions
- Location at gray/white matter junction
- High ratio of vasogenic edema to tumor size

If imaging modalities and clinical history do not provide sufficient information to render a diagnosis, a biopsy of the lesion is indicated.

BRAIN METASTASIS WITH UNKNOWN PRIMARY

Imaging

- Sixty percent of patients with brain metastasis of unknown primary have a lung mass from a pulmonary malignancy or pulmonary metastasis of a primary in a different location. Therefore, a chest radiograph should be obtained in any patient with a new brain mass.
- If the chest radiograph is nondiagnostic, a CT scan of the chest is indicated.
- To determine the extent of metastatic disease, CT scans of the abdomen and pelvis and a bone scan should be performed.

Treatment

Symptomatic Therapy

- To reduce symptomatic edema, give a loading dose of dexamethasone 10 mg followed by 4 mg 4 ×/day.
- Symptomatic improvement should be seen within 24 to 72 hours.
- Imaging studies may not show a decrease of cerebral edema for up to 1 week.
- Steroid use should be tapered after completion of irradiation or earlier if cerebral edema is minimal.

Seizure Management

- Because infratentorial metastases have a very low risk of seizures, anticonvulsant therapy is usually not indicated.
- In patients with supratentorial brain metastasis and no surgery or prior seizures, prophylactic anticonvulsant therapy is controversial and not routinely recommended. Generally, phenytoin is initiated after seizure activity has occurred or after a patient has undergone craniotomy.
- Close monitoring is advised because dexamethasone and phenytoin mutually increase the clearance of phenytoin, and an increasing number of reports suggest a correlation between Stevens-Johnson syndrome and palliative whole-brain irradiation in patients taking phenytoin.
- Because phenytoin (like most older antiepileptic drugs) induces hepatic cytochrome P450 isoenzymes, thereby considerably altering the metabolism and pharmacology of agents such as paclitaxel

and irinotecan, some physicians are initiating seizure prophylaxis with newer agents that do not induce hepatic enzymes, such as levetiracetam, lamotrigine, or topiramate.

Surgery

Before recommending surgical resection, the following factors should be considered:

- Interval between diagnosis of primary cancer and finding of brain metastasis
- Type of primary cancer
- Extent of systemic disease
- Number and location of cerebral metastases
- Patient's neurologic status

Several controlled studies suggest a benefit for surgery combined with whole-brain irradiation for patients with single brain metastasis and stable extracranial disease. The benefit of resection of multiple brain metastases with therapeutic intent has not been established. For patients with multiple brain metastases, the role of surgery is generally limited to the following:

- Large, symptomatic, or life-threatening lesions
- Tissue diagnosis in unknown primary
- Differentiation of metastasis from primary brain tumor–like meningioma

Radiation Therapy

- Considered first-line therapy for brain metastasis
- Whole-brain irradiation increases median survival to 3 to 6 months.
- Overall response rate is 64% to 85%
- Cranial nerve deficit improvement is seen in 40% of patients.
- Fractionation schedule: from 30 to 50 Gy in 1.5- to 4-Gy fractions
- Most common schedule: 30 Gy in 10 fractions over 2 weeks
- For patients with good prognosis, more prolonged fractionation, such as 40 Gy in 2-Gy fractions, may reduce long-term morbidity.

POSTOPERATIVE RADIATION THERAPY

Patients who receive postoperative radiation therapy (50.4 Gy in 28 fractions) have demonstrated:

- 62% reduction in treatment failure
- A 30% reduction in risk of death from neurologic causes
- No improvement in overall survival or duration of functional independence

LATE TOXICITIES

Dementia is seen in 11% of patients receiving a total dose of >30 Gy. Recommended dose is 40 to 45 Gy in 1- to 2-Gy fractions.

REIRRADIATION

- Radiosurgery is recommended for patients with 1 or 2 metastatic lesions.
- Whole- or partial-brain irradiation is for patients ineligible for radiosurgery/chemotherapy.
- Clinical response: 42% to 75%.
- Median survival: 3.5 to 5 months.
- Dosing schedules vary, with no established consensus.

RADIOSURGERY

Indications include:

- Young age

- Good performance status
- Limited extracranial disease
- Up to 3 lesions <3.5 cm
- Recurrent brain metastasis after whole-brain irradiation

Adverse prognostic indicators include:

- Poor performance status
- Progressive systemic disease
- Infratentorial location
- Large tumor size
- Multiple lesions

INTERSTITIAL BRACHYTHERAPY

There is presently no indication for interstitial brachytherapy.

Chemotherapy

- In select malignancies, brain metastases may respond to systemic treatment of the underlying cancer.
- In breast cancer, regimens of combined chemotherapeutic agents are generally directed at the systemic disease. Responses have been seen in 50% to 70% of cases, and there appears to be a survival advantage in patients who respond. Common breast cancer regimens include:
  - Cyclophosphamide/5-fluorouracil/cisplatin (CFP) *plus*
  - Cyclophosphamide/methotrexate/5-fluorouracil (CMF) *plus*
  - Doxorubicin (Adriamycin)/cyclophosphamide (AC)
- In small cell lung cancer, regimens including etoposide and platinating agents have been used. Overall response rates for primary brain metastasis approach 76%. Response rates decrease to 43% on CNS relapse.

Prognosis

Median survival is 2.3 to 7.1 months depending on prognostic indicators (Table 32.12) that include:

- Karnofsky Performance Status >70
- Age <65 years
- Controlled primary disease
- No extracranial metastasis

TABLE 32.12. *Prognostic indicators and median survival in metastatic brain tumors*

Indicator	Median survival (mo)
Untreated brain metastasis	1
Treated with steroids	2
Treated with whole-brain irradiation	3–6
Single metastasis, limited extracranial disease, surgery, and whole-brain irradiation	10–16

SUGGESTED READINGS

Batchelor T, Carson K, O'Neill A, et al. Treatment of primary CNS lymphoma with methotrexate and deferred radiotherapy: a report of NABTT 96-07. *J Clin Oncol.* 2003;21:1044–9.

Black PM. Meningiomas. *Neurosurgery.* 1993;31:643–57.

Cavaliere R, Wen PY, Schiff D. Novel therapies for malignant gliomas. *Neurol Clin.* 2007;25(4): 1141–71.

DeAngelis LM, Seiferheld W, Schold SC, Fischer B, Schultz CJ. Combination chemotherapy and radiotherapy for primary central nervous system lymphoma: Radiation Therapy Oncology Group Study 93–10. *J Clin Oncol.* 2002;20:4643–8.

DeVita VT Jr, Hellman S, Rosenberg SA. *Cancer: Principles and Practice of Oncology.* 8th ed. Philadelphia: Lippincott Williams & Wilkins; 2008.

Duran I, Raizer JJ. Low-grade gliomas: management issues. *Expert Rev Anticancer Ther.* 2007;7(12 Suppl):S15–21.

Gerstner E, Batchelor T. Primary CNS lymphoma. *Expert Rev Anticancer Ther.* 2007;7(5):689–700.

Haskell CM, ed. *Cancer Treatment.* 5th ed. Philadelphia: WB Saunders; 2001.

Hoffman HJ. Brainstem gliomas. *Clin Neurosurg.* 1997;44:549–58.

Jaeckle KA, Ballman KV, Rao RD, Jenkins RB, Buckner JC. Current strategies in treatment of oligodendroglioma: evolution of molecular signatures of response. *J Clin Oncol.* 2006;24(8):1246–52.

Kim L, Glantz M. Chemotherapeutic options for primary brain tumors. *Curr Treat Options Oncol.* 2006;7(6):467–78.

Levin VA, Silver P, Hannigan J, et al. Superiority of post-radiotherapy adjuvant chemotherapy with CCNU, procarbazine, and vincristine (PCV) over BCNU for anaplastic astrocytoma: NCOG 6G61 final report. *Int J Radiat Oncol Biol Phys.* 1990;18:321–4.

Maldjian JA, Patel RS. Cerebral neoplasms in adults. *Semin Roentgenol.* 1999;34(2):102–22.

Packer RJ, Gajjar A, Vezina G, et al. Phase III study of craniospinal radiation therapy followed by adjuvant chemotherapy for newly diagnosed average-risk medulloblastoma. *J Clin Oncol.* 2006;24(25):4202–8.

Packer RJ. Brain tumors in children. *Arch Neurol.* 1999;56(4):421–5.

Peacock KH, Lesser GJ. Current therapeutic approaches in patients with brain metastases. *Curr Treat Options Oncol.* 2006;7(6):479–89.

Perez CA, Brady LW, eds. *Principles and Practice of Radiation Oncology.* 4th ed. Philadelphia: Lippincott–Raven; 2004.

Pizzo PA, Poplack DG, eds. *Principles and Practice of Pediatric Oncology.* 5th ed. Philadelphia: Lippincott–Raven; 2006.

Rasheed BK, Wiltshire RN, Bigner SH, BBigner DD. Molecular pathogenesis of malignant gliomas. *Curr Opin Oncol.* 1999;11(3):162–7.

Sanford RA, Gajjar A. Ependymomas. *Clin Neurosurg.* 1997;44:559–70.

Schiffer D. Classification and biology of astrocytic gliomas. *Forum (Genova).* 1998;8(3):244–55.

Schild SE, Haddock MG, Scheithauer BW, et al. Nongerminomatous germ cell tumors of the brain. *Int J Radiat Oncol Biol Phys.* 1996;36(3):557–63.

Shaw EG, Daumas-Duport C, Scheithauer BW, et al. Radiation therapy in the management of low-grade supratentorial astrocytomas. *J Neurosurg.* 1989;70:853–61.

Soffietti R, Cornu P, Delattre JY, et al. EFNS Guidelines on diagnosis and treatment of brain metastases: report of an EFNS Task Force. *Eur J Neurol.* 2006;13(7):674–81.

Stupp R, Mason WP, van den Bent MJ, et al. Radiotherapy plus concomitant and adjuvant temozolomide for glioblastoma. *N Engl J Med.* 2005;352(10):987–96.

Tomlinson FH, Kurtin PJ, Suman VJ, et al. Primary intracerebral malignant lymphoma: a clinicopathologic study of 89 patients. *J Neurosurg.* 1995;82(4):558–66.

33

Endocrine Tumors

Michael E. Menefee, Richard L. Piekarz, and Tito Fojo

Endocrine tumors are relatively uncommon (Table 33.1) and are often difficult to diagnose and treat effectively. They may cause morbidity and mortality not only by local and distant metastasis, but also through systemic effects caused by biologic mediators produced by the tumor cells. The most common endocrine tumors include:

- Thyroid carcinoma
- Parathyroid carcinoma
- Adrenocortical carcinoma
- Pheochromocytoma
- Carcinoid tumors
- Pancreatic endocrine tumors
- Multiple endocrine neoplasia (MEN)

TABLE 33.1. *Epidemiology of endocrine cancers in the United States*

	Incidence per year	% of total
All endocrine cancers		
Thyroid	18,100	91
Endocrine pancreas	800	4
Adrenal	550	2.8
Thymus	425	2.1
Pineal gland	128	0.6
Pituitary gland	77	0.4
Parathyroid	48	0.2
Carotid body, paraganglia	33	0.16
Primary thyroid cancers		
Well-differentiated		87–90
Papillary		75
Follicular		10
Hürthle cell		2–4
Anaplastic		1–2
Medullary		5–9
Sporadic		6
Familial		3
Lymphoma		1–3
Sarcoma/others		<1

Source: From DeVita VT Jr, Hellman S, Rosenberg SA, eds. *Cancer: Principles and Practice of Oncology.* 5th ed. Philadelphia: Lippincott-Raven; 1997, with permission.

THYROID CARCINOMA

While thyroid carcinoma is an uncommon type of cancer, it is the most common endocrine malignancy.

Epidemiology

- With more than 37,000 new cases diagnosed in the United States per year, thyroid carcinoma accounts for more than 90% of all endocrine tumors.
- The ratio of female to male patients is 2–3:1.
- Risk factors include irradiation to the head and neck during childhood and a family history of thyroid cancer.

Subtypes

Papillary

- This most common subtype of thyroid carcinomas (60–75%) is well differentiated and generally unilateral, but may be multifocal within a lobe.
- Variants include tall cell, columnar, and diffuse sclerosing.
- Metastasizes via lymphatic invasion; vascular invasion is uncommon.
- *RET* rearrangements are found in 3% to 33% of papillary carcinomas not associated with irradiation, and in 60% to 80% of those that occur post-irradiation.
- BRAF V600E mutation has been found in approximately 50% of papillary thyroid carcinomas.
- Prognosis depends on tumor stage and patient age. Ten-year survival in patients with distant metastases is 30% to 50%.

Follicular

- Metastasis to lung and bones occurs in late-stage disease via a vascular route.
- Lymph node involvement is rare and prognosis is only slightly less favorable than that of papillary thyroid carcinoma.
- PAX/PPARγ translocation is associated with follicular carcinoma.

Hürthle Cell

- Represents 4% of thyroid carcinomas.
- Also referred to as oxyphilic thyroid carcinoma; sometimes classified as a variant of follicular thyroid carcinoma.
- May be less responsive to radioactive iodine therapy.

Medullary

- This neuroendocrine, calcitonin-secreting tumor of the parafollicular (C) cells represents 3% to 5% of all thyroid carcinomas.
- May be associated with multiple endocrine neoplasia type 2 (MEN-2) syndrome, a germline mutation in the *RET* oncogene, although most tumors are sporadic.
- Sporadic tumors tend to be solitary, whereas familial tumors tend to be bilateral and multifocal.
- Approximately 50% of patients present with regional lymphadenopathy.
- Distant metastases typically occur in late-stage disease and usually involve lung, liver, bones, and adrenal glands.

Anaplastic

- This subtype accounts for 2% to 5% of all thyroid carcinomas. Up to 50% of patients have antecedent or concurrent history of well-differentiated thyroid carcinoma.

• All anaplastic thyroid carcinomas are high-grade and often have lymphovascular invasion and regional or distant spread at diagnosis.

Other Thyroid Cancers

• Primary thyroid lymphoma
• Metastasis to the thyroid

Clinical Presentation

Most patients present with an asymptomatic thyroid nodule. Clinical symptoms may include the following:

• Hoarseness caused by invasion of the recurrent laryngeal nerve or by direct compression of the larynx
• Cervical lymphadenopathy
• Dysphagia
• Horner syndrome (miosis, partial ptosis, hemifacial anhidrosis).

Diagnosis and Staging

• Palpable thyroid nodules are routinely evaluated by fine-needle aspiration and biopsy (FNAB) (Fig. 33.1 and Table 33.2). Ultrasonography is warranted in patients with a history of neck irradiation.
• FNAB is inappropriate for definitive diagnosis of thyroid carcinoma (see Table 33.2). Most well-differentiated thyroid carcinomas are diagnosed at surgery; however, some are not diagnosed until after initial resection or until local recurrence or metastasis.
• Carcinoma is suggested by a large neck mass and markedly elevated calcium levels.
• Differential includes parathyroid adenoma and hyperplasia.
• TNM classification and staging of thyroid carcinomas are outlined in Tables 33.3 and 33.4.
• Increased use of advanced diagnostic testing had led to a noted increase in incidentalomas of the thyroid, which are predominantly papillary microcarcinomas.

Treatment

Surgery

• Total thyroidectomy for papillary lesion >1 cm, lesion that extends beyond thyroid, or for patient with history of prior exposure to ionizing radiation to head/neck.

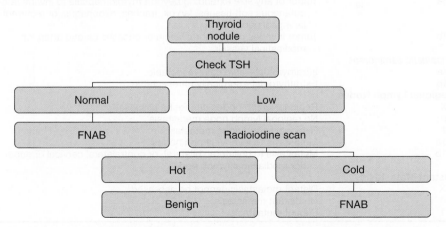

Fig. 33.1. Evaluation of a palpable thyroid nodule. TSH, thyroid-stimulating hormone; FNAB, fine-needle aspiration and biopsy.

TABLE 33.2.   *Follow-up for thyroid nodules based on results of fine-needle aspiration and biopsy (FNAB)*

Diagnosis at FNAB	% of thyroid nodules	Recommendation	% of thyroid nodules found to be malignant at surgery following FNAB
Benign	60–70	Routine follow-up	1–2
Malignant	5–10	Surgery/excisional biopsy	98
Suspicious	20	Surgery/excisional biopsy in most cases	20–30
Inconclusive	5–10	Repeat FNA using ultra- sound guidance	5–10

- Unilateral lobectomy with en bloc resection of tumor may be considered for papillary lesion <1 cm or for follicular lesion with no evidence of multicentric disease.
- Modified radical neck dissection for regional lymph node metastasis.
- Consider aggressive local resection for anaplastic carcinoma.
- Following thyroid resection, treatment with iodine-131 (a radioisotope of iodine) may be used to ablate normal residual thyroid tissue; treat micrometastases; and decrease cancer-related death, tumor recurrence, and development of distant metastases. Table 33.5 outlines indications for iodine-131 treatment after surgery.

TABLE 33.3.   *TNM classification of thyroid carcinomas*

Primary Tumor	
TX	Primary tumor cannot be assessed.
T0	No evidence of primary tumor
T1	Tumor ≤2 cm in greatest dimension; limited to thyroid
T2	Tumor >2 cm but ≤4 cm in greatest dimension; limited to thyroid
T3	Tumor >4 cm in greatest dimension; limited to thyroid or with minimal extension
T4a	Tumor of any size extending beyond thyroid capsule to invade sub-cutaneous soft tissues, larynx, trachea, esophagus, or recurrent laryngeal nerve.
T4b	Tumor invades prevertebral fascia or encases carotid artery or mediastinal vessels.
Anaplastic carcinomas	
T4a	Intrathyroidal—surgically resectable.
T4b	Extrathyroidal—surgically unresectable.
Regional Lymph Nodes	
NX	Regional lymph nodes cannot be assessed.
N0	No regional lymph node metastasis
N1	Regional lymph node metastasis
N1a	Metastasis to level VI lymph nodes
N1b	Metastasis to unilateral, bilateral, or contralateral cervical or supe-rior mediastinal lymph nodes
Distant Metastasis	
MX	Distant metastasis cannot be assessed.
M0	No distant metastasis
M1	Distant metastasis

Source: From *American Joint Committee on Cancer Staging Manual*. 6th ed. New York: Springer; 2002, with permission.

TABLE 33.4. *Staging of thyroid cancer*

| | Papillary or follicular (well differentiated) | | | |
Stage	Age <45 yr	Age >45 yr	Medullary	Anaplastic
1	Any T, any N, M0	T1	T1	—
2	M1	T2–T3	T2–T4	—
3	—	T4 or N1	N1	—
4	—	M1	M1	Any

Chemotherapy

- Limited efficacy: Partial responses have been reported with newer tyrosine kinase inhibitors.
- Paclitaxel is single most effective agent for anaplastic carcinoma.
- Clinical trials should be considered when possible.

Radiation

- Thyroid tumors are generally radioinsensitive.
- Radiation has mainly palliative benefit.

Recommended Follow-up

- Ultrasound, especially with extrathyroid invasion or locoregional nodal metastasis
- Thyroglobulin. Use caution in patients with TSH suppression, nontotal thyroidectomy, or dedifferentiated disease.
- Thyroid replacement with added goal of suppressing TSH to avoid stimulation of thyroid cancer cell growth.

Prognosis

- Overall survival at 10 years for middle-aged adults is 80% to 95%
- Local or regional recurrence: 5% to 20%
- Distant metastases: 10% to 15%
- Prognostic indicators for recurrent disease and death: age at diagnosis, histologic subtype, extent of tumor

TABLE 33.5. *Indications for post-surgical treatment with iodine-131 in patients with thyroid cancer*

| | Iodine-131 | |
Finding	Indicated	Not indicated
Low risk of cancer-specific mortality or relapse		X
Incomplete excision of tumor	X	
Complete excision of tumor but high risk of mortality	X	
Complete excision of tumor but high risk of relapse due to:	X	
Age (<16 yr or >45 yr)		
Histologic subtype (tall cell, columnar cell, diffuse sclerosing papillary variants; widely invasive or poorly differentiated follicular subtypes; Hürthle cell carcinomas)		
Extent of tumor (large tumor mass, extension beyond thyroid capsule, lymph node metastases)		
Distant metastases	X	
Elevated serum thyroglobulin >3 mo post-surgery	X	

PARATHYROID CARCINOMA

Clinically, it is important to distinguish this disease from other benign disorders that cause hyperparathyroidism. Parathyroid carcinoma accounts for more than 1% of cases of hyperparathyroidism.

Epidemiology and Natural History

- Occurs in 0.015 per 100,000 individuals, predominantly diagnosed in the fifth or sixth decade of life.
- 10-year survival: 49%
- Morbidity and mortality usually related to hypercalcemia rather than complications of metastases.

Clinical Presentation

- Symptoms of hypercalcemia, with calcium levels usually >14 mg/dL
- Elevated parathyroid hormone levels
- Vocal cord paralysis in more advanced disease
- Metastases to lungs, cervical lymph nodes, and liver

Diagnosis

Large neck mass (>3 cm) and markedly elevated calcium levels are suggestive of carcinoma.

- Differential includes parathyroid adenoma and hyperplasia.
- Most parathyroid carcinomas are diagnosed at surgery; however, some are not diagnosed until after initial resection or until local recurrence or metastases.
- FNAB is inappropriate for diagnosis.

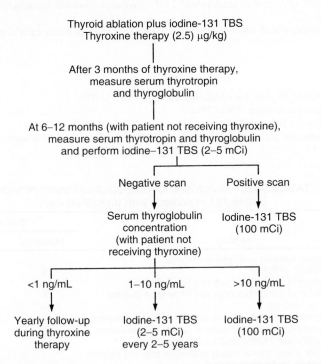

Fig. 33.2. Recommended follow-up after total thyroid ablation based on serum thyroglobulin assessment and iodine-131 total body scanning (TBS). (Used with permission from Schlumberger MJ. Papillary and follicular thyroid carcinoma. *N Engl J Med.* 1998;338:297–308.)

TABLE 33.6. *Potential clinical manifestations of pheochromocytomas*

Mild labile hypertension to hypertensive crisis; sustained hypertension also common
Myocardial infarction
Cerebral infarction
Classic pattern of paroxysmal hypertension (30–50% of cases)
Spells of paroxysmal headache
Pallor or flushing
Tremor
Apprehension
Palpitation
Orthostasis
Mild weight loss
Diaphoresis

Treatment

Surgery

- Primarily en bloc resection of tumor and involved structures and of the ipsilateral lobe of thyroid.
- Recurrent tumor and oligometastases should also be resected.

Medical

- Chemotherapy is of limited value. Agents with activity include dacarbazine, 5-fluorouracil, and cyclophosphamide.
- Management of hypercalcemia is essential while treating parathyroid carcinoma.

Radiation

- Parathyroid tumors are generally radioinsensitive.
- Radiation has only palliative benefit.

ADRENOCORTICAL CARCINOMA

Epidemiology

- Adrenocortical carcinoma is rare, accounting for 0.05% to 0.2% of all cancers.
- It has a bimodal age distribution, with a first peak in children younger than 5 years and a second peak in adults in their fourth to fifth decade.

Pathology

- Histological differentiation of adrenocortical adenomas and carcinomas is challenging. However, carcinomas tend to display mitotic activity, aneuploidy, and venous invasion. Carcinomas may also secrete abnormal amounts of androgens and 11-deoxysteroids.

Clinical Presentation

Symptoms may arise from the effects of local mass or distant metastases. Approximately 50% of patients present with evidence of hormonal excess. Other endocrine dysfunctions may include:

- Hypercortisolism
- Virilization/feminization
- Mineralocorticoid excess

Stage I – Tumor <5 cm without regional extension

Stage II – Tumor >5 cm without regional extension

Stage III – Regional extension ± lymph node

Stage IV – Distant metastases (e.g., liver, lung, and bone)

Fig. 33.3. MacFarlane classification of adrenocortical carcinomas. (Used with permission from DeVita VT Jr, Hellman S, Rosenberg SA, eds. *Cancer: Principles and Practice of Oncology*. 5th ed. Philadelphia: Lippincott-Raven; 1997.)

Diagnosis and Staging

- MacFarlane classification and staging of adrenocortical carcinoma is shown in Fig. 33.3.
- Better quality and more frequent use of imaging technologies have led to increased incidental detection of adrenal tumors (Fig. 33.4).
- Biochemical evaluation (urinary steroids, suppression tests) should be conducted if clinically warranted.

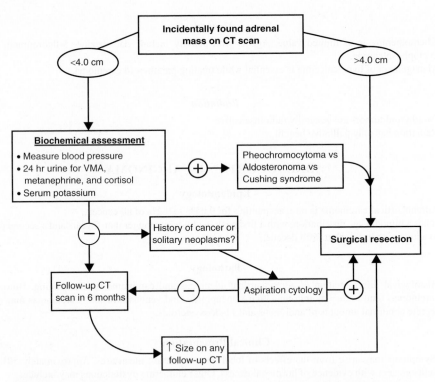

Fig. 33.4. Evaluation of adrenal mass in a patient with suspected pheochromocytoma. CT, computed tomography; VMA, vanillylmandelic acid. (Used with permission from DeVita VT Jr, Hellman S, Rosenberg SA, eds. *Cancer: Principles and Practice of Oncology*. 5th ed. Philadelphia: Lippincott-Raven; 1997.)

Treatment

- En bloc resection is initially appropriate for all stages; local recurrence and metastatic disease require further resection when feasible.
- Tumors >6 cm (or <6 cm but suspected of being malignant) should not be resected laparascopically.
- Radiofrequency ablation may be implemented for local control or metastases in patients with unresectable disease.
- Mitotane induces hormonal response rates in up to 75% of patients with functional tumors, with no change in overall survival.
- Other active agents include doxorubicin, etoposide, and cisplatin.

Prognosis

- 5-year survival rate: 23%
- 10-year survival rate: 10%
- Prognosis is better in children.
- Common sites of distant metastasis are liver, lung, lymph nodes, and bone.

PHEOCHROMOCYTOMA

Epidemiology

- Approximately 10% of cases are associated with a familial genetic syndrome such as MEN-2 or von Hippel-Lindau disease.
- Found in <0.2% of patients with hypertension

Clinical Presentation and Progression

- Pheochromocytomas are generally indolent, with morbidity and mortality related to the tumors' secretory products.
- Approximately 10% of pheochromocytomas are bilateral, with occurrence more frequent in familial syndromes.
- Approximately 10% of pheochromocytomas are extra-adrenal; these tumors are more likely to be malignant.
- Metastasis is most common in lung, brain, and bone.
- Clinical features of pheochromocytomas are summarized in Table 33.6.

Pathology

- Pheochromocytomas arise from chromaffin cells, most of which nest in the adrenal medulla.
- Vascular invasion and extension into the cortex may be seen with both benign and malignant tumors.
- The only absolute criterion for malignancy is the presence of secondary tumors in sites where chromaffin cells do not usually exist.

Diagnosis

Metabolic

- Vanillylmandelic acid test for catecholamine-secreting tumors performed on a 24-hour urine specimen. Vanillylmandelic acid is the major urinary metabolite of norepinephrine and epinephrine.
- Measurement of urinary metanephrine is the most specific tool for diagnosis of pheochromocytoma.
- Clonidine suppression test is recommended for intermediate catecholamine levels. Catecholamine levels will not be suppressed in patients with pheochromocytoma.

Radiologic

- CT and MRI are equally sensitive diagnostic tools for pheochromocytoma.
- Labeled metaiodobenzylguanidine (^{131}I-MIBG), which is structurally similar to norepinephrine, is taken up and concentrated in adrenergic tissue. It is highly sensitive and specific for malignant tumors and familial syndromes, but is inferior to bone scan for detecting bone metastases.

Treatment

SURGERY

- Surgery is the mainstay of treatment and should be considered for primary, recurrent, and metastatic disease.
- Appropriate preoperative evaluation and α ± β-blockade are required to minimize risk of hypertensive crisis.
- Laparoscopy is acceptable if no obvious tumor invasion or metastases are seen by imaging (Fig. 33.5).

CHEMOTHERAPY

- In a small study (14 patients), the combination of cyclophosphamide, vincristine, and dacarbazine had a biochemical response of 79%, with a 57% reduction in measurable disease and median duration of response >20 months.

RADIATION

- Radiation has a limited role in the treatment of pheochromocytoma, but may be used for bone and soft-tissue metastases.

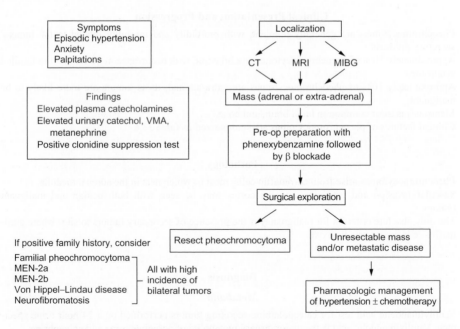

Fig. 33.5. Diagnosis and treatment of pheochromocytoma. (Used with permission from Abeloff M, Armitage J, Niederhuber J, Kastan M, McKenna W, eds. *Abeloff: Clinical Oncology.* 3rd ed. Philadelphia: Elsevier; 2004.)

NEUROENDOCRINE TUMORS

Neuroendocrine tumors are cancers of the interface between the endocrine system and the nervous system. These rare tumors are distinguished from most other solid tumors by their ability to secrete biologically active molecules that can produce systemic syndromes. The primary subgroups of neuroendocrine tumors are carcinoid tumors and pancreatic endocrine tumors.

Carcinoid Tumors

- Incidence in the United States is 1–2/100,000 individuals.
- Carcinoids are slow-growing malignant tumors that arise from enterochromaffin cells throughout the gut. They are most commonly found in the foregut and small intestine.
- Foregut (15%): patients present with symptoms of atypical hormonal excesses. Bronchial lesions: pulmonary symptoms; gastric or pancreatic lesions: abdominal pain or bleeding.
- Midgut (65%): small intestine (less frequent, metastases common) or appendix (more common, metastases rare). Symptomatic when metastatic or bulky.
- Hindgut (20%): colon or rectum. Patients present with bleeding or pain. Hormonal production is uncommon.
- Carcinoid syndrome observed in 10% of patients, especially those with liver metastases, retroperitoneal disease, or disease outside of the GI tract where excessive hormones can bypass metabolism in liver.

Treatment

- Abdominal and rectal carcinoids tend to be small (2 cm). Surgery involves segmental resection with mesenteric lymphadenectomy.
- Hepatic carcinoid is treated with surgical debulking, cryotherapy, or radiofrequency ablation. Transplantation may benefit patients with no extrahepatic disease.
- Carcinoids are resistant to most chemotherapeutic agents. Active agents include 5-fluorouracil, doxorubicin, and interferon α-2a and α-2b (10–20% response rates). Combining chemotherapeutic agents offers minimal clinical and survival benefit while increasing toxicity.
- Symptoms of hormonal excess may be mitigated with somatostatin analogs, steroids, and other agents.
- Radiation therapy is for palliation only.

Pancreatic Endocrine Tumors

Gastrinoma (Zollinger-Ellison Syndrome)

Gastrinoma is a tumor that secretes gastrin. Primary tumors predominate in the pancreatic head but may also develop in the small intestine or stomach.

Epidemiology

- Gastrinoma is the most common pancreatic endocrine tumor.
- Gastrinoma occurs in 0.1% to 1% of patients with peptic ulcer disease.
- Usually diagnosed between the third and sixth decades but can occur at any age.
- 20% of gastrinomas are familial and 20% of patients develop MEN-1.
- Approximately one-third of patients with gastrinoma have metastatic disease at diagnosis.

Pathology

- Gastrinomas are well differentiated, with few mitoses.
- Most gastrinomas are malignant. Malignant potential is determined by the presence of distant metastases, not by histologic grade.

CLINICAL PRESENTATION

- Increased secretion of gastric acid due to excess production of gastrin
- Severe, often refractory peptic ulcer disease
- Secretory diarrhea
- Abdominal pain

DIAGNOSIS

- Gastric acid pH <3.0 in the setting of hypergastrinemia (1,000 pg/mL) indicates gastrinoma.
- Gastrin level that increases by >200 pg/mL within 15 minutes of i.v. infusion of secretin is suggestive of gastrinoma.
- Other common diagnostic procedures include ultrasonography, CT scan, MRI, endoscopic ultra-sonography, angiography, and octreotide scan.

TREATMENT

- With the advent of more effective medical therapies, surgery has a limited role. It is an option in only 20% of patients and is controversial for patients with MEN-1. Resection of the primary tumor can reduce the rate of liver metastases.
- Medical therapies include proton pump inhibitors, somatostatin analogs (e.g., octreotide), and tumor embolization. Active chemotherapeutic agents include 5-fluoruracil, etoposide, doxorubicin, dacar-bazine, streptozotocin, and interferon-α.
- The role of radiation in the adjuvant setting is undefined. It may be effective for palliation in patients with unresectable disease.

Insulinoma

EPIDEMIOLOGY

- Insulinoma is the most common type of hormone-secreting tumor, accounting for 60% of pancreatic endocrine tumors.
- It occurs most commonly in the fifth decade of life, with a slight female predominance.
- Most insulinomas are solitary and approximately 10% are malignant, as defined by the presence of metastases.

CLINICAL PRESENTATION

Three criteria, known as Whipple's triad, suggest hypoglycemia:

- Symptoms known or likely to be caused by hypoglycemia
- Neuroglycopenic and/or adrenergic symptoms
- Relief of symptoms when glucose is raised to normal

DIAGNOSIS

- An inappropriately high level of insulin during an episode of hypoglycemia establishes the presence of insulinoma.
- Asymptomatic patients may be diagnosed after prolonged fasting by testing levels of serum glucose, insulin, and C-peptide every 6 to 12 hours.

TREATMENT

- Surgery is the treatment of choice for insulinoma and may be completely curative.
- Hypoglycemia may be managed with small, frequent meals.
- Oral diazoxide inhibits pancreatic secretion of insulin and stimulates release of catecholamine and glucose from the liver.
- Streptozotocin, 5-fluorouracil, and doxorubicin are active in patients with malignant disease.

VIPoma (Verner-Morrison Syndrome)

- VIPoma is a rare neuroendocrine tumor that usually originates in the pancreas and produces vasoactive intestinal peptide (VIP).
- Elevated serum VIP establishes the presence of VIPoma.
- Patients present with watery diarrhea, hypokalemia, and achlorhydria.
- Surgery is the treatment of choice; chemotherapy and radiation have limited roles. Diarrhea may be treated effectively with somatostatin analogs.

Glucagonoma

- Glucagonoma is a rare tumor of the pancreas that results in overproduction of the hormone glucagon.
- Serum levels of glucagon >500 pg/mL are diagnostic of glucagonoma.
- Glucagonoma leads to diabetes, weight loss, anemia, and increased risk of thromboembolism.
- Patients commonly present with ecrolytic migratory erythema, which may be treated with zinc supplements and amino acid infusion.
- Surgery, somatostatin analogs, anticoagulants, and chemotherapy are therapeutic options for glucagonomas.

Somatostatinoma

- Somatostatinoma is a tumor of the endocrine pancreas that secretes excess somatostatin. The tumor inhibits secretion of insulin and pancreatic enzyme and increases production of gastric acid.
- Surgery is the treatment of choice, but chemotherapy is indicated for unresectable disease.

MULTIPLE ENDOCRINE NEOPLASIA TYPES I AND II

MENs are characterized by the occurrence of tumors in two or more endocrine glands. MENs are uncommon, but are inherited as autosomal-dominant traits, thus giving first-degree relatives about a 50% risk of developing the disease (Table 33.7 and Fig. 33.6).

TABLE 33.7. *Syndromes of multiple endocrine neoplasias*

MEN-1 (Wermer syndrome)
Pituitary adenomas
Pancreatic islet cell tumors (insulinoma, gastrinoma)
Parathyroid hyperplasia/adenomas
Peptic ulcers (with Zollinger-Ellison syndrome)
Bronchial and thymic carcinoid
Adrenocortical adenoma
Thyroid follicular adenoma
MEN-2a (Sipple syndrome)
Thyroid C-cell hyperplasia and medullary carcinoma of the thyroid
Adrenal pheochromocytomas and medullary hyperplasia
Parathyroid hyperplasia/adenoma
MEN-2b
Thyroid C-cell hyperplasia and medullary carcinoma of the thyroid
Adrenal medullary hyperplasia
Multiple mucosal neuromata
Marfanoid body habitus
Megacolon

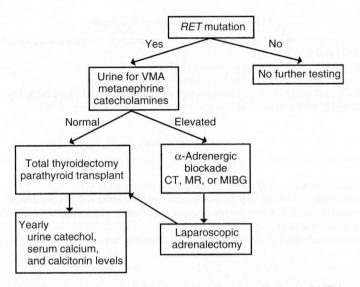

Fig. 33.6. Suggested treatment of individuals from kindreds of MEN-
2a. VMA, vanillylmandelic acid. (Used with permission from DeVita VT
Jr, Hellman S, Rosenberg SA, eds. *Cancer: Principles and Practice of
Oncology*. 5th ed. Philadelphia: Lippincott-Raven; 1997.)

SUGGESTED READINGS

Abeloff M, Armitage J, Niederhuber J, Kastan M, McKenna W, eds. *Abeloff: Clinical Oncology*. 3rd ed.
    Philadelphia: Elsevier; 2004.

Bellantone R, Lombardi CP, Raffaelli M, et al. Is routine supplementation therapy (calcium and vitamin
    D) useful after total thyroidectomy? *Surgery.* 2002;132(6):1109–12.

Grant CS, Hay ID, Gough IR, Bergstralh EJ, Goellner JR, McConahey WM. Local recurrence in papil-
    lary thyroid carcinoma: is extent of surgical resection important? *Surgery.* 1998;104:954–62.

Hundahl SA, Fleming ID, Fremgen AM, Menck HR. A National Cancer Data Base report on 53,856
    cases of thyroid carcinoma treated in the U.S., 1985–1995. *Cancer.* 1998;83:2638–48.

Icard P, Chapuis Y, Andreassian B, Bernard A, Proye C. Adrenocortical carcinoma in surgically treated
    patients: a retrospective study on 156 cases by the French Association of Endocrine Surgery. *Surgery*
    1992;112:972–9.

Ladenson PW. Recombinant thyrotropin for detection of recurrent thyroid cancer. *Trans Am Clin Cli-
    matol Assoc.* 2002;113:21–30.

Lairmore TC, Ball DW, Baylin SB, Wells SA Jr. Management of pheochromocytomas in patients with
    multiple endocrine neoplasia type 2 syndromes. *Ann Surg.* 1993;217:595–603.

Luton JP, Cerdas S, Billaud L, et al. Clinical features of adrenocortical carcinoma, prognostic factors,
    and the effect of mitotane therapy. *N Engl J Med.* 1990;322:1195–201.

Mazzaferri EL. Treating differentiated thyroid carcinoma: where do we draw the line? *Mayo Clin Proc.*
    1991;66:105–11.

Neumann HP, Berger DP, Sigmund G, et al. Pheochromocytomas, multiple endocrine neoplasia type 2,
    and von Hippel-Lindau disease. *N Engl J Med.* 1993;329:1531–8.

Norton JA. Adrenal tumors. In: DeVita VT Jr, Hellman S, Rosenberg SA, eds. *Cancer: Principles and Practice of Oncology*. 5th ed. Philadelphia: Lippincott-Raven; 1997:1659–77.

Sanders LE, Cady B. Differentiated thyroid cancer: reexamination of risk groups and outcome of treatment. *Arch Surg*. 1998;133:419–25.

Schlumberger MJ. Papillary and follicular thyroid carcinoma. *N Engl J Med*. 1998;338:297–308.

Sclafani LM, Woodruff JM, Brennan MF. Extraadrenal retroperitoneal paragangliomas: natural history and response to treatment. *Surgery*. 1990;108:1124–9.

Sherman SI. Thyroid carcinoma. *Lancet*. 2003;231:501–11.

SECTION 11

Supportive Care

34

Hematopoietic Growth Factors

Mahsa Mohebtash and Philip M. Arlen

BACKGROUND

- Hematologic toxicity (leukopenia, anemia, and thrombocytopenia) is the most common side effect of chemotherapy. It can lead to serious complications, such as neutropenic fever, which may require hospitalization.
- Hematopoietic growth factors are the regulatory molecules that stimulate the proliferation, differentiation, and survival of hematopoietic progenitor and stem cells. They were originally called colony-stimulating factors (CSFs) because of their role in colony formation in bone marrow cell cultures.
- Several hematopoietic growth factors are currently available for clinical use and are synthesized mainly by DNA recombinant technology.
- Recommendations in this chapter come primarily from the evidence-based clinical practice guidelines of the American Society of Clinical Oncology (ASCO) and the American Society of Hematology (ASH).

MYELOID GROWTH FACTORS

- Currently, two myeloid growth factors, filgrastim and sargramostim, have been approved for clinical use by the U.S. Food and Drug Administration (FDA) and there is no firm evidence indicating the superiority of one agent over another; both effectively increase absolute neutrophil count (ANC). However, their side effect profiles differ.
- Filgrastim is a granulocyte colony-stimulating factor (G-CSF) and is more specific for production of neutrophils, but has immunomodulatory effects on lymphocytes, monocytes, and macrophages. Anti-inflammatory effects have also been described for G-CSF. A pegylated form (pegfilgrastim) with a longer half-life is also available.
- Sargramostim is a granulocyte-macrophage colony-stimulating factor (GM-CSF) that stimulates the production of monocytes and eosinophils, in addition to neutrophils, and prolongs their half-lives. It also enhances their function through activation of chemotaxis, phagocytosis, oxidative activity, and antibody-dependent cellular cytotoxicity.

INDICATIONS

Primary Prophylaxis

CSFs are recommended for use with first- and subsequent-cycle chemotherapy to prevent febrile neutropenia (FN) when risk of FN is >20%. Most commonly used chemotherapy regimens have FN risks of <20%. However, CSFs can be used in special circumstances when the risks of prolonged neutropenia are high. Risk factors include:

- Age above 65
- Poor performance status
- Extensive prior treatments, including large-port radiation
- Previous episodes of FN

- Bone marrow involvement
- Advanced cancer
- Active infections or other serious comorbidities.

"Dose-dense" regimens of G-CSF have shown efficacy in the adjuvant treatment of node-positive breast cancer and may be beneficial in the treatment of elderly patients with aggressive lymphoma. Based on a recent meta-analysis of 3,439 patients, CSFs reduce the relative risk of FN and infection-related mortality by 46% and 45%, respectively. However, there is no evidence to date that they have any effect on overall or disease-free survival.

Secondary Prophylaxis

ASCO guidelines recommend administering CSFs to patients who have developed neutropenic complications from a prior cycle of chemotherapy when no CSFs were given. Dose reduction and treatment delay are reasonable alternatives, especially in the palliative setting.

Neutropenic Fever

Routine adjunctive use of CSFs for uncomplicated neutropenia is not recommended. However, in expected prolonged (>10 days) and profound (ANC $<100/\mu L$) neutropenia, CSFs should be considered. They should also be considered in patients with high-risk features for poor clinical outcome, including:

- Age above 65
- Sepsis syndrome
- Invasive fungal infection
- Uncontrolled primary disease

CSF in this setting has been shown to shorten hospital stay and duration of neutropenia, with no effect on its grade. CSF has no favorable impact on mortality from FN.

Hematopoietic Stem Cell Transplantation

CSFs are used routinely for peripheral blood stem cell (PBSC) mobilization and after autologous PBSC transplantation to shorten the duration of neutropenia and hospitalization, and to reduce costs. However, their use shortly after allogeneic transplantation may be associated with increased risk of graft-versus-host disease and worse survival.

Leukemia and Myelodysplastic Syndromes

- In patients with acute myeloid leukemia (AML), use of G-CSF shortly after completion of induction chemotherapy can lead to a modest decrease in neutropenia duration, but has no effect on remission rate and duration or survival. However, administration of G-CSF after completion of consolidation chemotherapy seems to have a more pronounced impact on neutropenia duration and infection rate, with no effect on complete response duration or overall survival. Currently there are insufficient data to support the use of long-acting CSF (pegfilgrastim) in AML, and its use should be confined to clinical trials.
- In myelodysplastic syndrome (MDS), intermittent use of CSFs may be considered in patients with severe neutropenia complicated by recurrent infections. There are no data on the safety of long-term use.
- In acute lymphoblastic leukemia (ALL), CSFs are recommended after the initial induction or first postremission chemotherapy course to shorten the duration of neutropenia. They can be given along with continued corticosteroids/antimetabolites; there is no evidence that this may prolong the myelosuppressive effects of chemotherapy. Their effects on the duration of hospital stay or incidence of serious infection are less prominent and have no impact on survival.

SIDE EFFECTS

Bone pain is frequently encountered with the use of myeloid growth factors. Rarely, splenic rupture and severe thrombocytopenia have been reported. CSFs may cause a transient acute respiratory distress syndrome or inflammatory pleuritis and pericarditis, which are thought to be secondary to neutrophil influx or capillary leak syndrome. In patients with sickle cell disease, use of CSFs has led to severe sickle cell crisis, resulting in death in some cases. Concurrent use of CSFs with chemotherapy and radiation therapy should be avoided because of the potential sensitivity of rapidly dividing myeloid cells to cytotoxic chemotherapy.

GM-CSF

- May cause flulike symptoms, fever, and rash.
- There is in vitro evidence that GM-CSF may stimulate HIV replication; however, clinical studies have not shown adverse effects on viral load among patients on antiretroviral therapy.
- The liquid form of sargramostim was withdrawn from the market in January 2008 because of increased reports of syncope, which was not seen with the lyophilized formulation.

G-CSF

- In general, G-CSF is better tolerated than GM-CSF and is used more commonly.
- May rarely cause pathologic neutrophil infiltration (Sweet syndrome).
- Antibodies to growth factors have been detected with some preparations, but are not neutralizing.
- Fragmentary evidence has raised concerns for increased risk of late monosomy 7-associated MDS and AML in patients with aplastic anemia treated with long-term G-CSF.

DOSING

- Recommended dosing of CSFs is listed in Table 34.1.
- In chemotherapy patients, transient increase in neutrophil count is typically observed in the first 1 to 2 days after initiation of CSFs. Treatment should continue until post-nadir ANC reaches 10,000/mm^3. Check complete blood count twice weekly.
- Pegfilgrastim should not be administered from 14 days before to 24 hours after myelosuppressive chemotherapy.
- Sargramostim is licensed for use after autologous or allogeneic bone marrow transplant and for AML.

ERYTHROPOIESIS-STIMULATING AGENTS

Erythropoiesis-stimulating agents (ESAs) are semisynthetic agents that simulate the effects of erythropoietin (EPO), an endogenous hormone produced by the kidneys. By binding to EPO receptors, ESAs stimulate the division and differentiation of committed erythroid progenitors in bone marrow. ESAs are manufactured by recombinant DNA technology and are available as epoetin alfa and darbepoetin alfa. Darbepoetin alfa has a half-life around three times longer than that of epoetin alfa; however, they are considered equivalent in terms of effectiveness and safety.

EFFECTS

- ESAs were first used to manage anemia in patients with chronic renal failure (CRF). Several randomized clinical trials have demonstrated that ESAs decrease blood transfusion requirements and improve quality of life in patients on hemodialysis.
- In cancer patients, ESAs have been shown to reduce the need for transfusion, but their effects on anemia symptoms and quality of life have not been proven.
- A growing body of evidence has raised serious concerns about the safety of ESAs.

TABLE 34.1. *Growth factors for transplant or nonmyeloid cancer patients only:
FDA-approved dosing and indications*

Drug	Dosing	Indications
Filgrastim (Neupogen)	5 μg/kg SC daily 24 h after completion of chemotherapy until ANC reaches 2,000 to 3,000/mm^3 10 μg/kg SC daily at least 4 d before the first leukapheresis; continue until the last leukapheresis	Myelosuppressive chemo-therapy PBSC mobilization
Pegfilgrastim (Neulasta)	Single 6-mg fixed dose SC 24 h after com-pletion of chemotherapy	Myelosuppressive chemo-therapy
Sargramostim (Leukine)	250 μg/mm^2 i.v. daily until ANC reaches 1,500/mm^3 for 3 consecutive days; reduce dose by 50% if ANC increases to >20,000/mm^3	Auto/allo BMT, after AML induction chemotherapy
Epoetin alfa (Epo-gen; Procrit)	Start at 150 U/kg SC TIW or 40,000 U SC weekly Escalate dose to 300 U/kg TIW or 60,000 U SC weekly if no reduction in transfusion requirements or rise in Hb after 8 wk (for TIW dosing) or if no rise in Hb by ≥1 g/dL after 4 wk (for weekly dosing) Reduce dose by 25% when Hb reaches level needed to avoid transfusion or Hb rises >1 g/dL in 2 wk • Hold if Hb >12 g/dL; withhold until Hb falls to a level where transfusions may be required; resume at 25% below previous dose	Chemotherapy-induced anemia
Darbepoetin alfa (Aranesp)	Start at 2.25 mcg/kg SC weekly or 500 mcg SC Q3W Escalate dose to 4.5 mcg/kg if Hb rises <1 g/dL after 6 wk Reduce dose by 40% of previous dose when Hb reaches level needed to avoid transfusion or Hb rises >1 g/dL in 2 wk Hold if Hb >12 g/dL; withhold until Hb falls to a level where transfusions may be required. Resume at 40% below previous dose	Chemotherapy-induced anemia
Oprelvekin (Neumega)	50 mcg/kg SC daily; start 6 to 24 h after completion of chemotherapy and con-tinue until post-nadir platelet count is >50,000/mm^3	Nonmyeloablative chemo-therapy-induced thrombo-cytopenia

AML, acute myeloid leukemia; ANC, absolute neutrophil count; auto/allo BMT, autologous/allogeneic bone marrow transplant; d, days; ESA, erythropoiesis-stimulating agent; FDA, U.S. Food and Drug Administration; h, hours; Hb, hemoglobin; i.v., intravenously; PBSC, peripheral blood stem cell; Q3W, every 3 weeks; SC, subcutaneously; TIW, three times per week; wk, weeks.

Transfusion Requirements and Quality of Life

A recent systematic review summarized the results of 57 trials involving 9,353 cancer patients ran-domly assigned to receive ESA plus RBC transfusion or transfusion alone. This meta-analysis included patients who did and patients who did not receive concurrent antineoplastic therapy. Results showed a 36% reduction in transfusion requirement in those receiving ESA. Although there was a positive overall effect on quality of life, the report could not draw definite conclusions because of different parameters used by the various studies.

Survival, Mortality, and Disease Control

- Observational studies have suggested that anemia in cancer patients is associated with shorter survival and that increasing hemoglobin (Hb) levels may improve survival and tumor response in some cancers. Because radiation and some chemotherapy agents are dependent on tissue oxygenation for their effect, it was speculated that improving oxygen delivery by increasing Hb levels may optimize the effects of antineoplastic treatments. Based on this hypothesis, several randomized trials in head and neck, breast, non–small cell lung, lymphoid, and cervical cancers were conducted to evaluate the effect of ESAs on survival and disease control. Most of these studies were terminated prematurely because of disease progression and increased mortality. Poor outcomes could not be consistently attributed to thromboembolic events, which minimally increased in some of these trials. Furthermore, thromboembolic events would not explain shortened time-to-tumor progression (TTP). A preliminary report of a study using ESAs in cancer patients not receiving chemotherapy showed no reduced need for blood transfusions; it did show increased mortality. Based on this report, the FDA released a black box safety alert in February 2007 warning against the use of ESAs for anemia in cancer patients not receiving chemotherapy. The FDA also recommended a minimum effective dose of ESAs that would gradually increase Hb levels sufficient to avoid transfusion, but not to exceed 12 g/dL. Most of the ESA trials had set a goal of Hb >12 g/dL; however, the risks of shortened survival and TTP have persisted even when ESAs are dosed to achieve Hb levels <12 g/dL.
- It has been suggested that shorter TTP could be attributed to EPO receptor-positive tumors. However, currently available assays to detect EPO receptors are nonspecific and their validity has not been determined.
- In July 2007, the Centers for Medicare and Medicaid Services revised their national coverage guidelines to limit reimbursement of ESAs. Coverage of ESAs in cancer patients is now restricted to those receiving chemotherapy whose Hb level is <10 g/dL prior to initiation of ESA treatment.
- Increased mortality and adverse events have also been observed in CRF patients, which has led to lower Hb targets in this patient population.

INDICATIONS

ASCO and ASH Guidelines

In nonmyeloid cancers, ESAs should only be considered in patients receiving chemotherapy whose anemia is symptomatic and thought to be due to chemotherapy. ESAs can be initiated if Hb approaches or falls below 10; Hb should not exceed 12. For Hb levels between 10 and 11, use of ESAs should be based on symptoms and clinical circumstances. If there is no response after 6 to 8 weeks with appropriate dose modification, treatment should be discontinued. Blood transfusion is a therapeutic option.

FDA-Approved Indications

ESAs are approved for chemotherapy-related anemia in nonmyeloid malignancies, CRF, HIV (zidovudine) therapy, and to reduce the need for blood transfusion in elective noncardiac and nonvascular surgeries.

Off-Label/Investigational Use

- There is evidence supporting the use of ESAs for anemia related to MDS. However, patients may require higher doses and response may be delayed. Predictors of response include low-risk MDS and low EPO levels (<200 U/L). Combining ESAs and G-CSF in MDS patients has resulted in improved response rates.
- Other indications include multiple myeloma, non-Hodgkin's lymphoma, chronic lymphocytic leukemia, beta thalassemia, radiation therapy, rheumatoid arthritis, paroxysmal nocturnal hemoglobinuria, Castleman's disease, congestive heart failure, critical illnesses, hepatitis C (in patients treated with interferon-alfa and ribarvirin), and blood-unit collection for autotransfusion.

DOSING

Recommended dosing and dose adjustments of ESAs in chemotherapy-induced anemia are listed in Table 34.1. After initiation or dose modification of ESAs, Hb should be monitored weekly until it stabilizes.

SIDE EFFECTS

- The most serious side effects of ESAs are thromboembolic events, defined as transient ischemic attack, stroke, pulmonary emboli, deep vein thrombosis, and myocardial infarction. A meta-analysis showed that thromboembolic events increased 67% in cancer patients; for a population with baseline risk of 20%, the number needed to harm would be 7.5 patients (95% CI, 3.1–15.6). There is evidence for increased risk of thromboembolic events in CRF and surgical patients, especially with higher Hb targets. Preliminary analysis of a trial in spinal surgery patients given ESAs to decrease postsurgery transfusion requirements showed increased incidence of thromboembolic events in the ESA arm. Notably, patients received no prophylactic anticoagulants postoperatively.
- ESAs are contraindicated in uncontrolled hypertension, more commonly seen in CRF patients who receive i.v. ESAs.
- Other side effects include headache, fatigue, fever, rash, pruritis, hypersensitivity reactions, arthralgia and myalgia, nausea, seizures, and pure red-cell aplasia due to neutralizing antibodies to native EPO.

OTHER CONSIDERATIONS

- Iron supplementation should be considered in patients receiving ESAs, especially those with borderline iron stores, because iron deficiency can develop soon after initiation of ESAs and can adversely affect response to ESAs.
- Measuring serum EPO levels may help to identify patients more likely to respond to ESAs. Patients with baseline EPO levels <100 U/L are more likely to respond to ESAs than those with levels >100 U/L.

PLATELET GROWTH FACTORS

- Thrombocytopenia can be a life-threatening consequence of antineoplastic treatments. Platelet transfusions are required to prevent or mitigate hemorrhagic complications. Patients at high risk for bleeding or who experience delays in receiving planned chemotherapy include the following:
  - Patients with poor bone marrow reserve or a history of bleeding
  - Patients on treatment regimens highly toxic to bone marrow
  - Patients with a potential bleeding site (e.g., necrotic tumor)
- Fortunately, iatrogenic thrombocytopenia that requires platelet transfusion or causes major bleeding is relatively uncommon, although occurrence tends to increase with cumulative cycles of chemotherapy that are toxic to hematopoietic progenitor cells. At present, formal guidelines for the use of thrombopoietic growth factors are under development.
- Although several thrombopoietic agents are in clinical development, oprelvekin is the only thrombocytopoietic agent FDA-approved for clinical use. Oprelvekin is a product of recombinant DNA technology and is nearly homologous with native IL-11. Oprelvekin stimulates megakaryocytopoiesis and thrombopoiesis, and has been shown to modestly shorten the duration of thrombocytopenia and reduce the need for platelet transfusions in patients who develop platelet counts $<20 \times 10^3$ per μL after prior antineoplastic treatments. Oprelvekin is not indicated following myeloablative chemotherapy. Major side effects include fluid retention and atrial arrhythmias. Hypersensitivity reactions, including anaphylaxis, have also been reported. Table 34.1 provides the recommended dose of oprelvekin.

- Recombinant thrombopoietins (TPOs) are no longer being developed because of antibody production. TPO mimetics (TPO receptor agonists) are currently under investigation.

SUGGESTED READINGS

Bohlius J, Wilson J, Seidenfeld J, et al. Erythropoietin or darbepoetin for patients with cancer. *Cochrane Database Syst Rev* 2006;3:CD003407.

Boneberg EM, Hareng L, Gantner F, Wendel A, Hartung T. Human monocytes express functional receptors for granulocyte colony-stimulating factor that mediate suppression of monokines and interferon-gamma. *Blood* 2000;95(1):270–6.

Caro JJ, Salas M, Ward A, Goss G. Anemia as an independent prognostic factor for survival in patients with cancer: a systemic, quantitative review. *Cancer* 2001;91(12):2214–21.

Citron ML, Berry DA, Cirrincione C, et al. Randomized trial of dose-dense versus conventionally scheduled and sequential versus concurrent combination chemotherapy as postoperative adjuvant treatment of node-positive primary breast cancer: first report of Intergroup Trial C9741/Cancer and Leukemia Group B Trial 9741. *J Clin Oncol* 2003;21(8):1431–9.

Cwirla SE, Balasubramanian P, Duffin DJ, et al. Peptide agonist of the thrombopoietin receptor as potent as the natural cytokine. *Science* 1997;276(5319):1696–9.

Elliott S, Busse L, Bass MB, et al. Anti-Epo receptor antibodies do not predict Epo receptor expression. Blood 2006;107(5):1892–5.

Eschbach JW, Kelly MR, Haley NR, Abels RI, Adamson JW. Treatment of the anemia of progressive renal failure with recombinant human erythropoietin. *N Engl J Med* 1989;321(3):158–63.

Gribben JG, Devereux S, Thomas NS, et al. Development of antibodies to unprotected glycosylation sites on recombinant human GM-CSF. *Lancet* 1990;335(8687):434–7.

Henke M, Mattern D, Pepe M, et al. Do erythropoietin receptors on cancer cells explain unexpected clinical findings? *J Clin Oncol* 2006;24(29):4708–13.

Henry DH, Dahl NV, Auerbach M, Tchekmedyian S, Laufman LR. Intravenous ferric gluconate significantly improves response to epoetin alfa versus oral iron or no iron in anemic patients with cancer receiving chemotherapy. *Oncologist* 2007;12(2):231–42.

Koyanagi Y, O'Brien WA, Zhao JQ, Golde DW, Gasson JC, Chen IS. Cytokines alter production of HIV-1 from primary mononuclear phagocytes. *Science* 1988;241(4873):1673–5.

Kuderer NM, Dale DC, Crawford J, Lyman GH. Impact of primary prophylaxis with granulocyte colony-stimulating factor on febrile neutropenia and mortality in adult cancer patients receiving chemotherapy: a systematic review. *J Clin Oncol* 2007;25(21):3158–67.

Ludwig H, Fritz E, Leitgeb C, Pecherstorfer M, Samonigg H, Schuster J. Prediction of response to erythropoietin treatment in chronic anemia of cancer. *Blood* 1994;84(4):1056–63.

Osterborg A, Brandberg Y, Molostova V, et al. Randomized, double-blind, placebo-controlled trial of recombinant human erythropoietin, epoetin Beta, in hematologic malignancies. *J Clin Oncol* 2002;20(10):2486–94.

Pajkrt D, Manten A, van der Poll T, et al. Modulation of cytokine release and neutrophil function by granulocyte colony-stimulating factor during endotoxemia in humans. *Blood* 1997;90(4):1415–24.

Ringden O, Labopin M, Gorin NC, et al. Treatment with granulocyte colony-stimulating factor after allogeneic bone marrow transplantation for acute leukemia increases the risk of graft-versus-host disease and death: a study from the Acute Leukemia Working Party of the European Group for Blood and Marrow Transplantation. *J Clin Oncol* 2004;22(3):416–23.

Rizzo JD, Somerfield MR, Hagerty KL, et al. Use of epoetin and darbepoetin in patients with cancer: 2007 American Society of Clinical Oncology/American Society of Hematology clinical practice guideline update. *J Clin Oncol* 2008;26(1):132–49.

Singh AK, Szczech L, Tang KL, et al. Correction of anemia with epoetin alfa in chronic kidney disease. *N Engl J Med* 2006;355(20):2085–98.

Smith RE Jr, Aapro MS, Ludwig H, et al. Darbepoetin alfa for the treatment of anemia in patients with active cancer not receiving chemotherapy or radiotherapy: results of a phase III, multicenter, randomized, double-blind, placebo-controlled study. *J Clin Oncol* 2008;26(7):1040–50.

Smith TJ, Khatcheressian J, Lyman GH, et al. 2006 update of recommendations for the use of white blood cell growth factors: an evidence-based clinical practice guideline. *J Clin Oncol* 2006;24(19):3187–205.

Stasi R, Abruzzese E, Lanzetta G, Terzoli E, Amadori S. Darbepoetin alfa for the treatment of anemic patients with low- and intermediate-1-risk myelodysplastic syndromes. *Ann Oncol* 2005;16(12):1921–7.

Tepler I, Elias L, Smith JW II, et al. A randomized placebo-controlled trial of recombinant human interleukin-11 in cancer patients with severe thrombocytopenia due to chemotherapy. *Blood* 1996;87(9):3607–14.

Wright JR, Ung YC, Julian JA, et al. Randomized, double-blind, placebo-controlled trial of erythropoietin in non-small-cell lung cancer with disease-related anemia. *J Clin Oncol* 2007;25(9):1027–32.

35

Infectious Complications in Oncology

Nilofer S. Azad, Sarah W. Read, and Juan C. Gea-Banacloche

FEVER IN THE NEUTROPENIC CANCER PATIENT

Neutropenia is the most important risk factor for bacterial infection in cancer patients. The risk of infection increases with the rapidity of onset, degree, and duration of neutropenia. Febrile neutropenic patients require immediate evaluation and prompt initiation of empirical antibiotics (Fig. 35.1). Empirical broad-spectrum antibiotics with activity against *Pseudomonas aeruginosa* must be initiated as soon as the clinical evaluation is completed. Antifungal treatment should be considered with prolonged neutropenic fever (>4 days) and/or worsening clinical course.

DEFINITION

- Fever: one oral temperature greater than 38.3°C or two oral temperatures greater than 38°C measured 1 hour apart.
- Neutropenia: an absolute neutrophil count (ANC) <500/mm³, or ANC ≤1,000/mm³, with a predicted decline to <500/mm³ within 48 hours.
- Afebrile patients with neutropenia and clinical signs of infection (e.g., abdominal pain, hypotension) should be treated empirically as well, especially if they have been treated with corticosteroids, which blunt the febrile response.

ETIOLOGY

- In 10% to 20% of patients with fever and neutropenia an infection is documented microbiologically (most commonly bacteremia).
- In 20% to 30% of patients with fever and neutropenia there is clinical evidence of infection.
- In 50% of patients with fever and neutropenia no infection is found, but the response to empirical management with antibiotics is the same as the others.
- Gram-positive and gram-negative bacteria are isolated with similar frequency.
- Empirical treatment is targeted to cover gram-negative pathogens, particularly *Pseudomonas* species.
- *Candida* and *Aspergillus* species are the most common causes of fungal infections in neutropenic patients and increase in frequency with longer duration of neutropenia.

EVALUATION

- History and physical exam should be performed with special attention to potential sites of infection: skin, mouth, perianal region, and intravenous catheter exit site.
- Routine complete blood count, chemistries, urinalysis, blood and urine cultures, and chest x-ray should be obtained.
- Any accessible sites of possible infection should be sampled for gram stain and culture (catheter site, sputum, etc.).

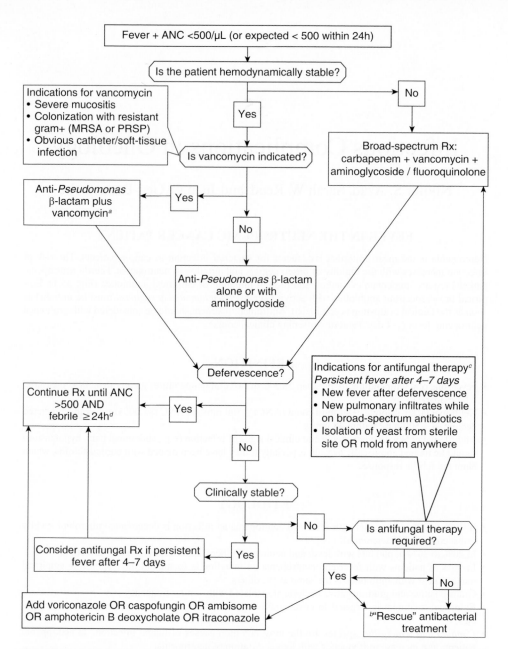

Fig. 35.1. Approach to patients with fever and neutropenia without clinically or microbiologically documented infection. For specific infections, see text and Table 35.2. [a]Vancomycin should be discontinued after 48 to 72 hours if there is no bacteriological documentation of a pathogen requiring its use, except in soft-tissue or tunnel infections. Linezolid may be substituted instead of vancomycin if there is suspicion of VRE. [b]This "rescue" antibacterial regimen will vary between institutions, depending on the local patterns of antibiotic resistance. Carbapenem + fluoroquinolone/aminoglycoside + vancomycin is typical. [c]For a detailed discussion of antifungal therapy options, see text. [d]May consider switching responding low-risk patients to oral antibiotics; see text. MRSA, methicillin (oxacillin)-resistant *Staphylococcus aureus*; PRSP, penicillin-resistant *Streptococcus pneumoniae*.

- Ideally, cultures should be obtained prior to starting antibiotics, but failure to do so should not delay antibiotic administration.

EMPIRICAL ANTIBIOTIC THERAPY

Monotherapy

Monotherapy with selected broad-spectrum beta-lactams with activity against *Pseudomonas* species is as effective as combination antibiotic regimens (beta-lactam plus aminoglycoside) for empirical therapy of uncomplicated fever and neutropenia, and has fewer toxicities. Antibiotics recommended by the Infectious Disease Society of America include the following; doses are for adults with normal renal function:

- Ceftazidime, 2 g i.v. every 8 hours
- Cefepime, 2 g i.v. every 8 hours
- Imipenem-cilastatin, 500 mg i.v. every 6 hours
- Meropenem, 1 g i.v. every 8 hours
- Piperacillin-tazobactam, 4.5 g i.v. every 6 hours

The choice of one agent over another should be guided mainly by institutional susceptibilities, which may make one or more of the aforementioned agents a poor choice. By meta-analysis, they seem to offer similar efficacy, but carbapenems (imipenem and meropenem) seem to result in increased pseudomembranous colitis and cefepime seems to be linked to increased overall mortality (see FDA Early Communication http://www.fda.gov/cder/drug/early_comm/cefepime.htm).

Combination Therapy

Combination therapy can be used empirically to broaden the antibacterial spectrum in certain clinical circumstances, although there are no definitive data showing clinical benefit. Combination therapy should be used in cases of:

- severe sepsis or septic shock, or
- high prevalence of multidrug-resistant gram-negative bacilli.

Effective antibiotic combinations include one of the aforementioned beta-lactams plus an aminoglycoside (choice based on local resistance, typically amikacin). Ciprofloxacin may be used instead of an aminoglycoside if the prevalence of quinolone-resistant bacteria is low or in patients with renal insufficiency.

Febrile neutropenic patients with candiduria or oral thrush should initially be covered with antifungal therapy empirically.

Role of Vancomycin

Vancomycin should *not* be part of the initial empirical regimen unless one or more of the following circumstances applies:

- Clinically suspected catheter-related infections (not the mere presence of an intravascular device)
- Positive blood cultures for gram-positive bacteria prior to identification of species or susceptibility Linezolid may be considered where there is high prevalence of vancomycin-resistant enterococcus (VRE).
- Known colonization with penicillin-resistant *Streptococcus pneumoniae* (PRSP) or methicillin-resistant *Staphylococcus aureus* (MRSA)
- Severe mucositis
- Soft-tissue infection
- Severe sepsis or septic shock
- Consider in patients treated with quinolones or TMP/SMX prophylaxis, due to potential selective pressure for resistant viridans streptococcal organisms.

TABLE 35.1.   *The MASCC index*

Characteristics	Score
Burden of illness	
No or mild symptoms	5
Moderate symptoms	3
No hypotension	5
No chronic obstructive pulmonary disease	4
Solid tumor or no previous fungal infection	4
No dehydration	3
Outpatient status	3
Age <60 yr	2

Scoring system based on patient characteristics and symptoms used for selecting patients who are suitable candidates for oral therapy (score ≥21 of 26 possible points).

Source: From Multinational Association for Supportive Care in Cancer risk index: a multinational scoring system for identifying low-risk febrile neutropenic cancer patients. *J Clin Oncol.* 2000;18(16):3038–51.

Adding vancomycin to the initial regimen because of persistent fever alone does not improve the outcome and is not recommended.

Oral Therapy

Oral therapy may be acceptable for initial empirical therapy in certain low-risk febrile neutropenic patients. A scoring system based on patient characteristics and clinical symptoms may be useful in selecting eligible patients (Table 35.1). Patients with a score of ≥21 of 26 possible points, indicating low risk, can be considered for oral therapy.

We recommend:

- ciprofloxacin, 750 mg P.O. every 12 hours, plus
- amoxicillin/clavulanate, 875 mg (amoxicillin component) P.O. every 12 hours.

We recommend starting oral antibiotics on an inpatient basis. Following discharge, patients should be seen in clinic daily and instructed to call or come in to clinic for new or worsening symptoms or persistent high fever.

Low-risk patients with no discernable source of neutropenia who respond to empirical i.v. antibiotics can be switched to oral antibiotics until their neutropenia resolves based on clinical judgment. We recommend observing these patients on oral therapy as inpatients for at least 24 hours before discharge.

Modifications of the Initial Antibiotic Regimen

After patients are started on empirical antibiotics for fever and neutropenia, their course must be monitored closely for development of signs or symptoms of infection; antibiotic therapy should be modified accordingly. Therapy modification is necessary in 30% to 50% of cases during the course of neutropenia. Specific modifications are dictated by specific clinical syndromes (Table 35.2) or by microbiologic isolates.

Empirical Antifungal Therapy

Candida and *Aspergillus* infections are most common and increase in frequency with increased duration of neutropenia. An antifungal agent should be added empirically for neutropenic patients with persistent or recurrent fever after 4 to 7 days of broad-spectrum antibiotic therapy. Treatment options include:

TABLE 35.2. *Specific infectious disease syndromes in oncology patients and approach to diagnosis and management*

Clinical syndrome	Diagnostic considerations	Management
Intravascular catheter-associated infections	Infections can be local involving the exit site or subcutaneous tunnel, or systemic causing bacteremia For local infections, check culture of exit-site discharge as well as blood cultures	For tunnel and systemic infections, empirical therapy should include vancomycin as well as gram-negative coverage (e.g., ceftazidime, cefepime, ciprofloxacin) Intravascular catheters should be removed in certain situations: Tunnel infections Blood cultures remain positive after 72 h of therapy regardless of pathogen Specific pathogens: *Mycobacteria* spp, *Bacillus* spp, *S. aureus*, fungi; case-by-case decision for *C. jekeium* VRE and gram-negative organisms Consider antibiotic lock if feasible
Skin/soft-tissue infections	Prompt biopsy with histologic staining and culture for bacteria, mycobacteria, viruses, and fungi Pathogens: *S. aureus*, *S. pyogenes*, gram-negative bacilli (e.g., *Pseudomonas*), VZV, HSV, *Candida* For vesicular lesions, scrape base for DFA for VZV and culture for HSV	Ecthyma gangrenosum: include coverage of *Pseudomonas* (e.g., ceftazidime, cefepime, ciprofloxacin) Infections with *S. pyogenes*: treat aggressively with penicillin G, clindamycin, IVIG, and surgical debridement Perianal cellulitis: broad-spectrum coverage including anaerobes (e.g., imipenem) VZV, HSV: acyclovir
Sinusitis	Evaluate with CT scan and examination by otolaryngologist Tissue should be biopsied if there is suspicion of fungal infection or no response to antibiotic therapy after 72 h Pathogens: *S. pneumoniae*, *H. influenzae*, *M. catarrhalis*, *S. aureus*, gram-negative bacilli (e.g., *Pseudomonas*), fungi including zygomycetes	Non-neutropenic: levofloxacin or amoxicillin/clavulanate Neutropenic: broad-spectrum coverage including *Pseudomonas* (e.g., imipenem) and consider fungal coverage (e.g., amphotericin B, voriconazole)
Pulmonary infections	CT scan and BAL should be performed early Pneumonias in any cancer patient are often caused by gram-negative bacilli and *S. aureus* as well as community-acquired pneumonia pathogens: *S. pneumoniae*, *H. influenzae*, *Legionella* spp, *Chlamydia pneumoniae*	For all patients, ensure adequate coverage of community-acquired pneumonia (e.g., newer generation fluoroquinolone) Neutropenic: include coverage of *S. pneumoniae* and *Pseudomonas* (e.g., newer generation fluoroquinolone and ceftazidime); add antifungal coverage if pneumonia develops on antibiotics (e.g., amphotericin B, voriconazole)

(Continued)

TABLE 35.2. *(Continued)*

	Neutropenic patients are at risk for invasive fungal infections, particularly aspergillosis	Cell-mediated immunodeficiency: consider coverage of *Pneumocystis* with TMP/SMX, CMV with ganciclovir, and *Nocardia* with TMP/SMX
	Patients with cell-mediated defects are at risk for infections with PCP, viruses (CMV, VZV, HSV), and *Nocardia* spp and *Legionella*	
	Mycobacteria should also be considered, particularly in patients with previous exposure	
Gastrointestinal tract infections	Lesions associated with mucositis can be superinfected with HSV or *Candida*	Mucositis or esophagitis: acyclovir and fluconazole
	Esophagitis can be caused by *Candida*, HSV, CMV	*C. difficile*: metronidazole or vancomycin if refractory
	Diarrhea is most commonly caused by *C. difficile* (send toxin assay) but can also be caused by *Salmonella*, *Shigella*, *Aeromonas*, *E. coli*, viruses, parasites, etc.	Neutropenic enterocolitis: broad-spectrum coverage including *Pseudomonas* (e.g., imipenem)
	Enterocolitis in neutropenic patients is most commonly caused by a mix of organisms including *Clostridium* spp and *Pseudomonas*	
Urinary tract infections	Pathogens: gram-negative bacilli, *Candida*	Remove catheter to clear colonization
	Consider whether candiduria may represent disseminated candidiasis	Neutropenic patient: treat bacteriuria/candiduria regardless of symptoms
		Nonneutropenic patient: reserve treatment for symptomatic episodes
		Antibiotic treatment should be tailored to organism
CNS infections	Bacteria cause most cases of meningitis (*S. pneumoniae*, *Listeria*, *N. meningitides*)	Bacterial meningitis: ceftriaxone, vancomycin, and ampicillin
	In patient with cell-mediated immunodeficiency, also consider *Listeria* or *Cryptococcus*	Cryptococcal meningitis: amphotericin B with flucytosine
	Encephalitis is most commonly caused by HSV but consider other viruses	Encephalitis: acyclovir (consider ganciclovir)
	Brain abscesses may be confused with tumor	

VZV, varicella zoster virus; HSV, herpes simplex virus; IVIG, intravenous immunoglobulin; CMV, cytomegalovirus.

- Amphotericin B deoxycholate, 0.6 to 1 mg/kg/day i.v.
- A lipid formulation of amphotericin B such as liposomal amphotericin B (Ambisome) or amphotericin B lipid complex (Abelcet), 3 to 5 mg/kg/day i.v.
- Voriconazole, 6 mg/kg i.v. every 12 hours for 24 hours followed by 4 mg/kg i.v. every 12 hours
- Posaconazole, 200 mg P.O. every 8 hours with food.
- Caspofungin, 70 mg i.v. loading dose followed by 50 mg i.v. daily.

Although there is reasonable evidence to suggest all of these may work as empirical additions during persistent fever, an effort should be made to rule out the presence of active invasive fungal infection by performing a thorough physical exam and obtaining CT studies as clinically indicated. Some authorities recommend serological testing for fungal infection (galactomannan and/or beta-glucan) in this setting, but its role has not been clearly defined.

Duration of Antibiotic Therapy

- Documented bacterial infection: antibiotics should be continued for the standard amount of time for that infection or until resolution of neutropenia, whichever is longer.
- Uncomplicated fever and neutropenia of uncertain etiology: antibiotics should be continued until the fever has resolved and the ANC is above 500 for 24 hours.
- If there was no documented fungal infection, antifungal agents can also be discontinued at this time.

FEVER IN THE NON-NEUTROPENIC CANCER PATIENT

Cancer patients may have fever for many reasons besides infection, including the underlying malignancy, deep venous thrombosis and pulmonary embolism, medications, blood products and, in allogeneic stem cell transplant, graft-versus-host disease. Infections, however, are a significant problem in patients with all types of malignancies in all stages of treatment. In addition to neutropenia, there are several other factors that contribute to increased susceptibility to infection.

- Local factors: breakdown of barriers (mucositis, surgery) that provide a portal of entry for bacteria, and obstruction (biliary, ureteral, bronchial) that facilitates local infection (cholangitis, pyelonephritis, postobstructive pneumonia).
- Intravascular devices, drainage tubes, or stents may become colonized and lead to local infection, bacteremia, or fungemia.
- Splenectomy increases susceptibility to infection due to *S. pneumoniae* and other encapsulated bacteria.
- Deficiencies of humoral immunity (multiple myeloma, chronic lymphoid leukemia) lead to increased susceptibility to encapsulated organisms such as *S. pneumoniae* and *Haemophilus influenzae*.
- Defects in cell-mediated immunity (lymphoma, hairy cell leukemia, treatment with steroids, fludarabine and other drugs, T cell-depleted hematopoietic stem cell transplant [HSCT]) increase susceptibility to opportunistic infections from *Legionella pneumophila*, *Mycobacteria* species, *Cryptococcus neoformans*, *Pneumocystis jirovecii*, cytomegalovirus (CMV), varicella zoster virus (VZV), and other pathogens.

Antibiotic Therapy in the Non-neutropenic Cancer Patient

- Antibiotics should be administered empirically in the setting of fever only when a bacterial infection is considered likely.
- In the absence of localizing signs and symptoms, consider bacteremia, particularly in patients with intravascular devices. Many authorities recommend empirical antibiotics (levofloxacin, ceftriaxone) until bacteremia is ruled out.
- Clinically documented infections and sepsis should be treated with antibiotics as warranted by the clinical scenario.
- Whenever antibiotics are started, a plan with specific endpoints should be formulated to avoid unnecessary toxicity, superinfection, and development of resistance.

SPECIFIC INFECTIOUS DISEASE SYNDROMES

If a patient presents with clinical signs and symptoms of a specific infection, with or without neutropenia, the workup and therapy are guided by the clinical suspicion (see Table 35.2).

Bacteremia/Fungemia

- A positive blood culture should prompt immediate initiation of appropriate antibiotics in a neutropenic patient or in a non-neutropenic patient who is febrile or clinically unstable.
- If the isolated organism is one that is commonly pathogenic, such as *S. aureus* or gram-negative bacilli, antibiotics should be started even if the patient is afebrile and clinically stable.
- If the isolate is a common contaminant, such as a coagulase-negative *Staphylococcus*, and the patient is afebrile, clinically stable, and non-neutropenic, it may be appropriate to repeat the cultures and observe before starting antibiotics.
- Whenever bacteremia has been documented, blood cultures should be repeated to confirm the effectiveness of therapy, and the source of the infection should be sought.

Gram-Positive Bacteremia

Gram-Positive Cocci

- Coagulase-negative *Staphylococcus* species is the most common cause of bacteremia. In the setting of neutropenia or clinical instability, the patient should be treated with vancomycin.
- *S. aureus* bacteremia is associated with a high likelihood of metastatic complications if not treated adequately. Intravascular devices should be removed and transesophageal echocardiogram performed to rule out endocarditis.
- Oxacillin and nafcillin are the drugs of choice for treating methicillin-susceptible *S. aureus*; vancomycin should be reserved for MRSA or the treatment of penicillin-allergic patients.
- Bacteremia with viridans group streptococci may cause overwhelming infection with sepsis and acute respiratory distress syndrome (ARDS) in the neutropenic patient; vancomycin therapy should be used until susceptibility results are known (most, but not all, isolates are susceptible to ceftriaxone and carbapenems).
- Risk factors for viridans group streptococci bacteremia include severe mucositis (particularly following treatment with cytarabine), active oral infection, and prophylaxis with trimethoprim/sulfamethoxazole (TMP/SMX) or a fluoroquinolone.
- Enterococci often cause bacteremia in debilitated patients who have had prolonged hospitalization and have been on broad-spectrum antibiotics.
- Vancomycin-resistant enterococci (VRE) are an increasingly common cause of bacteremia and should be treated with linezolid (600 mg every 12 hours I.V.), daptomycin (6 mg/kg every 12 hours I.V.), or quinupristin-dalfopristin (7.5 mg/kg every 8 hours I.V.). Empiric treatment with these agents should be initiated in febrile neutropenic patients with known VRE colonization.

Gram-Positive Bacilli

- *Clostridium septicum* is associated with sepsis and metastatic myonecrosis during neutropenia. Treat with high-dose penicillin or a carbapenem.
- *Listeria monocytogenes* may cause bacteremia with or without encephalitis/meningitis in patients with defects in cell-mediated immunity. Ampicillin plus gentamicin is the treatment of choice.
- Other gram-positive bacilli such as *Bacillus*, *Corynebacterium*, and *Lactobacillus* species are common contaminants of blood cultures, but in the setting of neutropenia can cause true infection that is usually catheter-related. *Propionibacterium* is almost always a contaminant, but it can cause infection of Ommaya reservoirs.

Gram-Negative Bacteremia

- Gram-negative bacteria in the blood should never be considered contaminants and should be treated immediately.
- Therapy should be initiated with two antimicrobials to ensure adequate coverage until susceptibility results are available. Combination therapy offers no convincing benefit once susceptibilities are known.

- *Escherichia coli* and *Klebsiella* species are the most prevalent gram-negative pathogens in neutropenic patients; however, the use of prophylactic antibiotics such as ciprofloxacin or TMP/SMX may increase the prevalence of more resistant enteric organisms such as *Enterobacter, Citrobacter,* and *Serratia* species. Some of these have practical importance, as they may carry an inducible beta-lactamase that may result in treatment failure with third-generation cephalosporins like ceftazidime. Carbapenems, fluoroquinolones, and piperacillin-tazobactam may be used in this setting.
- The prevalence of strains of *Klebsiella* and *E. coli* that produce extended-spectrum beta-lactamases is increasing; carbepenems are the drugs of choice for these organisms.
- *P. aeruginosa* is one of the most lethal agents of gram-negative bacteremia in the neutropenic patient. Combination therapy should be started to ensure the patient is receiving at least one agent to which the isolate is susceptible.
- *Stenotrophomonas maltophilia* is an increasingly common cause of infection in patients who have been on broad-spectrum antibiotics or who have intravascular catheters; TMP/SMX is the treatment of choice. For the allergic patient, ticarcillin-clavulanate or moxifloxacin may be effective.
- *Acinetobacter baumanii* bacteremia is frequently associated with infected intravascular catheters in cancer patients and is often resistant to multiple antibiotics, including imipenem-cilastatin. Ampicillin-sulbactam, tigecyclin, or colistin may be effective, but consultation with an infectious diseases specialist should be sought.

Fungemia

- *Candida* species cause most cases of fungemia in cancer patients. The frequency of non-*albicans* candidemia is increasing, probably as a consequence of the widespread use of fluconazole prophylaxis.
- Non-*albicans* species are likely to be resistant to fluconazole and should be treated with caspofungin, anidulafungin, micafungin, amphotericin B, or a lipid formulation of amphotericin B.
- All patients with candidemia should undergo ophthalmologic evaluation with fundoscopic exam. In most cases, intravascular catheters should be removed.
- *C. neoformans, Fusarium,* and *Trichosporon* species can also rarely cause fungemia in the cancer patient.

Intravascular Catheter-Associated Infections

Definitions

- Exit-site infections are diagnosed clinically by the presence of erythema, induration, and tenderness within 2 cm of the catheter exit site.
- A tunnel infection is characterized by erythema along the subcutaneous tract of a tunneled catheter that extends 2 cm beyond the exit site.
- Catheter-associated bloodstream infection is defined by positive blood cultures or a positive catheter-tip culture.

Management

- If a local infection is suspected, a swab of exit-site discharge should be sent for culture, in addition to blood cultures.
- Uncomplicated catheter-site infections (no signs of systemic infection or bacteremia) can be managed with local care and oral antibiotics such as dicloxacillin.
- If the patient has fever or there is significant cellulitis around the catheter site, vancomycin should be used empirically while awaiting culture results.
- Tunnel infections require i.v. antibiotics and removal of the catheter; empirical therapy should include vancomycin, as well as coverage of gram-negative bacilli such as ceftazidime, cefepime, or ciprofloxacin. Therapy can then be modified if an organism is identified.

- Septic thrombophlebitis also necessitates catheter removal, and anticoagulation can be considered. Surgical drainage is occasionally necessary.
- Catheter-related bloodstream infections caused by coagulase-negative *Staphylococcus* or gramnegative bacilli should be treated for 14 days with antibiotics. After the cultures are negative, therapy may be completed with oral antibiotics (linezolid or a fluoroquinolone) in stable non-neutropenic patients.
- Management of catheter-site infections with fever and tunnel infections is outlined in Fig. 35.2.

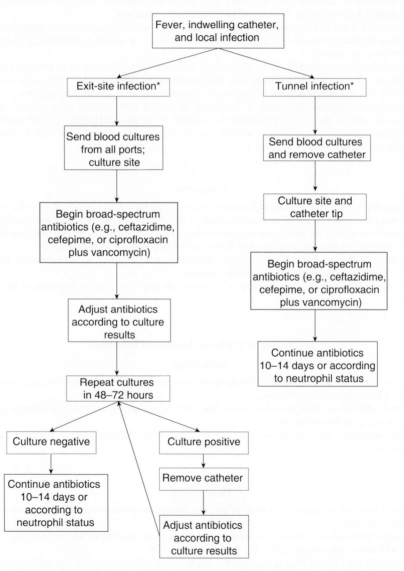

Fig. 35.2. Management of catheter-related infections. *Exit-site infection: erythema, induration, and tenderness within 2 cm of the catheter exit site; tunnel infection: erythema, induration, and tenderness along the subcutaneous tract of a tunneled catheter that extends 2 cm beyond the exit site.

Indications for Removal of Intravascular Catheters

Indwelling intravascular catheters should be removed in the following situations:

- Tunnel infections
- Blood cultures remain positive after 48 to 72 hours of therapy, regardless of the pathogen
- Septic thrombophlebitis
- Blood cultures positive for:
  - *S. aureus*
  - *Bacillus* species
  - *Mycobacteria* species
  - *Candida* species

In the case of catheter-related infections due to vancomycin-resistant enterococci, *Corynebacterium jekeium*, and gram-negative pathogens like *Pseudomonas* and *Stenotrophomonas*, the decision to remove the catheter should be made on a case-by-case basis.

Skin and Soft Tissue Infections

- Soft tissue infections may represent local or disseminated infection.
- A biopsy for staining and culture for bacteria, mycobacteria, viruses, and fungi should be considered early in the evaluation of skin and soft tissue infections.
- Ecthyma gangrenosum often presents in neutropenic patients as a dark, necrotic lesion but can be quite variable in appearance. Typically a manifestation of *P. aeruginosa* bacteremia, it may also be caused by bacteremia due to other gram-negative bacilli. Antibiotic therapy with coverage of *Pseudomonas* should be initiated and early surgical involvement for possible debridement is imperative.
- VZV and herpes simplex virus (HSV) generally present as vesicular lesions and may be indistinguishable. Scrapings from the base of vesicles should be sent for direct fluorescent antibody (DFA) testing to diagnose VZV and for shell-vial culture to diagnose HSV. Treatment of VZV in the immunocompromised host is acyclovir 10 mg/kg i.v. every 8 hours, and for HSV acyclovir 5 mg/kg i.v. every 8 hours. We prefer to use i.v. acyclovir in immunocompromised hosts. In immunocompetent patients, oral acyclovir, valacyclovir, and famciclovir have been used successfully.
- Cancer patients are at increased risk for streptococcal toxic shock syndrome and severe soft tissue infections caused by *Streptococcus pyogenes*. Treatment is aggressive surgical debridement as needed and antibiotic therapy with penicillin G and clindamycin, as well as, in the case of shock, i.v. immunoglobulin (IVIG).
- Perianal cellulitis may develop in neutropenic patients. Antibiotic therapy should include gram-negative and anaerobic coverage (e.g., imipenem-cilastatin or meropenem as single agents or ceftazidime plus metronidazole). A CT scan should be obtained to rule out a perirectal abscess. Incision and drainage may also be required in the setting of abscess or unremitting infection, but if possible should be delayed until resolution of neutropenia.
- Rash, including skin breakdown, is a common side effect of many new small molecule targeted therapies. Patients should have a detailed skin examination at each visit to evaluate for superinfections of their rash, as well as dermatology involvement as needed.

Sinusitis

- In the immunocompetence setting, the common pathogens of acute sinusitis are *S. pneumoniae, H. influenzae*, and *Morexella catarrhalis*, as well as *S. aureus*. Treatment is levofloxacin 500 mg daily or amoxicillin-clavulanate 875 mg twice daily.
- Sinusitis in immunocompromised hosts can also be caused by aerobic gram-negative bacilli, including *Pseudomonas*. Neutropenic patients are at high risk for fungal sinusitis.
- During neutropenia, sinusitis should be treated with broad-spectrum antibiotics, including coverage of *Pseudomonas*, and sinus CT scan and otolaryngology consult should be obtained. Biopsy should be obtained if there is any suspicion of fungal infection (e.g., bony erosion on CT scan, necrotic eschar of nasal turbinates) or if there is no response to antibiotic therapy within 72 hours.

- *Aspergillus* is the most common cause of invasive fungal sinusitis, but other molds such as Zygomycetes (which are resistant to voriconazole, the treatment of choice for aspergillosis) are increasingly recognized.
- If fungal sinusitis is confirmed, treatment is with surgical debridement and antifungal treatment, which should be started at maximum dosing:
  - Amphotericin B 1 to 1.5 mg/kg/day.
  - Lipid formulation of amphotericin B 5 to 7.5 mg/kg/day.
  - Voriconazole may be substituted only after it is certain the infection is not caused by Zygomycetes (*Mucor, Rhizopus*), which are not susceptible to voriconazole.
  - Posaconazole is a new oral-azole that has some activity against Zygomycetes and can be a possible treatment alternative once diagnosis is made. The two main obstacles for its consideration (besides lack of comparative data in this setting) are the fact that it is only available as an oral formulation that requires food to be absorbed, and the relatively long time required to achieve therapeutic levels.

Pneumonia

Pulmonary infiltrates in the immunocompromised host can be due to infectious or noninfectious causes. It is important to obtain an etiologic diagnosis. We recommend early use of bronchoalveolar lavage (BAL) if a diagnostic sputum specimen cannot be obtained.

Pulmonary Infiltrates in the Neutropenic Patient

- Adequate coverage for community-acquired pneumonia should be added to the antibiotic regimen (e.g., newer generation fluoroquinolone like levofloxacin or moxifloxacin, or macrolide like azithromycin in addition to ceftazidime).
- CT scan and bronchoscopy for BAL should be performed early, particularly if there is no prompt improvement.
- If pulmonary infiltrates appear while the patient is on broad-spectrum antibiotic therapy, the likelihood of fungal pneumonia is high. Empirical antifungal coverage with voriconazole, liposomal amphotericin B, or amphotericin B should be started immediately. Echinocandins should not be used for empiric fungal therapy for pulmonary infiltrates in neutropenic patients, as they have no activity against non-*Aspergillus* molds.

Fungal Pneumonia

- *Aspergillus* species are the most common disease-causing molds in cancer patients. Neutropenia is the most important risk factor, followed by use of corticosteroids.
- Clinical presentation:
  - Persistent or recurrent fever
  - Development of pulmonary infiltrates while on antibiotics
  - Chest pain, hemoptysis or pleural rub
- In the setting of allogeneic HSCT, most cases of *Aspergillus* pneumonia occur after engraftment, when the patient is no longer neutropenic. The most important risk factors in this setting are graft-versus-host disease, corticosteroid use, and CMV disease.
- Demonstration of fungal elements in biopsy tissue is necessary for definitive diagnosis. When a biopsy is not possible, positive respiratory cultures (sputum or BAL fluid) are highly predictive of invasive disease in a high-risk patient.
- Galactomannan (*Aspergillus*) and β-D-glucan are assays used to diagnose invasive fungal infections. A negative test *does not* rule out invasive fungal infection.
- Options for treatment of *Aspergillus* pneumonia include:
  - Voriconazole 6 mg/kg i.v. every 12 hours for 24 hours, then 4 mg/kg i.v. every 12 hours (preferred).
  - High-dose lipid formulation of amphotericin B (5 mg/kg/day).

– Amphotericin B (1–1.5 mg/kg/day).
– Caspofungin/micafungin (70 mg loading dose followed by 50 mg/day i.v.) has been approved for patients with invasive aspergillosis who are unresponsive to or intolerant of the above-mentioned antifungal agents.
- Zygomycetes such as *Rhizopus*, *Mucor*, and *Cunninghamella* species are less common causes of pulmonary infection in neutropenic patients. They are voriconazole-resistant but have variable susceptibility to posaconazole. Treatment should include high-dose amphotericin B (deoxycholate or lipid formulation). Early consideration should be given to surgical excision where feasible.
- *Fusarium* is a less common cause of pulmonary infection in neutropenic patients. Voriconazole or high-dose amphotericin can be tried. Response is usually contingent on neutrophil recovery.
- Dematiaceous fungi such as *Scedosporium, Alternaria, Bipolaris, Cladosporium*, and *Wangiella* species are rare causes of pneumonia in neutropenic patients. The best treatment is not well established, and consultation with an infectious diseases specialist is strongly advised.

Pulmonary Infiltrates in Patients With Defects in Cell-Mediated Immunity

- In addition to the common bacterial causes of pneumonia, patients with defects in cell-mediated immunity are at risk for infections with *P. jiroveci*, *Nocardia* species and viruses (see below), as well as *Legionella*, mycobacteria, and fungi.
- Bronchoscopy for BAL should be performed to aid in diagnosis.
- Empirical antibiotics should include newer generation fluoroquinolone for coverage of bacterial pathogens including *Legionella* and TMP/SMX for coverage of *Pneumocystis*. Consideration should also be given to antifungal and antiviral agents, depending on the clinical presentation.

Pneumocystis Pneumonia (PCP)

- Patients with pneumonia from *P. jirovecii* usually present with rapid onset of dyspnea, nonproductive cough, hypoxemia, and fever. PCP may have a more indolent presentation in HIV-infected patients.
- Radiologic studies generally show diffuse bilateral interstitial infiltrates but can show focal infiltrates. Pleural effusion is uncommon.
- Treatment should be started based on clinical suspicion: TMP/SMX 5 mg/kg i.v. every 8 hours (prednisone should be added if the pO2 is <70 mmHg).
- In TMP/SMX-allergic/intolerant patients, alternatives for serious disease include i.v. pentamidine, and for moderate disease dapsone-trimethoprim, atavaquone, or clindamycin-primaquine.

Nocardia

- Pneumonia from *Nocardia* species can cause a dense lobar infiltrate or multiple pulmonary nodules with or without cavitation.
- Diagnosis is made from material obtained at bronchoscopy, either by pathology or culture.
- Treatment is with TMP/SMX with or without ceftriaxone. Depending on the species, imipenem-cilastatin + amikacin may also be used.

Viral Pneumonia

- Pneumonia due to respiratory viruses (respiratory syncytial virus [RSV], influenza, parainfluenza, adenovirus) is more common in patients with defects in cell-mediated immunity.
- Treatment with ribavirin (RSV, parainfluenza) with or without immunoglobulins or cidofovir (adenovirus) has not been shown to change outcome. Some authorities recommend early use of ribavirin in cases of upper respiratory infection caused by RSV after allogeneic stem cell transplant, with the aim of preventing the development of pneumonia.
- Oseltamivir and zanamivir are effective in HSCT and immunocompromised patients with influenza and are recommended in documented or suspected influenza infections.

- CMV pneumonia is a significant complication of allogeneic stem cell transplants that typically develops between 40 and 100 days post-transplant and typically presents with fever, dyspnea, hypoxemia, and diffuse interstitial infiltrates. CMV pneumonia after day 100 is becoming more common and should be considered in patients with a history of previous CMV reactivation.
- After allogeneic stem cell transplant, the presence of CMV in the BAL culture is considered sufficient to establish the diagnosis. In other settings, tissue is required.
- Treatment of CMV pneumonia is with ganciclovir 5 mg/kg i.v. every 12 hours with IVIG 500 mg/kg every 48 hours for 3 weeks. Foscarnet (90 mg/kg every 12 hours) may be substituted for ganciclovir.
- Human herpes virus-6 (HHV-6), VZV, and (very rarely) HSV have also been associated with pneumonitis in the immunocompromised patient.

Gastrointestinal Infections

Mucositis

- The shallow, painful ulcerations of the tongue and buccal mucosa caused by chemotherapy can become superinfected with HSV or *Candida*.
- If severe, HSV infection is treated with acyclovir 5 mg/kg i.v. every 8 hours for 7 days. If the infection is less severe, valacyclovir 1,000 mg P.O. every 12 hours or famciclovir 500 mg P.O. every 12 hours can be used.
- Candidiasis can be treated locally with clotrimazole troches 10 mg dissolved in the mouth 5 ×/day, or systemically with fluconazole 200 mg P.O./i.v. once, then 100 mg daily.
- Patients with fever and neutropenia with thrush should be covered empirically with systemic antifungals with activity against *Candida* species.

Esophagitis

- Odynophagia, dysphagia, and substernal chest discomfort can be a result of chemotherapy but may also be due to herpes or candidal infections.
- Endoscopy with biopsy should be performed when possible.
- If endoscopy and biopsy are not possible, empirical therapy with fluconazole for *Candida* and acyclovir for HSV is recommended. In neutropenic patients with fever and clinical symptoms of esophagitis, antibacterial therapy appropriate for upper GI flora should be added (e.g., ceftazidime + vancomycin or piperacillin-tazobactam or imipenem or meropenem).
- CMV can also cause esophagitis.

Diarrhea

- *Clostridium difficile* is the most common pathogen to cause diarrhea in cancer patients.
- Diagnosis is usually made by detecting *C. difficile* toxin in the stool.
- Treatment is with metronidazole 250 mg P.O. four times a day or 500 mg P.O. three times a day. The antiparasitic agent itazoxanide (500 mg P.O. twice a day) may offer similar efficacy. In severe and/or refractory cases, vancomycin 125 to 250 mg P.O. four times a day should be used. Metronidazole can be given i.v. in patients who are unable to tolerate oral therapy. Treatment is continued for 10 to 14 days. The stool should not be retested for *C. difficile* toxin, as many patients may remain asymptomatic carriers.
- Recurrent infection after metronidazole therapy should be treated with longer course of metronidazole before oral vancomycin therapy is initiated.
- Bacteria such as *E. coli, Salmonella, Shigella, Aeromonas*, and *Campylobacter* species, as well as parasites and viruses, are less common causes of diarrhea in cancer patients. Stool should be sent for culture of bacterial pathogens and examined for ova and parasites. Specific therapy should be directed against recovered pathogens.

Neutropenic Enterocolitis (Typhlitis)

- Typhlitis typically presents as abdominal pain, rebound tenderness, bloody diarrhea, and fever in the setting of neutropenia. The diagnosis should be entertained in every case of abdominal pain during neutropenia.

- The diagnosis is frequently made based on characteristic CT scan findings: a fluid-filled, dilated, and distended cecum, often with diffuse cecal-wall edema and possibly air in the bowel wall (pneumatosis intestinalis). However, the CT may be unremarkable in the early stages; it has a reported sensitivity of only 80%.
- Pathogens are typically mixed aerobic and anaerobic gram-negative bacilli (including *Pseudomonas*) and *Clostridium* species.
- Treatment is with broad-spectrum antibiotics including coverage of *Pseudomonas* (e.g., imipenem or meropenem or the combination ceftazidime plus metronidazole plus vancomycin).
- Patients should be monitored closely for development of complications that may require surgical intervention, such as bowel perforation, bowel necrosis, or abscess formation.

Perforations/Fistulas

- Bevacizumab, a monoclonal antibody to vascular endothelial growth factor, has been associated with a gastrointestinal perforation/fistula rate of 1% to 5%.
- Patients with colon cancer and ovarian cancer have been found to be at greatest risk.
- Other risk factors may include prior abdominal/pelvic irradiation, bowel involvement by tumor, or unresected colon cancer.
- Any patient on bevacizumab with abdominal pain or new rectal bleeding should have prompt evaluation for perforation/fistula with imaging, as well as broad-spectrum antibiotic therapy covering gram-negative bacteria and anaerobes.

Hepatosplenic Candidiasis

- Hepatosplenic candidiasis typically presents as neutropenic fever without localizing signs or symptoms.
- When neutropenia resolves, the patient may continue to have fever, develop right upper quadrant pain and hepatosplenomegaly, and have significant elevation in alkaline phosphatase.
- CT scan, ultrasound, or MRI will show hypoechoic and/or bulls-eye lesions in the liver and spleen and sometimes the kidneys.
- Stable patients can be treated empirically without biopsy if suspicion is high. Blood cultures are typically negative. If the diagnosis is in question, an open liver biopsy is recommended. The diagnosis will be established by pathology showing granulomatous inflammation and yeast, as biopsy culture results are usually negative.
- Treatment consists of a prolonged course of fluconazole 400 to 800 mg daily. Caspofungin has also been effective.

Hepatitis B

- Hepatitis B reactivation can occur in chronic carriers who are undergoing cytotoxic chemotherapy, with lymphoma patients being at highest risk.
- Risk factors include positive hepatitis B DNA, HBsAg, HBeAg, and young age.
- Lamivudine prophylaxis is recommended, 100 mg daily beginning 1 week prior to chemotherapy and for 8 weeks after completion of treatment.

Urinary Tract Infections

- In the presence of neutropenia, it is reasonable to treat bacteriuria even in the absence of symptoms. In the non-neutropenic patient, treatment should be reserved for symptomatic episodes.
- Patients with indwelling stents may have persistent microbial colonization and pyuria. Treatment should be initiated in neutropenic patients with pyuria even with a history of chronic asymptomatic pyuria.
- Candiduria may represent colonization in a patient with an indwelling urinary catheter, particularly in the setting of broad-spectrum antibiotics. Removal of the catheter is frequently sufficient to clear it.
- Persistent candiduria can occasionally cause infections such as pyelonephritis or disseminated candidiasis in immunocompromised patients. Additionally, candiduria can be indicative of disseminated

candidiasis. However, treatment of asymptomatic candiduria with systemic antifungals has not been associated with improved outcomes overall.
- If a decision is made to treat, fluconazole 400 mg/day for 1 to 2 weeks is the treatment of choice. In the case of non-*Albicans* candiduria, another -azole or amphotericin should be used. Caspofungin is minimally present in the urine, and there is no clinical experience in this setting.

Central Nervous System Infections
- Changes in mentation or level of consciousness, headache, or photophobia should be evaluated promptly with MRI and lumbar puncture.
- In addition to the usual bacterial causes of meningitis (*S. pneumoniae, Nisseria meningitides*), *Listeria* and *Cryptococcus* should also be considered, particularly when a defect in cell-mediated immunity is present.
- For *Listeria*, the treatment of choice is ampicillin 2 mg i.v. every 4 hours in combination with gentamicin.
- For *Cryptococcus*, treatment is with liposomal amphotericin B 3 mg/kg/day or amphotericin B 0.5 to 0.7 mg/kg/day in combination with flucytosine 37.5 mg/kg every 6 hours for 2 weeks. If the patient improves (afebrile, cultures negative), therapy can be changed to fluconazole 400 mg daily.
- Encephalitis in patients with cancer is most commonly caused by HSV. Diagnosis is made by the presence of viral DNA in CSF and should be treated with acyclovir 10 mg/kg i.v. every 8 hours. Potential clinical indications for empiric HSV treatment include predominance of altered mentation symptoms and focal changes on EEG or MRI, especially in the temporal lobes.
- VZV, CMV, and HHV-6 are other less common causes of encephalitis.
- Progressive multifocal leukoencephalopathy (OML), caused by JC virus, presents with multiple non-enhancing white matter lesions and has been associated with rituximab and mycophenolate mofetil (MMF).
- Brain abscesses that develop during neutropenia are typically caused by fungi (most commonly *Aspergillus* and *Candida*). Bacterial abscesses may also be a local extension of infection (sinusitis, odontogenic infection), caused by mixed aerobic and anaerobic flora (streptococci, *Staphylococcus, Bacteroides*). Pending results from biopsy and cultures, we recommend empirical treatment with ceftazidime plus vancomycin plus metronidazole plus voriconazole.

Infectious Issues Secondary to Monoclonal Antibody Therapy
- The increased use of monoclonal antibodies, in particular those targeting leukocytes, has important implications for infectious disease.
- Alemtuzumab, an anti-CD52 antibody approved for chronic lymphocytic leukemia, results in profound depletion of cell-mediated immunity and places patients at risk for viral reactivation and infection with intracellular pathogens. *Pneumocystis*, HSV, and EBV infection, as well CMV reactivation, are being seen regularly.
- Rituximab, a monoclonal antibody against CD20 used in lymphoma and leukemia treatment, causes B-cell depletion from 6 to 9 months and can also result in prolonged hypogammaglobulinemia and reactivation of viral hepatitis.
- Perforation and fistula are rare but serious side effects of bevacizumab.

PROPHYLAXIS

Antibacterial Prophylaxis
- Fluoroquinolones are the most commonly used antibiotics for prophylaxis against bacterial infections in neutropenic patients and can significantly reduce the frequency of gram-negative infections. However, they may increase the frequency of gram-positive infections and could conceivably result in the emergence of resistance among enteric gram-negative bacteria. Meta-analyses suggest fluoroquinolone prophylaxis may be associated with improved overall survival in patients with prolonged neutropenia, and this approach is currently recommended in a variety of practice guidelines.

Antiviral Prophylaxis

HSV and VZV

- Prophylaxis against HSV should be considered in patients who are seropositive or have a history of herpetic stomatitis and are undergoing allogeneic stem cell transplant or highly immunosuppressive chemotherapy, including high-dose steroids and alemtuzumab.
- Prophylaxis should be given beginning with the conditioning chemotherapy prior to transplant and continued 100 days post-transplant and until immunosuppressants are discontinued. This approach is effective for VZV prophylaxis, which is not recommended by all experts. In general, it is not considered necessary to routinely administer prophylaxis for HSV beyond the immediate peritransplant period.
- The drugs of choice are valacyclovir 500 mg P.O. once or twice daily or acyclovir 250 mg/m² i.v. every 12 hours or 800 mg P.O. twice daily.

CMV

- Prophylactic ganciclovir can reduce the incidence of CMV disease, but its use is limited by myelosuppressive toxicity.
- Patients who have undergone allogeneic stem cell transplant should be monitored for CMV replication by following CMV antigenemia or PCR weekly.
- If positive, patients should be treated with ganciclovir 5 mg/kg i.v. every 12 hours for 7 days followed by 5 mg/kg i.v. daily until CMV antigenemia or PCR results are negative one week apart.
- Alternative treatments include (a) foscarnet 90 mg/kg i.v. every 12 hours for 7 days followed by 90 mg/kg daily, (b) valganciclovir 900 mg i.v. every 12 hours for 7 days followed by 900 mg daily, or (c) cidofovir 5 mg/kg i.v. weekly for 2 weeks followed by 5 mg/kg i.v. every other week (very limited evidence is available regarding use of cidofovir for this indication).

Pneumocystis jirovecii Pneumonia Prophylaxis

- Prophylaxis against *Pneumocystis* is generally administered to patients during the 6-month poststem cell transplant period or after being treated with alemtuzumab. Patients with a history of PCP or with brain tumors on high-dose steroids should also receive prophylaxis.
- The regimen of choice is 160 mg trimethoprim/800 mg sulfamethoxazole P.O. daily 3 days a week.
- Alternative treatments include (a) dapsone 100 mg P.O. daily (rule out G6PDH deficiency before using dapsone), (b) inhaled pentamidine 300 mg every 4 weeks, or (c) atovaquone 1,500 mg daily.

Antifungal Prophylaxis

- Fluconazole 400 mg P.O./i.v. daily has been the regimen of choice.
- An alternative regimen is itraconazole 200 mg i.v. every 12 hours for 2 days followed by 200 mg i.v. daily for 12 days followed by 200 mg P.O. every 12 hours.
- Posaconazole 200 mg P.O. three times a day has been shown to be more effective than fluconazole in patients with prolonged neutropenia or on intensive immunosuppression for graft-versus-host disease. It is reasonable to prefer posaconazole when the risk of mold infection is considered significant.
- Prophylaxis should be continued until 100 days post-transplant and until immunosuppressants have been discontinued.
- Use of fluconazole has led to increased frequency of fluconazole-resistant infections such as *Candida tropicalis*, *C. parapsilosis*, and *C. krusei*.

SUGGESTED READINGS

Gea-Banacloche J, Palmore T, Walsh T, et al. Infections in the cancer patient. In: DeVita VT, Hellman S, Rosenberg SA, eds. *Cancer: Principles and Practice of Oncology*. 8th ed. Philadelphia, PA: Lipincott Williams and Wilkins; 2008.

Klastersky J, Paesmans M, Rubenstein EB, et al. The Multinational Association for Supportive Care in Cancer Risk Index: a multinational scoring system for identifying low-risk febrile neutropenic cancer patients. *J Clin Oncol.* 2000;18:3038–3051.

Mermel LA, Farr BM, Sherertz RJ, et al. Guidelines for the management of intravascular catheter-related infections. *Clin Infect Dis.* 2001;32(9):1249–1272.

NCCN Practice Guidelines. Prevention and Treatment of Cancer-Related Infections.v.1.2008. Available at: http://www.nccn.org/professionals/physician_gls/f_guidelines.asp.

Picazo JJ. Management of the febrile neutropenic patient: a consensus conference. *Clin Infect Dis.* 2004;39:S1–S6.

Pizzo PA. Fever in immunocompromised patients. *N Engl J Med.* 1999;341:893–900.

Vidal L, Paul M, Ben dor I, Soares-Weiser K, Leibovici L. Oral versus intravenous antibiotic treatment for febrile neutropenia in cancer patients: a systematic review and meta-analysis of randomized trials. *J Antimicrob Chemother.* 2004;54:29–37.

Walsh TJ, Pappas P, Winston DJ, et al. National Institute of Allergy and Infectious Diseases Mycoses Study Group. Voriconazole compared with liposomal amphotericin B for empirical antifungal therapy in patients with neutropenia and persistent fever. *N Engl J Med.* 2002;346:225–234.

Walsh TJ, Teppler H, Donowitz GR, et al. Caspofungin versus liposomal amphotericin B for empirical antifungal therapy in patients with persistent fever and neutropenia. *N Engl J Med.* 2004;351:1391–1402.

Wingard JR. Empirical antifungal therapy in treating febrile neutropenic patients. *Clin Infect Dis.* 2004;39:S38–S43.

36

Oncologic Emergencies and Paraneoplastic Syndrome

Susan L. Bever and Richard A. Messmann

SPINAL CORD COMPRESSION

- Spinal cord compression (SCC) is a true oncologic emergency, as delay in evaluation and treatment can result in permanent bowel and bladder dysfunction or paralysis.
- Most cord compression cases involve tumor or collapsed bone fragments in the epidural space, a few cases are subdural, and intramedullary metastases are very rare.
- The thoracic spine is most often involved (60–70%), followed by the lumbosacral (20–30%) and cervical spine (10%) (1).

Etiology of Spinal Cord Compression

- Hematogenous seeding of tumor to vertebral bodies from primary breast, lung, and prostate cancer; lymphoma; multiple myeloma; renal and gastrointestinal tumors (1).
- SCC, infrequently, is the first sign of cancer.

Clinical Signs and Symptoms of Spinal Cord Compression

- Back or radicular pain
- Muscle weakness
- Acute or slowly evolving changes in bowel or bladder function
- Sensory loss or autonomic dysfunction

Any of these signs and symptoms should bring about the initiation of a prompt clinical evaluation for SCC (2,3).

A thorough physical and neurologic examination should be performed (4), including:

- Gentle percussion of the spinal column
- Evaluation for motor or sensory weakness
- Passive neck flexion
- Straight-leg raising
- Rectal examination (to evaluate the sphincter tone)
- Pinprick testing from toe to head to establish whether a "sensory level" is present.

A clinical suspicion of SCC should prompt the initiation of steroid therapy (see Treatment) (5).

Diagnostic Imaging

The choice of diagnostic imaging should be suggested by the results of the neurologic examination.

- Magnetic resonance imaging (MRI) with gadolinium contrast is the standard for diagnosis because of its high sensitivity and specificity for detecting SCC (2,4,5). The entire neuraxis is readily imaged such that the superior and inferior extent of the compression can be used to target radiotherapy.
- Some limitations include limited availability in some communities, inability of the patient to lie absolutely still and supine for 30 to 60 minutes of imaging, and issues that preclude MRI [e.g., history of metallic vertebral stabilization surgery, earlier pacemaker/automatic implantable cardioverter–defibrillator (AICD) placement, or presence of certain other implanted devices].
- Computerized tomography (CT) scan of the spinal region combined with myelogram (CT-myelogram) provides an excellent assessment of the epidural space and surrounding soft tissue and is useful in diagnosis and therapy planning.
- It is generally more available than MRI and is an acceptable imaging modality when MRI is not possible.
- Technical limitations include the need for lumbar puncture to administer radiocontrast, as well as a requirement that the ordering physician identifies the expected spinal region to be imaged. The procedure is impractical for the entire neuraxis and may require supplemental studies to exclude a more superior level of compression.
- Conventional radiographs are readily obtained and are inexpensive. Radiographs exploit the finding that almost all SCC begins as vertebral bone metastases that lead to subsequent fracture and cord compression by the bone and tumor. The value of conventional radiographs is limited to verifying a diagnostic impression of SCC, assessing surgical options, and evaluating spinal stability. Radiographs do not exclude the diagnosis of SCC even if they are "normal" and are insufficient to plan radiotherapy.

Diagnosis of Spinal Cord Compression

Diagnosis of symptomatic patients with *abnormal* neurologic examination involves the following:

- Receive steroid therapy *at once*
- Conventional radiographs detect abnormalities in most patients with SCC, which aids prompt confirmation of the diagnosis.
- MRI is then done to define the proximal and distal extent of the compression to facilitate the therapeutic plan.

Diagnosis of symptomatic patients with *normal* neurologic examination involves the following:

- Conventional radiographs of the spine should be followed by MRI, if the conventional radiograph is abnormal (as for the patients with abnormal neurologic examination) or if clinical progression occurs or if the symptoms fail to resolve. It should be noted that a very small percentage of intradural tumor metastasis will be visible only in MRI.
- In addition, any abnormal radiological findings or progression of symptoms should prompt initiation of steroid therapy. Myelography (often assisted by simultaneous CT scan) may be useful if an MRI is not available.

Treatment of Spinal Cord Compression

The goals of treatment for SCC include pain control, recovery of normal neurologic function, local tumor control, and avoidance of complications.

Once SCC is suspected, administer steroids as follows:

- Begin treatment with a "loading" dose of dexamethasone, 10 mg by i.v. infusion.
- Six hours after the loading dose, and every 6 hours thereafter, administer dexamethasone, 4 mg by i.v. infusion (5,6).
- An alternative treatment strategy includes an initial bolus dose of dexamethasone, 100 mg by i.v. infusion, followed 6 hours later by dexamethasone, 4 mg by i.v. infusion every 6 hours; however, this regimen is associated with additional toxicities related to high-dose steroid administration (7) and no improvement has been seen compared to low-dose therapy with respect to pain, ambulation, and bladder function (8).

- Surgical and radiation oncology consultation(s) are required immediately after diagnosis, and further therapy is decided on the basis of the clinical signs and symptoms, availability of histologic diagnosis, spinal stability, and previous treatments. All symptomatic patients with SCC should be considered for decompression, and radical resection of metastatic tumor within 24 hours of onset of symptoms, regardless of spinal stability.
- In symptomatic patients with SCC caused by metastatic tumors other than lymphoma, initial debulking surgery followed by radiation results in a four times longer duration of maintained ambulation after treatment, and a three times higher chance of regaining ambulation for nonambulatory patients, than that with radiation alone. In addition, patients who receive combined-modality therapy achieve superior pain control and bladder continence. Patients treated with radiation therapy alone require more steroids and narcotics and are less likely to maintain continence (9).
- Patients with spinal instability even in the absence of clinical signs and symptoms should undergo surgery unless otherwise contraindicated.
- Additional surgical candidates include patients with relapsed compression at a site of earlier irradiation and patients with progression of deficits during radiation therapy.
- Radiotherapy is used to treat radiosensitive tumors in asymptomatic individuals and in those individuals who are symptomatic but are poor surgical candidates.
- Radiosensitive tumors include breast and prostate tumors, lymphoma, multiple myeloma, and neuroblastoma.
- Radiotherapy candidates may also include patients with multiple areas of compression.
- Standard radiation doses range from 2,500 to 4,000 cGy delivered in 10 to 20 fractions.
- Select patients with chemosensitive tumors may benefit from chemotherapy in addition to either radiation or surgical intervention (6,10).
- Chemotherapy may be an appropriate first-line therapy for patients with chemosensitive tumors (i.e., lymphoma, myeloma, germ cell tumors, and breast and prostate cancer) and in individuals who are not candidates for radiation or surgery. The reader is directed to a number of references for specific details (2, 11–18).

SUPERIOR VENA CAVA SYNDROME

- Superior vena cava syndrome (SVCS) is a common occurrence in cancer patients and may occur as a manifestation of either primary or metastatic tumor, or as a thrombosis associated with central venous access devices.
- Superior vena caval obstruction can result in life-threatening cerebral edema (increased intracranial pressure) or laryngeal edema (airway compromise).

Etiology of Superior Vena Cava Syndrome

SVCS is most often caused by extrinsic compression of the SVC by a tumor (intrathoracic) in the setting of (1,4):

- Lung cancer, especially right-sided bronchogenic carcinoma
- Non-Hodgkin lymphoma, especially diffuse large cell or lymphoblastic lymphoma in the anterior mediastinum
- Metastatic disease to the mediastinum, from primary
- Breast cancer
- Testicular cancer
- Gastrointestinal (GI) cancers
- Primary tumors:
  - Sarcomas (e.g., malignant fibrous histiocytoma)
  - Melanomas.

Other causes include:

- Central line thrombus and other iatrogenic causes

- Fibrosing mediastinitis, either idiopathic or secondary to infections like histoplasmosis, tuberculosis, actinomycosis, aspergillosis, blastomycosis, or bancroftian filariasis
- Retrosternal goiter

Clinical Signs and Symptoms of Superior Vena Cava Syndrome

- Clinical evolution of SVCS may occur acutely or gradually.
- Physical examination findings may include neck or chest wall superficial venous distension, facial and periorbital edema, cyanosis, facial plethora, mental status changes, lethargy, or edema of the upper extremities.
- SVCS symptoms include dyspnea, orthopnea, facial swelling, complaint of head "fullness," cough, arm swelling, chest pain, dysphagia, hoarseness, and positional worsening of symptoms (5).

Diagnosis of Superior Vena Cava Syndrome

A thorough physical examination may be sufficient to establish the diagnosis of SVCS (19). Noninvasive imaging that may facilitate the diagnosis of SVCS includes:

- Contrast-enhanced CT scan or MRI
- Chest radiograph that may show mediastinal widening with the presence of a mass often confirming the diagnosis
- Doppler ultrasonography examination of the jugular or subclavian vein may help differentiate thrombus from extrinsic obstruction.
- Radiocontrast or other injections into veins of the affected extremity are not recommended because of the risk of extravasation and the delayed entry of the contrast into central circulation.

Treatment of Superior Vena Cava Syndrome

- Options for the treatment of SVCS depend on the underlying etiology and on the pace of symptom progression (19,20).
- Emergent radiation therapy is required when respiratory compromise (e.g., stridor) or central nervous system (CNS) symptoms are present.
- The endpoints of the nonemergent treatment are symptom relief and treatment of the malignant or infectious or other process causing the SVCS.
- If SVCS is a presenting symptom (i.e., no history of cancer), and if time allows (i.e., no respiratory distress or changing neurologic status), tissue should be obtained to establish a diagnosis before treatment (21).
- Diagnostic strategies may be limited by the patient's inability to lie supine (i.e., worsened SVCS symptoms). Most malignancies that cause SVCS can be identified without major thoracic surgical procedures by using thoracentesis, bronchoscopy, lymph node biopsy, and bone marrow biopsy, or by analyzing sputum cytology. Limited thoracotomy and mediastinoscopy may be required in some cases.
- Conservative treatment includes elevation of the head of the bed, supplemental oxygen, and bed rest.

The emergent treatment of malignancy, or treatment once the histologic diagnosis is established, may include the following:

- Adjunct medical therapy with steroids can be used, but the benefit is not well established (22). For severe respiratory symptoms, hydrocortisone, 100 to 500 mg i.v., may be administered initially, followed by lower doses of hydrocortisone every 6 to 8 hours.
- Cautious use of loop diuretics may provide transient, symptomatic relief of edema. Overdiuresis may lead to dehydration and cardiovascular compromise.
- Endovascular stent insertion provides relief of symptoms more rapidly and in higher proportion of patients than that with radiation or chemotherapy (4,5,22,23). The use of a stent is limited when intraluminal thrombosis is present.

- Radiation therapy [especially for non–small cell lung cancer (NSCLC)]
- Chemotherapy (for lymphoma or germ cell tumor)
- Chemotherapy and radiation therapy is used for limited-disease small cell lung cancer.
- Anticoagulant or thrombolytic therapy (for caval thrombosis and in catheter-associated thrombosis).
- In cases of SVCS caused by catheter-associated thrombosis, removal of the catheter with a brief period of anticoagulant therapy remains an option. Alternatively, the catheter can be retained (if functional) and the patient can be treated indefinitely with therapeutic-dose warfarin.
- Surgery (especially in the setting of refractory disease or nonmalignant causes).

HYPERCALCEMIA

Etiology of Hypercalcemia

Hypercalcemia most often occurs in the setting of the following cancers:

- NSCLC: squamous cell/bulky disease
- Breast: adenocarcinoma/during hormonal therapy
- Genitourinary tumors: renal, small cell ovarian cancer
- Multiple myeloma
- Head and neck tumors
- Lymphoma: older patients with Hodgkin lymphoma who have bulky disease, intermediate or high-grade non-Hodgkin lymphoma/adult T-cell lymphoma
- Leukemias and unknown primary neoplasms (1,4)
- Patients with solid tumor metastasis to the bone comprise a large percentage of patients with cancer who have hypercalcemia (small cell lung and prostate cancers are seldom associated with hypercalcemia).

Clinical Signs and Symptoms of Hypercalcemia

The clinical signs and symptoms of hypercalcemia:

- May be general: dehydration, weakness, fatigue, and pruritus
- May involve many organ systems including CNS (i.e., hyporeflexia, mental status changes, seizure, coma, and proximal myopathy) and GI or genitourinary tract (GI: weight loss, nausea/vomiting, constipation, ileus, polyuria, polydipsia, azotemia, dyspepsia, and pancreatitis)
- May involve cardiac symptoms: bradycardia, short-QT interval, wide T wave, prolonged PR interval, arrhythmias, and arrest.

Diagnosis of Hypercalcemia

- It may be difficult to distinguish between hypercalcemia as a paraneoplastic syndrome and the hypercalcemia that results from metastatic disease to the bone.
- Hypercalcemia of malignancy: serum intact parathormone (iPTH) level is low or undetectable; serum parathormone-related peptide (PTH-RP) levels are elevated, whereas both 1,25-dihydroxyergocalciferol and inorganic phosphate levels are low or normal. Serum PTH-RP level has a high prevalence in malignancy-related hypercalcemia, which results from osteoclastic bone resorption and increased renal resorption of calcium.
- Osteolytic hypercalcemia is seen in the setting of multiple myeloma, NSCLC, and breast cancer.
- Calcitriol-mediated hypercalcemia is seen in relation to Hodgkin and non-Hodgkin lymphomas.
- In general terms, the degree of hypercalcemia can be characterized as follows: *Mild hypercalcemia* is characterized by a serum calcium level >10.5 mg/dL but <12 mg/dL, whereas in *moderate hypercalcemia*, serum calcium level ranges from 12 to 13.5 mg/dL, and *severe hypercalcemia* occurs at levels >13.5 mg/dL, although patients with chronic hypercalcemia may tolerate levels well in excess of 14 mg/dL without any apparent symptoms. The reader is cautioned, therefore, that the clinical manifestations and severity of hypercalcemia do not necessarily correlate with the absolute serum level of calcium but may be more directly related to the speed with which hypercalcemia develops (1).

- Albumin and certain serum proteins bind serum calcium and may distort "true" serum calcium levels; for example, in cases of myeloma, in which dramatic elevations in serum calcium levels simply reflect elevated concentrations of serum calcium–binding proteins as opposed to severe hypercalcemia. Approximation of the "corrected" serum calcium level can be calculated using one of several formulas that account for serum albumin levels, for example (15):

  Formulae for corrected serum calcium concentration:

$$(mg/dL) = serum\ Ca_{(measured)} + 0.8 \times [4.0\ serum\ albumin\ concentration\ (g/dL)]$$
$$(mEq/L) = serum\ Ca_{(measured)} + 0.4 \times [4.0\ serum\ albumin\ concentration\ (g/dL)]$$
$$(mmol/L) = serum\ Ca_{(measured)} + 0.2 \times [4.0\ serum\ albumin\ concentration\ (g/dL)]$$

General Principles of Treatment of Hypercalcemia

- The most effective treatment of hypercalcemia requires effective therapy directed at the underlying malignancy (i.e., the source of the hypercalcemia). Unfortunately, hypercalcemia most often occurs in advanced states of disease and in patients who have progressed through available standard chemotherapy. In patients with solid tumor primary cancers, survival is often <6 months.
- Any symptomatic patient with hypercalcemia, regardless of absolute serum calcium level, should be treated for correction of the hypercalcemia (24–27).
- Symptomatic patients with severely elevated calcium levels often require profound fluid volume replacement, which makes outpatient therapy impractical and unsafe.
- Mild asymptomatic hypercalcemia with serum calcium concentration in range of 11 to 12 mg/dL should be treated, when there is associated hypercalciuria, because of the risk of nephrolithiasis and nephrocalcinosis.

Practical Management of Hypercalcemia

- Therapy for mild chronic hypercalcemia usually includes observation and oral rehydration. Corticosteroids can be considered in select patients. Corticosteroid administration inhibits osteoclastic bone resorption and is useful in patients with tumors responsive to this steroid effect. These tumors include lymphoma, leukemia, myeloma (prednisone, 40–100 mg/day), and breast cancers (prednisone, 15–30 mg/day) during hormonal therapy (4,28–30). The hypocalcemic effect of corticosteroid administration is inconsistent, however, in steroid-resistant tumor types, and caution is advised (4). Oral phosphate (1–3 g/day) can also be considered as long as serum phosphate concentrations do not exceed 4 mg/dL. Oral phosphate usually lowers the serum calcium concentration by 0.5 to 1.0 mg/dL, but its use is frequently complicated by gastrointestinal symptoms.
- Acute therapy of patients with symptomatic or more severe hypercalcemia (i.e., serum calcium concentration exceeding 12 mg/dL) requires hospitalization. Therapy should be initiated by increasing urinary calcium excretion through vigorous hydration and by decreasing bone resorption through osteoclast inhibition (see subsequent text).
- The fluid and hemodynamic status should be assessed by evaluating blood pressure, pulse, orthostatics, urine volume, and appropriate laboratory values of the patient (4,27). Patients with hypercalcemia are often severely dehydrated (i.e., they need many liters of fluid) and require immediate administration of isotonic saline (1–2 L over 1 hour followed by 300–400 mL per hour, unless the patient has heart failure or renal failure) to increase renal blood flow and calcium excretion.
- During treatment, patients require frequent monitoring of clinical status and metabolic laboratory testing because forced diuresis may be complicated by hypomagnesemia, hypokalemia, fluid overload, or subsequent pulmonary edema.
- Once rehydration is complete and urinary output is optimized, the need for bisphosphonate administration should be assessed. These pyrophosphate analogs interfere with osteoclast function, thereby inhibiting calcium release.
- Intravenous zoledronic acid (4 mg i.v., infused over at least 15 minutes) or pamidronate (60 or 90 mg i.v., in 500 mL 0.9% saline or 5% dextrose in water, infused over 2–4 hours) is commonly used in malignancy-induced hypercalcemia (31,32). Zoledronic acid has replaced pamidronate as the agent

of choice. In a recent phase 3 trial, zoledronic acid was shown to normalize serum calcium level in 87% to 88% of patients as compared to 70% of patients who received pamidronate. The duration of response (32–43 days vs. 18 days) was also in favor of zoledronic acid (33). Bisphosphonate administration is well tolerated by patients except for occasional i.v. site irritation and fever during infusion. Its onset of action is within 24 to 48 hours of administration; the maximal effect may not be achieved until 72 hours after treatment.

- An additional and perhaps more effective intervention for hypercalcemia includes the use of gallium nitrate (not the radioisotope), which also inhibits bone resorption (4).
- Intravenous administration (100–200 mg/m^2/day over 24 hours or up to 5 days) of gallium nitrate in rehydrated nonoliguric (target urine output: 1,500–2,000 mL/day) patients is highly effective (70–90%) in the treatment of hypercalcemia. Care should be taken to discontinue gallium nitrate once normocalcemia is achieved, but close metabolic monitoring should be maintained because maximal drug effect occurs days after cessation of administration. The concomitant use of nephrotoxic drugs should be avoided when using gallium nitrate.
- Patients with hypercalcemia who do not respond to pamidronate may benefit from subsequent gallium nitrate administration. Conversely, patients who do not respond to gallium nitrate may benefit from pamidronate (1,4).
- Calcitonin has a rapid onset of action (within 4 hours) and is often useful in severe and symptomatic hypercalcemia until the more slowly acting agents become effective (e.g., zoledronic acid, pamidronate, and gallium nitrate).
- Salmon calcitonin is initially given at 4 units per kg (body weight) s.c. or i.m. every 12 hours. If response is not satisfactory after 1 to 2 days, the dosage may be increased to 8 units per kg s.c. or i.m. every 12 hours. If response is still not adequate after a 1- to 2-day trial at the higher dose, the dosing interval should be decreased to 8 units per kg s.c. or i.m. every 6 hours. Although many patients initially will respond to calcitonin, tachyphylaxis often develops rapidly, which renders patients refractory to its hypocalcemic effect (26–32,34).
- Plicamycin (mithramycin) also has a rapid onset of hypocalcemic activity (12 hours), with duration of response ranging from 3 to 7 days. Note that, due to associated toxicities, plicamycin is rarely used.
- The hypocalcemic effect of plicamycin is attributed to a direct cytotoxic effect on osteoclasts. Single doses of plicamycin, 0.025 mg/kg (body weight) in 150 to 250 mL of 0.9% sodium chloride injection or 5% dextrose injection by i.v. infusion over 30 to 60 minutes, are usually well tolerated. The duration of the hypocalcemic response with plicamycin is typically 3 to 7 days; however, it is essential to note that a maximal hypocalcemic effect may not be achieved until 48 hours after treatment. Consequently, repeated doses should not be given more frequently than every 48 hours if hypocalcemia is to be avoided. Higher doses and shorter treatment intervals also increase the risk of plicamycin-induced hepatic and renal toxicities, hemorrhagic diathesis, and thrombocytopenia (4,34).
- Hemodialysis should be considered, in addition to the other treatments listed for hypercalcemia, in patients who have serum calcium level in the range of 18 to 20 mg/dL and/or in those who have neurologic symptoms but are hemodynamically stable.

TUMOR LYSIS SYNDROME

Etiology of Tumor Lysis Syndrome

- The administration of antitumor agents can lead to cell death, with subsequent release of intracellular contents.
- Tumor lysis syndrome (TLS) occurs when cellular disruption results in life-threatening lactic acidosis, with concomitant hyperuricemia, hyperkalemia, hyperphosphatemia, and hypocalcemia (4). The patient rapidly develops renal failure or has renal insufficiency at presentation.

Clinical Setting, Signs, and Symptoms of Tumor Lysis Syndrome

- TLS is a complication of anticancer treatment that often occurs in patients with bulky disease treated with cytotoxic agents directed at rapidly proliferating tumors (1). Therapy (and the resultant killing of large numbers of neoplastic cells) results in the release of intracellular ions and metabolic byproducts into the systemic circulation.

- TLS occurs most often during the treatment of leukemia or high-grade lymphomas but may also occur during the treatment of other solid tumors (35).
- Cardiac arrhythmias may result from the severe hyperkalemia or hypocalcemia that accompanies the TLS.
- Hypocalcemia can result in tetany, whereas hyperphosphatemia and hyperuricemia can result in acute renal failure (ARF).

Clinically, the syndrome is characterized by rapid development of hyperuricemia, hyperkalemia, hyperphosphatemia, hypocalcemia, and ARF. The main principles of TLS management are (a) identification of high-risk patients with initiation of preventive therapy and (b) early recognition of metabolic and renal complications with prompt supportive care, including hemodialysis.

Prevention and Treatment of Tumor Lysis Syndrome

- Preventive measures include the a priori identification of individuals at risk; 24 to 48 hours of vigorous pretreatment volume expansion (3,000 mL/m^2/day), use of pretherapeutic allopurinol (300–600 mg, PO q day), and vigilant metabolic monitoring (every 3- to 4-hour laboratory tests) after institution of therapy. These actions are the hallmarks of TLS prevention and management (35,36). Elevated levels of lactate dehydrogenase (LDH), uric acid, or creatinine at presentation identify a particularly high-risk patient.
- Corrective measures should be directed toward any metabolic abnormalities that occur in patients after starting cytotoxic therapy, and particular care should be given to the appropriate monitoring of responses [e.g., continuous or serial electrocardiograms (ECGs)] and to the provision of early interventions while correcting hyperkalemia, while admitting the patient to the intensive care unit (ICU) for severe hemodynamic instability, and during hemodialysis, when the patient is faced with worsening or severely compromised renal function (4).
- The correction of metabolic abnormalities during TLS is similar to the general management of the ICU patient, with specific interventions for the following conditions.

Hyperphosphatemia

- In mild hyperphosphatemia, dietary phosphate is restricted to 0.6 to 0.9 g/day, and an oral phosphate binder such as calcium carbonate is added.
- Severe hyperphosphatemia with symptomatic hypocalcemia can be life-threatening. The hyperphosphatemia usually resolves within 6 to 12 hours if renal function is intact. Phosphate excretion can be increased by saline infusion, although this can further reduce the serum calcium concentration by dilution. Phosphate excretion can also be increased by administration of acetazolamide (15 mg/kg every 3–4 hours). Hemodialysis is often indicated in patients with symptomatic hypocalcemia, particularly if renal function is impaired.

Hypocalcemia

- The most appropriate treatment of hypocalcemia, in the absence of hypomagnesemia, is intravenous calcium, at a dose of 100 to 200 mg of elemental calcium (1–2 g of calcium gluconate) in 10 to 20 minutes. Such infusions do not raise the serum calcium concentration for more than 2 to 3 hours and, therefore, should be followed by a slow infusion of 10% calcium gluconate (90 mg of elemental calcium per 10 mL ampule) at the rate of 0.5 to 1.5 mg/kg i.v. per hour.
- Calcium chloride, 10% (272 mg of elemental calcium per 10 mL ampule) can also be used, with 5 to 10 mL given initially i.v. slowly over 10 minutes or diluted in 100 mL of 5% dextrose in water and infused over 20 minutes. This dosage should be repeated as often as every 20 minutes if the patient is symptomatic. Serum calcium levels should be monitored every 4 to 6 hours and hypomagnesemia be corrected as needed.

- Primary management of the hyperphosphatemia is critical to minimize metastatic deposition of insoluble calcium phosphate. Hemodialysis is almost always required by this time.

Hyperkalemia

- Confirm that the elevation in potassium level is genuine.
- *If the patient is asymptomatic,* with a plasma potassium concentration of 6.5 mEq/L and with an ECG that does not manifest signs of hyperkalemia, then withhold potassium and initiate the administration of cation exchange resins. *If the patient is symptomatic,* with peripheral neuromuscular weakness, electrocardiographic signs of hyperkalemia, or plasma potassium concentration above 7 mEq/L, consider calcium gluconate, 10% solution, 10 mL i.v. given over 2 to 5 minutes (dose can be repeated after 5 minutes if electrocardiographic changes persist), followed by glucose with insulin, sodium bicarbonate, or a nebulized β-agonist. Prepare for hemodialysis (37,38).
- Measures to reduce serum potassium level:
  1. Regular insulin, 10 U plus 50% glucose, 50 mL i.v. as a bolus (onset 15–60 minutes; duration 4–6 hours), followed by glucose infusion to prevent hypoglycemia. Insulin along with glucose lowers the potassium level by driving it into the cell.
  2. Adrenergic β_2-agonist such as nebulized albuterol, 10 to 20 mg in 4 mL normal saline, inhaled over 10 minutes (onset 15–30 minutes; duration 2–4 hours) is effective in reducing serum potassium concentration. Adrenergic β_2-agonists induce hypokalemia by stimulating the transport of potassium into skeletal muscle.
  3. Sodium bicarbonate, at the dose of is 45 mEq (1 ampule of a 7.5% sodium bicarbonate solution), is infused slowly over 5 minutes (onset 30–60 minutes; duration several hours); this dose can be repeated in 30 minutes if necessary. This also temporarily drives the potassium inside the cell.
  4. Kayexalate, orally or rectally, 15 to 50 g in 50 to 100 mL of 20% sorbitol solution, is repeated every 3 to 4 hours, as needed, for up to 5 times per day (onset, 1–3 hours, duration of several hours).
- Minimize administration of drugs that can cause or potentiate hyperkalemia [e.g., nonsteroidal antiinflammatory drugs (NSAIDs), β-blockers, angiotensin-converting enzyme (ACE) inhibitors, and potassium-sparing diuretics].

Hyperuricemia and Renal Failure

- Hyperuricemic ARF following chemotherapy may be avoided by (a) prechemotherapeutic identification of patients at risk for developing TLS and (b) administration of allopurinol at doses of 600 to 900 mg every day, starting several days before chemotherapy, with tapering doses to maintain uric acid levels of <7 mg/dL.
- The therapy for hyperuricemic ARF before chemotherapy consists of administering allopurinol (if it has not already been given) and attempting to wash out the obstructing uric acid crystals by a loop diuretic and by fluids. Sodium bicarbonate should not be given at this time because it is difficult to raise the urine pH in this setting. Hemodialysis to remove the excess circulating uric acid should be used in patients in whom a diuresis cannot be induced.
- Hyperuricemic ARF following chemotherapy is usually refractory to conservative intervention (hydration, diuretics, etc.), and patients require hemodialysis for supportive therapy and renal recovery.

In an effort to improve the control of hyperuricemia in patients with leukemia or lymphoma, Pui et al. tested the recombinant urate oxidase (rasburicase) by i.v. administration of the uricolytic agent for 5 to 7 consecutive days to children, adolescents, and young adults with newly diagnosed leukemia or lymphoma (39).

The recombinant enzyme produced a rapid and sharp decrease in plasma uric acid concentrations in all patients. Despite cytoreductive chemotherapy, plasma uric acid concentrations remained low throughout the treatment. The toxicity of the agent was negligible, and none of the patients required dialysis. The mean plasma half-lives of the agent were 16.0 ± 6.3 [standard deviation (SD)] hours and 21.1 ± 12.0 hours, respectively, in patients treated at doses of 0.15 and 0.20 mg/kg. Seventeen of the 121 assessable patients developed antibodies to the enzyme.

The authors concluded that rasburicase was a safe and effective prophylaxis for the treatment of hyperuricemia in patients with leukemia or lymphoma.

REFERENCES

1. Abeloff MD. *Clinical oncology*, 2nd ed. New York: Churchill Livingstone, 1999.
2. Boogerd W, van der Sande JJ. Diagnosis and treatment of spinal cord compression in malignant disease. *Cancer Treat Rev* 1993;19:129–150.
3. Talcott JA, Stomper PC, Drislane FW, et al. Assessing suspected spinal cord compression: a multidisciplinary outcomes analysis of 342 episodes. *Support Care Cancer* 1999;7:31–38.
4. DeVita VT, Hellman S, Rosenberg SA. *Cancer: principles and practice of oncology*, 6th ed. Philadelphia: Lippincott–Raven Publishers, 2001.
5. Djulbegovic B, Sullivan DM. *Decision making in oncology: evidence-based management*. New York: Churchill Livingstone, 1997.
6. Loblaw DA, Laperriere NJ. Emergency treatment of malignant extradural spinal cord compression: an evidence-based guideline. *J Clin Oncol* 1998;16:1613–1624.
7. Heimdal K, Hirschberg H, Slettebo H, et al. High incidence of serious side effects of high-dose dexamethasone treatment in patients with epidural spinal cord compression. *J Neurooncol* 1992;12:141.
8. Vecht CJ, Haaxma-Reiche H, van Putten WL, et al. Initial bolus of conventional versus high-dose dexamethasone in metastatic spinal cord compression. *Neurology* 1989;39:1255–1257.
9. Regine WF, Tibbs PA, Young A, et al. Metastatic spinal cord compression: a randomized trial of direct decompressive surgical resection plus radiotherapy vs. Radiotherapy alone. *Int J Radiat Oncol Biol Phys* 2003;57(Suppl. 2):S125.
10. Byrne TN. Spinal cord compression from epidural metastases. *N Engl J Med* 1992;327:614–619.
11. Burch PA, Grossman SA. Treatment of epidural cord compressions from Hodgkin's disease with chemotherapy: a report of two cases and a review of the literature. *Am J Med* 1988;84:555–558.
12. Clarke PR, Saunders M. Steroid-induced remission in spinal canal reticulum cell sarcoma: report of two cases. *J Neurosurg* 1975;42:346–348.
13. Cooper K, Bajorin D, Shapiro W, et al. Decompression of epidural metastases from germ cell tumors with chemotherapy. *J Neurooncol* 1990;8:275–280.
14. Friedman HM, Sheetz S, Levine HL, et al. Combination chemotherapy and radiation therapy: the medical management of epidural spinal cord compression from testicular cancer. *Arch Intern Med* 1986;146:509–512.
15. Payne RB, Carver ME, Morgan DB. Interpretation of serum total calcium: effects of adjustment for albumin concentration on frequency of abnormal values and on detection of change in the individual. *J Clin Pathol* 1979;32:56–60.
16. Sanderson IR, Pritchard J, Marsh HT. Chemotherapy as the initial treatment of spinal cord compression due to disseminated neuroblastoma. *J Neurosurg* 1989;70:688–690.
17. Sinoff CL, Blumsohn A. Spinal cord compression in myelomatosis: response to chemotherapy alone. *Eur J Cancer Clin Oncol* 1989;25:197–200.
18. Sasagawa I, Gotoh H, Miyabayashi H, et al. Hormonal treatment of symptomatic spinal cord compression in advanced prostatic cancer. *Int Urol Nephrol* 1991;23:351–356.
19. Ostler PJ, Clarke DP, Watkinson AF, et al. Superior vena cava obstruction: a modern management strategy. *Clin Oncol* 1997;9:83–89.
20. Patel V, Igwebe T, Mast H, et al. Superior vena cava syndrome: current concepts of management. *N Engl J Med* 1995;92:245–248.
21. Schraufnagel DE, Hill R, Leech JA, et al. Superior vena caval obstruction. Is it a medical emergency? *Am J Med* 1981;70:1169–1174.
22. Rowell NP, Gleeson FV. Steroids, radiotherapy, chemotherapy and stents for superior vena caval obstruction in carcinoma of the bronchus (Cochrane review). *Cochrane Database Syst Rev* 2001;4: CD001316.
23. Greenberg S, Kosinski R, Daniels J. Treatment of superior vena cava thrombosis with recombinant tissue type plasminogen activator. *Chest* 1991;99:1298–1301.

24. Chisholm MA, Mulloy AL, Taylor AT. Acute management of cancer-related hypercalcemia. *Ann Pharmacother* 1996;30:507–513.
25. Bilezikian JP. Management of acute hypercalcemia. *N Engl J Med* 1992;326:1196–1203.
26. Raisz LG, Trummel CL, Wener JA, et al. Effect of glucocorticoids on bone resorption in tissue culture. *Endocrinology* 1972;90:961–967.
27. Percival RC, Yates AJ, Gray RE, et al. Role of glucocorticoids in management of malignant hypercalcaemia. *Br Med J* 1984;289:287.
28. Kristensen B, Ejlertsen B, Holmegaard SN, et al. Prednisolone in the treatment of severe malignant hypercalcaemia in metastatic breast cancer: a randomized study. *J Intern Med* 1992;232:237–245.
29. Gucalp R, Theriault R, Gill I, et al. Treatment of cancer-associated hypercalcemia: double-blind comparison of rapid and slow intravenous infusion regimens of pamidronate disodium and saline alone. *Arch Intern Med* 1994;154:1935–1944.
30. Ralston SH, Gallacher SJ, Patel U, et al. Comparison of three intravenous bisphosphonates in cancer-associated hypercalcaemia. *Lancet* 1989;2:1180–1182.
31. Chan FK, Koberle LM, Thys-Jacobs S, et al. Differential diagnosis, causes, and management of hypercalcemia. *Curr Probl Surg* 1997;34:445–523.
32. Kiang DT, Loken MK, Kennedy BJ. Mechanism of the hypocalcemic effect of mithramycin. *J Clin Endocrinol Metab* 1979;48:341–344.
33. Major P, Lortholary A, Hon J, et al. Zoledronic acid is superior to pamidronate in the treatment of hypercalcemia of malignancy: a pooled analysis of two randomized, controlled clinical trials. *J Clin Oncol* 2001;19(2):558–567.
34. Green L, Donehower RC. Hepatic toxicity of low doses of mithramycin in hypercalcemia. *Cancer Treat Rep* 1984;68:1379–1381.
35. Jones DP, Mahmoud H, Chesney RW. Tumor lysis syndrome: pathogenesis and management. *Pediatr Nephrol* 1995;9:206–212.
36. Fleming DR, Doukas MA. Acute tumor lysis syndrome in hematologic malignancies. *Leuk Lymphoma* 1992;8:315–318.
37. Tierney LM, McPhee SJ, Papadakis MA, eds. Fluid and electrolyte disorders. *Current medical diagnosis and treatment*, 38th ed. Stanford, CT: Appleton & Lange, 1999:847.
38. Cogan MG. *Fluid and Electrolytes: Physiology and Pathophysiology*, 1st ed. Norwalk, CT: Appleton & Lange, 1991.
39. Pui C, Mahmoud H, Wiley J, et al. Recombinant urate oxidase for the prophylaxis or treatment of hyperuricemia in patients with leukemia or lymphoma. *J Clin Oncol*, 2001;19(3):697–704.

37

Psychopharmacologic Management in Oncology

Donald L. Rosenstein, Maryland Pao, and Daniel E. Elswick

Psychiatric syndromes, predominantly depression and anxiety, occur commonly in patients with cancer and, if misdiagnosed or poorly managed, can have a profoundly negative effect on optimal oncologic care. The comprehensive psychiatric care of patients with cancer includes psychosocial, behavioral, and psychoeducational interventions as well as appropriate pharmacologic and psychotherapeutic treatment. This chapter focuses on the psychopharmacologic management of the major psychiatric syndromes encountered in the oncology setting and includes information on specialist referral. The chapter concludes with specific recommendations for psychopharmacologic management in pediatric oncology.

CONSIDERATIONS PRIOR TO PRESCRIBING PSYCHOPHARMACOLOGIC AGENTS

1. Psychiatric symptoms are often manifestations of an underlying medical disorder or complications of its treatment (Table 37.1). For example, specific malignancies (e.g., lung, breast, gastrointestinal, and renal cancers) are prone to metastasize to the central nervous system (CNS). In addition, any advanced cancer can result in metabolic CNS insults that precipitate psychiatric symptoms. For

TABLE 37.1. *Medical conditions in oncologic and other disorders associated with anxiety and depression*

Neoplasms	**Cardiovascular diseases**
Brain tumors	Ischemic heart disease
Insulinoma	Arrhythmias
Lymphoma	Congestive heart failure
Small cell carcinoma	**Metabolic abnormalities**
Pancreatic cancer	Electrolyte disturbances
Leukemia	Uremia
Endocrinopathies	Vitamin B_{12} or folate deficiency
Cushing syndrome	**Other**
Adrenal insufficiency	Substance abuse and with-
Hypopituitarism	drawal
Pheochromocytoma	Pain (uncontrolled)
Thyroid dysfunction	Hematologic (e.g., anemia)
Medication adverse affects	
Interferon-alpha	
Corticosteroids	
Interleukin-2	
Dopamine-blocking antiemetics	

those patients whose psychiatric symptoms fail to respond to psychopharmacologic treatment, CNS involvement should be reconsidered, even in malignancies that do not commonly metastasize to the brain.

2. Medically ill patients are particularly susceptible to adverse effects of medications on the CNS. Specific examples of medications associated with mood, cognitive, and behavioral symptoms include the following: corticosteroids, interleukin-2, interferon-α, opiates, and dopamine-blocking antiemetics. For patients who develop psychiatric symptoms after treatment with such agents, it is often more prudent to lower the dose or to discontinue the use of a currently prescribed medication than to introduce yet another agent (i.e., a psychotropic) that might exacerbate psychiatric symptoms.

3. Polypharmacy is often unavoidable in patients with cancer; however, most clinically significant interactions with psychotropic agents are predictable and can be avoided by choosing alternative agents or by making dose adjustments. The use of monoamine oxidase inhibitors (MAOIs) with either meperidine (Demerol) or selective serotonin reuptake inhibitors (SSRIs) can be life threatening. Up-to-date drug interaction resources can be found at several Internet websites (e.g., http://medicine. iupui.edu/flockhart/).

4. Inadequate pain control frequently induces symptoms of anxiety, irritability, or depression. It is essential to have pain well-controlled so that the appropriate psychiatric diagnosis and treatment can proceed (see Chapter 40). One note of caution in this regard concerns the combined use of SSRIs and tricyclic antidepressants (TCAs), which are frequently used in the treatment of neuropathic pain. Some SSRIs (e.g., fluoxetine, paroxetine, and fluvoxamine) inhibit the metabolism of TCAs, which can in turn prolong the corrected QT (QTc) interval.

COMMON PSYCHIATRIC SYNDROMES IN THE ONCOLOGY SETTING

Adjustment Disorder

This is a time-limited, maladaptive reaction to a specific stressor that typically involves symptoms of depression, anxiety, or behavioral changes and impairs psychosocial functioning. The diagnostic criteria include the onset of symptoms within 3 months of the stressor but the duration of symptoms is no more than 6 months. The differential diagnosis includes the following disorders:

- Bereavement
- Post-traumatic stress disorder
- Other mood and anxiety disorders

Management

The initial treatment approach consists of crisis intervention and brief psychotherapy. Time-limited symptom management with medications may be indicated. For example, anxiety, tearfulness, and insomnia are frequent reactions to the diagnosis of a new or recurrent malignancy. Short-term treatment of these symptoms with benzodiazepines (BZDs) (e.g., lorazepam and clonazepam) is appropriate, effective, and rarely associated with the development of abuse or dependence. Short-term use of non-benzodiazepine sleep agents (e.g., zolpidem) is also commonplace in clinical practice (Table 37.2).

TABLE 37.2 *Commonly used hypnotic agents*

Generic	Brand	Dose range (mg)	Half-life
Eszopiclone	Lunesta	1–3 PO	Short
Temazepam	Restoril	7.5–30 PO	Med
Zaleplon	Sonata	5–20 PO	Short
Zolpidem	Ambien,	2.5–10 PO	Short
	Ambien CR	6.25–12.5 PO	Extended release

TABLE 37.3. *Risk factors for suicide in patients with cancer*

Historical considerations	Clinical descriptors
Prior suicide attempts	Elderly males
Family history of suicide	Recent loss and poor social support
Prior psychiatric illness	Current depression, anxiety, substance abuse
History of substance abuse	Advanced cancer, pain, poor prognosis
Impulsive behavior	Delirium, psychosis, illogical thoughts
	Access to firearms or other lethal means of suicide

Major Depression

Major depression and subsyndromal depressive disorders are common in patients with cancer. Prevalence rates vary between 5% and 50% depending on how depression is defined, whether study samples are drawn from outpatient clinics or hospital wards, and the type of cancer involved. Untreated depression has been correlated with poor adherence to medical care, increased pain and disability, and a greater likelihood of considering euthanasia and physician-assisted suicide.

A frequent diagnostic task in the oncology setting is differentiating symptoms of major depression from those symptoms that are caused by the underlying cancer or its treatment. The patient with disseminated cancer who is undergoing chemotherapy is likely to experience fatigue, anorexia, weight loss, and insomnia, whether a major depression is present or absent. Our practice is to institute empiric trials of antidepressants using a targeted symptom reduction approach. In questionable cases, a personal or family history of depression and the presence of symptoms of excessive guilt, poor self-esteem, anhedonia, and ruminative thinking strengthen the argument for a medication trial. Furthermore, because the number of well-tolerated, safe, and effective antidepressants has grown, we have lowered our threshold for treating subsyndromal depression in the oncology setting.

Because patients with cancer have an increased risk of suicide compared with the general population, particular attention should be paid to symptoms of hopelessness, helplessness, suicidal ideation, and intense anxiety (Table 37.3). The incidence of cancer at certain sites (e.g., head and neck, lung, gastrointestinal tract, urogenital tract, and breast) is associated with an even greater risk of suicide.

Differential diagnosis of major depression includes:

- Adjustment disorder
- Dysthymic disorder
- Delirium (hypoactive)
- Dementia
- Substance abuse
- Bipolar disorder
- Bereavement
- Mood disorder caused by a medical disorder or medication (Table 37.4)

Management

Treatment modalities include pharmacotherapy (Table 37.4), psychotherapy, and electroconvulsive therapy (ECT). Selection of an antidepressant should be based on a number of considerations such as active medical problems, the potential for drug interactions, prior treatment response, and an optimal match between the patient's target symptoms and the side-effect profile of the antidepressant (e.g., using a sedating agent for the patient with anxiety and insomnia). Potential interactions with cancer therapeutics should also be considered. For example, several antidepressants are inhibitors of cytochrome P-450 2D6. This inhibition may reduce the metabolism of tamoxifen to its active metabolite. Medications with less inhibitory effect at 2D6, such as venlafaxine (Effexor) or citalopram (Celexa), are preferred in breast cancer patients taking tamoxifen. Mirtazapine (Remeron) has several properties that make it a particularly attractive antidepressant choice in patients with cancer: it is sedating, causes weight gain, has few significant drug interactions, and is a partial 5HT-3 receptor antagonist, which gives it some antiemetic properties. Mirtazapine may also potentiate the antidepressant effect of SSRIs.

TABLE 37.4. *Commonly used antidepressants in patients with cancer*

Generic names (brand names)	Dose range (mg)	Common adverse effects and unique traits
SSRIs		
Fluoxetine (Prozac)[a,c,d]	5–60	GI symptoms, weight changes, sleep disruption, sexual dysfunction, agitation, anxiety, hyponatremia
Sertraline (Zoloft)[a,d]	12.5–200	GI symptoms, weight changes, sleep disruption, sexual dysfunction, hyponatremia
Paroxetine (Paxil)[c,d]	10–60	GI symptoms, weight changes, sleep disruption, sexual dysfunction, hyponatremia, anticholinergic effects, withdrawal syndrome
Citalopram (Celexa)[d]	10–60	GI symptoms, sleep disruption, sexual dysfunction, dry mouth
Escitalopram (Lexapro)[a,b]	5–40	GI symptoms, sleep disruption, sexual dysfunction, dry mouth
Fluvoxamine (Luvox)[a,c]	25–300	GI symptoms, sexual dysfunction, headache
Novel antidepressants		
Venlafaxine (Effexor)[c]	18.75–300	GI symptoms, sexual dysfunction, anticholinergic effects, hypertension at dose >225 mg/d, reduces hot flashes
Mirtazapine (Remeron)[b]	7.5–45	Sedation, dry mouth, increased appetite and weight gain, constipation, dizziness
Bupropion (Wellbutrin)[c]	37.5–450	GI symptoms, tremor, seizures at high dose or with CNS lesions
Trazodone (Desyrel)	25–200	Sedation, orthostatic hypotension, priapism
Duloxetine (Cymbalta)[c]	20–60	GI symptoms, headache, dizziness; also indicated for diabetic neuropathy
CNS stimulants		
Methylphenidate (Ritalin)[a,b,c]	2.5–40	Insomnia, agitation, GI symptoms, headache, tics, rebound depression
Dextroamphetamine (Dexedrine)[a,b,c]	2.5–30	Insomnia, agitation, confusion, GI symptoms, headache, tics, rebound depression, delusions, psychosis
Tricyclic antidepressants		
Amitriptyline (Elavil)[a]	25–150	Dry mouth, sedation, weight gain, GI symptoms, headache, ECG changes, orthostatic hypotension, anticholinergic effects
Desipramine (Norpramin)	25–150	Dry mouth, tachycardia, ECG changes
Nortriptyline (Pamelor)[a,d]	25–150	Tremor, confusion, anticholinergic effects
Doxepin (Sinequan)[a,d]	10–150	Potent antihistamine, anticholinergic effects, used for itching

SSRI, selective serotonin reuptake inhibitor; GI, gastrointestinal; CNS, central nervous system; ECG, electrocardiogram.

[a]FDA approval for use in children/adolescents.
[b]Orally disintegrating tablets or wafers available.
[c]Sustained-release and extended-release formulations available.
[d]Liquid formulation available.

Anxiety Disorders

Many medical conditions seen in the oncology setting, such as heart failure, respiratory compromise, seizure disorders, pheochromocytoma, and chemotherapy-induced ovarian failure, may cause anxiety. Additional conditions that may cause both anxiety and depression are listed in Table 37.1. Similarly, anxiety is an adverse effect of numerous medications. In particular, dopamine-blocking antiemetics such as metoclopramide (Reglan), prochlorperazine (Compazine), and promethazine (Phenergan) frequently cause akathisia, an adverse effect characterized by subjective restlessness and increased motor activity, which is commonly misdiagnosed as anxiety. Initiation of treatment with an antidepressant may also induce a transient anxiety state. It is important to inform patients of this potential side effect in order to improve adherence.

The differential diagnosis of anxiety disorders in the oncology setting includes the following:

- Exacerbation of medical illness
- Delirium
- Agitated depression
- Adverse effects of medications
- Substance or alcohol abuse or withdrawal
- Adjustment disorder

Management

In addition to behavioral therapy and psychotherapy, BZDs are the medications that are most frequently used for the short-term treatment of anxiety (Table 37.5). For anxiety that persists beyond a few weeks, treatment with an antidepressant (see Table 37.4) is indicated. If the patient has already been taking an SSRI, it is important not to discontinue it abruptly (with the exception of fluoxetine because of its long half-life) to avoid rebound anxiety. Low-dose, atypical antipsychotics are often useful for severe and persistent anxiety or for conditions such as anxiety secondary to steroids and delirium (Table 37.6).

The following issues associated with BZDs require attention:

- Although BZDs are the treatment of choice for delirium caused by alcohol or sedative–hypnotic withdrawal, their use predictably worsens other types of delirium.
- In patients with hepatic failure, lorazepam, temazepam, or oxazepam are the preferred BZDs.
- BZDs may result in "disinhibition," especially in delirium, substance abuse, organic disorders, and preexisting personality disorders. Disinhibition is more common in children and elderly patients.
- The abrupt discontinuation of BZDs with short half-lives (e.g., alprazolam [Xanax]) can cause rebound anxiety and precipitate a withdrawal syndrome.
- Long-term use of BZDs may lead to cognitive problems, tolerance, and dependence. Time-limited use is recommended.

Delirium

Delirium is an acute confusional state characterized by a fluctuating course of cognitive impairment, perceptual disturbances, mood changes, delusions, and sleep–wake cycle disruption. Patients can have a hyperactive (agitated) or hypoactive (quiet) delirium. Approximately 25% of delirium is hypoactive. Virtually any psychiatric symptom can be a manifestation of delirium. Anxiety and/or labile mood are common presentations often misdiagnosed as "depression." Patients who are elderly, who are on multiple medications, or who have underlying brain pathology are more prone to delirium. Delirium in terminally ill patients is common and often underdiagnosed. Several cancer-related therapies can

TABLE 37.5. *Preferred BZDs in the oncology setting*

	Lorazepam (Ativan)[a]	Clonazepam (Klonopin)
Dose equivalency	1 mg	0.25 mg
Dose range	0.25–2 mg PO, sublingual, i.m. or i.v. routes, every 1–6 h (maximum daily dose, 8 mg)	0.25–1 mg PO route only, every 8–12 h
Advantages	Rapid onset of action	Less frequent dosing than with lorazepam

BZD, benzodiazepines; PO, orally; i.m., intramuscularly; i.v., intravenously.
[a]Liquid formulation available.

TABLE 37.6.   *Commonly used neuroleptics in the oncology setting*

	Initial dose (mg)	Administrative routes and schedules	Maximum daily dose (mg)
Haloperidol[a,b,d] (Haldol)	0.25–1 PO, or i.v.	every 2–12 h s.c., i.m.	20
Chlorpromazine (Thorazine)	12.5–50 PO, i.m. or i.v.	every 4–12 h	300
Risperidone[a,b,c,d] (Risperdal)	0.25–3 PO	every 12 h	6
Olanzapine[b] (Zyprexa)	2.5–10 PO	every 12–24 h	20
Quetiapine[c] (Seroquel)	25–50 PO	every 12–24 h	800

PO, orally; s.c., subcutaneously; i.m., intramuscularly; i.v., intravenously.
[a]FDA approval for use in children/adolescents.
[b]Orally disintegrating tablets or wafers available.
[c]Sustained-release and extended-release formulations available.
[d]Liquid formulation available.

induce delirium. Chemotherapeutics associated with delirium include methotrexate, ifosfamide, and cytosine arabinoside. Immunotherapies including interferon-alpha and interleukin-2 can also contribute to delirium. Total brain radiation may cause cognitive changes and delirium.

The differential diagnosis includes the following:

- Dementia
- Affective disorders with psychosis (mania or depression)
- Psychotic disorders
- Medication effects or substance abuse or withdrawal

Management

The first steps in the management of delirium are the identification and treatment of precipitating factors and the discontinuation of nonessential medications. Haloperidol (Haldol) continues to be the treatment of choice for delirium in most cases (see Table 37.6). Common adverse effects of typical antipsychotics include sedation, EPS, and hypotension. Newer atypical antipsychotics such as olanzapine (Zyprexa), quetiapine (Seroquel), and risperidone (Risperdal) are associated with sedation, weight gain, and metabolic syndrome. Recent concerns have been raised about an increased risk of sudden death associated with antipsychotic use in elderly patients. These data suggesting a small increase in the relative risk of death must be weighed against the substantial risks of untreated delirium. Delirium secondary to BZD, or sedative–hypnotic and alcohol withdrawal should be treated with BZDs. Nonpharmacologic interventions such as reorientation and providing a sitter should also be initiated along with pharmacotherapy.

ADDITIONAL CONSIDERATIONS FOR PSYCHOPHARMACOLOGIC MANAGEMENT IN PEDIATRIC ONCOLOGY

Cancer is the fourth leading cause of death and the leading cause of nonacute death among children. Life-threatening illness in a child or an adolescent is traumatic and can be associated with anxiety and depression. Although many patients cope well with and adapt to the trauma, symptoms of depression such as fatigue, cognitive impairment, decreased social interaction and exploration, and anorexia may be part of a cytokine or immunologic response to cancer and its treatments. Psychotropic medications can dramatically improve the quality of life for children with cancer. These medications do not replace comprehensive, multimodal, multidisciplinary care, but are adjuncts to decrease discomfort and improve functioning of medically ill children.

Assessment and Diagnosis in Pediatric Oncology

A thorough psychiatric assessment is needed to make a correct diagnosis and to institute treatment. Typically, this assessment is based on multiple, brief examinations of the child and information gathered from additional sources including family, staff, and teachers. A patient's biologic vulnerability to depression and anxiety may be inferred from (a) a family history of a mood or anxiety disorder, or other psychiatric disorder, and (b) previous psychiatric symptoms or psychiatric treatment.

Common complaints in medically ill children include:

- Anxiety
- Pain
- Difficulty sleeping
- Fatigue
- Feeling "bored"

Adult psychiatric syndromes of adjustment disorder, major depression, anxiety, and delirium apply to children as well, but anxiety, rather than depression, is the most frequent diagnosis. Important determining factors for pharmacologic intervention are severity and duration of psychiatric symptoms.

Psychopharmacologic Treatment of Pediatric Patients

In 1994, manufacturers and federally funded researchers were mandated to study medications such as antidepressants in children. Although there have been no controlled antidepressant trials in depressed medically ill children, and the dose of psychiatric medications for children with cancer has not been systematically studied, antidepressants have been useful for treating anxiety and depression. Body weight, Tanner staging, clinical status, and potential for medications to interact are weighed in deciding doses. See Tables 37.4 and 37.6 for psychotropics with U.S. Food and Drug Administration (FDA) approval for use in children and adolescents.

BZDs, such as lorazepam, used in low doses in conjunction with nonpharmacologic distraction techniques, may be appropriate for procedures that induce considerable anxiety in children. Clonazepam is longer acting and may be helpful with more pervasive and prolonged anxiety symptoms. BZDs can cause sedation, confusion, and behavioral disinhibition. Their use should be carefully monitored, especially in those patients with CNS dysfunction. BZD withdrawal precipitated by abrupt discontinuation occurs most frequently on transferring the patient from intensive care settings.

Antihistamines have been used to sedate anxious children. Diphenhydramine, hydroxyzine, and promethazine may be helpful for occasional insomnia. However, antihistamines are not helpful for persistent anxiety and their anticholinergic properties can precipitate or worsen delirium. Intravenous diphenhydramine may be misused because it can induce euphoria when given by i.v. push. Very high doses of i.v. diphenhydramine can also provoke seizures.

Fluoxetine is the only FDA-approved SSRI for depression in children older than 6 years. Fluoxetine and sertraline are approved for obsessive-compulsive disorder in children older than 6 years; fluvoxamine is approved for those who are 8 years and older. Fluoxetine, with its active metabolite norfluoxetine, and fluvoxamine are potent inhibitors of cytochrome P-450 (CYP) 3A3 and 3A4. They are contraindicated with macrolide antibiotics, azole antifungal agents, and several other medications. Amitriptyline is approved for depression in children who are 12 years or older. TCAs are useful for treating insomnia, weight loss, anxiety, and some pain syndromes.

Some antidepressants may contribute to suicidal thinking in children and adolescents. This possibility mandates careful monitoring of all children treated with antidepressants. Use of non-FDA–approved psychopharmacologic agents in children with cancer may be considered in extreme or prolonged distress and poor functioning, but must be monitored closely. It is unusual for children with cancer to be suicidal in the absence of premorbid depression or adequate pain management.

Children and adolescents who cannot tolerate antidepressants may benefit from stimulants for depression and apathy. Psychostimulants are generally well tolerated and have a rapid onset of action. Children with delirium, hallucinations, severe agitation, or aggression may be safely treated with low-dose antipsychotics such as haloperidol or atypical neuroleptics such as risperidone and olanzapine.

Although there is a dearth of research in pediatric cancer psychopharmacology, child psychiatry consultation may considerably improve the quality of life for children undergoing cancer treatment and dealing with cancer survival. Routine psychological screening of children with cancer and survivors can detect ongoing distress. Psychopharmacologic consultation may also help children with postradiation or postchemotherapy conditions related to attention, mood, and anxiety disorders.

SPECIALIST REFERRAL

Many psychiatric symptoms can be readily addressed by the primary oncologist or oncology service through counseling and pharmacotherapy. Sometimes it is helpful to involve a psychiatric specialist to assist with psychopharmacology and other supportive interventions. There are a growing number of practitioners working within oncology centers who focus on issues associated with cancer diagnosis, treatment, and survivorship. The subspecialty of Psychosocial Oncology (or Psycho-Oncology) has existed in some centers since the 1970s. There is a great deal of variability of access to psychosocial specialists at cancer centers and in the community. Some centers have dedicated services while others utilize practitioners from palliative, general psychiatric, or psychosomatic medicine services. It may be beneficial for oncologists to establish relationships with local community mental health providers in settings where a dedicated service is not available.

Determining the appropriateness of a referral to assist with psychopharmacology can be difficult for some oncology providers. The National Comprehensive Cancer Network (NCCN) has established guidelines for management and referral for psychosocial issues in The Clinical Practice Guidelines in Oncology. There is a section on Distress Management (current version 1.2008) that includes referral and treatment algorithms for psychiatric, social, pastoral, and substance related issues. A simple screening tool called the "Distress Thermometer" exists to help determine the need for referral to supportive services including referral to psychiatric care. The NCCN guidelines are available online at http://www.nccn.org/professionals/physician_gls/PDF/distress.pdf. Additionally, a recent report from the Institute of Medicine establishes the standard of care for addressing psychosocial issues in the oncology setting (http://www.iom.edu/CMS/3809/34252/47228.aspx).

SUMMARY

Psychiatric syndromes are frequently misdiagnosed and poorly treated in patients with cancer. Before initiating psychopharmacologic therapy, underlying medical disorders and adverse effects of medication must be addressed and potential drug interactions anticipated. Psychiatric symptoms should then be treated promptly and aggressively. Consultation from a psychiatrist is indicated when the patient (a) has a complex psychiatric history and is taking multiple psychotropic medications; (b) exhibits depressive symptoms associated with extreme guilt, anxiety, and/or suicidal thoughts; (c) is confused, hallucinating, agitated, or violent; and (d) is nonadherent with care or rejects treatment and seeks physician-assisted suicide.

SUGGESTED READINGS

Academy of Psychosomatic Medicine. Psychiatric aspects of excellent end-of-life care: a position statement of the Academy of Psychosomatic Medicine. Available at: http://www.apm.org/eol-care.html. Accessed March 14, 2005.

American Psychiatric Association. *Diagnostic and statistical manual of mental disorders*, 4th ed. (Text Revision). Washington, DC: American Psychiatric Association, 2000.

Cassem EH. Depressive disorders in the medically ill: an overview. *Psychosomatics* 1995;36:S2–S10.

Cleeland CS, Bennett GJ, Dantzer R, et al. Are the symptoms of cancer and cancer treatment due to a shared biologic mechanism? A cytokine-immunologic model of cancer symptoms. *Cancer* 2003;97:2919.

Coyle N, Adelhardt J, Foley KM, et al. Character of terminal illness in the advanced patient with cancer: pain and other symptoms during the last four weeks of life. *J Pain Symptom Manage* 1990;5:83.

Emanuel EJ, Fairclough DL, Daniels ER, et al. Euthanasia and physician-assisted suicide: attitudes and experiences of oncology patients, oncologists, and the public. *Lancet* 1996;347:1805.

Endicott J. Measurement of depression in patients with cancer. *Cancer* 1984;53:2243.

Fawzy I, Greenburg D. Oncology. In Wise MG, and Rundell, JR, ed. *Textbook of Consultation-Liaison Psychiatry 2nd edition.* Washington, DC: American Psychiatric Press, 2002.

Goldman LS, Wise TN, Brody DS. *Psychiatry for Primary Care Physicians.* Washington, DC: American Psychiatric Press, 1997.

Gothelf D, Rubinstein M, Shemesh E, et al. Pilot study: fluvoxamine treatment for depression and anxiety disorders in children and adolescents with cancer. *J Am Acad Child Adolesc Psychiatry* 2005;44:1258–62.

Holland J, Greenberg D, Hughes M, et al. *Quick Reference for Oncology Clinicians: The Psychiatric and Psychological Dimensions of Cancer Symptom Management.* Charlottesville: IPOS Press, 2006.

Holland J. *Psycho-oncology.* New York: Oxford University Press, 1998.

Kersun LS, Shemesh E. Depression and anxiety in children at the end of life. *Pediatr Clin N Am* 2007;54:691–708.

Lipsett DR, Payne EC, Cassem NH. On death and dying. Discussion. *J Geriatr Psychiatry* 1974;7:108.

Lynch ME. The assessment and prevalence of affective disorders in advanced cancer. *J Palliat Care* 1995;11:10.

McDaniel JS, Musselman DL, Porter MR, et al. Depression in patients with cancer: diagnosis, biology, and treatment. *Arch Gen Psychiatry* 1995;52:89.

Pao M, Ballard E, Rosenstein DL, Wiener L, Wayne AS. Psychotropic medication use in pediatric patients with cancer. *Arch Pediatr Adolesc Med* 2006;160:818–822.

Portteus A, Ahmad N, Tobey D, Leavey P. The prevalence and use of antidepressant medication in pediatric cancer patients. *J Child Adolesc Psychopharmacol* 2006;16:467–473.

Recklitis C, O'Leary T, Diller L. Utility of routine psychological screening in the childhood cancer survivor clinic. *J Clin Oncol* 2003;21:787.

Rodin G, Lloyd N, Katz M, et al. The treatment of depression in cancer patients: a systematic review. *Support Care Cancer* 2007:15:123.

Spiegel D, Sands S, Koopman C. Pain and depression in patients with cancer. *Cancer* 1994;74:2570.

Wise TN. The physician and his patient with cancer. *Prim Care* 1974;1:407.

38

Management of Emesis in Oncology

David R. Kohler

RADIATION- AND CHEMOTHERAPY-ASSOCIATED EMETIC SYMPTOMS

Radiation- and chemotherapy-associated emetic symptoms are categorized by the period in which they occur in relation to emetogenic treatment (Fig. 38.1). Although "acute" and "delayed" are useful terms for describing clinical events and approaches to symptom management, they were arbitrarily assigned before the principal neural mechanisms that elicit acute- and delayed-phase symptoms were elucidated.

Acute-Phase Symptoms

Emetic symptoms that occur within 24 hours after treatment are classified as acute-phase symptoms (see Fig. 38.1). Acute-phase symptoms correlate with serotonin (5-HT$_3$) release from enterochromaffin cells. Emetic signals are propagated at local 5-HT$_3$ receptors and transmitted along afferent vagus nerve fibers. They activate a diffuse series of effector nuclei in the medulla oblongata (the so-called

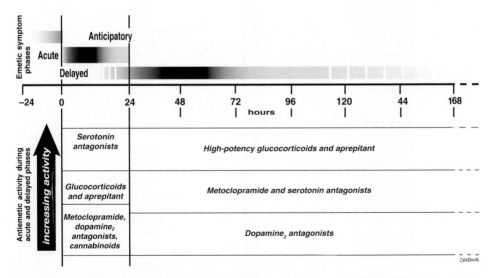

Fig. 38.1. Comparison of emetic symptom phases and antiemetic activity. *Top:* Temporal relation between the start of emetogenic treatment (hour 0) and emetic symptom phases. For each phase, shaded bars indicate the general periods during which nausea and emesis occur; depth of shading indicates incidence of symptoms. *Bottom:* Most highly active drug categories ranked by relative effectiveness in prophylaxis against acute-phase (0–24 h) and delayed-phase (>24 h) emetic symptoms.

479

"vomiting center"), which integrates afferent emetic signals and subsequently activates and coordinates motor nuclei that produce the physiologic changes associated with vomiting.

- Greatest incidence is 2 to 6 hours after treatment.
- Onset is generally within 1 to 3 hours after commencing chemotherapy. Notable exceptions are mechlorethamine (nitrogen mustard), which generally induces rapid symptom onset, and cyclophosphamide and carboplatin, which have long latency periods before acute-phase onset.
- Symptoms may persist or intermittently recur for ≥12 hours after treatment.

Delayed-Phase Symptoms

Delayed-phase symptoms occur >24 hours after treatment (Table 38.1) and are associated with central activation of neurokinin type 1 (NK_1) receptors, for which substance P is the natural ligand.

TABLE 38.1. *Onset and duration of emesis with selected chemotherapy agents*

Drug	Onset of emesis (h)	Duration of emesis (h)
Aldesleukin	0–6	
Altretamine	3–6	
Asparaginase	1–3	
Bleomycin	3–6	
Carboplatin	6–8	>24
Carmustine	2–6	4–24
Chlorambucil	48–72	
Cisplatin	1–6	24 to >48
Cyclophosphamide	6–18	6 to >24
Cytarabine	6–12	3–5
Dacarbazine	1–5	1–24
Dactinomycin	2–6	12–24
Daunorubicin	2–6	24
Doxorubicin	4–6	6 to >24
Etoposide	3–8	6–12
Fluorouracil	3–6	3–4
Hydroxyurea	6–12	
Ifosfamide	1–6	6–12
Irinotecan	2–6	6–12
Lomustine	2–6	4–12
Mechlorethamine	0.5–2	1–24
Melphalan	6–12	
Mercaptopurine	4–8	
Methotrexate	4–12	3–12
Mitomycin	1–6	3–12
Mitotane	Long latency	Persistent
Paclitaxel	3–8	3–8
Pentostatin	Long latency	Persistent (>24)
Plicamycin	4–6	12–24
Procarbazine	24–27	Variable
Streptozocin	1–4	12–24
Teniposide	3–8	6–12
Thioguanine	4–8	—
Thiotepa	6–12	Variable
Vinblastine	4–8	
Vincristine	4–8	
Vinorelbine	4–8	

Source: Adapted from Borison HL, McCarthy LE. Neuropharmacology of chemotherapy-induced emesis. *Drugs.* 1983;25(Suppl 1):8–17; and Aapro M. Methodological issues in antiemetic studies. *Invest New Drugs.* 1993;11(4):243–53.

TABLE 38.2. *Antineoplastic drugs implicated in delayed emesis*

Carboplatin ≥300 mg/m^2 (± other cytotoxic agents)
Cisplatin ≥50 mg/m^2
Cyclophosphamide ≥600 mg/m^2
Cyclophosphamide + anthracycline ("AC") combinations
Cyclophosphamide ± other cytotoxic agents
Doxorubicin ≥50 mg/m^2

Chemotherapy regimens with a high potential for emetic symptoms during the acute phase are often associated with delayed-phase symptoms as well (Table 38.2). Symptoms may occur as early as 16 to 18 hours after emetogenic treatment, with a period of greatest incidence between 24 and 96 hours after treatment. Delayed emesis may occur in patients who do not experience symptoms acutely, but incidence characteristically decreases in patients who achieve complete control during the acute phase. Although emesis is typically less severe during the delayed phase than during the acute phase, the reported severity of nausea is similar during both phases.

Anticipatory Events

Anticipatory emetic symptoms occur before exposure to an emetogenic treatment as an aversive conditioned response. They often develop after repeated antineoplastic treatments characterized by poor emetic control. Complete control throughout antineoplastic treatment is the best preventive strategy against developing symptoms. Although anxiolytic amnestic drugs are helpful in preventing and delaying anticipatory symptoms, behavioral therapy including relaxation techniques and systematic desensitization is recommended if symptoms occur. After symptoms develop, medical intervention during subsequent emetogenic treatment is limited to preventing conditioned stimulus reinforcement, which may exacerbate anticipatory symptoms.

EMETIC (EMETOGENIC) POTENTIAL

Emetogenic potential and symptom patterns vary among chemotherapy and radiation therapy techniques.

Chemotherapy

Among antineoplastic drugs, dosage is the most significant factor in emetogenic potential and duration of symptoms. The number of emetogenic drugs used in combination, dose schedule, treatment duration, and route of administration are also mitigating factors. Emetic potential may be lessened or eliminated by spreading drug delivery over hours or days; emetic potential is increased by rapid administration, repeated emetogenic treatment, and short intervals between repeated doses (Table 38.3).

Radiation

The emetic potential of ionizing radiation correlates directly with the amount of radiation administered per dose and rate of administration (dose rate). Large treatment volumes and fields, including the upper abdomen, upper hemithorax, and whole body, are prominent risk factors for severe emesis. Emetic potential is often increased when radiation and chemotherapy are administered concomitantly.

PATIENT RISK FACTORS

Patients at greatest risk for emetic symptoms include:

• Women, particularly those with a history of persistent and/or severe emetic symptoms during pregnancy

TABLE 38.3. *Emetic risk for single agents as a function of drug, dosage, and route of administration*

Drugs and combinations[b]	Acute-phase emetic potential[a]			
	NCCN	MASCC	ASCO	ESMO
Aldesleukin	moderate ($>$12–15 million IU/m^2)			
Alemtuzumab	minimal			
Altretamine (oral)	high	high		
Amifostine	moderate ($>$300 mg/m^2); low ($\leq$300 mg/m^2)			
Arsenic trioxide	moderate			
Asparaginase	minimal			
Azacitidine	moderate			
Bendamustine				
Bevacizumab	minimal	minimal	minimal	
Bexarotene (oral)	low			
Bleomycin	minimal	minimal	minimal	low
Bortezomib	minimal	low	low	
Busulfan	moderate ($>$4 mg/day); otherwise, minimal	minimal	minimal	low
Capecitabine (oral)	low	low		
Carboplatin	moderate	moderate	moderate	moderate to high
Carmustine	high ($>$250 mg/m^2); moderate ($\leq$250 mg/m^2)	high	high	high ($>$250 mg/m^2); moderate to high ($\leq$250 mg/m^2)
Cetuximab	minimal	low	low	
Chlorambucil (oral)	minimal	minimal		low
Cisplatin	high ($\geq$50 mg/m^2); moderate ($<$50 mg/m^2)	high	high	high ($\geq$50 mg/m^2); moderate to high ($<$50 mg/m^2)
Cladribine	minimal	minimal	minimal	
Cyclophosphamide	high ($>$1,500 mg/m^2); moderate ($\leq$1,500 mg/m^2)	high ($\geq$1,500 mg/m^2); moderate ($<$1,500 mg/m^2)	high ($\geq$1,500 mg/m^2); moderate ($<$1,500 mg/m^2)	high ($>$1,500 mg/m^2); moderate to high ($\leq$1,500 mg/m^2)
Cyclophosphamide (oral)	moderate	moderate		low to moderate
Cyclophosphamide + doxorubicin or epirubicin ("AC" regimens)	high	high	high	
Cytarabine	moderate ($>$1,000 mg/m^2); low (100–200 mg/m^2)	moderate ($>$1,000 mg/m^2); low ($\leq$100 mg/m^2)	moderate ($>$1,000 mg/m^2); low ($\leq$1,000 mg/m^2)	moderate to high ($>$1,000 mg/m^2)
Dacarbazine	high	high	high	high
Dactinomycin	moderate		high	
Dasatinib	minimal			
Daunorubicin	moderate	moderate	moderate	
Daunorubicin, liposomal				
Decitabine	minimal			
Denileukin diftitox	minimal			
Dexrazoxane	minimal			
Docetaxel	low	low	low	low to moderate

(Continued)

TABLE 38.3. *(Continued)*

Drugs and combinations[b]	Acute-phase emetic potential[a]			
	NCCN	MASCC	ASCO	ESMO
Doxorubicin	moderate	moderate	moderate	moderate to high ($\geq$60 mg/m^2)
Doxorubicin, lipo-somal	low	low		
Epirubicin	moderate	moderate	moderate	moderate to high ($\geq$90 mg/m^2)
Erlotinib	minimal			
Estramustine				
Etoposide	low	low	low	low to moderate
Etoposide (oral)	moderate	moderate		
Fludarabine	minimal	minimal	minimal	low
Fludarabine (oral[c])	low	low		
Floxuridine				
Fluorouracil	low	low	low	low to moderate ($<$1,000 mg/m^2)
Gefitinib (oral)	minimal	minimal		
Gemcitabine	low	low	low	low to moderate
Gemtuzumab ozo-gamicin	minimal			
Hydroxyurea (oral)	minimal	minimal		low
Idarubicin	moderate	moderate	moderate	
Ifosfamide	moderate	moderate	moderate	moderate to high
Imatinib (oral)	moderate	moderate		
Interferon alfa	minimal			
Irinotecan	moderate	moderate	moderate	low to moderate
Lapatinib (oral)	minimal			
Lenalidomide	minimal			
Lomustine	moderate			
Mechlorethamine	high	high	high	high
Melphalan	moderate ($>$50 mg/m^2)			
Melphalan (oral)	minimal ("low dose")	minimal		
Mercaptopurine				
Methotrexate	moderate ($\geq$250 mg/m^2); low ($>$50 to $<$250 mg/m^2); minimal ($\leq$50 mg/m^2)	low	low	low to moderate (50–250 mg/m^2); low ($\leq$50 mg/m^2)
Methotrexate (oral)		minimal		
Mitomycin	low	low	low	low to moderate
Mitoxantrone	low	low	low	low to moderate
Nelarabine	minimal			
Oxaliplatin	moderate ($>$75 mg/m^2)	moderate	moderate	moderate to high
Paclitaxel	low	low	low	low to moderate
Paclitaxel protein (albumin)-bound particles	low			
Panitumumab	minimal			
Pemetrexed	low	low	low	
Pentostatin	minimal			
Plicamycin[d]				
Procarbazine (oral)	high	high		low to moderate
Rituximab	minimal		minimal	
Sorafenib (oral)	minimal			

(Continued)

TABLE 38.3.   *(Continued)*

Drugs and combinations[b]	Acute-phase emetic potential[a]			
	NCCN	MASCC	ASCO	ESMO
Streptozocin	high	high	high	high
Sunitinib (oral)	minimal			
Tegafur + uracil (oral)[d,e]		low		
Temozolomide (oral)	moderate	moderate		
Temsirolimus	minimal			
Teniposide				low to moderate
Thalidomide (oral)	minimal			
Thioguanine (oral)	minimal	minimal		
Thiotepa				
Topotecan	low	low	low	low to moderate
Trastuzumab	minimal	low	low	
Valrubicin[d]	minimal			
Vinblastine	minimal	minimal	minimal	low
Vincristine	minimal	minimal	minimal	low
Vinorelbine	minimal	minimal	minimal	low
Vinorelbine (oral[c])	moderate	moderate		
Vorinostat (oral)	low			

[a]Estimated emetogenicity based on use as single agent at FDA-approved dose and schedule, without antiemetic prophylaxis. NCCN, National Comprehensive Cancer Network; MASCC, Multinational Association of Supportive Care in Cancer; ASCO, American Society of Clinical Oncology; ESMO, European Society for Medical Oncology. High: >90%; moderate: 30% to 90%; low: 10% to 30%; minimal: ≤10%.

[b]Unless otherwise indicated, route of administration is i.v.

[c]Neither FDA-approved nor commercially available in a formulation for oral administration.

[d]Not currently marketed in the United States.

[e]Not FDA-approved for commercial use.

- Children and young adults
- Patients with a history of acute- or delayed-phase emetic symptoms during prior cancer treatments are at increased risk for poor emetic control during subsequent treatments.
    - Patients with a history of acute- and delayed-phase emetic symptoms during prior cancer treatments are at greatest risk for developing emesis during subsequent treatments.
- Patients with low performance status and a predisposition to motion sickness
- Nondrinkers are at greater risk than patients with a history of chronic alcohol consumption (>100 g ethanol/day for several years).
- Intercurrent pathologies, such as gastrointestinal (GI) inflammation, compromised GI motility or obstruction, constipation, brain metastases, metabolic abnormalities (hypovolemia, hypercalcemia, hypoadrenalism, uremia), visceral organs invaded by tumor, and concurrent medical treatment (opioids, bronchodilators, aspirin, NSAIDS), may predispose to and exacerbate emetic symptoms during treatment and complicate good emetic control.

PRIMARY ANTIEMETIC PROPHYLAXIS

- Primary prophylaxis is indicated for all patients whose antineoplastic treatment presents at least a low risk of producing emetic symptoms (i.e., more than 10% of persons receiving similar chemotherapy or radiation therapy without antiemetic prophylaxis are predicted to experience emetic symptoms) (see Table 38.3).
- Planning effective antiemetic prophylaxis for chemotherapy entails evaluating each agent's emetic potential; the severity, onset, and duration of symptoms (see Table 38.1); and how drug dosage, schedule, and route of administration may affect those factors (see Table 38.3).

- Fig. 38.2 integrates evidence-based guidelines for treatment-appropriate antiemetic prophylaxis recommended by the National Comprehensive Cancer Network, the Multinational Association of Supportive Care in Cancer, the American Society of Clinical Oncology, and the consensus of experts in oncology. Recommendations are based on assessment of emetic risk and generally apply to adult patients. They may not be appropriate in all clinical situations. Use of particular drugs must be based on professional judgment, patient circumstances, and available resources.
- Treatment-appropriate antiemetic prophylaxis should precede each emetogenic treatment and proceed on a fixed schedule. Patients should not be expected to recognize prodromes and to rely on unscheduled antiemetics.
- Antiemetics should be given at the lowest fully effective dose.
- A minority of patients do not respond to treatment-appropriate antiemetic prophylaxis. Undertreatment puts patients at risk for emesis and debilitating morbidity, which may adversely affect their safety, comfort, and quality of life, and complicate their care. Treating these patients requires a rational empiric approach. Unfortunately, empiric antiemetic strategies often include drugs that are less safe at effective or clinically useful doses and schedules (e.g., dopaminergic antagonists, cannabinoids) than agents recommended for primary prophylaxis. These drugs may increase treatment costs and the risk of overtreatment and adverse effects.

BREAKTHROUGH SYMPTOMS

Up to 50% of patients who receive highly emetogenic therapy may experience breakthrough symptoms after primary prophylaxis. Breakthrough symptoms require rapid intervention. Patients who receive moderately or highly emetogenic treatment should be given a supply of medication to treat

(text continues on page 491)

Fig. 38.2. (See page 486.) Algorithms for antiemetic prophylaxis and treatment. (IM, intramuscular; IV, intravenous; PO, oral; PR, rectal; SL, sublingual.)

[a]Medications are not listed in order of preference. Pharmacologically similar alternatives are bounded by broken lines.

[b]Oral prophylaxis should begin 1 hour before commencing cytotoxic treatment; i.v. prophylaxis may be given minutes before emetogenic treatment.

[c]Antiemetic prophylaxis should be repeated each day emetogenic treatment is administered.

[d]When administered with i.v., phenothiazines should be given over 30 minutes to prevent hypotension.

[e]Aprepitant is recommended as prophylaxis for antineoplastic regimens containing cyclophosphamide and an anthracycline (e.g., doxorubicin, epirubicin), and for other combination chemotherapy regimens employing carboplatin, cisplatin, doxorubicin, epirubicin, ifosfamide, irinotecan, or methotrexate.

[f]Generally, regimens containing D_2 receptor antagonists and metoclopramide doses ≥20 mg should include primary prophylaxis with anticholinergic agents against acute dystonic extrapyramidal reactions; for example, diphenhydramine 25 to 50 mg PO or IV every 6 hours. Benztropine and trihexyphenidyl are alternatives. Parenteral administration is preferred for prompt treatment of extrapyramidal symptoms, as well as interrupting or discontinuing the drug that provoked the adverse reaction.

[g]When administered with i.v., dexamethasone should be given as a short infusion over 10 to 15 minutes to prevent uncomfortable sensations of warmth.

[h]Medications identified for breakthrough symptoms are not alternatives to primary prophylaxis, but should be added to a patient's antiemetic regimen.

[i]Delayed-phase prophylaxis may begin 12 to 24 hours after the start of emetogenic treatment.

[j]The maximum FDA-approved dose of ondansetron is 32 mg.

[k]Dexamethasone 12 mg or 20 mg if used with or without aprepitant or fosaprepitant, respectively.

[l]The recommended schedule for dexamethasone is twice daily if used without aprepitant and once daily if used with aprepitant.

Emetic Potential

High risk

Acute phase—primary prophylaxis[a,b,c]

• *Oral route available*
dexamethasone   12 mg or 20 mg[k] PO once
+ aprepitant   125 mg PO once
dolasetron   100 mg PO once; or
granisetron   2 mg PO once, or
    1 mg PO every 12 h for 2 doses; or
ondansetron   16–24 mg PO once
± lorazepam   0.5–2 mg PO or SL every 6–12 h

• *Oral route not available*
dexamethasone   10–12 mg IV once[g]
+ fosaprepitant   115 mg IV infusion once
dolasetron   1.8 mg/kg or 100 mg IV once; or
granisetron   0.01 mg/kg or 1 mg IV once; or
ondansetron   8–12 mg or 0.15 mg IV once; or
palonosetron   0.25 mg IV once
± lorazepam   0.5–2 mg IV or SL every 6–12 h

Moderate risk

• *Oral route available*
dexamethasone   12 mg PO once
+ aprepitant   125 mg PO once[e]
dolasetron   100 mg PO once; or
granisetron   2 mg PO once, or
    1 mg PO every 12 h
    for 2 doses; or
ondansetron   16–24 mg PO once
± lorazepam   0.5–2 mg PO or SL
    every 6–12 h

Delayed phase—primary prophylaxis[a,b,i]

• *Oral route available*
dexamethasone   8 mg twice daily or 8 mg once daily PO[l], or
    4 mg PO every 12 h for 2–4 days
+ aprepitant   80 mg PO daily, for 2 days
± lorazepam   0.5–2 mg PO or SL every 6–12 h for up to 3
    days after completing chemotherapy

• *Oral route not available*
dexamethasone   8 mg IV daily for 2–3 days[g]
± lorazepam   0.5– 2 mg IV or SL every 6–12 h for up to 3
    days after completing chemoherpy

• *Oral route available*
dexamethasone   8 mg PO daily or 4 mg PO every 12 h[l] for 1–3 days
+ aprepitant   80 mg PO daily, for 2 days (if aprepitant or
    fosaprepitant was given on day 1)[e]
± lorazepam   0.5–2 mg PO or SL every 6–12 h
    OR
dexamethasone   8 mg PO daily or 4 mg PO every 12 h for 1–3 days
± lorazepam   0.5–2 mg PO or SL every 6–12 h
    OR
dolasetron   100 mg PO daily; or
granisetron   2 mg PO daily or 1 mg PO every 12 h; or
ondansetron   16 mg PO daily or 8 mg PO every 12 h
± lorazepam   0.5–2 mg PO or SL every 6–12 h

Fig. 38.2.   Algorithms for antiemetic prophylaxis and treatment.

Emetic Potential	Acute phase—primary prophylaxis [a,b,c]	Delayed phase—primary prophylaxis [a,b,i]
	• *Oral route not available*	• *Oral route not available*
	dexamethasone 8–12 mg IV once[g] + fosaprepitant 115 mg IV infusion once[e]	dexamethasone 8 mg IV daily *or* 4 mg IV every 12 h for 1–3 days[g] ± lorazepam 0.5–2 mg IV *or* SL every 6–12 h
		OR
	dolasetron 1.8 mg/kg *or* 100 mg IV once; *or* granisetron 0.01 mg/kg IV once; *or* ondansetron 8–12 mg IV once; *or* palonosetron 0.25 mg IV once ± lorazepam 0.5–2 mg IV *or* SL every 6–12 h	dolasetron 1.8 mg/kg IV daily; *or* granisetron 0.01 mg/kg IV (maximum, 1 mg) IV daily, *or* ondansetron 8 mg *or* 0.15 mg/kg[j] IV daily ± lorazepam 0.5–2 mg IV *or* SL every 6–12 h
Low risk	• *Oral route available* dexamethasone 4–12 mg PO once; *or* prochlorperazine 10 mg PO every 4–6 h[f]; *or* metoclopramide 20–40 mg PO every 4–6 h[f] + diphenhydramine 25–50 mg PO every 4–6 h ± lorazepam 0.5–2 mg PO *or* SL every 6–12 h • *Oral route not available* dexamethasone 4–12 mg IV once; *or* prochlorperazine 10 mg IV every 4–6 h[d,f]; *or* metoclopramide 1–2 mg/kg IV every 3–4 h[f] + diphenhydramine 25–50 mg IV every 4–6 h ± lorazepam 0.5–2 mg IV *or* SL every 6–12 h	*Primary prophylaxis is not indicated*
Minimal risk	*Routine primary antiemetic prophylaxis is not indicated* • If emetic symptoms occur, follow the guidelines for breakthrough symptoms acutely. Consider using primary prophylaxis with antiemetics appropriate for low emetic risk during subsequent emetogenic treatments.[c]	*Primary prophylaxis is not indicated*

Fig. 38.2. (Continued)

Prophylaxis during second and subsequent emetogenic treatments

Control achieved during previous cycle

Intervention

No emetic symptoms   ⟶   No change in initial antiemetic regimen.

Nausea without emesis

Emetic symptoms controlled by rescue ("breakthrough") medications

⟶ Include in prophylaxis for repeated emetogenic treatment medications used for breakthrough symptoms during the previous cycle. Antiemetic prophylaxis should be given as scheduled medications.

Uncontrolled emetic symptoms ⟶

Acute management
- Implement fluid and electrolyte support.
- Escalate antiemetic doses or shorten administration intervals with agents currently in use, or add agents from other pharmacologic classes.
- Add nonpharmacologic interventions.

Management during repeated treatments
- Escalate antiemetic primary prophylaxis to the next greater emetic potential level

Prophylaxis for Radiation Therapy

Emetic potential

Primary prophylaxis[b,c]

Treatment for breakthrough symptoms[h]

High risk
Total body irradiation

A $5HT_3$ receptor antagonist
e.g.: **granisetron** 2 mg PO daily; *or*
ondansetron 8 mg PO every 8–12 h
± **dexamethasone** 2 mg PO every 8 h
- before each RT fraction
- continue for at least 24 h after RT is completed

Add agents from other pharmacologic classes (see guidance for Treatment for Breakthrough Symptoms Following Chemotherapy)

Moderate risk ⟶
Fields that include the abdomen, hemibody, mantle

A $5HT_3$ receptor antagonist
- before each RT fraction
- an optimal duration for prophylaxis after RT has not been identified

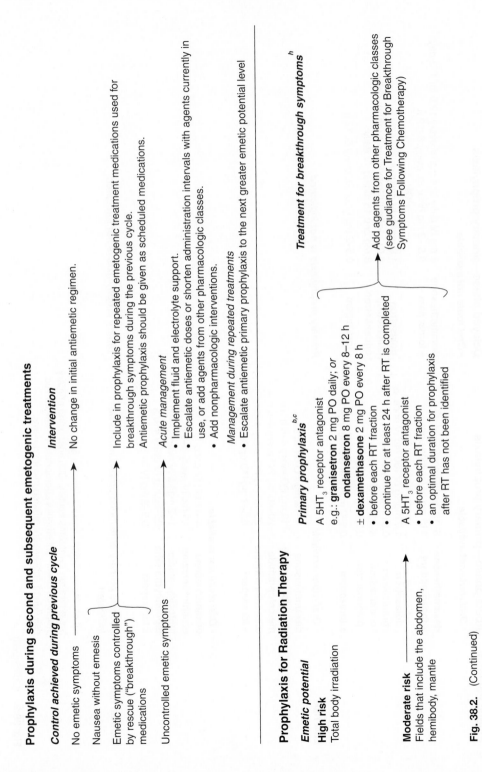

Fig. 38.2. (Continued)

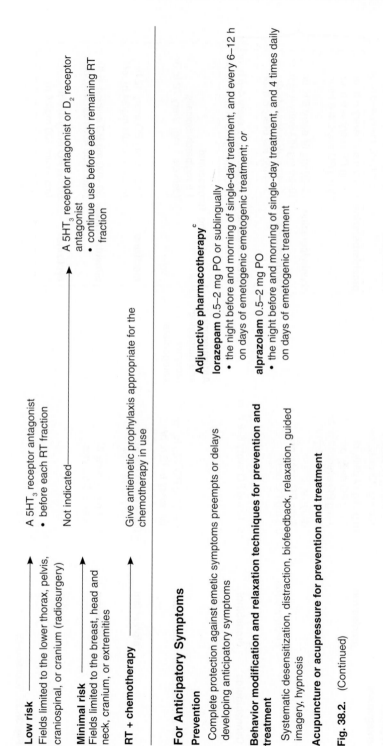

Low risk
Fields limited to the lower thorax, pelvis, craniospinal, or cranium (radiosurgery)

A 5HT$_3$ receptor antagonist
• before each RT fraction

Minimal risk
Fields limited to the breast, head and neck, cranium, or extremities

Not indicated

A 5HT$_3$ receptor antagonist or D$_2$ receptor antagonist
• continue use before each remaining RT fraction

RT + chemotherapy

Give antiemetic prophylaxis appropriate for the chemotherapy in use

For Anticipatory Symptoms

Prevention

Complete protection against emetic symptoms preempts or delays developing anticipatory symptoms

Behavior modification and relaxation techniques for prevention and treatment

Systematic desensitization, distraction, biofeedback, relaxation, guided imagery, hypnosis

Acupuncture or acupressure for prevention and treatment

Adjunctive pharmacotherapy[c]

lorazepam 0.5–2 mg PO or sublingually
• the night before and morning of single-day treatment, and every 6–12 h on days of emetogenic emetogenic treatment; *or*

alprazolam 0.5–2 mg PO
• the night before and morning of single-day treatment, and 4 times daily on days of emetogenic treatment

Fig. 38.2. (Continued)

Treatment for Breakthrough Symptoms with Emetogenic Treatment[a,h]

• Add to the current regimen a drug that is pharmacologically different from drugs already in use[c]:

Class	Drug	Dosing
Glucocorticoids	dexamethasone	12 mg PO daily, or 12 mg IV daily[g]; or
	methylprednisolone	125 mg IV daily
Serotonin receptor antagonists	dolasetron	100 mg IV daily, or 1.8 mg/kg IV daily, or 100 mg PO daily; or
	granisetron	10 µg/kg IV daily, or 2 mg PO daily, or 1 mg PO every 12 h; or
	ondansetron	8 mg or 0.15 mg/kg IV daily, or
	palonosetron	8 mg PO daily; or 0.5 mg PO daily
Cannabinoids	dronabinol	5–10 mg PO every 6–8 h; or
	nabilone	1–2 mg PO twice daily
Benzodiazepines	lorazepam	0.5–2 mg PO, SL, IV, or IM, every 6–12 h; or
	alprazolam	0.5–2 mg PO or SL, every 6–12 h; or
	midazolam	0.04 mg/kg slow IV over 3–5 minutes
Dopamine receptor antagonists[f]	metoclopramide	20–40 mg, or 0.5–2 mg/kg IV every 6 h, or 20–40 mg PO every 6 h; or
	haloperidol	1–3 mg IV every 4–6 h, or 1–5 mg PO every 4–6 h; or
	prochlorperazine	10–30 mg IV every 6 h, or 25 mg PR every 4–6 h, or 10 mg PO every 4–6 h; or
	thiethylperazine	10–20 mg IV every 6 h, or 10–20 mg PO every 4–6 h; or
	perphenazine	2–4 mg IV every 8 h, or 2–4 mg PO every 8 h; or
	promethazine	12.5–25 mg IV every 4–6 h, or 12.5–25 mg PO every 8 h; or
Antimuscarinic and histamine receptor antagonists	scopolamine transdermal	1.5 mg/patch topically, (delivers 1 mg) every 72 h; or
	meclizine	12.5–50 mg PO every 12 h (maximum 100 mg/24 h); or
	dimenhydrinate	50–100 mg PO every 4–6 h (maximum 400 mg/24 h); or
	cyclizine	50 mg PO every 4–6 h (maximum 200 mg/24 h)

[d] (brace grouping prochlorperazine through promethazine)

Fig. 38.2. (Continued)

breakthrough symptoms and clear instructions about how to supplement or modify their prophylactic regimen. If needed, breakthrough treatment should be administered at scheduled intervals and continued at least until after emetogenic treatment is completed.

A patient's poor response to antiemetic prophylaxis raises the following questions:

- Was the prophylactic strategy given an adequate trial?
- Were the drugs, doses, and administration schedules appropriate for the emetogenic challenge?
- Did the patient comply with the planned strategy?
- Would higher doses or shorter administration intervals improve the drug's effectiveness?

If it becomes necessary to "rescue" a patient from a suboptimal response:

- Add one or more agents from pharmacologic classes different from the drugs in use.
- Replace drugs that appear ineffective or poorly tolerated with more potent or longer-acting agents from the same pharmacologic class or with better adverse effect profiles.

Either or both strategies may be utilized with cyclical treatment or to intervene when response to prophylaxis is unsatisfactory.

Caveats

- Emetic symptoms may impair GI motility and drug absorption from the gut.
- Some patients may be too ill to swallow and retain oral medications.
- Rectal suppositories are a practical alternative, but absorption may vary among drugs and patients. Clinicians should ascertain patients' willingness to comply with this route of administration.
- Sustained- and extended-release products should not be given for acute symptoms.

ANTIEMETIC DRUGS

Serotonin (5-HT$_3$) Receptor Antagonists

Acute Phase

- 5-HT$_3$ antagonists are safer and more effective against acute-phase symptoms than other types of antiemetics.
- All 5-HT$_3$ antagonists provide equal benefit at maximally effective dosages. Doses greater than a maximally effective dose do not substantially improve emetic control.
- Single-dose prophylaxis is preferred for acute-phase symptoms. Additional doses of dolasetron, granisetron, or ondansetron within the first 24 hours after emetogenic treatment have not been shown to improve emetic control.
- Dolasetron, granisetron, ondansetron, and palonosetron have excellent oral bioavailability and provide equivalent antiemetic protection with either oral or parenteral administration.

Delayed Phase

- Metoclopramide and prochlorperazine are less expensive but at least as effective as dolasetron, granisetron, and ondansetron at controlling emetic symptoms.
- Palonosetron injection has the longest half-life and is the only 5-HT$_3$ antagonist FDA-approved for use in delayed-phase prophylaxis of emetic symptoms associated with moderately emetogenic chemotherapy. A single dose before starting chemotherapy is recommended, but other doses and schedules have proven safe (see below).

Potential Side Effects

Side effects common to all 5-HT$_3$ antagonists include:

- Headache
- Constipation

- Diarrhea
- Transiently increased hepatic transaminase concentrations
- Transient ECG changes, decreased cardiac rate, and cardiovascular adverse effects

Dolasetron

- Frequency and magnitude of side effects are related to serum concentration of hydrodolasetron, dolasetron's active metabolite.
- ECG changes are generally transient but may persist for >24 hours. ECG interval prolongation may lead to heart block or cardiac arrhythmias. Risk factors for ECG changes include:
  - Hypomagnesemia or hypokalemia
  - Diuretic use associated with aberrant serum electrolyte concentrations
  - Congenital long QT syndrome
  - Concomitant use of drugs that prolong the QT/QTc interval
  - Cumulative high doses of anthracycline drugs.

Ondansetron and Palonosetron

- Risk of adverse side effects varies directly with dose.
- Low risk of adverse effects at FDA-approved dosages and schedules.
- Product labeling for palonosetron injection indicates a single dose before starting chemotherapy, but safety has been demonstrated with other doses and schedules:
  - 10 mcg/kg single dose (healthy subjects)
  - 0.75 mg single dose before chemotherapy
  - 0.25 mg/dose every second day for 3 doses with dexamethasone before chemotherapy
  - 0.25 mg/day for 3 consecutive days (healthy subjects)
- Oral palonosetron is FDA-approved for prevention of acute symptoms associated with initial and repeated courses of moderately emetogenic chemotherapy. It is not approved for prevention of emetic symptoms associated with highly emetogenic chemotherapy or for delayed-phase symptoms.

Granisetron

- ECG abnormalities are rare with FDA-approved dosages and schedules.
- Granisetron transdermal system (Sancuso; ProStrakan, Inc., Bedminster, NJ) contains 34.3 mg of granisetron and delivers 3.1 mg/24 hours for up to 7 days.
- Used as prophylaxis with moderately or highly emetogenic chemotherapy for treatment durations up to 5 consecutive days in adults ≥18 years.
- A patch is applied to clean, dry, intact, healthy skin on the outer upper arm 24 to 48 hours before administration of emetogenic chemotherapy and remains in place for a minimum of 24 hours after chemotherapy is completed, or for up to 7 days.
- During clinical development, patients who received 3.1 mg granisetron/day transdermally experienced a slightly greater incidence of constipation than patients who received 2 mg/day granisetron p.o. (5.4% vs. 3%, respectively) and a lesser incidence of headache than patients who received 2 mg/day granisetron p.o. (0.7% vs. 3%, respectively).
- Continuous administration of transdermal granisetron may increase the potential for 5-HT$_3$ receptor antagonists to mask progressive ileus and gastric distention attributable to malignancy or other pathology.
- Granisetron may degrade with exposure to natural or artificial sunlight, and an in vitro study has suggested a potential for photogenotoxicity. Patients must be instructed to keep the transdermal patch covered with clothing at all times, and to keep the application site covered for 10 days after the patch is removed.
- Pharmacogenomic evaluation may help to identify patients at risk for suboptimal responses to 5-HT$_3$ receptor antagonists, which are substrates for catabolism by cytochrome P450 (CYP) enzymes (Table 38.4).

TABLE 38.4. *Catabolism of 5-HT$_3$ receptor antagonists by cytochrome P450 (CYP) enzymes*

5-HT$_3$ receptor antagonists	CYP catalysts for metabolism	Metabolites (activity vs. parent drug)
Hydrodolasetron (primary, highly active dolasetron metabolite)	Primarily CYP2D6, also CYP3A subfamily	Oxidation (inactive)
Granisetron	CYP3A subfamily	Oxidation, then conjugation (inactive)
Ondansetron	Primarily CYP3A4, also CYP1A2 and CYP2D6	Hydroxylation, then conjugation (inactive)
Palonosetron	Primarily CYP2D6, also CYP3A4 and CYP1A2	N-oxide-palonosetron (<1%), 6-S-hydroxypalonosetron (<1%)

- CYP2D6 is polymorphically expressed among human populations. Persons with more than two functionally competent (wild type) *CYP2D6* alleles may have increased metabolic capacity (extensive or ultra-rapid metabolizers), which has been associated with diminished emetic control in patients given 5-HT$_3$ receptor antagonists for which metabolism by CYP2D6 predominates.
- Patients who lack one or both *CYP2D6* alleles or express one or more variant alleles generally have altered functional capacity for CYP2D6 substrates and may have high concentrations and attenuated elimination of 5-HT$_3$ receptor antagonists for which CYP2D6 metabolism predominates (so-called poor metabolizers).
- Patients who express genetic polymorphism for the 5-HT$_3$ receptor may experience suboptimal antiemetic responses with 5-HT$_3$ receptor antagonists.

Glucocorticoids

- Effective as single agents against mild to moderate acute-phase symptoms
- Active against delayed-phase symptoms
- Parenteral and oral dexamethasone and methylprednisolone are equally effective.
- Prophylaxis and treatment are empirically based; safety and efficacy comparisons are lacking.
- Single doses are as effective as multiple-dose schedules. Optimal dosages and schedules have not been determined, but there is no evidence that dexamethasone >20 mg improves antiemetic response.
- Potential for adverse effects after a single dose is generally low and limited to activating psychogenic effects such as insomnia and sleep disturbances. Administering steroids early in a patient's waking cycle may minimize these effects.
- Adrenocortical suppression is generally not a problem when high-potency glucocorticoids are used for brief periods.
- Glycemic control may be a problem in patients with incipient or frank diabetes.

Neurokinin (NK$_1$) Receptor Antagonists

- Currently, aprepitant and the prodrug fosaprepitant dimeglumine are the only NK$_1$ receptor subtype antagonist antiemetics approved for use in patients ≥18 years of age. Approval was based on studies with emetogenic chemotherapy given on a single day.
- Aprepitant is recommended for use in combination with a glucocorticoid; a 5-HT$_3$ receptor antagonist is added for acute-phase emetic symptoms.
- Dosing:
  - Initial dose: Aprepitant 125 mg p.o. 60 minutes before emetogenic chemotherapy, or fosaprepitant dimeglumine 115 mg i.v. over 15 minutes
  - Subsequent doses: Aprepitant 80 mg/d p.o. on the second and third days after chemotherapy
  - May be given safely for 5 days: an initial dose of 125 mg p.o. (day 1), followed by daily doses of 80 mg/day p.o. for 4 consecutive days (days 2–5)

- Use with multiple-day chemotherapy regimens or for >5 consecutive days has not been adequately studied.
- Potential drug interactions:
  - Aprepitant is a substrate and moderate inhibitor of the cytochrome P450 (CYP) enzyme CYP3A4 and a moderate inducer of CYP3A4 and CYP2C9. Inhibition may occur after a single dose; induction occurs after repeated doses.
  - The potential for interaction with many CYP3A4 substrates is unknown.
  - Inhibits CYP3A4 in the gut and liver
  - Increases the bioavailability of concomitantly administered dexamethasone and methylprednisolone. When either dexamethasone or methylprednisolone is used in combination with aprepitant for antiemetic prophylaxis, decrease oral glucocorticoids by 50% and i.v. doses by 25%.
  - Do not modify steroid doses when they are used as components of a chemotherapy regimen.
  - Aprepitant metabolism and elimination may be affected by drugs that inhibit or induce CYP3A4.
- Common side effects of aprepitant in combination with a 5-HT$_3$ receptor antagonist and high-potency glucocorticoids include:
  - Abdominal pain
  - Epigastric discomfort
  - Hiccups
  - Anorexia
  - Dizziness
  - Asthenia
  - Fatigue

Dopamine (D$_2$) Receptor Antagonists

- Optimal doses and schedules have not been established.
- Overall, antiemetic activity varies directly with D$_2$ receptor antagonism.
- Adverse effects correlate with dose and frequency of administration, and include:
  - Sedation: Varies among structural classes (phenothiazines > butyrophenones; among phenothiazines, aliphatics >> piperazines)
  - Extrapyramidal reactions (dystonias, akathisia, dyskinesias): incidence correlates with drug dose and antagonistic potency at D$_2$ receptors
  - Anticholinergic effects: varies among structural classes (aliphatics >> piperazines)
  - ECG changes (haloperidol, droperidol)
  - Hypotension with rapid i.v. administration (phenothiazines).
- Anecdotal evidence supports the use of D$_2$ receptor antagonists with 5-HT$_3$ antagonists ± steroids for acute-phase symptoms, and with steroids, metoclopramide, or lorazepam for delayed-phase symptoms.

Metoclopramide

- A D$_2$ receptor antagonist; at high doses, acts as a competitive antagonist at 5-HT$_3$ receptors.
- Activity against delayed-phase symptoms is equivalent to that of ondansetron.
- Gastrointestinal prokinetic effects may benefit patients with intercurrent gastrointestinal motility disorders or gastroesophageal reflux disease.

Benzodiazepines

- Important adjuncts to antiemetics for their anxiolytic and anterograde amnestic effects.
- Clinically useful for mitigating akathisias associated with D$_2$ receptor antagonists.
- Many clinically useful agents are available in oral and/or injectable formulations. Lorazepam and alprazolam tablets are rapidly absorbed after sublingual administration.

- Primary liability is dose-related sedation.
- Pharmacodynamic effects are exaggerated in elderly patients.

Cannabinoids

- Cannabinoids are controlled substances (Schedule II) in the United States, but antiemetic benefit may be achieved without producing psychotropic effects. Use is empiric since optimal doses and administration schedules have not been determined.
- Dronabinol is an oral formulation of Δ^9-tetrahydrocannabinol (Δ^9-THC) with activity similar to low doses of prochlorperazine. Nabilone is a synthetic cannabinoid (CB_1) receptor agonist formulated for oral administration. Incidence of adverse effects associated with dronabinol and nabilone is greater than with phenothiazines at doses and schedules that produce comparable antiemetic effects.
- Adverse effects occur within the range of clinically useful doses; incidence and severity vary with dose and correlate inversely with the interval between successive doses. Adverse effects include:
  - Sedation
  - Confusion/decreased cognition
  - Dizziness
  - Short-term memory loss
  - Euphoria/dysphoria
  - Ataxia
  - Dry mouth
  - Orthostatic hypotension $\pm$ increased heart rate

Anticholinergic (Antimuscarinic) Agents and Histamine (H_1) Receptor Antagonists

- Utility in preventing and treating emetic symptoms is not defined. Most effective as prophylaxis; less effective after emetic symptoms develop.
- Antimuscarinics are most useful in patients whose symptoms are referable to movement.
- Agents have antihistaminic, anticholinergic, and antidopaminergic avidities in different proportions and, in some cases, agonistic or antagonistic activities at other neuroreceptors.
- Adverse effects correlate directly with dose and frequency of administration, and include:
  - Sedation
  - Dry mouth
  - Loss of visual accommodation/blurred vision
  - Deceased GI motility with constipation or diarrhea
  - Urinary retention or frequency
  - Mydriasis $\pm$ photophobia
  - Increased heart rate

COMBINATION STRATEGIES

Antiemetics in combination can be more effective than single agents by targeting two or more operative neural pathways.

- Numerous studies have demonstrated that control of acute-phase emetic symptoms improves significantly with the combination of 5-HT$_3$ receptor antagonists and high-potency glucocorticoids. Acute-phase symptom control is further augmented when aprepitant is used in combination with a 5-HT$_3$ receptor antagonist and a glucocorticoid.
- Delayed-phase symptom control is improved by either a high-potency glucocorticoid or aprepitant, and is further enhanced when both drugs are used in combination. However, aprepitant may compromise the safety of concomitantly administered medications due to its effects on cytochrome P450 metabolizing enzymes. In cases where prophylaxis against delayed-phase symptoms is indicated but concurrent medications make the use of aprepitant problematic, glucocorticoids alone or in

combination with either metoclopramide or a 5-HT$_3$ or D$_2$ receptor antagonist may improve control of symptoms.

SUGGESTED READINGS

Aapro M. Methodological issues in antiemetic studies. *Invest New Drugs.* 1993;11(4):243–53.

Aapro MS, Molassiotis A, Olver I. Anticipatory nausea and vomiting. *Support Care Cancer.* 2005;13(2):117–21.

Borison HL, McCarthy LE. Neuropharmacology of chemotherapy-induced emesis. *Drugs.* 1983;25 (Suppl 1):8–17.

D'Acquisito R, Tyson LB, Gralla RJ, et al. The influence of a chronic high alcohol intake on chemo-therapy-induced nausea and vomiting [abstract]. *Proc Am Soc Clin Oncol.* 1986;5:257.

de Wit R, Herrstedt J, Rapoport B, et al. Addition of the oral NK1 antagonist aprepitant to standard an-tiemetics provides protection against nausea and vomiting during multiple cycles of cisplatin-based chemotherapy [see comments]. *J Clin Oncol.* 2003;21(22):4105–11. Comment in: *J Clin Oncol.* 2003;21:4077–80.

Einhorn LH, Brames MJ, Dreicer R, Nichols CR, Cullen MT Jr, Bubalo J. Palonosetron plus dex-amethasone for prevention of chemotherapy-induced nausea and vomiting in patients receiving multiple-day cisplatin chemotherapy for germ cell cancer. *Support Care Cancer.* 2007;15(11): 1293–300.

Eisenberg P, Figueroa-Vadillo J, Zamora R, et al. Improved prevention of moderately emetogenic chemotherapy-induced nausea and vomiting with palonosetron, a pharmacologically nov-el 5-HT3 receptor antagonist: results of a phase III, single-dose trial versus dolasetron. *Cancer.* 2003;98(11):2473–82.

Eisenberg P, MacKintosh FR, Ritch P, Cornett PA, Macciocchi A. Efficacy, safety and pharmacokinet-ics of palonosetron in patients receiving highly emetogenic cisplatin-based chemotherapy: a dose-ranging clinical study. *Ann Oncol.* 2004;15(2):330–7.

European Society for Medical Oncology. ESMO recommendations for prophylaxis of chemotherapy-induced nausea and vomiting (NV). *Ann Oncol.* 2001;12(8):1059–60.

Gralla R, Lichinitser M, Van Der Vegt S, et al. Palonosetron improves prevention of chemotherapy-induced nausea and vomiting following moderately emetogenic chemotherapy: results of a double-blind randomized phase III trial comparing single doses of palonosetron with ondansetron. *Ann Oncol.* 2003;14(10):1570–7.

Hickok JT, Roscoe JA, Morrow GR, et al. 5-Hydroxytryptamine-receptor antagonists versus prochlo-rperazine for control of delayed nausea caused by doxorubicin: a URCC CCOP randomised control-led trial. *Lancet Oncol.* 2005;6(10):765–72.

Hunt TL, Gallagher SC, Cullen MR Jr, Shah AK. Evaluation of safety and pharmacokinetics of con-secutive multiple-day dosing of palonosetron in healthy subjects. *J Clin Pharmacol.* 2005;45(5): 589–96.

Italian Group for Antiemetic Research. Cisplatin-induced delayed emesis: pattern and prognostic fac-tors during three subsequent cycles. *Ann Oncol.* 1994;5(7):585–9.

Kaiser R, Sezer O, Papies A, et al. Patient-tailored antiemetic treatment with 5-hydroxytryptamine type 3 receptor antagonists according to cytochrome P-450 2D6 genotypes [see comments]. *J Clin Oncol.* 2002;20(12):2805–11. Comment in: *J Clin Oncol.* 2002;20:2765–7.

Kris MG, Gralla RJ, Clark RA, et al. Incidence, course, and severity of delayed nausea and vomiting following the administration of high-dose cisplatin. *J Clin Oncol.* 1985;3(10):1379–84.

Kris MG, Hesketh PJ, Somerfield MR, et al. American Society of Clinical Oncology guideline for an-tiemetics in oncology: update 2006. *J Clin Oncol.* 2006;24(18):2932–47.

Kris MG, Roila F, De Mulder PH, Marty M. Delayed emesis following anticancer chemotherapy. *Sup-port Care Cancer.* 1998;6(3):228–32.

Morrow GR, Hickok JT, Burish TG, Rosenthal SN. Frequency and clinical implications of delayed nausea and delayed emesis. *Am J Clin Oncol.* 1996;19(2):199–203.

Multinational Association of Supportive Care in Cancer. Perugia International Cancer Conference VII, Antiemetic Guidelines. Available at: http://www.mascc.org/content/127.html

National Comprehensive Cancer Network. NCCN Clinical Practice Guidelines in Oncology, Antiemesis. Available at: http://www.nccn.org/default.asp

Stoltz R, Parisi S, Shah A, Macciocchi A. Pharmacokinetics, metabolism and excretion of intravenous [l4C]-palonosetron in healthy human volunteers. *Biopharm Drug Dispos.* 2004;25(8):329–37.

Sullivan JR, Leyden MJ, Bell R. Decreased cisplatin-induced nausea and vomiting with chronic alcohol ingestion. *N Engl J Med.* 1983;309(13):796.

Tremblay PB, Kaiser R, Sezer O, et al. Variations in the 5-hydroxytryptamine type 3B receptor gene as predictors of the efficacy of antiemetic treatment in cancer patients. *J Clin Oncol.* 2003;21(11): 2147–55.

39

Medical Nutrition Therapy

Marnie Dobbin

While only effective cancer treatment can reverse the symptoms of cancer cachexia, nutritional deficits and weight loss in patients with cancer can be minimized with timely nutritional intervention and pharmacologic management.

INCIDENCE AND IMPACT OF MALNUTRITION

- More than 40% of oncology patients develop signs of malnutrition during treatment.
- Malnourished patients incur higher costs for their care, have impaired responses to treatment, greater risk of drug toxicity, and increased rates of morbidity and mortality compared to patients with normal nutritional status.
- As many as 20% of oncology patients die from nutritional complications rather than from their primary diagnosis.

CANCER CACHEXIA

- Nealy two-thirds of patients with cancer develop cancer cachexia characterized by systemic inflammation, anorexia, immunosuppression, and metabolic derangements. These can lead to unintentional weight loss and failure to preserve muscle and fat mass.
- There is no consistent relationship between tumor type, tumor burden, anatomic site of involvement, and cancer cachexia.
- Hypermetabolism is not uniformly present.
- Tumor-induced changes in host production of proinflammatory cytokines (TNF, IL-1, IL-6, and IFN) can lead to hypermetabolism and to anorexia due to changes in gherlin, seratonin, and leptin production. Tumor production of proteolysis-inducing factor and lipid-mobilizing factor contribute to loss of muscle and fat mass. Inefficient energy metabolism and insulin resistance lead to further depletion of lean body mass.
- Even patients with cancer cachexia who presumably maintain adequate nutritional intake may not be able to sustain their weight.
- Overfeeding will lead to further metabolic dysregulation and will not result in weight gain.

SCREENING FOR NUTRITIONAL RISK

- Nutritional deterioration can be minimized if patients are screened at each visit, so that problems can be identified and interventions provided when they can have the most impact. The Joint Commission on Healthcare Accreditation standards state that in-patients are to be screened for nutritional risk within 1 day of admission. Validated screening tools such as the Subjective Global Assessment (SGA) form, developed by Jeejeebhoy et al. (1987) and adapted for use with oncology patients by Dr. Faith Ottery (www.ons.org/webcasts/downloads/pg-sga.pdf), may be especially helpful in the out-patient setting. Patients can complete the form in a few minutes during their medical appointments. The form covers questions about weight change, dietary intake, gastrointestinal symptoms, and functional capacity.

- Members of the healthcare team then gather additional data about metabolic demand (presence of fever, use of corticosteroids, etc.) and complete a nutrition-related physical assessment. The patient-generated tool (PG-SGA) not only aids in identifying the need for nutritional counseling and/or pharmacologic intervention, but can also convey to the patient that nutrition is a primary concern of the medical team.

NUTRITIONAL ASSESSMENT

- Registered dietitians use anthropometric data, biochemical indices, nutritional physical assessment, and dietary and medical histories to assess the nutritional status of patients and to determine appropriate intervention.
- Rate of weight change is the most useful parameter for identifying patients at nutritional risk. An unintentional weight loss of >5% per month, >2% per week, >7.4% in 3 months, or >10% in 6 months is associated with severe risk of malnutrition. Comparison of current weight to usual weight is more useful than comparing current weight to an ideal or desirable weight. Loss of more than 15% of usual weight may indicate a risk of protein-energy malnutrition.

BODY COMPOSITION

- Obtaining baseline measurements of body composition and comparing these measurements over time can be helpful for monitoring nutritional status. Measures of muscle mass include the use of skin calipers to measure mid-arm circumference (MAC) and mid-arm muscle circumference (MAMC). Triceps skinfold measurements can be used to estimate fat stores.
- Bioelectric impedance (BIA) is an inexpensive, noninvasive method for measuring body fat and fat-free mass, based on the principle that lean tissue has greater conduction and lower impedance than fatty tissue.
- Body mass index (BMI) correlates well with body fat, morbidity, and mortality (Table 39.1). However, BMI could incorrectly categorize highly muscled patients or those with edema or ascites as having excess fat stores. A BMI correlation of <18.5 is associated with protein-energy malnutrition.

PROTEIN

- If energy intake is inadequate, catabolism of protein will occur, especially as tumors preferentially metabolize protein. Limiting cancer patients' protein intake has not been shown to interfere with tumor growth and may lead to protein malnutrition and impaired immunity.
- Protein turnover in patients with cancer is similar to that of patients with infection or injury, and their protein requirements are 50% above those of healthy individuals.
- Transport proteins (such as albumin and thyroxin-binding prealbumin) are negative acute-phase proteins that decrease in the presence of inflammation, regardless of a patient's protein status. Earlier studies incorrectly correlated these proteins with nutritional status, not accounting for their role as inflammatory markers. Inflammatory processes can lead to loss of lean body mass, and low levels of transport proteins are correlated with poor clinical outcome, but the relationship with nutritional status is indirect. Dietary history and nitrogen balance measurements are more reliable measures of protein adequacy.

NUTRITIONAL REQUIREMENTS

- Indirect calorimetry, the preferred method for estimating resting energy expenditure, measures O_2 consumed (VO_2) and volume of carbon dioxide produced (VCO_2) to determine respiratory quotient (RQ). This can be done with a portable metabolic cart operated by a respiratory therapist, or by a handheld device recently approved by the FDA.
- There are a variety of recommended calculations for estimating energy, fluid, and protein requirements (Table 39.2). However, formulas that rely on stress and activity factors, or calculations such as

TABLE 39.1. *Body mass index (BMI)*

Height (cm)	Weight (kg)									
	45	50	55	60	65	70	75	80	85	95
150	20	22.2	24.4	26.7	28.9	31.1	33	35.6	37.8	42.2
155	18.7	20.8	22.9	25.0	26	29.1	31.2	33.3	35.4	39.5
160	17.6	19.5	21.5	23.4	25.4	27.3	29.3	31.3	33.2	37.1
165	16.5	18.4	20.2	22.0	23.9	25.7	27.5	29.4	31.2	34.9
170	15.6	17.3	19.0	20.8	22.5	24.2	26.0	27.7	29.4	32.9
175	14.7	16.3	18.0	19.6	21.2	22.9	23.8	26.1	27.8	31.0
180	13.9	15.4	16.3	18.5	20.1	21.6	23.2	24.7	26.2	29.3
185	12.8	14.6	16.1	17.5	19.0	20.5	21.9	23.4	24.8	27.8
190	12.5	13.9	15.2	16.6	18.0	19.4	20.8	22.2	23.6	26.3

BMI	
≥40	Obesity grade III
35–39.9	Obesity grade II
30–14.9	Obesity grade I
25–29.9	Overweight
18.5–25	Normal weight
17–18.4	Protein-energy malnutrition grade I
16–16.9	Protein-energy malnutrition grade II
<16	Protein-energy malnutrition grade III

% Usual weight[a]	
85–95%	Mild malnutrition
75–84%	Moderate malnutrition
0–74%	Severe malnutrition

[a]Rate of weight loss associated with severe risk of malnutrition: >5% per month, >2% per week, >7.4% in 3 months, or >10% in 6 months.

>45 kilocalories (kcals)/kg "for stress," have been shown to overestimate requirements. It is important not to overfeed cancer patients. Overfeeding can increase infection and induce respiratory distress, hyperglycemia, and fatty liver.
- The initial calorie goal for critically ill patients should be to meet their estimated resting energy expenditure (Table 39.3).

NUTRITIONAL INTERVENTION

- Nutritional counseling by a registered dietitian (RD) is associated with improvement in quality of life scores and nutritional parameters, and with success of oral nutritional intervention for oncology patients. Continual reassessment, pharmacologic management, and nutritional counseling can often help avoid costly, risky nutritional support options.
- Nutritional intervention by an RD may include education on individualized nutritional goals for energy, protein, and micronutrients, modification of foods and feeding schedules, fortification of foods

TABLE 39.2. *Recommendations for nutritional therapy*

Patient/condition	Kilocalories[a]
Acutely ill; obese (BMI 30–50)	21/kg
Inactive; cancer	25–30/kg
Hypermetabolism; malabsorption	35/kg
Stem cell transplant	30–35/kg

[a]Fever increases energy needs by ~14%/F°.

TABLE 39.3. *Mifflin-St. Jeor formula for estimating resting energy expenditure (REE)*

Males	REE = 10W + 6.25H − 5A + 5
Females	REE = 10W + 6.25H − 5A - 161

W = weight (kg); H = height (cm); A = age (yr).

with modular nutritional products, supplementation with meal-replacement products, or recommendations for appropriate nutritional support (Table 39.4). Overfeeding will lead to further metabolic dysregulation and will not result in weight gain.

- Self-imposed diets and the use of dietary supplements should be evaluated by an RD for possible risks to the patient and for their potential to confound protocol results.
- A national registry of RDs is available from the American Dietetics Association.

MICRONUTRIENT CONSIDERATIONS

- Although two-thirds of American adults are overweight or obese (BMI >25), the majority do not meet their requirements for magnesium, vitamin B_6, zinc, and calcium. Optimal dietary intake of vitamins A, C, and E is rare, and patients often take excessive amounts of supplementary antioxidants. Use of dietary supplements should be evaluated as part of a nutritional assessment.
- When treatment involves oxidation (such as radiation therapy), pharmacologic doses of antioxidants might interfere with the treatment objective and may protect the tumor. A diet including foods that are good sources of antioxidants, along with a multivitamin providing 100% to 200% of recommended levels for most nutrients, has not been shown to be harmful and is recommended for patients on limited diets who are undergoing cancer treatment.
- Patients with low levels of ionized calcium, elevated AlkP, and a history of corticosteroid use and risk for osteoporosis should have their vitamin D levels assessed by measuring levels of cholecalciferol [25(OH)D]. Calcitrol, the 1,25 dihydroxy form of vitamin D, is not a reliable indicator of vitamin D status due to its short half-life and dysregulation in the presence of deficiency. The best available current data indicate that a serum 25(OH)D level of >32 ng/mL (80 mmol/L) is a supportable goal.
- Repleting vitamin D stores is associated with improved insulin sensitivity, enhanced immunity, improved musculoskeletal function (reduced falls and fractures), and a beneficial effect on bone mineral density. Vitamin D has an inhibitory effect on leukemia and cancer of the breast, colon, and prostate. Low levels of cholecalciferol are commonly found in the elderly, dark-skinned individuals, the obese, and those with malabsorption syndromes and osteoporosis.

NUTRITIONAL SUPPORT

Although tumor growth is stimulated by a variety of nutrients, limiting the nutrients preferred by tumors can be detrimental to the patient, while maintenance of good nutritional status does not appear to have deleterious effects on tumor growth. For example, among more than 200 patients with Hodgkin's disease, malnourished patients had higher rates of tumor growth (demonstrated by incorporation of [³H] thymidine-labeling index in the tumor tissue) than well-nourished patients.

Enteral Nutrition

- Reviews of nutritional support practices indicate that parenteral nutrition (PN) is often instituted even when safer, more physiologic enteral nutritional support could have been provided. The benefits of enteral over PN have been well demonstrated, including fewer infections, decreased catabolic hormones, improved wound healing, shorter hospital stay, and maintenance of gut integrity. In other words, if the gut works, use it.
- To be successful, enteral nutrition should be implemented as soon as possible. Surgeons may approve of enteral feeding within 4 hours of placement of gastrostomy tubes and immediately after jejunostomy (because bowel sounds are not needed). Prophylactic placement of gastrointestinal tubes can

TABLE 39.4. *Common oral nutrition recommendations for patients (by condition)*

Condition	Recommendations
Diabetes/ hyperglycemia	Begin by familiarizing patients with the carbohydrate content of foods. Most men need 45 to 75 g of carbohydrate per meal; most women need 45 to 60 g per meal. If a snack is taken, 15 to 30 g of carbohydrate is usually recommended. One ounce of bread product, ½ cup cooked starch, ½ cup fruit or juice, and 8 oz. milk (regardless of fat content) each provide ~15 g of carbohydrate.
Diarrhea	↓ lactose, ↓ fat, ↓ insoluble fiber (wheat bran, skin and seeds of produce), ↑ soluble fiber (peeled fruit, oat bran, guar gum products). Cheese has insignificant carbohydrate/lactose content (<2 g/100 g of cheese) and yogurt is naturally low in lactose due to microorganisms consuming the lactose as milk is converted into yogurt. Probiotics may be helpful.
Early satiety	Calorically dense foods/nutrition products (e.g., medical nutrition beverages with >1.5 kcals/mL); foods such as nuts, cheese, seeds, modular kcal or protein supplements that can be added to foods without significantly altering the flavor or volume of foods.
Fat malabsorption	↓ fat diet and MCT–oil fortified foods/products. A diet with <30% of kcals from fat or <40 g of fat/day may be unrealistic long-term. A trial of pancreatic enzymes and bile acid sequestrants may significantly improve symptoms.
Hypercalcemia of malignancy	Does not respond to low-calcium diet. Often, crucial sources of protein and kcals are limited by such a diet.
Magnesium and potassium status	Refractory hypokalemia is often related to limited Mg stores, even when serum Mg levels are within normal range. Repletion of Mg may help normalize K levels. Increased intake of dietary Mg, K, and P can reduce reliance on supplements and will not cause the gastrointestinal side effects associated with supplementation.
Malabsorption	Semi-elemental palatable products, trials of pancreatic enzymes, bile acid sequestrants, and medium-chain triglycerides (MCT) may reduce symptoms.
Neutropenia	Many bone marrow transplant centers emphasize prevention of food-borne illness (verifying temperatures of cooked foods with a thermometer, avoiding unpasteurized dairy products and juices, etc.) over encouraging strict diets that limit fresh produce, have poor compliance rates, and have no proven benefit in reducing infection rates.
Poor appetite/ fatigue	Recommend >5 scheduled feedings/day to lessen dependence on appetite, with use of nutritious liquids for high % of kcals (milk, lactose-treated milk, soup, soy milk, fruit smoothies made with nut butters, or meal replacement beverages) since liquids may improve nutrient intake better than solid meals alone. Discourage patients from relying on water alone to meet fluid requirement, as nutritious beverages such as milk contain >90% water and could provide nutrition as well; excess water intake may blunt appetite.
Sodium-restricted diets	The relationship between K and Na influences hypertension. Increasing K intake, even if Na intake remains high, can improve blood pressure. A diet emphasizing high-K foods, such as employed in the Dietary Approaches for Stopping Hypertension (DASH) study, can be effective.

considerably reduce weight loss during radiotherapy and may reduce the need for hospitalization due to dehydration, weight loss, or other complications of mucositis.

Parenteral Nutrition

- Total parenteral nutrition (TPN) (Table 39.5) can be beneficial to cancer patients when response to treatment is good but associated nutritional morbidity is high, and when the GI tract is unavailable to support nutrition. Perioperative TPN should be limited to patients who are severely malnourished, with surgery expected to prevent oral intake for more than 10 days after surgery.

TABLE 39.5. *Sample parenteral nutrition recommendations*

	Infants/Children (3–30 kg)	Adolescents (≥30 kg)	Adults
Water	1,500–1,800 mL/m²/d 1,500 mL/kg for first 20 kg 25 mL/kg for remaining weight	1,500 mL/m²/d	1,500 mL/m²/d 35 mL/kg or 1 mL/kcal
Energy	70–110 cal/kg/d	40–60 cal/kg/day	20–35 cal/kg/d
Dextrose (3.4 kcals/g for the hydrated form)			
Initial	5–10% (50–100 g/L)	5–10% (50–100 g/L)	10–15% (100–150 g/L)
Advance	5% (50 g/L)	5% (50 g/L)	5–10% (50–100 g/L)
Max dextrose oxidation rate	12–15 mg/kg/min	5–13 mg/kg/min	4–5 mg/kg/min
Max dextrose concentration	20–35% (200–350 g/L)	20–35% (200–350 g/L)	20–35% (200–350 g/L) for central access; 10% for peripheral
Protein			
Initial	1 g/kg/d	1 g/kg/d	At goal
Advance	0.5–1 g/kg/d	1 g/kg/d	—
Max	2–3 g/kg/d	1.5–2 g/kg/d	2 g/kg/d
IVFE	20% lipid provides 2 kcals/mL. Due to glycerol in fat emulsions, 1 g of fat in 20% emulsions = 10 kcals; ~1 g of fat per 5 mL of 20% IVFE		
Initial	1 g/kg/d	1 g/kg/d	At goal; usually ≥250 mL 20% IVFE for ~30% of total kcals
Advance	1 g/kg/d	1 g/kg/d	—
Minerals			
Max	2–3 g/kg/d	2 g/kg/d	2 g/kg/d (60% of total kcals)
Sodium	2–4 mEq/kg/d	2–3 mEq/kg/d	1–2 mEq/kg 60–150 mEq/d max 155 mEq/L
Potassium	2–3 mEq/kg/d	1.5–3 mEq/kg/d	1–2 mEq/kg 40–240 mEq/d max 80 mEq/L
Magnesium	0.3–0.5 mEq/kg/d	0.2–0.3 mEq/kg/d	8–24 mEq/d
Calcium	0.5–2.5 mEq/kg/d	0.5–1 mEq/kg/d	10–40 mEq/d max 30 mEq/L
Phosphorus	0.5–2 mM/kg/d	0.5–1.3 mM/kg/d	20–40 mM/d max 30 mM/L
Selenium	2 mcg/kg/d (40 mcg/max)	2 mcg/kg/d (40 mcg/max)	40 mcg
Trace metals and multivitamins	daily	daily	daily

IVFE, intravenous fat emulsion.

• For the families of cancer patients, feeding is synonymous with caring. Provision of nominal support-ive care for preterminal patients can reduce family tension as well as readmissions for hydration and electrolyte maintenance. Data indicate that PN can improve quality of life and functional status for pre-terminal patients with a Karnofsky Performance Status score >50. The risks and benefits of nutritional support must be addressed individually and evaluated for each case with patient and family input.

COMPLICATIONS OF NUTRITIONAL SUPPORT

Refeeding Syndrome

Feeding after starvation is associated with increased intravascular volume, cardiopulmonary com-promise, and plummeting levels of phosphorus, magnesium, and potassium due to the intracellular movement of electrolytes during anabolism. Malnourished individuals with severe weight loss, negligi-ble intake for >7 days, a history of alcoholism, recent surgery, electrolyte losses due to diarrhea, high-output fistulas, or vomiting are especially vulnerable. Initially, no more than 50% of estimated needs (~15 kcals/kg/day and no more than 150 g dextrose/day) is recommended. Because thiamin is an impor-tant coenzyme for carbohydrate metabolism, the addition of 10 to 100 mg of thiamin is warranted.

Hypertriglyceridemia

For individuals with preexisting hyperlipidemia and obesity, or for those taking sirolimus, cy-closporine, and other medications associated with increased triglyceride (TG) levels, the goal is to keep TG <300 mg/dL. Ensure that blood is drawn 4 hours after lipid infusion or before lipids are hung, as this will falsely elevate TG. Lipid dose should be reduced if TG is >300 mg/dL (but <600 mg/dL), as stopping lipid altogether can worsen liver dysfunction. Slowing the rate of infusion of intravenous fat emulsion (IVFE) to between 6 and 12 hours may help with TG clearance.

Parenteral Nutrition–Associated Liver Disease (PNALD)

Hepatic fat accumulation is most common in adults and usually resolves within 2 weeks, even if PN continues. It typically presents within 2 weeks of PN with moderate elevations in serum aminotran-ferase concentrations. PNALD is usually a complication of overfeeding; it has become less common in the last 10 years, since calories provided via PN have become more appropriate.

Parenteral Nutrition–Associated Cholestasis (PNAC)

• PNAC is primarily a result of excess calories. Overfeeding contributes to fat deposition in the liver by stimulating insulin release, which promotes lipogenesis and inhibits fatty acid oxidation. PNAC occurs most often in children. It is associated with elevated serum conjugated bilirubin (>2 mg/dL) and may progress to cirrhosis and liver failure. Factors unrelated to PN that have been implicated in PNAC include bacterial and fungal infections.
• Fat-free PN formulations have also been implicated in the development of fatty liver, since a high percentage of calories from carbohydrates can lead to fat deposition in the liver. Providing a balance of calories from dextrose and fat seems to decrease the incidence of steatosis, possibly by decreasing hepatic TG uptake and promoting fatty oxidation.
• IVFE exceeding 1 g/kg/day is associated with chronic PNAC and severe PNALD. Cyclic TPN (gener-ally 8–12 hours) has shown better results in terms of improved liver enzymes and conjugated bilirubin concentrations compared to continuous PN infusions. Fat emulsions containing a combination of medium-chain and long-chain TGs (not yet available in the United States) may reduce liver complica-tions as well.

SUGGESTED READINGS

Adrogue HJ, Madias NE. Sodium and potassium in the pathogenesis of hypertension. *N Engl J Med.* 2007;356:1966–1978.

Aker SN. Oral feedings in the cancer patient. *Cancer.* 1979;43(5 Suppl):2103–2107.

Ambrus J, Ambrus CM, Mink IB, Pickren, JW. Causes of death in cancer patients. *J Med.* 1975;6: 61–64.

American Diabetes Association. What Can You Eat? Available at: http://www.diabetes.org/home.jsp

American Dietetic Association. Find a Nutrition Professional: Registered Dietitians and Dietetic Technicians, Registered. Available at: http://www.eatright.org/cps/rde/xchg/ada/hs.xsl/home_4874_ENU_HTML.htm

Bischoff-Ferrari HA. Optimal serum 25-hydroxyvitamin D levels for multiple health outcomes. *Adv Exp Med Biol.* 2008;624:55–71.

Bowman LC, Williams R, Sanders M, Ringwald-Smith K, Baker D, Gajjar A. Algorithm for nutritional support: experience of the Metabolic and Infusion Support Service of St. Jude Children's Research Hospital. *Int J Cancer Suppl.* 1998;11:76–80.

Bozzetti F, Boracchi P, Costa A, et al. Relationship between nutritional status and tumor growth in humans. *Tumori.* 1995;81:1–6.

Caba D, Ochoa JB. How many calories are necessary during critical illness? *Gastrointest Endosc Clin N Am.* 2007;17(4):703–710.

Elliott L, Molseed LL, McCallum PD, Grant B, eds. *The Clinical Guide to Oncology Nutrition.* 2nd ed. Oncology Nutrition Dietetic Practice Group. Chicago: American Dietetic Association; 2006.

Gariballa S. Refeeding syndrome: a potentially fatal condition but remains underdiagnosed and under-treated. *Nutrition.* 2008;24:604–606.

Gottschlich MM, ed. *The A.S.P.E.N. Nutrition Support Core Curriculum: A Case-Based Approach—The Adult Patient.* Silver Spring, MD: American Society for Parenteral and Enteral Nutrition; 2007.

Guglielmi FW, Regano N, Mazzuoli, et al. Cholestasis induced by total parenteral nutrition. *Clin Liver Dis.* 2008;12(1):97–110.

Heaney RP. The vitamin D requirement in health and disease. *J Steroid Biochem Mol Biol.* 2005;97: 13–19.

Jeejeebhoy KN. Permissive underfeeding of the critically ill patient. *Nutr Clin Pract.* 2004;19(5):477–480.

Johnson G, Salle A, Lorimier G, et al. Cancer cachexia: measured and predicted resting energy expenditures for nutritional needs evaluation. *Nutrition.* 2008;24:443–450.

Kelly CJ, Daly JM. Perioperative care of the oncology patient. *World J Surg.* 1993;17:199–206.

Lee JH, Machtay M, Unger LD, et al. Prophylactic gastrostomy tubes in patients undergoing intensive irradiation for cancer of the head and neck. *Arch Otolaryngol Head Neck Surg.* 1998;124: 871–875.

Mercadante S. Parenteral versus enteral nutrition in cancer patients: indications and practice. *Support Care Cancer.* 1998;6:85–93.

Moynihan T, Kelly DG, Fisch MJ. To feed or not to feed: is that the right question? *J Clin Oncol.* 2005;23:6256–6259.

National Ag Safety Database. A Consumer Guide to Safe Handling and Preparation of Ground Meat and Ground Poultry. Available at: http://www.cdc.gov/nasd/docs/d001201-d001300/d001229/d001229.html

National Heart Lung and Blood Institute. Calculate Your Body Mass Index. Available at: http://www.nhlbisupport.com/bmi/bmicalc.htm

Osoba D. Current applications of health-related quality-of-life assessment in oncology. *Support Care Cancer.* 1997;5:100–104.

Ottery FD. Nutritional oncology: a proactive, integrated approach to the cancer patient. In: Chernoff R, ed. *Nutrition Support: Theory and Therapeutics.* New York: Chapman & Hall; 1997:395–409.

Ottery FD. Supportive nutrition to prevent cachexia and improve quality of life. *Semin Oncol.* 1995;22 (2 Suppl 3):98–111.

Tisdale MJ. Pathogenesis of cancer cachexia. *J Support Oncol.* 2003;1:159–168.

United States Department of Agriculture, Food Safety and Inspection Service. Fact Sheets. Available at: http://www.fsis.usda.gov/Fact_Sheets/At_Risk_&_Underserved_Fact_Sheets/index.asp

Villet S, Chiolero RL, Bollmann MD, et al. Negative impact of hypocaloric feeding and energy balance on clinical outcome in ICU patients. *Clin Nutr.* 2005;24:502–509.

40

Pain and Palliative Care

Eric Bush and Ann Berger

DEFINITIONS

- Palliative care is based on a holistic model of symptom management. It concerns improving the quality of life (including end-of-life care) for patients and their families facing life-threatening illnesses by preventing and/or identifying and relieving suffering associated with physical, psychosocial, and spiritual problems. For cancer patients, pain is the most common reason for palliative care consultation.
- Acute pain is the predictable physiologic response to an adverse chemical, thermal, or mechanical stimulus. It is normally associated with surgery, trauma, and acute illness. It is generally time-limited and responsive to a variety of pharmceutical and nonpharmaceutical therapies.
- When acute pain persists over time, it is classified as chronic pain.
- Pain is usually, but not always, associated with tissue damage. It is always subjective and may be influenced by emotional, psychological, social, and spiritual factors, as well as financial concerns and fear of death.
- Neuropathic (stimulus-independent) pain is characterized by dysesthesia, allodynia, or hyperpathia. It may be secondary to direct tumor involvement or may arise postsurgery or postradiation. Agents associated with chemotherapy-related neuropathic pain include vincristine, cisplatin, and procarbazine. Neuropathic pain may be treated effectively with antidepressants or anticonvulsants.

EPIDEMIOLOGY

- Most cancer patients experience some degree of pain, especially in the advanced and metastatic phases of disease. In advanced cancer, the prevalence of pain is about 70%, but varies with the type and stage of disease.
- There are several published guidelines for cancer pain management recommended by the World Health Organization (WHO), and effective treatments are available for 70% to 90% of cases.
- Nevertheless, an estimated 40% of cancer patients remain undertreated for reasons related to the health care provider, the patient and family, or cultural mores. The most frequent cause of undertreatment is misconceptions about the use of opioids.

ASSESSMENT

- Proper pain assessment can help to establish a good doctor/patient relationship, guide the therapeutic regimen, improve pain management, maximize patient comfort and function, and increase patient satisfaction with therapy. Failure to fully assess pain in the cancer patient may result in inadequate pain management, regardless of the amount or type of analgesia and adjuvants used.
- Patients' self-reports should be the main source of pain assessment. For infants and the cognitively impaired, physicians must rely on behavioral observation.

506

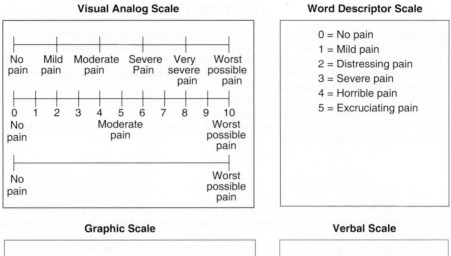

Visual Analog Scale

No pain   Mild pain   Moderate pain   Severe Pain   Very severe pain   Worst possible pain

0   1   2   3   4   5   6   7   8   9   10
No pain   Moderate pain   Worst possible pain

No pain   Worst possible pain

Word Descriptor Scale

0 = No pain
1 = Mild pain
2 = Distressing pain
3 = Severe pain
4 = Horrible pain
5 = Excruciating pain

Graphic Scale

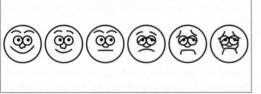

Verbal Scale

"On a scale of 0 to 10, with 0 meaning no pain and 10 meaning the worst pain you can imagine, how much pain are you having now?"

Functional Pain Scale

0 = No pain
1 = Tolerable and pain does not prevent any activities
2 = Tolerable and pain prevents some activities
3 = Intolerable and pain does not prevent use of telephone, TV viewing, or reading
4 = Intolerable and pain prevents use of telephone, TV viewing, or reading
5 = Intolerable and pain prevents verbal communication

Fig. 40.1. Common tools for assessment of pain intensity. [Adapted from the American Geriatrics Society (AGS) Panel on Chronic Pain in Older Persons. The management of chronic pain in older persons. *J Am Geriat Soc.* 1998;46:635–651; Gloth FM III, Scheve AA, Stober CV, et al. The functional pain scale (FPS): Reliability, validity, and responsiveness in a senior population. *J Am Med Direct Assoc.* 2001;3:110–114; and Gloth FM III. Assessment. *Handbook of Pain Relief in Older Adults: An Evidence-Based Approach.* Totowa, NJ: Humana Press; 2003:17.]

- For rapid assessment of acute pain, select a simple measurement of pain intensity (Fig. 40.1) and record the measurement for treatment evaluation.
- Patients should be reassessed frequently by inquiring how much their pain has been relieved after each treatment. A consistent disparity between patient's self-report of pain and their ability to function necessitates further assessment to ascertain the reason for the disparity.
- Underlying anxiety and depression can increase patient suffering. Inadequate assessment of these factors may result in under- or overtreatment with analgesics.

CHAPTER 40

TREATMENT

- Severe pain should be considered a medical emergency; timely and aggressive management should be provided until the pain becomes tolerable. Aggressive pain management, with the goal of attaining maximal functional ability, is especially important with cancer patients.
- Sedatives and anxiolytics alone should not be used to manage pain as they can mask the behavioral response to pain without providing analgesia.
- NSAIDs or acetaminophen should be used to manage mild to moderate pain, unless contraindicated.
- Opiates are the foundation of management for severe pain.
- For cancer-related anxiety and depression, treatment approaches include tricyclic antidepressants, SSRIs, and psychosocial intervention.

OPIATES

- Opiate therapy should be tailored to each patient, based on the type and expected duration of pain, as it is impossible to predict which patients will achieve adequate analgesia or develop intolerable adverse effects from a given opiate.
- Tolerance and physical dependence are expected with long-term opiate treatment and should not be confused with psychologic dependence (addiction).
- Equianalgesic doses of oral opiates (Table 40.1) should be prescribed when necessary.
- Begin administration of opiates at lowest effective dose and titrate as necessary. No maximal therapeutic dose for analgesia has been established.
- Immediate-release opiates (mu receptor agonists) are short-acting and may be appropriate for acute incidental pain, or to initiate and titrate opiate therapy. Long-acting opiates are used around the clock for baseline pain and to maintain analgesia.
- Titration of opiates: Start at lower doses and titrate as tolerance to side effects develops. Increase dose in increments of 30% to 50%. For severe uncontrolled pain, increase 100% and reassess at peak effect.
- Early side effects often improve or resolve with repeated doses. With the exception of constipation, tolerance often develops rapidly to most of the common opiate-related adverse effects.

Common Adverse Effects

- Constipation
- Sedation
- Nausea/vomiting
- Pruritus
- Sweating
- Dry mouth
- Weakness

Uncommon Adverse Effects

- Dyspnea
- Urinary retention
- Confusion
- Hallucinations
- Nightmares
- Myoclonus
- Dizziness
- Dysphoria
- Hypersensitivity/anaphylaxis

TABLE 40.1. *Opiate doses equianalgesic to morphine 10 mg intramuscular[a] for treatment of chronic pain in cancer patients*

Drug	mg PO	mg i.m.	Half-life (h)	Duration (h)	Considerations
Morphine	20–30[b]	10	2–3	2–4	Standard for comparison
Morphine CR	20–30	10	2–3	8–12	Various formulations are not bioequivalent.
Morphine SR	20–30	10	2–3	24	
Oxycodone	20		2–3	3–4	
Oxycodone CR	20		2–3	8–12	
Hydromorphone	7.5	1.5	2–3	2–4	Potency may be greater, i.e., i.v. hydromorphone:i.v. morphine = 3:1 rather than 6.7:1 during prolonged use.
Methadone	20	10	12–190	4–12	Although 1:1 ratio with morphine was used in a single-dose study, there is a change with repeated administration. Dose reduction of 75–90% needed when switching to methadone.
Oxymorphone	10 (rectal)	1	2–3	2–4	Available in rectal and injectable forms.
Levorphanol	4	2	12–15	4–6	
Fentanyl			7–12		Can be administered as continuous i.v. or subQ infusion; based on clinical experience, 10 mcg i.v. = 1 mg i.v. morphine.
Fentanyl TS			16–24	48–72	Based on clinical experience, 100 mcg/h is roughly equianalgesic to morphine 200 mg PO per day.

CR, controlled release; i.m., intramuscular; PO, oral; i.v., intravenous; subQ, subcutaneous; SR, sustained release; TS, transdermal system.

[a]Studies to determine equianalgesic doses of opiates have used i.m. morphine. In clinical practice, i.m. and i.v. routes are considered equivalent and the i.v. route is most common.

[b]Although the PO:i.m. morphine ratio was 6:1 in a single-dose study, other observations indicate a ratio of 2–3:1 with repeated administration.

Source: Adapted from Derby S, Chin J, Portenoy RK. Systemic opioid therapy for chronic cancer pain: practical guidelines for converting drugs and routes of administration. *CNS Drugs.* 1999;9:99–109.

Long-Term Opiate Use

- Physicians have an ethical and regulatory duty to inform the patient of the risks and benefits of long-term opiate use, particularly when initiating treatment in patients at high risk for misuse of opiates.
- Certain factors, such as personal or family history of substance abuse, risk of diversion of opiates, or lack of compliance, dictate a multidisciplinary approach, including the involvement of a pain specialist.
- Long-term use of opiates should always be supported by maximal use of coanalgesics and adjuvants, psychological therapy, and appropriate follow-up.

Risks of Long-Term Opiate Use

- Addiction: extremely rare in cancer patients
- Physical dependence: manifested by withdrawal syndrome at cessation or dose reduction

- Tolerance: diminution of one or more of the opiate's effects over time
- Pseudoaddiction: iatrogenic syndrome that develops in response to inadequate pain management

Termination of Opiate Therapy

- When opiates are no longer required for pain management, appropriate tapering is essential to reduce the risk of withdrawal syndromes. The recommended regimen involves reducing dosage by 10% to 20% daily, or more slowly if symptoms such as anxiety, tachycardia, sweating, or other autonomic symptoms arise.
- Symptoms may be relieved by clonidine 0.1 to 0.2 mg/day PO or 1.5 mg transdermal patch/3 days.

ADJUVANT ANALGESICS

- An adjuvant analgesic is any drug with a primary indication other than pain, but with proven analgesic effect in specific circumstances.
- Indications include poor response to opiate, opiate toxicity, or pain that is more responsive to adjuvant (i.e., neuropathic, bone, visceral, or myofascial pain).
- Adjuvants should be tried one at a time until analgesia is achieved or side effects become intolerable. If only partial analgesia is reached at maximal dose of one adjuvant, consider adding a second adjuvant.
- Potential benefits of adjuvant analgesia include:
  - Targeting of multiple pain pathways
  - Complementary pharmacokinetic activity
  - Potentially synergistic analgesic effects
  - Reduced adverse events with comparable efficacy

NONPHARMACOLOGIC THERAPY

- Psychologic and behavioral interventions may enhance the benefits of pain medications or help to reduce their use.
- Integration of these modalities into treatment should be culturally sensitive and tailored to patients' individual needs.
- Modalities include, among others:
  - Acupuncture
  - Relaxation/biofeedback
  - Recreation/art/music therapy
  - Reiki/healing touch
  - Transcutaneous electrical nerve stimulation (TENS)
  - Myofascial trigger release
  - Behavioral counseling

SUGGESTED READINGS

Benjamin LJ, Dampier CD, Jacox A, et al. Guideline for the management of acute and chronic pain in sickle-cell disease. American Pain Society. APS Clinical Practice Series. 1999;1:xi.

Cherny N. The management of cancer pain. *Cancer J Clin.* 2000;50:70–116.

Cohen MZ, Easley MK, Ellis C, et al. Cancer pain management and the JCAHO's pain standards: an institutional challenge. *J Pain Symptom Manage.* 2003;25:519–527.

Hearn J, Higginson IJ. Cancer pain epidemiology: a systematic review. In: Bruera ED, Portenoy RK, eds. *Cancer Pain, Assessment and Management.* New York: Cambridge University Press; 2003.

Jennings AL, Davies A, Higgins JP, Broadley K. Opioids for the palliation of breathlessness in terminal illness. *Cochrane Database Syst Rev.* 2001;4:CDE002066.

National Heart, Lung, and Blood Institute. *The Management of Sickle Cell Disease.* 4th ed. Publication no. 02-2117. Bethesda, MD: National Institutes of Health; 2002.

Qaseem A, Snow V, Shekelle P, et al. Evidence-based interventions to improve the palliative care of pain, dyspnea, and depression at the end of life: a clinical practice guideline from the American College of Physicians. *Ann Intern Med.* 2008;148(2):141–146.

Ripamonti C, De Conno F, Blumhuber H, Ventafridda V. Morphine for relief of cancer pain. *Lancet.* 1996;347:1262–1263.

Throm MJ, Fudin J, Otis JA. Managing chronic pain: an analysis of the use of opioids. *Pharm Times.* July 2005:88.

WHO Cancer Pain Relief: With a Guide to Opioid Availability. 2nd ed. Geneva: WHO; 1990.

Zenz M, Willweber-Strumpf A. Opiophobia and cancer pain in Europe. *Lancet.* 1993;341:1075–1076.

41

Complementary and Alternative Medicine

Patrick J. Mansky, Dawn B. Wallerstedt, Scott Miller, and Jamie Stagl

During the last decade, patients with cancer have increasingly turned to complementary and alternative medicine (CAM) resources in an attempt to cure cancer, to provide relief from cancer-related symptoms, or to improve overall well-being and quality of life. CAM, as defined by the National Center for Complementary and Alternative Medicine (NCCAM), is a group of diverse medical and health care systems, practices, and products that are not presently considered to be part of conventional medicine (1,2). Complementary medicine approaches are used in combination with conventional medicine, while alternative medicine approaches are considered by patients and practitioners as therapeutic alternatives to conventional therapy. Although some scientific evidence exists about some CAM therapies, for most therapies there are key questions that are yet to be answered through well-designed scientific studies—questions such as whether these therapies are safe and whether they work for the diseases or medical conditions for which they are used.

The list of what is considered to be CAM changes continually, as those therapies that are proven to be safe and effective become adopted into conventional health care and as new approaches to health care emerge (see http://nccam.nih.gov/health/whatiscam/).

Scientific assessments of safety, efficacy, and mode of action are either fragmented or totally lacking for many CAM modalities and approaches.

THE DOMAINS OF COMPLEMENTARY AND ALTERNATIVE MEDICINE

The NCCAM groups CAM modalities into five major domains that are applicable to cancer-related CAM:

- Whole medical systems
- Mind–body medicine
- Biologically based practices
- Manipulative and body-based practices
- Energy medicine

USE OF COMPLEMENTARY AND ALTERNATIVE MEDICINE IN PATIENTS WITH CANCER

CAM use in patients with cancer varies according to region, geographic location, gender, and disease diagnosis. This chapter focuses on the data available on cancer patients in the United States. The prevalence of CAM use in patients with cancer has been estimated to be between 7% and 54% (1).

Predictors of use of CAM in patients with cancer include the following:

- Higher educational status
- White ethnicity
- Deteriorating health status
- Female gender

The following is a list of CAM modalities used frequently by cancer patients:

- Herbs, dietary supplements, and minerals
- Special diets
- Spirituality
- Meditation or mind–body work
- Relaxation or guided imagery
- Acupuncture
- Healing touch
- Support groups
- Yoga
- Patients often utilize several CAM modalities concurrently.

Most patients with cancer use CAM in an effort to

- boost the immune system,
- relieve pain, or
- control side effects related to disease or treatment.

Only a few patients include CAM in the treatment plan with curative intent (2).

CAM APPROACHES TO CANCER TREATMENT

A diverse array of CAM approaches has been used in clinical practice for the treatment of cancer and cancer-related symptoms. A comprehensive review of existing CAM practices used in cancer is beyond the scope of this chapter. Here we focus on a set of CAM modalities and approaches based on the following selection criteria:

- Accessibility and availability within the United States
- Existence of peer-reviewed, published information on efficacy or treatment-associated clinical benefit
- Components of the CAM cancer treatment spectrum commonly employed (based on published demographic data) as complementary modalities by health care professionals or requested by patients

Alternative medical systems approaches are not included in this chapter. There is a paucity of published data from controlled clinical trials on the efficacy of these approaches in the treatment of cancer. The interested reader is referred to the available literature and is encouraged to seek advice from trained experts in the field (3,4).

Emerging evidence for the use of botanicals for cancer symptom management has been included in this chapter. However, biologics employed in the treatment of cancer are not discussed in detail. Most biologics would be considered experimental from the perspective of available scientific evidence of activity in cancer treatment. Some fall into the category of alternative medical systems. For some of the agents the interested reader is referred to the information available in the PDQ Cancer Information Summaries: CAM of the National Cancer Institute (NCI) at http://www.nci.nih.gov/cancerinfo/pdq/cam.

A separate section has been included in this chapter to address some emerging data on interactions between botanicals and drugs and on resources regarding ongoing clinical trials that are investigating the efficacy of CAM.

CAM therapies discussed in this chapter are grouped into two categories: cancer symptom management and diet, nutrition, and supplements.

CANCER SYMPTOM MANAGEMENT

Acupuncture for Cancer Symptom Management

Acupuncture, acupressure, and electroacupuncture are all widely used in cancer symptom management. A number of acupuncture approaches are being practiced, including Chinese, Japanese, Korean, and French acupuncture. Mainly used in the context of traditional Chinese medicine, acupuncture stimulates points along the meridians of the body to balance the *qi* (energy flow) (5). Scientific evidence validates the use of acupuncture for relief from the following cancer-related symptoms:

Chemotherapy-Induced Nausea and Vomiting

According to the 1997 NIH Consensus Conference on Acupuncture existing evidence based on clinical trials suggests a beneficial role for acupuncture in the areas of chemotherapy-induced nausea/vomiting.

- Commonly used acupuncture points include P6, Neiguan point of the pericardium meridian of hand (jueyin), and St 36, Zunsali point of the stomach meridian of foot (yang ming) (6).
- Acupuncture and electroacupuncture are effective in the reduction of acute vomiting (7).
- Acupressure, by administration on point P6, can reduce intensity of nausea, retching experience, and frequency of vomiting in breast cancer patients receiving chemotherapy (8).
- Acupuncture may be administered before the first dose and during the course of treatment. Antiemetic agents may be used in conjunction with acupuncture.

Fatigue

- Preliminary evidence suggests that by stimulating certain energy points along the meridians, acupuncture and acupressure may be effective in alleviating fatigue associated with chemotherapy treatment (9).

Cancer-Related Pain

- Evidence exists supporting the use of electroacupuncture to relieve cancer-related neuropathic pain (10).
- Recent data suggests a role for auricular acupuncture in patients experiencing ongoing cancer-related neuropathic pain managed with a stable analgesic pain regimen (11).

Side Effects

Acupuncture is generally a well-tolerated and safe procedure when administered by an experienced practitioner. In fact, a recent study in Germany revealed only six cases of serious adverse events in patients receiving acupuncture out of a total of 97,733 patients treated (12).

- The most frequent side effects include minimal local bleeding/bruising and mild pain (13,14).
- Other less common, minor side effects include nausea and fainting.

Caveats

Acupuncture is not advisable in patients with the following:

- Arrhythmia or pacemakers
- Thrombocytopenia
- Bleeding disorders
- Aplasia
- Valvular heart disease
- Infection
- Severe polyneuropathy or paraplegia
- Conditions of unknown medical origin

Botanicals for Cancer Symptom Management

Various botanicals and herbs have been found to be possibly effective in cancer symptom management. While the area is in need of more rigorous clinical trials, there is some supporting evidence for the use of ginger, ginseng, and certain Chinese herbal medicines.

Chemotherapy-Induced Nausea and Vomiting

- There is some evidence to suggest that ginger root is as effective as the antiemetic metoclopramide in controlling nausea and vomiting. However, ginger root is not more effective than the antiemetic ondasetron (15).
- A Cochrane Review concluded that Huangqi decoctions (a Chinese herbal medicine) are effective in reducing chemotherapy-induced nausea and vomiting (16).
- Evidence suggests that a Chinese herbal preparation of seven different herbs, known as Aifukang capsules, are effective in reducing nausea and vomiting (17).

Fatigue

- In a recent study, patients taking Aifukang capsules during chemotherapy treatment experienced a significant relief in symptoms of fatigue (18). A similar effect was found in patients taking Huangqi decoctions (19).
- Preliminary evidence suggests that ginger root has a role in stimulating energy and decreasing fatigue (16).

Cancer-Related Pain

The Chinese herbal remedy known as nourishing yin and unblocking meridians recipe (NUR), when used in addition to opioid analgesics has been found to be more effective than analgesics alone in relieving cancer-related pain (18).

Insomnia

Literature points to a possible decrease in treatment-related insomnia through the use of valerian, St. John's wort, chamomile, hops, passionflower, lavender, and lemon balm. Evidence is preliminary and these botanicals need more exploration (20).

Mucositis

Some preliminary evidence exists for the use of aloe vera to reduce radiation-related mucositis (21). More research is needed for mucositis relief.

Menopausal Symptoms

A number of botanical products including soy and soy extracts, black cohosh (*Cimicifuga racemosa*), chaste tree berry (*Vitex agnus-cactus*), don quai (*Angelica sinensis*), ginseng (*Panax ginseng*), evening primrose oil (*Oenothera biennis*), red clover (*Trifolium pratense*), motherwort (*Leonurus cardiaca*), and licorice (*Glycyrrhiza glabra*) have been widely used as adjunct treatments for menopausal symptoms including hot flashes, considered to be mostly due to the effects of the isoflavone components.

A recent review of 29 randomized clinical trials (RCTs) of CAM therapies for menopausal symptoms (22) concluded the following:

- Black cohosh and phytoestrogen-containing foods show promise in the treatment of menopausal symptoms.
- Clinical trials do not support the use of other herbs or CAM therapies for menopausal symptoms.

Limited data based on two RCTs of soy beverage (23) or phytoestrogen tablets (24) specifically used by postmenopausal women with breast cancer concluded, respectively, that:

- soy phytoestrogens administered as a soy beverage do not alleviate hot flashes, and
- pure isoflavones administered as tablets do not alleviate menopausal symptoms.

Quality of Life

- Sun ginseng shows benefits for improving aspects of mental and physical functioning on quality-of-life scales in patients with gynecological or hepatobiliary cancer (25).
- Some evidence suggests that the Chinese herbal Huachansu injection may be beneficial in improving overall quality of life in esophageal cancer patients; however, more research is needed (26).

Side Effects

It is important to be aware of the characteristics of certain botanicals and their potential for interaction with other botanicals and drugs (Table 41.1).. Concern has been raised about liver toxicity from black cohosh. Further research is needed to determine safety and efficacy. Herbals and botanicals should only be taken under an oncologist's supervision and with prior review of the product, contents, dosing, and possible contraindications. Refer to the Natural Standard (www.naturalstandard.com) for more information on safety, side effects, and possible complications.

Mind–Body Therapies

Mind–body interventions utilize the processes of the mind to impact the health of the body (27). These approaches encompass a wide spectrum of modalities, including relaxation, hypnosis, guided imagery, meditation, biofeedback, tai chi, and cognitive-behavioral therapies. In the therapeutic setting, mind–body interventions have been used to reduce psychological distress, change physiologic symptoms, alter perceptions (e.g., anticipatory nausea), and change unhealthy behaviors (e.g., smoking cessation, weight loss).

Hypnotherapy

Hypnosis is a state of inner absorption, concentration, and focused attention in which the individual is more receptive to suggestion. While its mechanism of action remains to be elucidated, it has been used in therapeutic settings to effectively treat anxiety, pain, irritable bowel syndrome, and tension headaches.

CHEMOTHERAPY-INDUCED NAUSEA AND VOMITING (CINV) AND ANTICIPATORY NAUSEA AND VOMITING (ANV)

- Hypnosis is effective in reducing CINV and ANV, particularly in pediatric groups (28) and painful medical procedures (lumbar puncture, bone marrow aspirate).
- Hypnosis is more effective than no-treatment control or therapist attention in reducing self-reported pain and anxiety in pediatric oncology patients (29).

POSTOPERATIVE OUTCOMES

- Hypnosis decreased emotional upset and anxiety during excisional breast biopsies in two studies (30,31).
- Hypnosis resulted in decreased pain intensity, less intraoperative anesthetics, and shorter operative time versus attention-control group in women undergoing excisional biopsy or lumpectomy (32).

CHRONIC CANCER PAIN

- Hypnosis is effective in decreasing metastatic bone pain in several studies (33,34).

PALLIATIVE CARE SETTING

- Hypnotherapy may be effective in the palliative care setting to decrease physical distress and pain; evidence is hampered by lack of well-designed RCTs (35).

ADVERSE EVENTS

- Distressing emotions or thoughts may occur.
- Strong emotional response (abreaction) possible, especially with history of trauma.
- Paradoxical anxiety reactions can rarely occur.

TABLE 41.1. *Safety, side effects, and interactions of selected botanicals*

Botanical	Safety	Possible side effects	Possible interactions
Ginseng	Avoid ginseng if known allergy to plants in the Araliaceae family. There has been a report of a serious life-threatening skin reaction, possibly caused by contaminants in the ginseng formulation.	Altered blood cell counts, alteration in blood clotting, alteration in menstrual cycle or blood pressure, altered hearth rhythm, blurred vision, cessation of menstruation in younger women, breast tenderness chest pain, delayed ejaculation, diarrhea, difficulty sleeping, dizziness, drowsiness, erectile dysfunction, fever, headache, increased breast growth, increased sex drive, irritation and burning, loss of appetite, mild pain, nausea, nervousness, nosebleeds, rapid and pounding heartbeats, skin disturbances (such as itching or rose spots), stomach discomfort, swelling, throat irritation, vaginal bleeding in postmenopausal women, vomiting, water retention.	Anticoagulants/blood thinners like warfarin (Coumadin®), drugs that are broken down by the liver, HIV drugs like protease inhibitors, drugs that lower blood sugar levels, digoxin (Lanoxin®), nifedipine (Procardia®), blood pressure drugs, over-the-counter drugs for treating cold symptoms (like pseudoephedrine), diuretics and central nervous system stimulants such as methylphenidate (Ritalin®), corticosteroids, hormonal drugs, antipsychotics, opioids like morphine, phenelzine (Nardil®), alcohol, metronidazole (Flagyl®), and disulfiram (Antabuse®), herbs or supplements with similar effects.
Ginger	Avoid if allergic to ginger or other members of the Zingiberaceae family (like red ginger, Alpinia purpurata, shell ginger, Alpinia zeru, green cardamom, and balsam of Peru). Caution if driving or operating machinery. Stop 2 weeks prior to surgery/dental/diagnostic procedures due to risk of bleeding. Avoid if history of irregular heartbeat (arrhythmia). Caution if history of ulcers, acid reflux, heart conditions, inflammatory bowel disease, blocked intestines or bleeding disorders. Caution if pregnant or breastfeeding.	Bleeding, bruising skin rash, altered taste, bloating, gas, stomach discomfort, blocked intestines, increased urination, irregular heartbeat (arrythmmia), altered blood pressure, heartburn, nausea, menstrual changes, depression, altered blood sugar levels, drowsiness, sleepiness.	Drugs that alter stomach acid (like Pepcid® or omeprazole), drugs that increase bleeding risk (anticoagulants/ "blood thinners," like warfarin (Coumadin®), aspirin), calcium, digoxin, blood pressure drugs, drugs that alter blood sugar levels, drugs that cause drowsiness (like some allergy drugs, Lorazepam®, barbiturates, narcotics, alcohol), drugs broken down by the liver, xanthine oxidase drugs, and herbs or supplements with similar effects.

(Continued)

TABLE 41.1. *(Continued)*

Botanical	Safety	Possible side effects	Possible interactions
Huangqi (Astragalus)	Avoid if allergic to astragalus, peas, or any related plants or with a history of Quillaja bark-induced asthma. Avoid with aspirin or aspirin products or herbs or supplements with similar effects. Avoid with inflammation (swelling) or fever, stroke, transplant or autoimmune diseases (like HIV/AIDS). Stop use 2 weeks before surgery/dental/diagnostic procedures with a risk of bleeding and avoid use immediately after these procedures. Use cautiously with bleeding disorders, diabetes, high blood pressure, lipid disorders or kidney disorders. Use cautiously with blood-thinners, blood sugar drugs, or diuretics or herbs and supplements with similar effects. Avoid if pregnant or breastfeeding.	Abdominal discomfort, bleeding, breathing problems, bruising, changes in blood sugar, changes in blood pressure or heartbeat, changes in the immune system, dehydration, diarrhea, growth hormone changes, increased urination, itching, neurological problems, pneumonia (aspiration), palpitations, poisoning, skin rash, upset stomach.	Drugs that increase the risk of bleeding (anticoagulants), antiplatelet drugs, blood pressure drugs, blood sugar/diabetes drugs, cholesterol-lowering drugs, colchicine, some weight-loss drugs, diuretics, ephedrine or epinephrine, drugs broken down by the liver, drugs that alter the immune system, hypnotics, intravenous calcium salts, nalbuphine, oral medications, pain relievers (like ibuprofen) naproxen (Aleve®), pancuronium, procarbazine, propoxyphene, rauwolfia alkaloids, sedatives (like phenobarbital), succinylcholine, and herbs or supplements with similar effects.

Source: Adapted from www.naturalstandard.com.

- Controversial in persons with severe psychiatric disease (e.g., psychoses), although this has not been very well studied

Guided Imagery and Relaxation Techniques

Guided imagery uses the imaginative ability of the mind to positively affect physical and/or emotional outcomes. As with hypnosis, a guided imagery therapist makes specific suggestions using a directive, permissive, or interactive approach.

- Progressive muscle relaxation and guided imagery significantly reduced cancer pain compared with a control group in two RCTs (36,37).
- Relaxation, guided imagery, and cognitive-behavioral training (such as deep breathing, muscle relaxation, and visualization) alleviate cancer pain and can reduce the need for nonopioid analgesics (38).

Adverse events related to guided imagery are similar to those seen with hypnosis.

Meditation

Cancer therapists and patients with cancer have employed a wide range of meditation methods to alleviate cancer symptoms. The two most widely studied techniques are transcendental meditation (TM) and mindfulness-based meditation. TM uses the repetition of a specific mantra with the intent of quieting and ultimately "transcending" the practitioner's internal mental dialogue. Mindfulness-based meditation strives to develop an objective "observer role" for the practitioner toward his own emotions, feelings, perceptions, and so on, thereby creating a nonjudgmental "mindful" state of conscious awareness. Other meditation practices are usually pursued in a religious or spiritual context.

Studies of TM in the management of cancer symptoms are lacking. There is weak evidence that TM may help with reduction of anxiety and stress (39), but it remains unclear how this information can be translated into the cancer setting. The mindfulness-based stress reduction (MBSR) program was developed by Jon Kabat-Zinn. The components of sitting meditation, body scan, and mindful movement are taught over a training period of 7 to 8 weeks (40).

Studies of MBSR in cancer populations (41–44) suggest that MBSR may result in:

- decrease in anxiety and in mood disturbances;
- decrease in depression, anger, and confusion; and
- change in post-treatment total stress scores.

MBSR is a highly structured, didactic program that may not be appropriate for patients of all educational levels.

Yoga

Deriving from the Ayurvedic medical system, yoga combines breath awareness and control with meditation, movement, and chanting. Studies have supported its beneficial role in stress management, anxiety reduction, and insomnia (45). Several RCTs have been conducted utilizing yoga as an intervention for cancer patients undergoing treatment (46,47) and in cancer survivors (48). From these several studies, there appear to be improvements in psychosocial outcomes in these groups. Additionally, yoga is likely a safe modality, except in patients with bone metastases who are at risk for pathologic fractures.

Therapeutic Massage

Therapeutic massage is generally practiced as a series of strokes and kneading movements aimed at treating the body without adjusting any body structures. Details of the array of massage techniques and approaches can be found in the literature. In general, patients should be treated only by experienced, trained, and (if applicable) licensed massage therapists.

- A Cochrane review of aromatherapy and massage for symptom relief in cancer patients found reductions in anxiety (four RCTs), depression (one RCT), pain (three RCTs), and nausea (two RCTs); there is conflicting evidence that aromatherapy adds any additional benefit (49).
- A large observational study of 1,290 cancer patients receiving various types of massage found immediate improvements in visual analogue symptom scores in pain, fatigue, anxiety, nausea, and depression (50).
- The efficacy of manual lymph drainage is unclear (51,52).

ADVERSE EVENTS

Although uncommon in the literature, there have been reports of adverse events associated with massage therapy, most often associated with massage administered by nonprofessionals and the use of forceful techniques such as shiatsu and Rolfing (53).

Potential adverse effects of massage in cancer patients include:

- Bruising
- Internal bleeding
- Fractures at sites of bone metastases

CAVEATS

Massage therapy should be modified with cancer patients who have any of the following conditions (54):

- Coagulation disorder (including low platelet count, medications such as warfarin, heparin, aspirin therapy)

- Thrombus
- Prosthetic devices/stents in the massage field
- Irradiated skin and tissues; open wounds
- Metastatic cancer at bony sites

Distant Healing Modalities

"Distant healing" interventions include such modalities as therapeutic touch, Reiki, spiritual healing, prayer, and external Qigong. Some of these interventions, such as Reiki, are based on the belief that the practitioner serves as a conduit of subtle vibrational energy flow by placement of hands on the recipient, while others, such as therapeutic touch, do not necessarily require direct contact with the recipient.

- The data claiming efficacy for these modalities is controversial from a scientific viewpoint.
- The mechanism by which potential benefit can be derived from these modalities has not been elucidated.
- A number of RCTs and several reviews of beneficial effects have been published. However, only a few studies have been conducted in cancer populations.

Available data from a recent meta-analysis conducted by Astin et al. (55) show the following results from sixteen double-blind studies of the total of 23:

- Ten positive studies using therapeutic touch versus a sham control
- Two positive studies using distant intercessory prayer
- Four positive studies using other forms of distant healing
- Only one of the studies included in this meta-analysis was conducted in a population of patients with cancer (56).

The only RCT utilizing Reiki as an intervention in a cohort of patients with cancer (57) reported no reduction in pain scores.

DIET/NUTRITION/SUPPLEMENTS

Dietary Supplements

The antioxidant vitamins A, C, and E are commonly used by patients with cancer in an attempt to improve disease outcome. There is currently no published information based on controlled clinical trials available that would suggest that a specific dietary supplement or a supplement combination is effective in curing cancer.

Vitamin A

Vitamin A may promote progression of latent prostate cancer (58) and may result in increased lung cancer incidence in high-risk populations (59). Based on the available evidence, vitamin A should not be administered in excess of the recommended daily allowance.

ADVERSE EFFECTS

- Hypervitaminosis A when administered in high doses

CAVEATS

- Prostate cancer
- Lung cancer risk or lung cancer

Vitamin C

Vitamin C is an essential nutrient. RCTs with oral vitamin C have failed to show clinical benefit in the treatment of cancer (60). Some of the observed anecdotal benefits of vitamin C may be related to the much higher bioavailability of vitamin C when administered intravenously than when administered orally (61,62). There is no scientific rationale for administering vitamin C orally in high doses.

Vitamin E

Vitamin E, in addition to acting as a free radical scavenger, may block gastric formation of carcinogenic nitrosamines and may enhance the immune function. Nonetheless, clinical trials and surveys that have attempted to demonstrate a relation between vitamin E and the incidence of cancer have been generally inconclusive. Vitamin E may prevent progression of latent prostate cancer (63). Increased vitamin E serum levels following dietary supplementation have been associated with decreased risk for esophageal and gastric cancer in high-risk populations (64,65). Vitamin E in high doses interferes with platelet function (26).

ADVERSE EFFECTS

• High doses of vitamin E can lead to thrombocytopenia.

CAVEATS

• Surgery
• Anticoagulant therapy

Diet

Many cancer patients are highly motivated to seek information about food choices, physical activity, dietary supplement use, and complementary nutritional therapies. Current scientific evidence suggests that diet is responsible for 30% to 40% of cancers worldwide, and accounts for up to 75% of colorectal cancer, in particular (66). The cancer prevention recommendations that follow are adapted from an American Institute for Cancer Research report released in 2007 and apply to cancer survivors (66). Anyone who has been diagnosed with cancer, from the time of diagnosis through the rest of life, is considered a cancer survivor (67). While these recommendations are from a conventional source, they nonetheless parallel many of the dietary suggestions made by CAM practitioners, who often recommend additional supplements.

1. Eat mostly foods of plant origin with a variety of vegetables, fruits, whole grains, and legumes.
2. Limit or avoid intake of red meats (such as beef, pork, and lamb) and avoid processed meats and charred meat.
3. Be as lean as possible without becoming underweight with a goal BMI to be between 21 and 23.
4. Be physically active for at least 30 minutes every day.
5. Avoid sugary drinks. Limit consumption of energy-dense foods (particularly processed foods high in added sugar, low in fiber, or high in fat).
6. Limit alcoholic drinks to two for men and one for women a day.
7. Limit consumption of salt to 2 g/day; avoid moldy grains and legumes.
8. Don't use supplements to protect against cancer; rather, obtain nutrients from a balanced diet.

Dietary counseling during cancer treatment for improving outcomes, such as fewer treatment-related symptoms, improved quality of life, and better dietary intake is an important consideration (67). Special considerations need to be tailored to individual needs such as consuming smaller, more frequent meals to help to increase food intake for those with a reduced appetite. For those who cannot meet their nutritional needs through foods alone, homemade or commercial nutrient-dense shakes may improve the intake of energy and nutrients, although plant-based preparations from whole foods would be preferable. Juicing vegetables and fruits can add variety to the diet and may help to overcome difficulties chewing or swallowing. Juicing also improves the body's absorption of some of the nutrients in vegetables and fruits (67).

Caveats

Achieving BMI goals should not occur during cancer treatment and should be deferred until successful treatment and recovery, as many cancer treatments and cancer itself can lead to unintentional weight loss.

The dietary recommendations above are generalized and an individual nutritional plan is the optimal approach in patients undergoing active cancer treatment.

Soy

Soy, a subtropical plant native to southeastern Asia, has been a main dietary component in Asian countries for at least 5,000 years. More easily digestible fermented forms of soy include tempeh, miso, and tamari soy sauce. Soy and the soy components, isoflavones (such as genistein), are believed to exert estrogenic effects (68,69). Although genistein has demonstrated anticancer effects in preclinical studies, the effects of genistein on cancer in humans in vivo have not been adequately determined (69). Preliminary research on humans suggests that soy isoflavones do not exert the same effects on the body as do estrogens (e.g., promoting the thickening of the endometrium) (68). It remains to be determined whether the consumption of soy by adults affects the risk of developing breast cancer, and whether soy consumption affects the survival of patients with breast cancer (70).

The role of soy and soy components in the prevention and treatment of prostate cancer in humans remains unclear (71,72).

Diet Composition

Whole Grains/Fiber

• Whole grains and fiber (73) are protective against cancer, especially gastrointestinal cancers such as gastric and colonic, and hormone-dependent cancers including cancers of breast and prostate.

Fruits and Vegetables

Published case-control and cohort studies are inconclusive about the protective effect of fruits and vegetables against cancer risk (74).

• Balanced diets rich in fresh fruits and vegetables can be recommended for patients with cancer (75).
• Extremes in diet may be associated with poorer survival rates (76).
• Ongoing research is investigating the benefit of a diet rich in fruits and vegetables for improving survival in cancer, however survivors of early stage breast cancer who followed a diet that was very high in vegetables, fruit, and fiber and low in fat did not experience a reduction in additional breast cancer events or mortality during a 7.3-year follow-up period (77).

Nutrition: Specialized Diets

Specialized diets have not been shown to improve cancer survival or cancer-related symptoms in controlled clinical trials, and may even be unsafe for use in some patients with cancer. Many of these diets are vegetarian based. If no animal products are used, occasional supplementation with vitamin B_{12} needs to be considered.

Gerson Diet

The Gerson diet is a metabolic treatment method based on the idea of detoxifying the body by eliminating commercially farmed fruits, vegetables, and prepared foods. The intake of numerous food items is restricted. The diet calls for 13 hourly glasses of juice from organically grown fruits and vegetables, supplemented by a specific regimen of supplements and coffee enemas (78). No prospective, controlled studies have been published that confirm the safety or effectiveness of the Gerson diet in the treatment of cancer.

Adverse Effects

• Pain, diarrhea, and cramping caused by the diet itself and from the coffee enemas
• Electrolyte imbalances
• Infections
• Colitis

Caveats

This is a very stringent and restrictive regimen that may require close monitoring for risks of side effects and complications.

Macrobiotics

Macrobiotic diets are among the most popular comprehensive, nutrition-based CAM treatment approaches to cancer. Macrobiotics is based on a predominantly vegetarian, whole-foods diet consisting of 20% to 30% vegetables, 50% to 60% cereal grains, and 5% to 10% beans and legumes. Sweets, fruits, seafood, and nuts or seeds are limited to a few times per week, whereas meats, eggs, and dairy products are consumed only once a week, if at all.
• The dietary components of the macrobiotic diet have been associated with decreased cancer risk.
• Macrobiotic diets may lower the levels of circulating estrogen in women.
• The role of macrobiotics in the treatment of cancer has not been investigated adequately (79).

ADVERSE EFFECTS

• The risk of nutritional deficiencies in poorly nourished patients
• Some components of the macrobiotic diet may alter the metabolism of certain drugs.

CAVEATS

• Caution is called for, especially in women with estrogen-receptor (ER)–positive breast cancer or endometrial cancer because of the high phytoestrogen content of some macrobiotic diets.
• Macrobiotic diets are a potentially useful adjunct to conventional treatment in well-nourished patients, if closely monitored by an experienced oncologist (63).

Gonzalez Regimen

Dr. Gonzalez's summary of the findings of Dr. William Donald Kelley, a Texas dentist, who for 20 years had been treating patients with cancer with a complicated nutritional therapy, suggested a marked survival advantage for patients with advanced pancreatic cancer, among other disease groups. An NCI-sponsored pilot study of 11 patients with advanced pancreatic cancer treated with this approach (regimen details: http://www.dr-gonzalez.com/regimen.htm) showed promising results (80). An NCI-sponsored clinical trial in advanced pancreatic cancer is currently closed.

At this point, no published prospective clinical trials have demonstrated the efficacy of the Gonzalez regimen in the treatment of cancer.

ADVERSE EFFECTS

• Diarrhea and cramping from engaging in a regimen that includes coffee enemas
• Electrolyte imbalances

CAVEATS

• Infectious risk associated with the ingestion of raw meat extracts

Weight Management

• Current evidence suggests a decreased risk for disease recurrence in women with breast cancer who follow a low-fat diet, which is associated with decrease in body weight (81).
• The combination of a healthy lifestyle including recommended intake of fruits and vegetables and moderate levels of physical activity increased survival in women with breast cancer, independent from obesity (82).
• Weight control and moderate exercise may reduce the risk for concomitant illnesses (e.g., cardiovascular disease).

COMPLEMENTARY AND ALTERNATIVE MEDICINE IN CANCER: INTERACTIONS AND CAVEATS

Botanical–Drug Interactions

The role of biologics in the CAM treatment of cancer is not discussed in detail in this chapter. However, the interaction of botanicals and nutritional supplements with pharmaceutical drugs is being reported with increasing frequency (83). Commonly used botanicals that affect the metabolism of pharmaceutical drugs in humans are listed in Table 41.2.

A number of caveats relating to the use of CAM therapies have been listed during the course of this chapter. Table 41.3 provides a summary of some important caveats for consideration when using complementary therapies in the treatment of cancer patients.

TABLE 41.2. *Drug interactions of five of the top-selling botanicals on the U.S. market*

Botanical	Drug interactions
St. John's wort	5-HT1 agonists (triptans), alprazolam, aminolevulinic acid, amitriptyline, analgesics with serotonergic activity, antidepressants, barbiturates, cyclosporine, digoxin, dextromethorphan, fenfluramine, fexofenadine, irinotecan, monoamine oxidase inhibitors, narcotics, nefazodone, NNRTIs, nortriptyline, oral contraceptives, paroxetine, phenobarbital, phenprocoumon, phenytoin, photosensitizing drugs, protease inhibitors, reserpine, sertraline, simvastatin, tacrolimus, theophylline, warfarin
Ginkgo biloba	Anticoagulant-antiplatelet drugs (aspirin, heparin, indomethacin), buspirone, fluoxetine, insulin, MAOIs, seizure-threshold–lowering drugs, thiazide diuretics, trazodone, warfarin, other drugs metabolized by cytochrome P-450: CYP1A2 (acetaminophen, diazepam, estradiol, ondansetron, propranolol, and warfarin), CYP2D6 (amitriptyline, codeine, fentanyl, fluoxetine, meperidine, methadone, ondansetron, and others) and CYP3A4 chemotherapeutic agents (etoposide, paclitaxel, vinblastine, vincristine, and vindesine), antifungals (ketoconazole and itraconazole), glucocorticoids, fentanyl, calcium channel blockers (diltiazem, nicardipine, and verapamil), and others
Panax ginseng	Anticoagulant-antiplatelet drugs (aspirin, heparin, indomethacin), antipsychotic drugs, caffeine, furosemide, immunosuppressants (azathioprine, cyclosporine, tacrolimus, prednisone, others), insulin, MAOIs, oral hypoglycemic agents (glimepiride, glyburide), stimulant drugs, warfarin, other drugs metabolized by cytochrome p450 CYP2D6 enzyme (amitriptyline, codeine, fentanyl, fluoxetine, meperidine, methadone, ondansetron, and others)
Allium sativum (garlic)	Anticoagulant–antiplatelet drugs (warfarin, aspirin, heparin, and indomethacin), cyclosporine, NNRTIs, saquinavir (potentially, other protease inhibitors), oral contraceptives, other drugs: preparations containing allicin may increase the activity of the cytochrome P450 CYP3A4. Drugs that might be affected include chemotherapeutic agents (etoposide, paclitaxel, vinblastine, vincristine, and vindesine), antifungals (ketoconazole and itraconazole), glucocorticoids, fentanyl, calcium channel blockers (diltiazem, nicardipine, and verapamil), and others
Piper methysticum (kava)	Alcohol, alprazolam, CNS depressants, hepatotoxic drugs (azathioprine, methotrexate, and tamoxifen), levodopa, other drugs metabolized by cytochrome p450 enzymes: CYP1A2, CYP2C9 (tamoxifen and warfarin); CYP 2C19 (cyclophosphamide), CYP2D6 (codeine, ondansetron, and paroxetine), and CYP3A4 (cyclosporine and others)

NNRTIs, nonnucleoside reverse transcriptase inhibitors; MAOI, monoamine oxidase inhibitors; CNS, central nervous system.

Source: From Jellin JM, Gregory PJ, Batz F, Hitchens K, et al. *Pharmacist's Letter/Prescriber's Letter Natural Medicines Comprehensive Database.* Stockton, CA: Therapeutic Research Faculty; www.naturaldatabase. com, accessed on December 5, 2003, with permission.

TABLE 41.3. *Caveats of CAM therapy*

Therapy	Caveat
Highly restrictive diets	Poor nutritional status
Antioxidants	Concurrent radio/chemotherapy
Supplements with anticoagulant activity	Low platelet count, surgery
Phytoestrogens	Breast cancer (ER+)
Acupuncture	Low platelet count, anticoagulation
Deep tissue/forceful massage	Low platelet count, anticoagulation
St. John's wort	Chemotherapy (see Table 41.2)
High-dose vitamin A	Try to avoid
High-dose vitamin C	Try to avoid

RESOURCES

CAM cancer research: http://www.cancer.gov/cam/research_information.html

CAM cancer research trials: http://www.nci.nih.gov/clinicaltrials

CAM in cancer: http://cancer.gov/cancerinfo/pdq/cam

Dietary supplement research: http://ods.od.nih.gov/research/research.aspx

Dietary supplements: http://ods.od.nih.gov/Health_Information/Health_Information.aspx

Information about CAM: http://nccam.nih.gov/health

Information about CAM cancer research: http://nccam.nih.gov/research

National Cancer Institute (NCI): http://www.cancer.gov

National Center for Complementary and Alternative Medicine (NCCAM): http://nccam.nih.gov

Office of Cancer Complementary and Alternative Medicine (OCCAM), NCI: http://www.cancer.gov/cam/index.html

Thinking about CAM: A guide for people with cancer: http://www.cancer.gov/cancertopics/thinking-about-CAM

REFERENCES

1. Ernst E, Cassileth BR. The prevalence of complementary/alternative medicine in cancer: a systematic review. *Cancer.* 1998;83(4):777–82.
2. Morris KT, Johnson N, Homer L, Walts D. A comparison of complementary therapy use between breast cancer patients and patients with other primary tumor sites. *Am J Surg.* 2000;179(5):407–11.
3. Beinfield H, Korngold E. Chinese medicine and cancer care. *Altern Ther Health Med.* 2003;9(5): 38–52.
4. Singh RH. An assessment of the ayurvedic concept of cancer and a new paradigm of anticancer treatment in Ayurveda. *J Altern Complement Med.* 2002;8(5):609–14.
5. Kundu A, Berman B. Acupuncture for pediatric pain and symptom management. *Pediatr Clin North Am.* 2007;54(6):885–9; x.
6. Shen J, Wenger N, Glaspy J, Hays RD, Albert PS, Choi C, et al. Electroacupuncture for control of myeloablative chemotherapy-induced emesis: a randomized controlled trial. *JAMA.* 2000;284(21):2755–61.
7. Ezzo JM, Richardson MA, Vickers A, Allen C, Dibble SL, Issell BF, et al. Acupuncture-point stimulation for chemotherapy-induced nausea or vomiting. *Cochrane Database Syst Rev.* 2006(2): CD002285.
8. Molassiotis A, Helin AM, Dabbour R, Hummerston S. The effects of P6 acupressure in the prophylaxis of chemotherapy-related nausea and vomiting in breast cancer patients. *Complement Ther Med.* 2007;15(1):3–12.
9. Molassiotis A, Sylt P, Diggins H. The management of cancer-related fatigue after chemotherapy with acupuncture and acupressure: a randomised controlled trial. *Complement Ther Med.* 2007;15(4):228–37.
10. Minton O, Higginson IJ. Electroacupuncture as an adjunctive treatment to control neuropathic pain in patients with cancer. *J Pain Symptom Manage.* 2007;33(2):115–7.

11. Alimi D, Rubino C, Pichard-Leandri E, Fermand-Brule S, Dubreuil-Lemaire ML, Hill C. Analgesic effect of auricular acupuncture for cancer pain: a randomized, blinded, controlled trial. *J Clin Oncol.* 2003;21(22):4120–6.

12. Melchart D, Weidenhammer W, Streng A, Reitmayr S, Hoppe A, Ernst E, et al. Prospective investigation of adverse effects of acupuncture in 97 733 patients. *Arch Intern Med.* 2004;164(1):104–5.

13. White A, Hayhoe S, Hart A, Ernst E. Adverse events following acupuncture: prospective survey of 32 000 consultations with doctors and physiotherapists. *BMJ.* 2001;323(7311):485–6.

14. MacPherson H, Thomas K, Walters S, Fitter M. The York acupuncture safety study: prospective survey of 34 000 treatments by traditional acupuncturists. *BMJ.* 2001;323(7311):486–7.

15. Sontakke S, Thawani V, Naik MS. Ginger as an antiemetic in nausea and vomiting induced by chemotherapy: a randomized, cross-over, double blind study. *Indian J Pharmacol.* 2003;35(1):32–36.

16. Elam JL, Carpenter JS, Shu XO, Boyapati S, Friedmann-Gilchrist J. Methodological issues in the investigation of ginseng as an intervention for fatigue. *Clin Nurse Spec.* 2006;20(4):183–9.

17. Zhang M, Liu X, Li J, He L, Tripathy D. Chinese medicinal herbs to treat the side-effects of chemotherapy in breast cancer patients. *Cochrane Database Syst Rev.* 2007(2):CD004921.

18. Zhang T, Ma SL, Xie GR, Deng QH, Tang ZZ, Pan XC, et al. Clinical research on nourishing yin and unblocking meridians recipe combined with opioid analgesics in cancer pain management. *Chin J Integr Med.* 2006;12(3):180–4.

19. Taixiang W, Munro AJ, Guanjian L. Chinese medical herbs for chemotherapy side effects in colorectal cancer patients. *Cochrane Database Syst Rev.* 2005(1):CD004540.

20. Block KI, Gyllenhaal C, Mead MN. Safety and efficacy of herbal sedatives in cancer care. *Integr Cancer Ther.* 2004;3(2):128–48.

21. Su CK, Mehta V, Ravikumar L, Shah R, Pinto H, Halpern J, et al. Phase II double-blind randomized study comparing oral aloe vera versus placebo to prevent radiation-related mucositis in patients with head-and-neck neoplasms. *Int J Radiat Oncol Biol Phys.* 2004;60(1):171–7.

22. Kronenberg F, Fugh-Berman A. Complementary and alternative medicine for menopausal symptoms: a review of randomized, controlled trials. *Ann Intern Med.* 2002;137(10):805–13.

23. Van Patten CL, Olivotto IA, Chambers GK, Gelmon KA, Hislop TG, Templeton E, et al. Effect of soy phytoestrogens on hot flashes in postmenopausal women with breast cancer: a randomized, controlled clinical trial. *J Clin Oncol.* 2002;20(6):1449–55.

24. Nikander E, Kilkkinen A, Metsa-Heikkila M, Adlercreutz H, Pietinen P, Tiitinen A, et al. A randomized placebo-controlled cross over trial with phytoestrogens in treatment of menopause in breast cancer patients. *Obstet Gynecol.* 2003;101(6):1213–20.

25. Kim JH, Park CY, Lee SJ. Effects of sun ginseng on subjective quality of life in cancer patients: a double-blind, placebo-controlled pilot trial. *J Clin Pharm Ther.* 2006;31(4):331–4.

26. Wei X, Chen ZY, Yang XY, Wu TX. Medicinal herbs for esophageal cancer. *Cochrane Database Syst Rev.* 2007(2):CD004520.

27. Hughes E, Barrows, K. Complementary & alternative medicine. In: McPhee S, Papadakis MA, Tierney LM Jr, eds. *Current Medical Diagnosis & Treatment 2009.* 48th ed. McGraw Hill; 2009.

28. Richardson J, Smith JE, McCall G, Richardson A, Pilkington K, Kirsch I. Hypnosis for nausea and vomiting in cancer chemotherapy: a systematic review of the research evidence. *Eur J Cancer Care (Engl).* 2007;16(5):402–12.

29. Richardson J, Smith JE, McCall G, Pilkington K. Hypnosis for procedure-related pain and distress in pediatric cancer patients: a systematic review of effectiveness and methodology related to hypnosis interventions. *J Pain Symptom Manage.* 2006;31(1):70–84.

30. Schnur JB, Bovbjerg DH, David D, Tatrow K, Goldfarb AB, Silverstein JH, et al. Hypnosis decreases presurgical distress in excisional breast biopsy patients. *Anesth Analg.* 2008;106(2):440–4.

31. Lang EV, Berbaum KS, Faintuch S, Hatsiopoulou O, Halsey N, Li X, et al. Adjunctive self-hypnotic relaxation for outpatient medical procedures: a prospective randomized trial with women undergoing large core breast biopsy. *Pain.* 2006;126(1-3):155–64.

32. Montgomery GH, Bovbjerg DH, Schnur JB, David D, Goldfarb A, Weltz CR, et al. A randomized clinical trial of a brief hypnosis intervention to control side effects in breast surgery patients. *J Natl Cancer Inst.* 2007;99(17):1304–12.

33. Elkins GR, Cheung A, Marcus J, Palamara L, Rajab H. Hypnosis to reduce pain in cancer survivors with advanced disease: a prospective study. *Journal of Cancer Integrative Medicine.* 2004;2(4):167–172.

34. Elkins G, Jensen MP, Patterson DR. Hypnotherapy for the management of chronic pain. *Int J Clin Exp Hypn.* 2007;55(3):275–87.

35. Rajasekaran M, Edmonds PM, Higginson IL. Systematic review of hypnotherapy for treating symptoms in terminally ill adult cancer patients. *Palliat Med.* 2005;19(5):418–26.

36. Sloman R, Brown P, Aldana E. The use of relaxation for the promotion of comfort and pain relief in persons with advanced cancer. *Contemp Nurse.* 1994;3:6–12.

37. Syrjala KL, Donaldson GW, Davis MW. Relaxation and imagery and cognitive-behavioral training reduce pain during cancer treatment: a controlled clinical trial. *Pain.* 1995;63:189–98.

38. Cassileth B, Trevisan C, Gubili J. Complementary therapies for cancer pain. *Curr Pain Headache Rep.* 2007;11(4):265–9.

39. Canter PH. The therapeutic effects of meditation. *BMJ.* 2003;326(7398):1049–50.

40. Barrows KA, Jacobs BP. Mind-body medicine. An introduction and review of the literature. *Med Clin North Am.* 2002;86(1):11–31.

41. Speca M, Carlson LE, Goodey E, Angen M. A randomized, wait-list controlled clinical trial: the effect of a mindfulness meditation-based stress reduction program on mood and symptoms of stress in cancer outpatients. *Psychosom Med.* 2000;62(5):613–22.

42. Carlson LE, Speca M, Patel KD, Goodey E. Mindfulness-based stress reduction in relation to quality of life, mood, symptoms of stress, and immune parameters in breast and prostate cancer outpatients. *Psychosom Med.* 2003;65(4):571–81.

43. Carlson LE, Ursuliak Z, Goodey E, Angen M, Speca M. The effects of a mindfulness meditation-based stress reduction program on mood and symptoms of stress in cancer outpatients: 6-month follow-up. *Support Care Cancer.* 2001;9(2):112–23.

44. Ott MJ, Norris RL, Bauer-Wu SM. Mindfulness meditation for oncology patients: a discussion and critical review. *Integr Cancer Ther.* 2006;5(2):98–108.

45. Ott MJ. Complementary and alternative therapies in cancer symptom management. *Cancer Pract.* 2002;10(3):162–6.

46. Moadel AB, Shah C, Wylie-Rosett J, Harris MS, Patel SR, Hall CB, et al. Randomized controlled trial of yoga among a multiethnic sample of breast cancer patients: effects on quality of life. *J Clin Oncol.* 2007;25(28):4387–95.

47. Banerjee B, Vadiraj HS, Ram A, Rao R, Jayapal M, Gopinath KS, et al. Effects of an integrated yoga program in modulating psychological stress and radiation-induced genotoxic stress in breast cancer patients undergoing radiotherapy. *Integr Cancer Ther.* 2007;6(3):242–50.

48. Culos-Reed SN, Carlson LE, Daroux LM, Hately-Aldous S. A pilot study of yoga for breast cancer survivors: physical and psychological benefits. *Psychooncology.* 2006;15(10):891–7.

49. Fellowes D, Barnes K, Wilkinson S. Aromatherapy and massage for symptom relief in patients with cancer. *Cochrane Database Syst Rev.* 2004(2):CD002287.

50. Cassileth BR, Vickers AJ. Massage therapy for symptom control: outcome study at a major cancer center. *J Pain Symptom Manage.* 2004;28(3):244–9.

51. Johansson K, Albertsson M, Ingvar C, Ekdahl C. Effects of compression bandaging with or without manual lymph drainage treatment in patients with postoperative arm lymphedema. *Lymphology.* 1999;32(3):103–10.

52. Johansson K, Lie E, Ekdahl C, Lindfeldt J. A randomized study comparing manual lymph drainage with sequential pneumatic compression for treatment of postoperative arm lymphedema. *Lymphology.* 1998;31(2):56–64.

53. Ernst E. The safety of massage therapy. *Rheumatology (Oxford).* 2003;42(9):1101–6.

54. Corbin L. Safety and efficacy of massage therapy for patients with cancer. *Cancer Control.* 2005;12(3):158–64.

55. Astin JA, Harkness E, Ernst E. The efficacy of "distant healing": a systematic review of randomized trials. *Ann Intern Med.* 2000;132(11):903–10.

56. Collipp PJ. The efficacy of prayer: a triple-blind study. *Med Times.* 1969;97(5):201–4.

57. Olson K, Hanson J, Michaud M. A phase II trial of Reiki for the management of pain in advanced cancer patients. *J Pain Symptom Manage.* 2003;26(5):990–7.

58. Heinonen OP, Albanes D, Virtamo J, Taylor PR, Huttunen JK, Hartman AM, et al. Prostate cancer and supplementation with alpha-tocopherol and beta-carotene: incidence and mortality in a controlled trial. *J Natl Cancer Inst.* 1998;90(6):440–6.

59. Omenn GS, Goodman GE, Thornquist MD, Balmes J, Cullen MR, Glass A, et al. Effects of a combination of beta carotene and vitamin A on lung cancer and cardiovascular disease. *N Engl J Med.* 1996;334(18):1150–5.

60. Weitzman S. Alternative nutritional cancer therapies. *Int J Cancer Suppl.* 1998;11:69–72.

61. Padayatty SJ, Levine M. Reevaluation of ascorbate in cancer treatment: emerging evidence, open minds and serendipity. *J Am Coll Nutr.* 2000;19(4):423–5.

62. Padayatty SJ, Katz A, Wang Y, Eck P, Kwon O, Lee JH, et al. Vitamin C as an antioxidant: evaluation of its role in disease prevention. *J Am Coll Nutr.* 2003;22(1):18–35.

63. Weiger WA, Smith M, Boon H, Richardson MA, Kaptchuk TJ, Eisenberg DM. Advising patients who seek complementary and alternative medical therapies for cancer. *Ann Intern Med.* 2002;137(11):889–903.

64. Blot WJ, Li JY, Taylor PR, Guo W, Dawsey SM, Li B. The Linxian trials: mortality rates by vitamin-mineral intervention group. *Am J Clin Nutr.* 1995;62(6 Suppl):1424S–6S.

65. Taylor PR, Qiao YL, Abnet CC, Dawsey SM, Yang CS, Gunter EW, et al. Prospective study of serum vitamin E levels and esophageal and gastric cancers. *J Natl Cancer Inst.* 2003;95(18):1414–6.

66. *Food, Nutrition, Physical Activity, and the Prevention of Cancer: A Global Perspective.* Washington DC: World Cancer Research Fund/American Institute for Cancer Research; 2007.

67. Doyle C, Kushi LH, Byers T, Courneya KS, Demark-Wahnefried W, Grant B, et al. Nutrition and physical activity during and after cancer treatment: an American Cancer Society guide for informed choices. *CA Cancer J Clin.* 2006;56(6):323–53.

68. Penotti M, Fabio E, Modena AB, Rinaldi M, Omodei U, Vigano P. Effect of soy-derived isoflavones on hot flushes, endometrial thickness, and the pulsatility index of the uterine and cerebral arteries. *Fertil Steril.* 2003;79(5):1112–7.

69. Dixon RA, Ferreira D. Genistein. *Phytochemistry.* 2002;60(3):205–11.

70. Messina MJ, Loprinzi CL. Soy for breast cancer survivors: a critical review of the literature. *J Nutr.* 2001;131(11 Suppl):3095S–108S.

71. Castle EP, Thrasher JB. The role of soy phytoestrogens in prostate cancer. *Urol Clin North Am.* 2002;29(1):71–81, viii–ix.

72. Morrissey C, Watson RW, Castle EP, Thrasher JB. Phytoestrogens and prostate cancer. The role of soy phytoestrogens in prostate cancer. *Curr Drug Targets.* 2003;4(3):231–41.

73. Slavin JL. Mechanisms for the impact of whole grain foods on cancer risk. *J Am Coll Nutr.* 2000;19(3 Suppl):300S–7S.

74. Riboli E, Norat T. Epidemiologic evidence of the protective effect of fruit and vegetables on cancer risk. *Am J Clin Nutr.* 2003;78(3 Suppl):559S–569S.

75. Rock CL, Demark-Wahnefried W. Nutrition and survival after the diagnosis of breast cancer: a review of the evidence. *J Clin Oncol.* 2002;20(15):3302–16.

76. Goodwin PJ, Ennis M, Pritchard KI, Koo J, Trudeau ME, Hood N. Diet and breast cancer: evidence that extremes in diet are associated with poor survival. *J Clin Oncol.* 2003;21(13):2500–7.

77. Pierce JP, Natarajan L, Caan BJ, Parker BA, Greenberg ER, Flatt SW, et al. Influence of a diet very high in vegetables, fruit, and fiber and low in fat on prognosis following treatment for breast cancer: the Women's Healthy Eating and Living (WHEL) randomized trial. *JAMA.* 2007;298(3):289–98.

78. Gerson M. The cure of advanced cancer by diet therapy: a summary of 30 years of clinical experimentation. *Physiol Chem Phys.* 1978;10(5):449–64.

79. Kushi LH, Cunningham JE, Hebert JR, Lerman RH, Bandera EV, Teas J. The macrobiotic diet in cancer. *J Nutr.* 2001;131(11 Suppl):3056S–64S.

80. Gonzalez NJ, Isaacs LL. Evaluation of pancreatic proteolytic enzyme treatment of adenocarcinoma of the pancreas, with nutrition and detoxification support. *Nutr Cancer.* 1999;33(2):117–24.

81. Chlebowski RT, Blackburn GL, Thomson CA, Nixon DW, Shapiro A, Hoy MK, et al. Dietary fat reduction and breast cancer outcome: interim efficacy results from the women's intervention nutrition study. *J Natl Cancer Inst.* 2006;98(24):1767–76.

82. Pierce JP, Stefanick ML, Flatt SW, Natarajan L, Sternfeld B, Madlensky L, et al. Greater survival after breast cancer in physically active women with high vegetable-fruit intake regardless of obesity. *J Clin Oncol.* 2007;25(17):2345–51.

83. Sorensen JM. Herb-drug, food-drug, nutrient-drug, and drug-drug interactions: mechanisms involved and their medical implications. *J Altern Complement Med.* 2002;8(3):293–308.

42

Central Venous Access Device

June L. Remick and Magesh Sundaram

Once the diagnosis of cancer has been made, the oncology patient will go through staging and management of the disease. Typically, a large battery of blood tests is drawn, often repeatedly, during staging and treatment to document the patient's clinical well-being and the progress of treatment. Added to this are a rigorous venous sampling schedule, the need for intravenous (i.v.) access, and contrast administration during radiologic imaging studies. Most of these exams can be instituted without establishing a long-term venous access device, however it is prudent to anticipate long-term needs early in treatment.

Factors to consider early on are the patient's age, as the elderly may have small, fragile, and damaged peripheral vessels; prior hospitalizations with peripheral or central i.v. access; past medical treatments where patients have been treated with vesicant i.v. medications such as antibiotics or chemotherapy agents; and surgical alteration of venous and lymphatic anatomy, as with a mastectomy, with resultant lymphedema. These patients begin therapy with compromised venous access and attempts should be instituted to preserve all vasculature. As with any procedure vascular access is not without risks and should be carefully considered to provide the most appropriate access device to meet the patient's needs while minimizing insertion or foreign body complications.

INDICATIONS

Indications for venous access placement in the oncology patient are guided by complex factors that evolve during the transition from diagnosis through treatment and into remission. Consideration is given to the composition of the infusates being administered; the frequency of treatment (monthly vs. daily); the size or number of lumens required; patient's ability to provide self-care of the device; patient's preference, which may be influenced by vanity (not an inappropriate consideration as part of the decision-making process); and cost of catheter including possible daily maintenance with flushes and dressing changes that may not be covered by insurance. A transplant patient, for example, may require a large bore multichannel catheter for stem cell collection initially, but will also need a long-term catheter for the transplant process. Historically, transplant patients require a rigid temporary catheter for retrieval of stem cells, which would be removed after adequate stem cell collection. This process would be followed by a tunneled central catheter placed surgically for treatment. New catheters such as the Trifusion catheter (Bard Access Systems) are now being introduced, which can accommodate both collection and transplantation in some patients. Ongoing evaluation and reevaluation are required to manage access in these complex situations.

Venous access devices can be categorized into five groups based on mechanism of insertion and catheter dwell. These categories include peripheral angiocatheters, peripherally inserted central catheters, percutaneous or nontunneled central catheters, tunneled central catheters, and implanted ports. Each category is then further defined by device-specific characteristics, such as flow rates, lumen size, catheter tip location, and dwell time. In utilizing this process, it is easier to identify which catheter meets the specific needs of the patient (Table 42.1).

Peripheral Angiocatheter

The simplest access utilized in patients is the standard peripheral angiocatheter also known as peripheral intravenous access (PIV). These devices are relatively easy to insert and discontinue.

TABLE 42.1. *Summary of types of venous access catheters*

Type of catheter	Indications	Limitations
Peripheral angiocatheters and midline catheters	Hydration, PPN, short-term access	Frequent infiltration/phlebitis; easily dislodged; short dwell time (up to 72° PIV, 2–4 weeks midline); cannot be used for solutions with extreme pH or osmolarity; not for home-going patients
Peripherally inserted central catheters	Hydration, antibiotic, blood infusion/withdrawal, chemotherapy, medication administration; dwell up to 1 year or more	Requires weekly dressing change and flushing, must keep dry at all times, limited flow rates, visible, easily dislodged, higher occlusion rate, avoid placement if potential dialysis in future
Nontunneled catheters: a) Central lines b) Temporary rigid dialysis catheters	a) Acute-care medication, large bore access, hydration, all i.v. medication, CVP measurements b) Hemodialysis, stem cell collection and transplant requiring only dual lumen access, plasmapheresis treatment	Short dwell time: 7–14 days central lines, 1–4 weeks rigid catheters; higher risk of infection than tunneled catheter; increased risk of dislodgement; uncomfortable on clavicle; highly visible
Tunneled catheters: a) Traditional tunneled catheter b) Tunneled dialysis catheters c) Hybrid triple lumen tunneled catheters	a) Long-term i.v. medication, hydration, chemotherapy b) Hemodialysis, plasmapheresis, stem cell collection/dual lumen transplant access c) Stem cell collection, transplantation requiring triple lumen	Requires routine dressing changes and flushing, must keep site dry at all times, may be visible to others
Implanted ports: a) Chest ports b) Arm ports	Intermittent i.v. access, chemotherapy, hydration, antibiotics, lab draws	Requires needle stick to access, difficult to access in obese patients

PPN, peripheral parenteral nutrition; i.v., intravenous; CVP, central venous pressure; PIV, peripheral intravenous catheter.

Specialized training/certification is not required for standard insertions and most practitioners are competent. They come in a variety of gauges and lengths to accommodate patients with small vasculature as well as large-bore peripheral catheters preferred for rapid infusion of large volumes such as venous contrast or blood infusions. Intermittent nonvesicant chemotherapy can be administered via peripheral access, however reliability of obtaining access during each treatment session may be unpredictable. Therapy with extremes of pH (normal pH = 7.35–7.45) or osmolarity (normal 280–295 mOsm/L) should not be administered through peripheral access as the concentration of material infused can lead to patient discomfort, infiltration, clotting, and infection (3). An exception is parenteral nutrition with dextrose contents under 10% and osmolarities >500 mOsm/L (INS), which are safe to administer peripherally. Limitations of these catheters include short dwell time (1–3 days), high thrombophlebitis rates, thrombosis and shear of the vessel, infiltration into the surrounding tissue, cellulitis, sepsis, and pain with infusions (3). As a result of these limitations, PIVs are reserved primarily for hospital/clinic use and management by health care professionals.

Midline Catheters

A subclass of peripheral angiocatheters include midline catheters. Midline catheters are peripherally inserted central catheters (PICC), usually inserted into the antecubital fossa or in brachial veins, with the guidance of a handheld ultrasound device. The catheter is then advanced proximally 8 to 10 inches, as far as the axillary region. In this position, the catheter is not considered central and should be treated as a peripheral angiocatheter with regard to infusates. However, since the catheter tip is in a larger vessel with increased blood flow the risk of phlebitis and infiltration is decreased as compared to peripheral angiocatheters. Typical dwell time for midline catheters is 1 to 2 weeks with careful monitoring for complications (3). In addition to extended dwell time, the midline, unlike a PICC, does not need radiographic verification for tip placement, since it is not advanced centrally. This benefit yields less costly insertion fees and simplification of insertion-related malpositioning.

Midline catheters do have limitations. First, their tips do not reside centrally so infusates are limited to those safe for PIV. Since the axillary veins lie deep it may be difficult to identify early phlebitis, infiltration, or infection. Frequently, a blood return is not achieved for confirmation of vascular patency or specimen collection. The short catheter length compared to the external component yields increased risk of dislodgement. Midline catheters require daily flushing to maintain patency and dressing changes at least weekly, which may require home health services.

Peripherally Inserted Central Catheter (PICC)

A PICC is a long, flexible catheter that is inserted into a peripheral vein and advanced into the central circulation. It is typically placed in a vein of the upper arm although it can also be introduced in the internal or external jugular veins, the long and short saphenous veins, or the temporal or posterior auricular veins. The saphenous vein, temporal vein, and posterior auricular veins are usually reserved for pediatric patients. Once the vein is cannulated, the catheter is digitally advanced until its distal tip resides in the superior vena cava (SVC) or the inferior vena cava (IVC) relative to the insertion site vessel. There is minimal risk to chest organs as seen in direct central vessel access. The tip location of the PICC is desired in the lower third of the SVC preferably at the junction of the right atrium and SVC or IVC. The external component is secured to skin, preferably with a removable locking device or sutures.

PICC catheters come in single, dual, or triple lumens in a variety of sizes. The catheters have a small outer diameter allowing for initial insertion into smaller vessels prior to advancement centrally and are radio-opaque for visualization of catheter tip placement on chest radiograph. These devices can be modified in length, specific to each patient. Some PICCs are approved for use with power injectors that can rapidly administer a radiologic contrast bolus. Insertion can be done during inpatient hospitalization, outpatient settings, and in the home by certified nurses.

PICC catheters are used for patients with poor venous access; infusions of solutions with extreme pH or osmolarity; extended i.v. medication use (1 week to several months in duration); intermittent blood sampling; and as a respite from long-term catheters. Patients with acute line infections who need extraction of the compromised catheter but still require central access are ideal candidates for PICCs. Power-injectable PICCs may be utilized in patients where frequent power injection procedures are likely.

The relatively small lumen and long length result in decreased flow rates, especially with infusions of viscous solutions such as blood products or i.v. nutrition therapy and often cannot be used for gravity-driven infusions when pumps are unavailable such as in home settings. Frequent flushing of the catheter with normal saline and/or heparin–lock, and dressing changes weekly or more frequently may be challenging for some patients. In addition, careful attention is required to protect the exposed catheter exit site from contamination or damage. The patient's modesty may be compromised due to visibility of the external component. There are activity limitations including no straining maneuvers such as heavy lifting or straining that could alter thoracic pressure leading to catheter malposition. Malpositioning can even occur with physiologic pressure changes during cough or forceful emesis. Submersion of the extremity in water when bathing in pools or hot tubs during catheter dwell is forbidden secondary to infection risks. Patients may not be candidates for PICCs if they have had surgical alteration of anatomy, lymphedema, ipsilateral radiation to the chest or arm, or loss of skin integrity at the anticipated insertion site, or anticipate future dialysis access needs (3).

However minimal, PICC-related complications can be anticipated. These include infection, phlebitis, vein thrombosis, catheter occlusion, catheter breakage/leaking, and inadvertent removal prior to completion of therapy (Table 42.2). Oncology patients are at increased risk for venous thrombus formation secondary to their malignancy, treatment regimen, and the trauma of catheter insertion and dwell (8).

TABLE 42.2.   *Tabulation of complications of various venous access approaches*

Complication	PICC (%)	Nontunneled central catheters (%)	Tunneled central catheters (%)	Implanted catheters (%)
Examples of access	PICC	Central line, rigid temporary catheter	Traditional, dialysis, hybrid	Peripheral port(s), chest port(s)
Arterial puncture				2.4
Malposition	5–10	5–10	5–10	0.5 5–10
Pneumothorax	0.2–6.0	0.2–6.0	0.2–6.0	0.3 0.2–6.0
Venous thrombosis: asymptomatic, symptomatic, cancer patient	3.4 AS = 23–39(L) S = 3.4–3.9(L)		AS = 30–74(L) S = 4.7–10(L)	0.8% (general venous thrombosis) AS = 2–30(L) S = 0–9 chest(L) S = 2–30 arm(L)
Bacteremia	0.4–20	20–22	10–20	
Pocket infection				0.5
Cardiac tamponade	0.25–1.4	0.25–1.4	0.25–1.4	0.25–1.4
Phlebitis	6.6			
Additional complications Hemothorax Tunnel infection Air embolism				
Comments	Tabulation from cancer patients			Tabulation from cancer patients
References	3, 7, 9–12	3, 6, 9–12, 15	6, 9–12, 15	6, 9–12, 15

PICC, peripherally inserted central catheters.

Percutaneous Central Venous Catheters

These catheters, either the thin flexible or the larger rigid variety, are inserted directly into the central circulation via the subclavian vein, the external jugular vein, the internal jugular vein, or the femoral vein. Catheters included in this category include standard central venous catheters (CVC) or temporary rigid hemodialysis/aphoresis catheters. The CVC is utilized in the hospital setting for acute central venous access with dwell time up to 14 days. CVCs are typically used for rapid infusion; multiple infusates needed simultaneously or for hemodynamic monitoring (central venous pressure measurement). CVCs may be exchanged over guidewire, using sterile technique, for longer dwell times. CVCs are for use in acute care settings, thus reserving them for hospitalized patients only.

Frequent assessment of the catheter for integrity, dislodgment, and site evaluation is required. Flushing of each catheter lumen is performed frequently for patency. Complications related to insertion include infection, bleeding, inadvertent arterial access, air embolism, pneumothorax, hemothorax, cardiac perforation and tamponade, and cardiac dysrhythmia. The cancer patient with cachexia cancer patient is at increased risk for insertion complications as are patients with large body habitus or coagulopathies. Utilization of image-guided placement with ultrasound technology for venipuncture and modified Seldinger approach helps to minimize these risks. During catheter dwell infection, thrombosis of the accessed vein, loss of catheter lumens patency, and dislodgment can occur.

The rigid nontunneled central catheters are typically used for acute hemodialysis; hemodialysis access post removal of an infected tunneled dialysis catheter; stem cell collection for autologous transplant or healthy donor collection; or therapeutic aphoresis. These catheters are placed by certified nurse practitioners, physician assistants, or physicians at the bedside, in a surgical suite, or in interventional radiology with image guidance. Unlike CVCs, the rigid catheters can dwell for up to 4 to 6 weeks if free of complications. Often in hemodialysis, temporary rigid catheters are exchanged over a guidewire for a new rigid catheter or exchanged for a tunneled dialysis catheter. Catheter exchange at the same venous site can indefinitely maintain a single access site, which may be limited in hemodialysis patients or oncology patients from prior access and thrombosis of other central access points.

The catheter exit site must by kept dry with an intact occlusive dressing changed biweekly to minimize infection risks. The lumens are given a high-dose heparin lock to maintain patency. Inadvertent flushing of the heparin lock can lead to bleeding. Accidental dislodgment of the rigid catheter can occur even though sutures are placed. Usage of these catheters and dressing changes are typically reserved for certified dialysis technicians to provide optimal consistent management. Dressing changes and flushing for patients undergoing stem cell collection are managed by nursing services.

Tunneled Catheters

A tunneled catheter is a larger bore catheter inserted by tunneling through the subcutaneous tissue prior to entrance into the central circulation with the tip of the catheter terminating in the SVC/right atrial junction or IVC/atrial junction. A retention cuff, which causes inflammation and ingrowth to the cuff, is integrated on the catheter. The cuff is positioned approximately 1 to 2 cm within the skin insertion point. The cuff serves as a barrier to bacteria migration along the tract into the central circulation. After tunnelling, the catheter is threaded into the central circulation via the internal/external jugular veins, subclavian vein, femoral vein, or lumbar vein access in vein-compromised patients. Tunneled catheters can be further divided into three types; tradition tunneled catheters best know as the Hickman or Broviac which is intended for infusions requiring long-term use such as total parenteral nutrition, chemotherapy, hydration or chronic medication administration, blood infusion or retrieval; dialysis catheters that are typically used for hemodialysis but more recently they are additionally utilized for stem cell collection and post-transplant venous access; and hybrid tunneled catheters that can be used for stem cell collection, transplant access, or photophoresis treatments in graft-versus-host disease of transplant patients. These catheters are available in single, double, or triple lumens and a variety of lumen sizes and lengths. Some catheters are also modifiable for size. These catheters are known for lower rate of infection as compared to nontunneled catheters.

Management of tunneled catheters requires flushing protocols, weekly dressing changes, and protection from inadvertent dislodgment. In addition, the patient is restricted from submersion of the catheter during bathing or swimming. Tunneled catheters with high-dose heparin lock solution require removal of the lock prior to catheter use to prevent inadvertent systemic heparinization. Catheters containing valve devices may only require saline flushes, thus simplifying this regime.

Complications of tunneled catheters include the expected ones associated with the insertion procedure (i.e., bleeding, air embolus, pneumothorax, cardiac dysrhythmia) as well as long-term issues (i.e., infection, migration, thrombosis, catheter shear). Most medical centers will stock catheter repair kits that allow salvage of a cracked or leaking part of these longer-term indwelling catheters. Extrusion of the cuff from the subcutaneous position is an indication for replacement or removal of the tunneled catheter (3,8).

Implanted Ports

Implanted ports are CVCs attached to a reservoir with a self-sealing septum. The reservoir is surgically implanted into a pocket in the subcutaneous tissue and the attached catheter is tunneled subcutaneously before advancement into the central venous circulation. The reservoir insertion site typically include the anterior chest wall, the arm, or thigh placement with the catheter advanced into the corresponding vein. The implanted port is ideal for patients undergoing intermittent or cyclic therapy when daily access is not required. Ports are well known for chemotherapy administration or venous access for lab draws in vein-compromised patients requiring chronic access. Newer models of implanted ports allow for use with power i.v. contrast injections for radiologic imaging. Medical device companies also promote ports with differing flow patterns or characteristics within the reservoir chamber (i.e., "the port") that claim to improve infusion, blood draws, and lower thrombosis rates.

Use of the port requires sterile preparation of the site and access with a noncoring Huber needle to prevent damage to the reservoir. The patient may feel a needle stick as the port is being accessed, but the discomfort may be minimized by applying topical anesthetics, or Emla cream, to the port site prior to the needle stick. While the port is accessed, it requires daily flushing; however, when it is not used at least monthly only intermittent flushes are required to maintain patency.

The port provides patient privacy as it is not visible once deaccessed. In addition, active patients may find more freedom during unaccessed periods. The port has the lowest incidence of infection related to implantation. These catheters have an extended dwell time of several years or longer depending on number of punctures into the septum. Consideration should be given to retaining the port for a period of time after completion of therapy for use in surveillance blood testing purposes.

Power Injection Catheters

Catheters, such as PICCs, have been studied in the past for safety in power injection with mixed results in efficacy depending on the gauge, length, and material of the catheter. In one study, silicone PICC catheters were found to have very low burst rates not conducive to power injection and polyurethane catheters varied greatly (1,14). Incidence of inadequate flow rates and catheter rupture due to limited PSI restrictions from manufacturers have limited the use of most catheters for power injection until recently. Optimal contrast imaging requires uniform contrast delivery, which is best achieved by power injection at 2 mL/sec (13). In fact, these limitations have led to current trends in catheter manufacturing in which some catheters can tolerate 300 pounds per square inch (Bard Access). Candidates for power injection catheters include those anticipated to have recurring contrast medium injection studies versus one-time usage. Herts et al. studied a variety of CVCs including standard CVC, tunneled catheters, and implanted ports finding successful injections without harm to the patients or catheter (2). Some vascular imaging limitations were noted. Their findings suggest usage of central lines as a possible alternative to peripheral angiocatheters. Institutional policies need to address these catheters for identification and usage as there may be additional training required of the staff prior to utilizing to prevent complications. Special equipment may be required for accessing power injection ports to prevent rupture or extravasation. In addition, the more rigid catheter required for power injection may lead to increased complications such as phlebitis or thrombosis.

Valve Technology

Ongoing clinical presentation of heparin allergies, specifically heparin-induced thrombocytopenia has led to marketing of catheters with valve technology. The valve remains closed unless acted upon by negative (aspiration) or positive (infusion) pressure. It is this technology that opposes central venous pressure preventing reflux of blood into the catheter tip during the cardiac cycle, or changes in intrathoracic pressure such as with straining of vomiting. Additionally, removal of a syringe after flushing or deaccessing the port can facilitate negative pressure drawing blood into the catheter (5). Without blood in the catheter tip, the risk of catheter occlusion related to internal clotting is thought to be eliminated as well as decreased infection rate (4). Lamont et al. found the PASV (Boston Scientific Corporation, Natick, Mass) valved implanted port had a lower incidence of difficulty in obtaining a blood return than the Groshong (Bard Access System, Salt Lake City, Utah) which resulted in less nursing time trouble shooting (5). Valve technology has been incorporated into some catheters at the distal tip or in the proximal end piece. This technology is also available as an "add-on" device for catheters. A saline-only flush is recommended however, heparin flushes are not a contraindication.

REFERENCES

1. Salis AI, Eclavea A, Johnson JS, Patel NH, Wong DG, Tennery G. Maximal flow rates possible during power injection through currently available PICCs: an in vitro study. *JVIR* 2004;15:275–281.
2. Herts BR, O'Malley CM, Wirht SL, Lieber ML, Pohlman B. Power injection of contrast media using central venous catheters. *AJR Am J Roentgenol* 2001;176:447–453.

3. Vanek VW. The Ins and outs of venous access: Part I. *Nutr Clin Pract* 2002 April;17:85–98.
4. Hoffer EK, Borsa JJ, Santulli P, Bloch RD, Fontaine AB. Prospective randomized comparison of valved versus nonvalved peripherally inserted central vein catheters. *AJR Am J Roentgeno* 1999;173:1393–1398.
5. Lamont JP, McCarty TM, Stephens JS, et al. A randomized trial of valved vs nonvalved implantable ports for vascular access. *BUMC Proceedings* 2003;16:384–387.
6. Ozyuvaci E, Kutlu F. Totally implanted venous access devices via subclavian vein: a retrospective study of 368 oncology patients. *Adv Therapy* 2006;23:574–581.
7. Walshe LJ, Malak SF, Eagan J, Sepkowitz KA. Complication rates among cancer patients with peripherally inserted central catheters. *J Clin Oncol* 2002;20(15):3276–3281.
8. Verso M, Agnelli G. Venous thromboembolism associated with long-term use of central venous catheters in cancer patients. *J Clin Oncol* 2003;21(19):3665–3675.
9. Linenberger ML. Catheter related thrombosis:risks, diagnosis and management. *J Natl Compr Canc Netw* 2006;4(9):889–901.
10. Kluger DM, Maki DG. A meta-analysis of the risk of intravascular device (IVD)-related blood stream infection (BSI) based on 223 published prospective studies. *Abstr intersci Conf Antimicrob agents chemother intersci conf antimicrob agents chemothery* 1999 Sep 26–29;39:647 (abstract no.1913).
11. Forauer AR. Pericardial tamponade in patients with central venous catheter. *J Infus Nurs* 2007 May/June;30(3):161–167.
12. Hamilton H. Complications associated with venous access devices: part one. *Nurs Stand* 2006 March;20(26):43–51.
13. Williamson EE, McKinnley JM. Assessing the adequacy of peripherally inserted central catheters for power injection of intravenous contrast agents for CT. *J Comput Assist Tomogr* 2001;25(6): 932–937.
14. Rivitz SM, Drucker EA. Power injection of peripherally inserted central catheters. *J Vasc Interv Radiol* September–October 1997;8(5):857–863.
15. Maecken T, Grau T. Ultrasound imaging in vascular access. *Crit Care Med* 2007;35(5):S178–S185.

SECTION 12

Common Office Procedures and Other Topics

43

Procedures in Medical Oncology

Suzanne G. Demko, Kerry Ryan, and George Carter

Procedures performed in oncology patients may serve both diagnosis and treatment. This chapter describes common procedures performed in medical oncology, along with special considerations and techniques to assist in performing them rapidly and confidently, and to keep the patient comfortable and well informed.

INFORMED CONSENT

Written informed consent, or a legally sufficient substitute, must be obtained before every procedure described here and filed in the patient's medical record.

ANESTHESIA

All procedures should be performed under local anesthesia. For certain patients and procedures, premedication with a narcotic (fentanyl) and a benzodiazepine (midazolam) should be considered. Lidocaine (1% mixed in a 3:1 or 5:1 ratio with $NaHCO_3$ to prevent the usual lidocaine sting) will ensure proper anesthetic effect.

INSTRUMENTS

Most medical facilities are equipped with sterile trays or self-contained disposable kits specific to each procedure. Additional instruments may be used at the operator's discretion or preference.

PROCEDURES

Bone Marrow Aspiration and Biopsy

Indications

- Diagnosis
- Analysis of abnormal blood cell production
- Staging of hematologic and nonhematologic malignancies

Contraindications

- Severe thrombocytopenia (<20,000); platelet transfusion may be given before procedure.
- Skin infection at proposed site of biopsy
- Biopsy at previously radiated site may cause fibrosis; consider alternative site.
- Avoid sternal aspirate in patients with thoracic aortic aneurysm or lytic bone disease of ribs or sternum.
- Heparin should be discontinued before procedure and resumed after hemostasis is achieved.

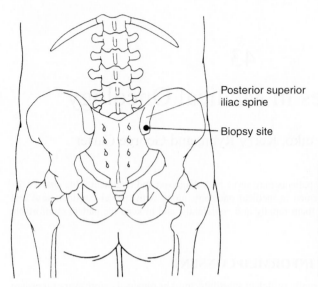

Posterior superior
iliac spine

Biopsy site

Fig. 43.1. Biopsy site in the posterior superior iliac spine. The needle should be directed toward the anterior superior iliac spine. (Used with permission from Chestnut MS, Dewar TN, Locksley RM. *Office and Bedside Procedures.* Norwalk, CT: Appleton & Lange; 1992:381.)

Anatomy

- Sternal aspiration
  - Patient is supine; head is not elevated.
  - Landmarks: sternal angle of Louis and lateral borders of sternum in second intercostal space
- Posterior superior iliac spine aspiration and biopsy (Fig. 43.1)
  - Patient is prone or in lateral decubitus position.
- Anterior iliac crest aspiration and biopsy (for patients with history of radiation to pelvis or extremely obese patients)
  - Patient is supine.

Procedure

- Sternal aspiration
  1. Identify landmarks, clean the area, and position a fenestrated drape using sterile technique.
  2. In the area to be aspirated, infiltrate the skin, subcutaneous tissues, and periosteum with 1% lidocaine for anesthesia. Using the infiltration needle, "sound" the surface of the bone to approximate the distance from skin to periosteum.
  3. Use a 16-gauge sternal aspiration needle with guard to prevent penetration of the posterior table of the sternum. Adjust needle guard based on the approximate distance from skin to periosteum.
  4. Make a 2 mm superficial skin incision with a surgical blade in the midsternum, medial at the second intercostal space.
  5. Introduce the aspiration needle with guard, using gentle, corkscrew-type pressure to advance the needle until fixed in bone. Remove obturator, attach a 10 to 12 mL syringe, and aspirate. The pain of this procedure cannot be prevented but lasts only a few seconds.
  6. Obtain 1 mL of aspirate. An amount >1 mL will be diluted by peripheral blood.
  7. Spicules of bone marrow will be present unless significant fibrosis is present or the marrow is packed with leukemia or other malignancy.
  8. If no specimen is obtained, replace the obturator and carefully advance the needle 2 to 3 mm to repeat aspiration.
  9. Prepare smears for evaluation.

- Posterior superior iliac spine aspiration and biopsy
  1. The technique described here is for the Jamshidi bone marrow needle. Other available needles, such as the HS Trapsystem Set and Goldenberg Snarecoil, are variations of the Jamshidi with their own specific instructions.

2. The patient may be prone, but the lateral decubitus position is more comfortable for the patient and better for identifying anatomic sites. These positions are suitable for all but the most obese patients. For extremely obese patients or for those who have had radiation to the pelvis, aspirate and biopsy may be taken from the anterior iliac crest.
3. Once the site has been prepared and anesthetized, make a small incision at the site of insertion, and advance the needle into the bone cortex until it is fixed. Attempt to aspirate 0.2 to 0.5 mL of marrow contents. If unsuccessful, advance the needle slightly and try again. Failure to obtain aspirate, known as a "dry tap," is often due to alterations within the marrow associated with myeloproliferative or leukemic disorders and less commonly due to faulty technique. In such case, a touch preparation of the biopsy often provides sufficient cellular material for diagnostic evaluation.
4. Biopsy can be performed directly after aspiration without repositioning to a different site on the posterior iliac crest. Advance the needle using a twisting motion, without the obturator in place, to obtain the recommended 1.5 to 2 cm biopsy specimen. To ensure successful specimen collection, rotate the needle briskly in one direction and then the other, then gently rock the needle in four directions by exerting pressure perpendicular to the shaft with the needle capped. Gently remove the needle while rotating it in a corkscrew manner. Remove the specimen from the needle by pushing it up through the hub with a stylet, taking care to avoid needlestick injuries. Jamshidi needle kits include a small, clear plastic guide to facilitate this process.

Aftercare

- Place a pressure dressing over the site and apply direct external pressure for 5 to 10 minutes to avoid prolonged bleeding and hematoma formation.
- The pressure dressing should remain in place for 24 hours.
- The patient may shower after the pressure dressing is removed, but should avoid immersion in water for 1 week after the procedure to avoid infection.

Complications

Infection and hematoma are the most common complications of bone marrow biopsy and aspiration. Careful technique during and after the procedure can minimize these effects.

Lumbar Puncture
Indications

- Analysis of cerebrospinal fluid (CSF), including pressure measurement, to assess adequacy of treatment
- Administration of intrathecal chemotherapy

Contraindications

- Increased intracranial pressure
- Coagulopathy
- Infection near planned site of lumbar puncture (LP)

Anatomy

- Avoid interspaces above L3 (Fig. 43.2), as the conus medullaris rarely ends below L3 (L1–L2 in adults, L2–L3 in children).
- The L4 spinous process or L4–L5 interspace lies in the center of the supracristal plane (a line drawn between the posterior and superior iliac crests).
- There are eight layers from the skin to the subarachnoid space: skin, supraspinous ligament, interspinous ligament, ligamentum flava, epidural space, dura, subarachnoid membrane, and subarachnoid space.

Procedure

1. Describe the procedure to the patient, with assurances that you will explain what you are about to do before you do it.

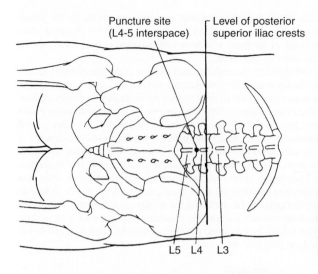

Puncture site
(L4-5 interspace)

Level of posterior
superior iliac crests

L5 L4   L3

Fig. 43.2. Anatomy of the lumbar spine. (Used with permission from Chestnut MS, Dewar TN, Locksley RM. *Office and Bedside Procedures.* Norwalk, CT: Appleton & Lange; 1992:391.)

2. Patient should be in a lateral decubitus or sitting position. The lateral decubitus position is preferable for obtaining opening pressures. The seated position may be used if the patient is obese or has difficulty remaining in the lateral decubitus position. Either seated or lying on one side, the patient should curl into a fetal position with the spine flexed to widen the gap between spinous processes (Fig. 43.3).
3. Identify anatomic landmarks and the interspace to be used for the procedure.
4. Using sterile technique, prepare the area and one interspace above or below it with povidone-iodine solution. Drape the patient, establishing a sterile field.
5. Using 1% lidocaine/bicarb mixture, anesthetize the skin and deeper tissues, carefully avoiding epidural or spinal anesthesia.
6. Insert the spinal needle through the skin into the spinous ligament, keeping the needle parallel to the bed or table. Immediately angle the needle 30 to 45 degrees cephalad. Data indicate that a Sprotte ("pencil-tipped") needle reduces the risk of post-LP headache. The bevel of the spinal needle should

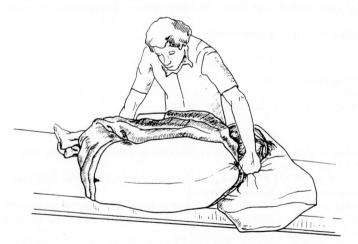

Fig. 43.3. Lateral decubitus position for lumbar puncture. (Used with permission from Chestnut MS, Dewar TN, Locksley RM. *Office and Bedside Procedures.* Norwalk, CT: Appleton & Lange; 1992:390.)

be positioned facing the patient's flank, allowing the needle to spread rather than cut the dural sac. Advance the needle through the eight layers in small increments. With practice, an experienced operator can identify the "pop" as the needle penetrates the dura into the subarachnoid space. Even so, it is wise to remove the stylet to check for CSF before each advance of the needle.

7. When the presence of CSF is confirmed, attach a manometer to measure opening pressure. Collect 8 to 15 mL of CSF. If special studies are required, 40 mL of CSF may be safely removed. Four sample tubes should be sent as follows: tube 1, cultures; tube 2, chemistries (especially glucose and protein); tube 3, cell count and differential; tube 4, cytopathology or other special studies (flow cytometry, cytogenetics, etc.).
8. Replace the stylet, withdraw the needle, observe the site for CSF leak or hemorrhage, and bandage appropriately.
9. Ease the patient into a recumbent position and maintain for 5 to 10 minutes.

Complications

- Spinal headache occurs in approximately 20% of patients after LP. Incidence appears to be related to needle size and CSF leak and not to postprocedure positioning. There is no evidence that increased fluid intake prevents spinal headache. It is characterized by pounding pain in the occipital region when the patient is upright. Incidence is highest in female patients, younger patients (peak 20–40), and patients with a history of headache prior to LP. Patients should be encouraged to remain recumbent if possible, drink plenty of fluids, and take over-the-counter analgesics. For severe, persistent spinal headache (up to 1 week is possible), stronger medication, caffeine, or an analgesic patch may be indicated.
- Nerve root trauma is possible but rare. A low interspace entry site reduces the risk of this complication.
- Cerebellar or medullary herniation occurs rarely in patients with increased intracranial pressure. If recognized early, this process can be reversed.
- Infection, including meningitis.
- Bleeding. A small number of red blood cells in the CSF is common. In approximately 1% to 2% of patients, serious bleeding can result in spinal compromise. Risk is highest in patients with thrompcytopenia or serious bleeding disorders, or patients given anticoagulants immediately before or after LP.

Paracentesis

Indications

- To confirm diagnosis or assess diagnostic markers
- As treatment for ascites resulting from tumor metastasis or obstruction

Contraindications

- The complication rate for this procedure is about 1%.
- The potential benefit of therapeutic paracentesis outweighs the risk of coagulopathy.

Anatomy

- Identify the area of greatest abdominal dullness by percussion, or mark the area of ascites via ultrasound. Take care to avoid abdominal vasculature and viscera.

Procedure

1. Place the patient in a comfortable supine position at the edge of a bed or table.
2. Identify the area of the abdomen to be accessed (Fig. 43.4).
3. Prepare the area with povidone-iodine solution and establish a sterile field by draping the patient.
4. Anesthetize the area with a 1% lidocaine/bicarb mixture.
5. For diagnostic paracentesis, insert a 22- to 25-gauge needle attached to a sterile syringe into the skin, then pull the skin laterally and advance the needle into the abdomen. Release the tension on the skin and withdraw an appropriate amount of fluid for testing. This skin-retraction method creates a "z" track into the peritoneal cavity, which minimizes the risk of ascitic leak after the procedure (Fig. 43.5).

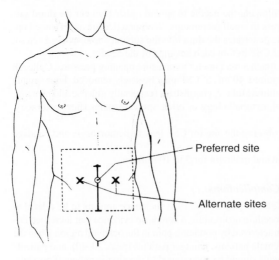

Preferred site

Alternate sites

Fig. 43.4. Sites for diagnostic paracentesis. (Used with permission from Chestnut MS, Dewar TN, Locksley RM. *Office and Bedside Procedures.* Norwalk, CT: Appleton & Lange; 1992:269.)

6. For therapeutic paracentesis, use the z-track method with a multiple-port flexible catheter over a guide needle. When the catheter is in place, the ascites may be evacuated into multiple containers. Make sure that the patient remains hemodynamically stable while removing large amounts of ascites.
7. When the procedure is completed, withdraw the needle or catheter and, if there is no bleeding or ascitic leakage, place a pressure bandage over the site.
8. Following therapeutic paracentesis, the patient should remain supine until all vital signs are stable. Offer the patient assistance getting down from the bed or table.
9. If necessary, standard medical procedures should be used to reverse orthostasis. The patient should be hemodynamically stable before being allowed to leave the operating area.

Complications
- Hemorrhage, ascitic leak, infection, and perforated abdominal viscus have been reported. Properly siting paracentesis virtually eliminates these complications.

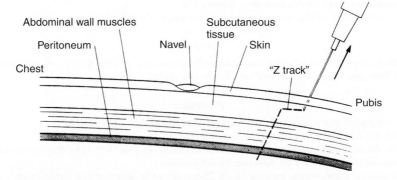

Abdominal wall muscles

Peritoneum

Navel

Subcutaneous tissue

Skin

Chest

"Z track"

Pubis

Fig. 43.5. "Z"-track technique for inserting needle into peritoneal cavity. (Used with permission from Chestnut MS, Dewar TN, Locksley RM. *Office and Bedside Procedures.* Norwalk, CT: Appleton & Lange; 1992:381.)

Thoracentesis

Indications

- Diagnostic or therapeutic removal of pleural fluid.

Contraindications

There are no absolute contraindications to diagnositic thoracentesis. Relative contraindications include the following:

- Coagulopathy
- Bullous emphysema (increased risk of pneumothorax)
- Cardiovascular disease
- Patients on mechanical ventilation with PEEP have no greater risk of developing a pneumothorax than nonventilated patients. However, mechanically ventilated patients are at greater risk of developing tension physiology or persistent air leak if a pneumothorax does occur.
- Patient unable to cooperate
- Cellulitis, if thoracentesis would require penetrating the inflamed tissue

Imaging

If chest radiographs suggest loculation of fluid, decubitus films and possibly computed tomography or ultrasound may be required before thoracentesis is attempted.

Anatomy

- Carefully ascertain the location of the diaphragm to avoid accidental injury to abdominal organs and viscera.
- Place the patient in a seated position facing a table, arms resting on a raised pillow. Have the patient lean forward 10 to 15 degrees to create intercostal spaces.
- Perform thoracentesis through the seventh or eighth intercostal space, along the posterior axillary line. With guidance from fluoroscopy, sonography, or computed tomography, the procedure may be performed below the fifth rib anteriorly, the seventh rib laterally, or the ninth rib posteriorly. Without radiographic guidance, underlying organs may be injured.
- The extent of pleural effusion is indicated by decreased tactile fremitus and dullness to percussion. Begin percussion at the top of the chest and move downward, listening for a change in sound. When a change is noted, compare to the percussive sound in the same interspace and location on the opposite side. This will denote the upper extent of pleural effusion.

Procedure

1. Position the patient, clean the site with antiseptic, and administer local anesthetic using 1% lidocaine and a 25-gauge needle. Infiltrate the deeper tissues using a 22-gauge needle, slowly advancing the needle at a right angle to the chest wall in the center of the intercostal space. Direct the needle into the space just above the lower rib to avoid injury to the intercostal nerve and vessels that may run just below the upper rib. Aspirate frequently to ensure that no vessel has been pierced and to determine the distance from the skin to the pleural fluid. When pleural fluid is aspirated, remove the anesthesia needle and note the depth of penetration.
2. A small incision may be needed to pass a larger gauge thoracentesis needle into the pleural space. Generally, a 16- to 19-gauge needle with intracath is inserted just far enough to obtain pleural fluid. Fluid that is bloody or different in appearance from the fluid obtained with the anesthesia needle may be an indication of vessel injury. In this case, the procedure must be stopped. If there is no apparent change in the pleural fluid aspirated, advance the flexible intracath and withdraw the needle to avoid puncturing the lung as the fluid is drained. Using a flexible intracath with a three-way stopcock allows for removal of a large volume of fluid with less risk of pneumothorax. If only a small sample of

pleural fluid is needed, a 22-gauge needle connected to an airtight three-way stopcock is sufficient. Attach tubing to the three-way stopcock and drain fluid manually or by vacutainer. Withdrawing more than 1,000 mL per procedure requires careful monitoring of the patient's hemodynamic status. As the needle is withdrawn, have the patient hum or do the Valsalva maneuver to increase intrathoracic pressure and lower the risk of pneumothorax.

3. After the procedure, obtain a chest radiograph to determine the amount of remaining fluid, to assess lung parenchyma, and to check for pneumothorax. Small pneumothoraces do not require treatment; pneumothoraces involving >50% lung collapse do (Fig. 43.6).

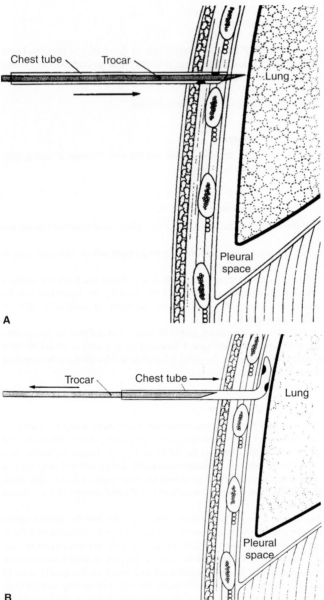

Fig.43.6. Trocar technique for inserting chest tube. (A) Insertion of chest tube. (B) Advancement of chest tube off trocar into pleural space. (Used with permission from Chestnut MS, Dewar TN, Locksley RM. *Office and Bedside Procedures.* Norwalk, CT: Appleton & Lange; 1992:221.)

Complications

- Pneumothorax
- Air embolism (rare)
- Infection
- Pain at puncture site
- Bleeding
- Splenic or liver puncture

SUGGESTED READINGS

Chestnut MS, Dewar TN, Locksley RM. *Office and Bedside Procedures.* Norwalk, CT: Appleton & Lange; 1992.

Ellenby MS, Tegtmeyer K, Lai S, Braner DA. Videos in clinical medicine. Lumbar puncture. *N Engl J Med.* 2006:355(13):e12.

Evans RW, Armon C, Frohman EM, Goodin DS. Assessment: prevention of post-lumbar puncture headaches: report of the Therapeutics and Technology Assessment Subcommittee of the American Academy of Neurology. *Neurology.* 2000;55(7):909–14.

Humphries JE. Dry tap bone marrow aspiration: clinical significance. *Am J Hematol.* 1990;35(4):247–50.

Kuntz KM, Kokmen E, Stevens JC, Miller P, Offord KP, Ho MM. Post-lumbar puncture headaches: experience in 501 consecutive procedures. *Neurology.* 1992;42(10):1884–7.

LeMense GP, Sahn SA. Safety and value of thoracentesis in medical ICU patients. *J Intensive Care Med.* 1998;13:144.

McCartney JP, Adams JW II, Hazard PB. Safety of thoracentesis in mechanically ventilated patients. *Chest.* 1993;103(6);1920–1.

Rohlfing BM, Webb WR, Schlobohm RM. Ventilator-related extra-alveolar air in adults. *Radiology.* 1976;121(1):25–31.

Runyon BA. Paracentesis of ascitic fluid. A safe procedure. *Arch Intern Med.* 1986;146(11):2259–61.

Strupp M, Schueler O, Straube A, Von Stuckrad-Barre S, Brandt T. "Atraumatic" Sprotte needle reduces the incidence of post-lumbar puncture headaches. *Neurology.* 2001;57(12):2310–2.

Wolff SN, Katzenstein AL, Phillips GL, Herzig GP. Aspiration does not influence interpretation of bone marrow biopsy cellularity. *Am J Clin Pathol.* 1983;80(1):60–2.

44

Basic Genomics for Practicing Oncologists

Vicky M. Coyle, Wendy L. Allen, Puthen V. Jithesh, Patrick G. Johnston

Cancer remains a leading cause of morbidity and mortality in the Western world. Despite recent advances in our understanding of the underlying molecular processes involved in tumor growth and associated therapeutic developments, management choices for individual patients are largely still based upon population risk stratification and empirical treatment strategies rather than on the molecular phenotype of their tumor.

Traditional laboratory techniques have allowed the identification and investigation of single genes. The classical adenoma-carcinoma sequence in colorectal cancer (CRC) described by Vogelstein (1) identified a series of genetic alterations in this process including allelic loss, mutations in tumor suppressor genes, and activation of oncogenes. Although these findings have greatly enhanced our understanding of tumor biology, the evaluation of these genomic abnormalities as markers of outcome and response to treatment has produced inconsistent results, highlighting the complexity of this disease and the diversity between tumors of comparable anatomic or pathologic stage.

Advances in genomic technologies have enabled researchers to investigate polymorphisms in single genes associated with chemotherapy toxicity or resistance and measure the expression levels of multiple genes simultaneously in different patient populations. The potential of such approaches is immense: the identification of characteristic gene expression patterns associated with prognosis, response to treatment and toxicity, the elucidation of molecular pathways underlying tumor development and growth, and the investigation of novel targets for therapeutic intervention.

This chapter will discuss novel high-throughput genomic technologies and their application in the clinical setting, results from early clinical studies evaluating these methodologies with particular reference to breast and CRC and the challenges to be overcome in implementing these techniques into routine clinical practice.

NOVEL GENOMIC TECHNOLOGIES

The introduction of new high-throughput technologies has allowed the simultaneous measurement of multiple biologic variables with major implications for both laboratory and clinical research. Three such technologies are well established: microarray-based gene expression profiling, single-nucleotide polymorphism analysis, and array-comparative genomic hybridization. In broad terms, these three methods have similar underlying technology based on linking thousands of nucleic acid sequences (cDNA or DNA) to a solid support such as glass or silicon. Of these methods, microarray-based gene expression profiling is the best investigated and validated in both laboratory and clinical settings.

SNP Analysis

Single-nucleotide polymorphisms (SNPs) are variations in single bases occurring at a particular genomic locus with a frequency of $>1\%$ in the population. They represent the most frequent variation in the human genome with an estimated occurrence of 1 in 300 base pairs (2). Such polymorphisms can have a wide range of effects on cellular processes such as gene transcription or translation or protein activity. The identification of an association between individual polymorphisms in genes or genomic regions and drug toxicity is now well established. One of the earliest reported was the association between a number of variant alleles in the thiopurine methyltransferase (TPMT) gene and significantly reduced enzyme activity resulting in profound, potentially fatal neutropenia in patients with acute lymphoblastic leukemia (ALL) receiving thiopurine therapy (3).

Such a finding can have a significant impact on patient management. Recently the U.S. Food and Drug Administration (FDA) altered the prescribing information for the topoisomoerase 1 inhibitor irinotecan to include consideration of a dose reduction when commencing treatment in patients with a UGT1A1*28 polymorphism following reports of an association between polymorphisms in the number of TA repeats (seven TA repeats in the case of the UGT1A1*28 polymorphism) and reduced UGT1A activity leading to decreased glucuronidation of the active metabolite of irinotecan and increased drug toxicity (4,5).

Identification of polymorphisms can now be performed both in higher densities and on a wider scale with new high-throughput SNP analysis techniques such as oligonucleotide microarrays or bead-based assays. Briefly, these employ fixed oligonucleotide probes that correspond to both alleles of a particular SNP. Hybridization of these to genomic DNA extracted from the experimental sample generates a signal image, which is used to determine the genotype of a specific SNP (6).

Novel cancer genes or candidate gene regions may be discovered by genotyping multiple SNPs in linkage and association studies, and this approach has been utilized in the evaluation of a number of different cancer types. Moreno et al. used a microarray platform to investigate the association between 28 polymorphisms in 15 genes from four DNA repair pathways and the risk of developing CRC and prognosis in 377 cases and 329 controls (7). One of the polymorphisms was significantly associated with an increased risk of CRC; the association between this same polymorphism and other cancer types has previously been reported (8). In a multivariate analysis, polymorphisms in XRCC1 and ERCC1 were significantly associated with better and worse prognosis respectively, particularly in patients who received chemotherapy suggesting enhanced sensitivity to chemotherapy.

Such studies highlight the power of this approach in identifying cancer genes and pathways associated with cancer development, drug response, and prognosis. However, these are largely small studies with limited patient numbers; prospective validation in larger cohorts would be needed to confirm associations between particular polymorphisms and cancer risk or assess the utility of polymorphisms as prognostic markers.

Array-Comparative Genomic Hybridization

Chromosomal DNA copy number changes can be identified on a genome-wide scale by array comparative genomic hybridization (CGH) (9). Experimental samples are hybridized to an array of genomic clones such as bacterial artificial chromosomes (BACs) or increasingly frequently, oligonucleotides, to identify genomic regions that are amplified or deleted in particular cancer types or tumor stages (10). This technology has been applied in a number of different cancer types to classify tumors and to identify markers of tumor progression and prognosis (11).

In CRC, high-resolution array-CGH has been used to investigate copy number changes in both CRC cell lines and primary tumors identifying consistent regions of copy number change (12). These included previously reported copy number changes but also novel chromosomal aberrations in regions containing genes of relevance to CRC, potentially enabling the identification of novel candidate genes.

In the setting of advanced CRC, Mehta et al. used genome-wide array-CGH of colorectal liver metastases to identify genomic markers predictive of recurrence after hepatic resection, demonstrating alterations in $30+/-14\%$ of the genome (13). Two scores were calculated for patients, a total fraction of genome-altered score (FGA) and a clinical risk score (CRS): A low CRS score and a high FGA score ($\geq 20\%$) was associated with a significantly longer median survival than a low CRS and low FGA score. This small study underscores the role of this methodology in identifying genomic markers predictive of outcome however the prognostic utility of these markers requires verification in larger patient cohorts.

Both array-CGH and SNP analysis techniques use genomic DNA isolated from tissue or tumor samples. In practical terms, this is advantageous given its stability, and, with recent reports demonstrating successful profiling of archived formalin-fixed paraffin embedded (FFPE) tumors (14,15), a large potential resource of archived diagnostic tissue. However, some challenges remain to be overcome before attempting to implement this technology in routine clinical management; these include the robustness of the arrays, difficulties in interpreting datasets generated on different array platforms and deficiencies in analytical software (16).

Finally, this technology is relatively immature and continues to evolve rapidly: the integration of oligonucleotide-based SNP arrays with CGH platforms has enabled the measurement of both changes in copy number and copy number-neutral changes such as loss of heterozygosity (17,18), which may render current platforms obsolete (19).

Microarray-Based Gene Expression Profiling

This is the most mature of the genomic technologies in terms of platform design and data analysis. The power of this approach lies in the ability to identify genome-wide transcriptional changes simultaneously in response to a stimulus or in comparison to another population of interest. There are two main types of arrays available, oligonucleotide and cDNA arrays which involve cross-linking of oligonucleotide and cDNA sequences respectively to a glass slide and detecting hybridization of reverse-transcribed total RNA from the sample of interest to these probes (20).

This approach has been used successfully to distinguish tumor from normal tissue, and in the classification of tumor subtypes, the identification of markers predictive of response to therapy, and outcome and the identification of specific transcriptional targets for further investigation; some relevant clinical studies in breast cancer and CRC will be discussed below.

In CRC, this approach has been used to identify both prognostic gene sets and gene sets predictive of chemotherapy response. These have been generally small, retrospective studies, however results are promising. A number of prognostic studies have identified several different candidate gene sets using gene expression profiling (21–23). Eschrich et al. generated a 43-gene set using a cDNA microarray platform which performed with 90% accuracy by cross-validation in predicting outcome in Duke's B and C tumors; a restricted 26-gene signature from this gene set was tested in an independent test set of 95 tumor samples profiled on an oligonucleotide microarray platform. This 26-gene signature outperformed conventional pathologic staging in predicting survival (22).

Barrier et al. reported a 30-gene signature predictive of recurrence in stage II CRC which had a predictive accuracy of 76.3% when tested in an independent validation set and proceeded to compare the performance of this signature to that of a previously reported prognostic gene signature; the predictive accuracy of the previously reported signature was maintained (23). Both the independent validation of a prognostic signature developed by another research group and the cross-platform validation are important when considering the clinical implementation of this technology.

The identification of gene sets associated with response to chemotherapy in CRC has been investigated in both the in vitro (24) and clinical settings (25). Del Rio et al. identified a 14-gene signature predictive of response to irinotecan/5-FU chemotherapy in patients with advanced CRC; this signature performed with an overall accuracy of 95% and high sensitivity and specificity (92% and 100% respectively) when assessed by cross-validation (25). Although this is a small study ($n = 21$) the authors are conducting a larger multicenter study to validate these findings, therefore this gene signature could potentially be a useful tool in selecting patients likely to benefit from chemotherapy avoiding unnecessary toxicity, time, and expense in patients unlikely to respond. An additional important aspect of this study is that the predictive gene signature was derived from colorectal primary tumor. Participants were chemotherapy-naïve patients with synchronous unresectable liver metastases who underwent resection of their primary tumor prior to commencing chemotherapy. A predictive signature based on gene expression in primary tumor would avoid the need to obtain metastatic tumor samples from patients and, for many patients with archived diagnostic primary tumor specimens, avoid any invasive tumor procurement procedures altogether.

The use of microarray-expression profiling to identify markers of prognosis is more advanced in breast cancer; a number of gene sets predictive of recurrence in early-stage breast cancer have been reported and two are currently under evaluation in prospective studies. These are a 70-gene good/poor outcome model derived from microarray profiling studies (26,27) and a 21 gene recurrence score, a reverse transcriptase polymerase chain reaction (RT-PCR) assay derived from the literature, gene databases, and microarray profiling studies (28). A comparison of the performance of these two predictors in an independent test set demonstrated a high level of concordance in their predictions of outcome for individual samples (77–81% agreement) (29). This finding is of interest not only in demonstrating the robustness of these datasets, but also in the fact these predictors contained only one gene in common, suggesting that the ability of such predictors to identify a particular molecular phenotype is of more importance than their content.

Two large prospective randomized trials of these predictors, the Trial Assigning Individualized Options for Treatment (TAILORx) and the Microarray in Node-Negative Disease May Avoid Chemotherapy (MINDACT) studies are underway; these will use the recurrence score and the 70-gene profile to identify which patients with ER-positive node-negative breast cancer are at most risk of recurrence and would benefit most from adjuvant chemotherapy (30). This exciting development demonstrates not only that this technology is sufficiently developed in terms of accuracy and reproducibility for introduction into patient management, but also a move away from traditional clinical trial design, allocating treatment based on genomic signatures rather than clinicopathologic variables.

IMPACT OF PHARMACOGENOMICS ON PATIENT MANAGEMENT AND DRUG DEVELOPMENT

Initial clinical studies utilizing these technologies have shown promising results and have prompted their further evaluation in larger retrospective validation studies and prospective trials. This process has been driven by a number of players: Regulatory bodies such as the FDA have developed guidelines regarding the submission of multiplex tests such as gene expression signatures in support of traditional clinical trial data, while the pharmaceutical industry is facing increasing economic pressure to bring effective new treatments to market, avoiding high profile failures at a late stage in the drug development process. Finally, in the academic setting there is a growing realization that traditional clinical trial design may be inadequate given the differences in mechanisms of action and effects of new targeted therapeutic agents in comparison with conventional cytotoxic agents.

A number of challenges must be overcome before these genomic technologies or derived genomic markers become implemented into routine clinical use. Further clinical studies should be adequately powered, use standardized protocols, and have clearly defined endpoints and study inclusion criteria. The major obstacle in achieving this has been the difficulty in obtaining suitable patient tumor samples. These technologies have required fresh frozen tissue to yield the high quality DNA and RNA required for analysis; the costs associated with sample procurement and storage and the general lack of coordinated tissue collection procedures have limited the numbers of samples obtained.

In contrast, FFPE samples are routinely prepared from the majority of tumor samples, but utilizing tumor samples prepared in this manner has proven technically challenging. Genetic material derived from FFPE tissue is generally partially degraded (particularly RNA) and often limited in terms of quantities obtained. However, this technology is rapidly evolving; several studies describe the use of RNA derived from FFPE tissue to measure gene expression changes by RT-PCR (31,32) and, as discussed earlier, successful use of DNA obtained from FFPE tissue for SNP and CGH arrays has also been reported (14,15). Additionally, it is likely that FFPE-derived RNA will also be utilized for high-throughput gene expression profiling in the near future. Early results of a new colorectal disease-specific array developed and optimized for analysis of expression profiling of FFPE tissues are very promising; a 48-gene prognostic signature derived using this technology has demonstrated high accuracy in predicting recurrence in stage II CRC (33).

Additional factors need to be considered when considering incorporating genomic technologies in the drug development process. The view that this should occur at an early stage must be tempered by the scarcity of clinical samples: use of in vitro cell line or xenograft models to generate genomic signatures for patient stratification in clinical studies might overcome this problem, however, evidence of strong correlation between effects observed in preclinical models relative to effects observed in clinical studies is lacking currently. An alternative approach is to reconsider clinical trial design, performing phase 1 and phase 2 clinical studies with the objective of collecting enough clinical material to derive statistically significant molecular signatures that can be used to preselect patients for phase 3 studies.

Finally, studies using the above technologies generate large amounts of data that often require complex bioinformatic analysis. It is argued that the lack of standard terminology for defining such datasets and the inadequate standards and infrastructure for the integration of patient data with bioinformatics data may limit meaningful interpretation or meta-analysis of the results. The introduction of standards in both reporting and sharing data will help to address this issue. These include the CONSORT Statement for reporting clinical studies (34), the REMARK guidelines for diagnostic marker studies (35), and the Minimum Information about a Microarray Experiment (MIAME) standard (36). Additionally, the development of international metadata representation standards by the U.S. National Cancer Institute's cancer Biomedical Informatics Grid project (caBIG) (https://cabig.nci.nih.gov) will facilitate the international exchange of knowledge, standards, and models.

CONCLUSION

The advent of high-throughput genomic technologies has enabled the simultaneous measurement of multiple biologic variables, greatly enhancing our understanding of the cellular processes occurring in tumor development. Early studies investigating these technologies in the clinical setting have shown promising results in diagnostic and prognostic classification of tumors and the potential of predicting response to therapy; validation in larger studies with well-defined patient populations using a standardized methodological approach will facilitate the routine clinical implementation of such markers.

The genomic era is now well established; the integration of the other "omic" technologies, proteomics and metabolomics, will herald a new "systems biology" era, bringing the goal of individualized patient therapy and improved outcomes even closer.

REFERENCES

1. Vogelstein B, Fearon ER, Hamilton SR, et al. Genetic alterations during colorectal-tumor development. *N Engl J Med* 1988;319(9):525–32.
2. Cargill M, Altshuler D, Ireland J, et al. Characterization of single-nucleotide polymorphisms in coding regions of human genes. *Nat Genet* 1999;22(3):231–8.
3. Weinshilboum RM, Sladek SL. Mercaptopurine pharmacogenetics: monogenic inheritance of erythrocyte thiopurine methyltransferase activity. *Am J Hum Genet* 1980;32(5):651–62.
4. Innocenti F, Undevia SD, Iyer L, et al. Genetic variants in the UDP-glucuronosyltransferase 1A1 gene predict the risk of severe neutropenia of irinotecan. *J Clin Oncol* 2004;22(8):1382–8.
5. Ando Y, Saka H, Ando M, et al. Polymorphisms of UDP-glucuronosyltransferase gene and irinotecan toxicity: a pharmacogenetic analysis. *Cancer Res* 2000;60(24):6921–6.
6. Engle LJ, Simpson CL, Landers JE. Using high-throughput SNP technologies to study cancer. *Oncogene* 2006;25(11):1594–601.
7. Moreno V, Gemignani F, Landi S, et al. Polymorphisms in genes of nucleotide and base excision repair: risk and prognosis of colorectal cancer. *Clin Cancer Res* 2006;12(7 Pt 1):2101–8.
8. Goode EL, Ulrich CM, Potter JD. Polymorphisms in DNA repair genes and associations with cancer risk. *Cancer Epidemiol Biomarkers Prev* 2002;11(12):1513–30.
9. Pinkel D, Albertson DG. Array comparative genomic hybridization and its applications in cancer. *Nat Genet* 2005;37 Suppl:S11–7.
10. Carvalho B, Ouwerkerk E, Meijer GA, Ylstra B. High resolution microarray comparative genomic hybridisation analysis using spotted oligonucleotides. *J Clin Pathol* 2004;57(6):644–6.
11. Kallioniemi A. CGH microarrays and cancer. *Curr Opin Biotechnol* 2008;19(1):36–40.
12. Douglas EJ, Fiegler H, Rowan A, et al. Array comparative genomic hybridization analysis of colorectal cancer cell lines and primary carcinomas. *Cancer Res* 2004;64(14):4817–25.
13. Mehta KR, Nakao K, Zuraek MB, et al. Fractional genomic alteration detected by array-based comparative genomic hybridization independently predicts survival after hepatic resection for metastatic colorectal cancer. *Clin Cancer Res* 2005;11(5):1791–7.
14. Jacobs S, Thompson ER, Nannya Y, et al. Genome-wide, high-resolution detection of copy number, loss of heterozygosity, and genotypes from formalin-fixed, paraffin-embedded tumor tissue using microarrays. *Cancer Res* 2007;67(6):2544–51.
15. Lips EH, Dierssen JW, van Eijk R, et al. Reliable high-throughput genotyping and loss-of-heterozygosity detection in formalin-fixed, paraffin-embedded tumors using single nucleotide polymorphism arrays. *Cancer Res* 2005;65(22):10188–91.

16. Lockwood WW, Chari R, Chi B, Lam WL. Recent advances in array comparative genomic hybridization technologies and their applications in human genetics. *Eur J Hum Genet* 2006;14(2): 139–48.

17. Rauch A, Ruschendorf F, Huang J, et al. Molecular karyotyping using an SNP array for genomewide genotyping. *J Med Genet* 2004;41(12):916–22.

18. Zhao X, Li C, Paez JG, et al. An integrated view of copy number and allelic alterations in the cancer genome using single nucleotide polymorphism arrays. *Cancer Res* 2004;64(9):3060–71.

19. Fan JB, Chee MS, Gunderson KL. Highly parallel genomic assays. *Nat Rev Genet* 2006;7(8): 632–44.

20. Harkin DP. Uncovering functionally relevant signaling pathways using microarray-based expression profiling. *Oncologist* 2000;5(6):501–7.

21. Wang Y, Jatkoe T, Zhang Y, et al. Gene expression profiles and molecular markers to predict recurrence of Dukes' B colon cancer. *J Clin Oncol* 2004;22(9):1564–71.

22. Eschrich S, Yang I, Bloom G, et al. Molecular staging for survival prediction of colorectal cancer patients. *J Clin Oncol* 2005;23(15):3526–35.

23. Barrier A, Boelle PY, Roser F, et al. Stage II colon cancer prognosis prediction by tumor gene expression profiling. *J Clin Oncol* 2006;24(29):4685–91.

24. Mariadason JM, Arango D, Shi Q, et al. Gene expression profiling-based prediction of response of colon carcinoma cells to 5-fluorouracil and camptothecin. *Cancer Res* 2003;63(24):8791–812.

25. Del Rio M, Molina F, Bascoul-Mollevi C, et al. Gene expression signature in advanced colorectal cancer patients select drugs and response for the use of leucovorin, fluorouracil, and irinotecan. *J Clin Oncol* 2007;25(7):773–80.

26. van de Vijver MJ, He YD, van't Veer LJ, et al. A gene-expression signature as a predictor of survival in breast cancer. *N Engl J Med* 2002;347(25):1999–2009.

27. van't Veer LJ, Dai H, van de Vijver MJ, et al. Gene expression profiling predicts clinical outcome of breast cancer. *Nature* 2002;415(6871):530–6.

28. Paik S. Development and clinical utility of a 21-gene recurrence score prognostic assay in patients with early breast cancer treated with tamoxifen. *Oncologist* 2007;12(6):631–5.

29. Fan C, Oh DS, Wessels L, et al. Concordance among gene-expression-based predictors for breast cancer. *N Engl J Med* 2006;355(6):560–9.

30. O'Shaughnessy JA. Molecular signatures predict outcomes of breast cancer. *N Engl J Med* 2006;355(6):615–7.

31. Lewis F, Maughan NJ, Smith V, Hillan K, Quirke P. Unlocking the archive—gene expression in paraffin-embedded tissue. *J Pathol* 2001;195(1):66–71.

32. Cronin M, Pho M, Dutta D, et al. Measurement of gene expression in archival paraffin-embedded tissues: development and performance of a 92-gene reverse transcriptase-polymerase chain reaction assay. *Am J Pathol* 2004;164(1):35–42.

33. Johnston PG, Mulligan K, Kay E, et al. A genetic signature of relapse in stage II colorectal cancer derived from formalin fixed paraffin embedded tissue (FFPE) tissue using a unique disease specific colorectal array. In: *Journal of Clinical Oncology, 2006 ASCO Annual Meeting Proceedings* Part I. Vol 24, No. 18S, 2006:3519.

34. Moher D, Schulz KF, Altman DG. The CONSORT statement: revised recommendations for improving the quality of reports of parallel-group randomised trials. *Lancet* 2001;357(9263):1191–4.

35. McShane LM, Altman DG, Sauerbrei W, Taube SE, Gion M, Clark GM. Reporting recommendations for tumor marker prognostic studies. *J Clin Oncol* 2005;23(36):9067–72.

36. Brazma A, Hingamp P, Quackenbush J, et al. Minimum information about a microarray experiment (MIAME)-toward standards for microarray data. *Nat Genet* 2001;29(4):365–71.

45

Basic Principles of Radiation Oncology

Jondavid Pollock

As one of the three widely accepted modalities in the management of cancer, radiotherapy (RT) maintains perhaps the most "alternative" form; it is neither chemical or invasive. Indeed, because of the general lack of understanding of the physics and biology underlying the principle and practice of RT, many clinicians and patients remain perplexed by its ability to cure disease and the constant evolution in its delivery to maintain the therapeutic window, ultimately designed to preserve quality of life and functionality while eradicating disease.

RADIATION BIOLOGY AND PHYSICS

Although radiobiology and physics are clearly separable in theory, and many textbooks have been written to focus on one or the other, a practical understanding of one subject cannot be easily delineated from the other.

Prior to discussing the biology and antineoplastic activity of RT, it is important to understand the basic physical properties of contemporary RT, both in terms of its activity as well as its production by a modern linear accelerator. The most common form of RT used today is a photon, or packet of x-rays. Discovered by Wilhelm Rontgen in 1895, photons were found to blacken photographic film; as these "new kinds of ray" were unable to be measured at the time, they were called "x rays." Shortly following their discovery, Wilhelm Freund treated a mole with the x-rays, giving birth in 1897 to the field of therapeutic radiology or radiation oncology. The following year, in 1898, Antoine Bequerel discovered radioactivity and the Curie family isolated radium. Indeed, because of the transportability and ease of administration, radioactive elements such as radium remained the preferred route of RT thereafter. Subsequent experiments demonstrated that the energy released by the radioactive decay of an element, so-called gamma ray, was identical to that artificially produced by a gas tube, an x-ray. Today, most modern RT consists of photons produced by linear accelerators, though there are many effective and curative applications from radioactive decay, generally termed brachytherapy.

Mechanism of Action

Radiotherapy, in any of its forms, represents ionizing radiation because the energy passed from RT to the tissues is sufficient to cause an outer orbital electron to be released, thus ionizing or charging the tissue's atom. Specifically, x-rays and gamma rays are forms of electromagnetic radiation, while the less commonly used forms of RT (protons, neutrons mesons, carbon ions) are generally termed particulate radiation because they have mass. Despite the fact that RT "excites" or ionizes tissue particles, and thus can be measured by calories, it does not increase the temperature of the recipient or induce a thermal effect. So-called radiation burns are not thermal; the erythema of the skin is a reflection of the denudement of the superficial layers of the skin, caused by the increased cellular turnover induced by RT, leaving behind the better-vascularized deeper dermal tissues to show through as red.

When RT is delivered it is either directly or indirectly ionizing. Particulate, charged, or heavy ions deliver their energy to the tissue by direct effect; that is, these particles have enough kinetic energy to alter the genetic material with which they make contact. On the other hand, electromagnetic RT (gamma and x-rays) affect cells by indirectly ionizing them. These rays give up their energy to the absorbed tissues, thus causing the formation of fast-moving charged particles. Typically, the energy of an x-ray or gamma ray is passed to many circulating electrons (often called free radicals), which then go on to interact with various host tissues, including the genetic material of cancer cells. It is this interaction with the DNA of cancer cells that underlies the biology of RT.

Linear Accelerator

Modern RT is manufactured by a complex machine called a linear accelerator. The basic premise of this technology is that electrons are accelerated to a frequency of 3,000 megacycles/second and then are shot at a tungsten steel target. The negatively charged electrons are then repelled by the orbiting electrons of the steel target and, as they are deflected away and change direction, they lose some energy. In the observation of Newton's laws regarding conservation of energy, the energy lost by the deflection of the electron interaction is gathered into a form, called an x-ray. The gathered x-rays (photons) are then shot out of the head of the linear accelerator into the patient. There are many beam-modifying devices (wedges, compensators, and blocks, among others) that can be placed between the accelerator and patient to conform the radiation to accomplish its goal of sparing normal tissues while targeting tumors.

Treatment Planning

In order to determine the methods and specifics by which the beam should be modified to accomplish its goals, the radiation oncologist works closely with several specialists. In fact, because of the complexity and ever-changing landscape of the field of radiation oncology, the days when the single clinician could consult a patient, set them up for treatment, calculate the physical parameters of the RT, and actually deliver the treatment are extinct. Many clinicians have been trained to operate all elements of the department, but this remains inefficient and the increasing volume of patients for whom radiation therapy is a necessary modality has relegated the clinician to consultation of the patient, prescription of the RT, and oversight of the various affiliated health care professionals responsible for the myriad of treatment responsibilities.

In today's modern department, a simulator technologist sets the patient on a fluoroscopy unit or CT-simulator to determine the site to be treated. The medical dosimetrist then takes the clinician's prescription and assists in determining the most appropriate beam arrangement to accomplish the goals of therapy. The medical physicist, whose main responsibility is to ensure the machines are properly referenced and operating without any problems on a daily basis, calculates the dose delivered by the machine to coincide with the prescription without error. The radiation technologists then actually deliver the radiation therapy, closely following all set-up data provided to them by the physician, dosimetrist, and simulator technologist. The radiation technologist may also be responsible for performing ultrasounds and CT scans of the patient prior to each treatment fraction to ensure that the location receiving treatment is without error. The radiation oncology nursing team then evaluates the patient every few days of treatment to ensure there are no concerning side effects that require attention and they, along with the physician, initiate the appropriate clinical response. Furthermore, with the increasing realization that RT is often improved by sensitizing tumors with targeted agents and cytotoxic and cytostatic chemotherapeutics, the nurse and physician need to be more aware of potential interactions, toxicities, and tumor-response parameters than previously encountered when RT alone was delivered. Because of the evolving combined- or multi-modality approach to many cancers, it is important to mention the pure biologic characteristics of tumors and normal tissues, to appreciate how and why RT alone has become less commonly used in the definitive and curative treatment of cancer.

FUNDAMENTALS OF RADIOBIOLOGIC PRINCIPLES

There are four fundamental radiobiologic principles that are considered by a radiation oncologist when determining the course of RT to be delivered: cellular repair, repopulation, redistribution, and reoxygenation.

CHAPTER 45

Cellular Repair

The ability of a cell to repair potentially lethal damage induced by RT remains one of the basic differences between malignant and normal tissues. Normal cells maintain an enhanced ability to repair RT damage, while malignant cells generally do not have that capacity. However, at a certain threshold dose of RT even normal, nonmalignant tissues lose the capacity to recover and therefore attention to dose is critically important to avoid permanent damage to uninvolved tissues. Several rather inexact estimates have been published to guide clinicians on total doses, daily doses, and volumes of tissue irradiated, beyond which normal tissue toxicities will be encountered.

Cellular Repopulation

Cellular repopulation is a phenomenon often observed following the initiation of RT. The often-recited theory to explain this event is that as a percentage of cells are destroyed by RT, the remaining living cells have access to greater relative blood supply, among other probable growth-related cytokines, resulting in greater growth of the remaining fraction of cells. Indeed, this is observed clinically in head and neck cancers, cervical cancers, and lung cancers prompting the standard that definitive RT be completed as soon as possible and without avoidable treatment breaks.

Cellular Redistribution

Cellular redistribution refers to the portion of the cell cycle within which a cell resides at a specific time. Tumors divide at varying rates and portions of the cell cycle are inherently more sensitive to antineoplastic agents. Notably, RT most effectively eradicates cells in the G2-M junction, while cells in the S1 portion of the cell cycle are relatively radiounresponsive. The benefits and purpose of exploiting cellular redistribution underlies the concept of fractionated RT. By dividing the RT dose daily over many weeks, there is a greater chance that RT delivery will coincide with cells in the responsive portion of the cell cycle, resulting in greater cell kill. As a corollary, cellular cytostatic agents thought to cause cellular arrest in a certain portion of the cell cycle (i.e., tamoxifen) have been theorized to potentially reduce the benefits of RT, though recent studies have demonstrated the absence of a clinical decrement.

Cellular Reoxygenation

Cellular reoxygenation remains one of the most critical elements of RT effect. The indirect ionization occurring when electromagnetic radiation (x-rays) enter target tissues, which results in the excitation of electrons to free radical status. These free radicals then directly affect the tumor's DNA, inflicting a potentially lethal injury. The main source of these electrons is circulating tissue concentrations of oxygen, and clear in vitro and clinical data demonstrate that relative tissue hypoxia reduces the killing effect of RT. In many tumor sites, including cervix and head and neck, low oxygen levels or relatively low hemoglobin levels significantly reduce the benefits of RT. Further evidence that electron free radicals are the "smart bombs" formed by RT is the clinical loss of local control when antioxidants (namely megadoses of vitamin C and E) are ingested concurrent with RT.

RADIOSENSITIZATION

Sensitization refers to the increased clinical response of a tumor to a combination of any agent delivered concurrently with RT. Almost every cytotoxic systemic agent has the ability to sensitize tumors to RT, while most targeted agents and cytostatic drugs do not typically increase the clinical response. Most potent in their ability to sensitize are the anthracyclines and platinum agents, though the newer taxanes and gemcitabine have clearly demonstrated an ability to increase both tumor and normal tissue response to RT. The mechanism behind chemotherapy-induced cellular sensitization to RT appears to be a result of the incorporation of halogenated pyrimidines into the tumor's DNA. The new analog weakens and damages the DNA, rendering it incapable of repairing RT-induced injury. Experiments have shown that only several generations of substitutions can inflict this type of DNA injury, thus the most effective sensitization occurs when the systemic agent is delivered concurrently with RT, or for several cycles prior to the RT. Because of the increased normal tissue effect of concurrent therapies, they are considered when monotherapies have proven inadequate or extenuating circumstances exist. There have been limited attempts to improve breast cancer response by temporally combining chemotherapy and RT; most studies have evaluated preoperative chemotherapy followed by but not concurrent with RT. Those studies have demonstrated a clinical response, though no phase 3, level 3 data exists suggesting an improvement over chemotherapy or RT alone. The few studies that have actually temporally combined chemotherapy and RT have clearly demonstrated increased acute morbidity, again without clear evidence of clinical benefit.

INTENSITY-MODULATED RADIOTHERAPY

Intensity-modulated radiotherapy (IMRT) refers to any technology wherein dose is modified to differentially treat target tumor and uninvolved normal tissues. Several different techniques are currently in use to accomplish IMRT, including customized brass-based tissue compensators and multileaf collimation, the latter of which is used in a dose delivery system that is either dynamic or static. The dynamic system arcs around the patient, delivering different beamlets from each beam's-eye view of the tumor, accomplishing this dose delivery from an almost limitless number of angles. The static systems aim and shoot x-rays from each angle and then the machine stops and rotates before targeting the tumor from a new angle; this dose delivery is usually accomplished from four to eight different angles.

PARTIAL-BREAST IRRADIATION

Partial-breast irradiation (PBI) refers to any technique used to irradiate a portion of the breast. The most commonly used technique includes intracavitary methods (Mammosite, Contura, Savi) wherein a balloon with 1 to 8 catheters jointly housed are postoperatively placed within the surgical tumor bed. High-dose–rate brachytherapy is then delivered remotely and directly to the tumor bed, typically twice daily for 1 week. To date, the greatest experience has been with the Mammosite applicator and results have generally been very good (excellent in-breast tumor control and favorable cosmesis), though a prospective phase 3 Intergroup trial comparing PBI to standard whole-breast RT is currently accruing patients to determine whether PBI is equal. Other forms of PBI include three-dimensional conformal RT (using external beam RT directed at the tumor bed with a noncoplanar beam arrangement of generally three to four beams), intraoperative electron beam teletherapy (mostly used in Europe where the exposed tumor bed is irradiated with a single high-dose beam), and low- or high-dose rate interstitial brachytherapy (where intraoperative catheters are placed within and surrounding the tumor bed cavity). Interstitial brachytherapy has the longest experience of PBI, though the operating room time, potential need for an inpatient admission, and risk of developing a pneumothorax has made this technique less favorable for patient and clinician.

PROTONS

The most commonly used form of electromagnetic radiation in the field of radiation oncology is photons, or x-rays. These particles are uncharged and their energy slowly dissipates when they enter the body. Depending upon the location of the tumor and the angle or beam perspective, other uninvolved structures receive radiation and this leads to side effects. Most photon beams require between 1 and 1.5 cm of normal tissue to traverse before enough dose has built up to achieve maximum dose effect, and the dose then regresses over a 2 to 5 cm length of tissue beyond the target tumor.

Protons are charged particles with very different physical characteristics than x-rays or photons. Protons enter the body at a very low energy level and can rapidly escalate to maximum energy over a few millimeters, deep within the body. This effect, called a Bragg peak, allows the length over which maximum dose is delivered to be minimized and thus less normal tissue receives a high dose. Protons have been shown to be effective when tumors are closely situated adjacent to critical structures, where any considerable radiation dose could be devastating, such as the spinal cord, brain, retina, or developing tissues in a child.

Because of the extraordinary expense associated with the creation of protons, their use has been limited to very few malignancies and few centers have maintained any degree of expertise with their use. Because of increasing pressure to maximize economic advantages, however, more centers have recently begun to develop their own proton beam facilities and the use of this special particle beam has started to evolve, with the more common prostate and lung cancers now being treated. To date, this author is unaware of any data demonstrating a benefit or widespread use of protons in breast cancer though one could imagine it as a potential competitor in the field of PBI.

SUGGESTED READINGS

Bartelink H, Horiot JC, Poortmans PM, Struikmans H, Van den Boagaert W, Fourquet A, et al. Impact of a higher radiation dose on local control and survival in breast-conserving therapy of early breast cancer: 10-year results of the randomized boost versus no boost EORTC 22881-10882 trial. *J Clin Oncol.* 25: 3259–3265, 2007.

Brade AM, Tannock IF. Scheduling of radiation and chemotherapy for limited-stage small-cell lung cancer: repopulation as a cause of treatment failure? *J Clin Oncol.* 24:1020–1022, 2006.

Buchholz TA. Treatment optimization using computed tomography-delineated targets should be used for supraclavicular irradiation for breast cancer. *Int J Radiat Oncol Biol Phys.* 69:711–715, 2007.

Chino JP, Marks LB. Prone positioning causes the heart to be displaced anteriorly within the thorax: implications for breast cancer treatment. *Int J Radiat Oncol Biol Phys.* 70:916–920, 2008.

Coen JJ, Taghian AG, Kachnic LA, Assaad SI, Powell SN. Risk of lymphedema after regional nodal irradiation with breast conservation therapy. *Int J Radiat Oncol Biol Phys.* 55:1209–1215, 2003.

Flanagan SA, Robinson BW, Krokosky CM, Shewach DS. Mismatched nucleotides as the lesions responsible for radiosensitization with gemcitabine: a new paradigm for antimetabolite radiosensitizers. *Mol Cancer Ther.* 6:1858–1868, 2007.

Fodor J. Interactions between radiation and hormonal therapy in breast cancer: simultaneous or sequential treatment. *Orv Hetil.* 147:121–125, 2006.

Hermann RM, Rave-Frank M, Pradier O. Combining radiation with oxaliplatin: a review of experimental results. *Cancer Radiother.* 12:61–67, 2008.

Liengsawangwong R, Yu TK, Sun TL, Erasmus JJ, Perkins GH, Tereffe W, et al. Randomized multicenter trial of sentinel node biopsy versus standard axillary treatment in operable breast cancer: the ALMANAC Trial. *J Natl Cancer Inst.* 98:599–609, 2006.

Lim K, Chan P, Dinniwell R, Fyles A, Haider M, Cho YB, et al. Cervical cancer regression measured using weekly magnetic resonance imaging during fractionated radiotherapy: radiobiologic modeling and correlation with tumor hypoxia. *Int J Radiat Oncol Biol Phys.* 70:126–133, 2008.

Malinen E, Sovik A, Hristov D, Bruland OS, Olsen DR. Adapting radiotherapy to hypoxic tumors. *Phys Med Biol.* 51:4903–4921, 2006.

Meyer F, Bairati I, Fortin A, Gelinas M, Nabid A, Brochet F, Tetu B. Interaction between antioxidant vitamin supplementation and cigarette smoking during radiation therapy in relation to long-term effects on recurrence and mortality: a randomized trial among head and neck cancer patients. *Int J Cancer.* 122:1679–1683, 2008.

Supiot S, Gouard S, Charrier J, Apostolidis C, Chatal JF, Barbet J, et al. Mechanisms of cell sensitization to alpha radioimmunotherapy by doxorubicin or paclitaxel in multiple myeloma cell lines. *Clin Cancer Res.* 11:7047–7052, 2005.

Stegman LD, Beal KP, Hunt MA, Fornier MN, McCormick B. Long-term clinical outcomes of whole-breast irradiation delivered in the prone position. *Int J Radiat Oncol Biol Phys.* 68:73–81, 2007.

Terhaard CH, Kal HB, Hordijk GK. Why to start the concomitant boost in accelerated radiotherapy for advanced laryngeal cancer in week 3. *Int J Radiat Oncol Biol Phys.* 62:62–69, 2005.

46

Anticancer Agents

Sakar M. Wahby and Thomas E. Hughes

Please note that all information has been obtained from current product labeling as of June 1, 2008. Doses listed are those from the package insert and apply when the agent is given alone, unless otherwise noted. Doses are expressed in accordance with nomenclature guidelines from Kohler et al. (1).

ADVERSE REACTIONS

Adverse reactions to anticancer agents involve the following:

- Cardiovascular system (CV)
- Skin and integument system (DERM)
- Electrolyte abnormalities (ELECTRO)
- Endocrine system (ENDO)
- Gastrointestinal system (GI)
- Genitourinary system (GU)
- Hematopoietic system (HEMAT)
- Hepatic system (HEPAT)
- Infusion-related reactions (INFUS)
- Neurologic system, central and peripheral (NEURO)
- Ocular system
- Pulmonary system (PULM)
- Liver function
- Serum creatinine (Cr)
- Creatinine clearance (CrCl)
- Nausea and vomiting (N/V). Classified on a four-level system. Emetogenic potential is based on the incidence of acute emesis in product labeling and/or based on classification by national chemotherapy-induced nausea and vomiting (CINV) guidelines: minimal, <10%; low, 10–30%; moderate, 30–90%; high, >90% (see Chapter 38).

ALDESLEUKIN (PROLEUKIN)

Mechanism of Action

- Cellular immunity activation

Food and Drug Administration (FDA)–approved Indications

- Metastatic renal cell carcinoma
- Metastatic melanoma

FDA-approved Dosage

- 600,000 IU/kg i.v. over 15 minutes every 8 hours for a maximum of 14 doses
- May be repeated after 9 days of rest for a maximum of 28 doses per course.

Dose Modification Criteria

- Withhold or interrupt a dose for toxicity

Adverse Reactions

- CV: hypotension, tachycardia, arrhythmia
- DERM: rash, pruritis
- GI: diarrhea
- N/V (moderate), mucositis, anorexia
- GU: oliguria, acute renal failure
- HEMAT: myelosuppression
- NEURO: confusion, somnolence, anxiety, dizziness
- PULM: dyspnea, pulmonary edema
- Other: pain, fever, chills, malaise

Comments

- Restrict use to patients with normal cardiac and pulmonary function.
- Monitor for capillary leak syndrome.
- Associated with impaired neutrophil function; consider antibiotic prophylaxis for patients with indwelling central lines.
- Withhold in patients developing moderate to severe lethargy or somnolence; continued administration may result in coma.

ALEMTUZUMAB (CAMPATH)

Mechanism of Action

- Humanized monoclonal antibody directed against the cell surface protein CD52. The CD52 antigen is expressed on the surface of normal and malignant B and T lymphocytes, NK cells, monocytes, macrophages, and a subpopulation of granulocytes. The proposed mechanism of action is antibody-dependent lysis of leukemic cells following cell-surface binding.

FDA-approved Indications

- B-cell chronic lymphocytic leukemia (CLL): second-line therapy in patients who have been treated with alkylating agents and who have failed fludarabine therapy.

FDA-approved Dosage

- Alemtuzumab is dose escalated in a stepwise format to a maintenance dose of 30 mg.
  The initial recommended dose is 3 mg i.v. over 2 hours daily. When this dose is tolerated (infusion-related toxicities ≤ grade 2), the daily dose should be escalated to 10 mg i.v. over 2 hours daily and continued until tolerated. When the 10 mg dose is tolerated, the maintenance dose of 30 mg may be initiated. The maintenance dose is 30 mg i.v. over 2 hours administered three times per week (i.e., Monday, Wednesday, Friday) for up to 12 weeks. In most patients, escalation to 30 mg can be accomplished in 3 to 7 days. If therapy is interrupted for 7 or more days, alemtuzumab should be reinitiated with gradual dose escalation.
- Single doses of Campath >30 mg or cumulative doses >90 mg per week should not be administered because these doses are associated with a higher incidence of pancytopenia.
- Premedicate patients with an antihistamine (e.g., diphenhydramine 50 mg p.o. or i.v.) and acetaminophen (650 mg p.o.) 30 minutes prior to alemtuzumab to ameliorate or avoid infusion-related toxicity. Antiemetics, meperidine, and corticosteroids have also been used to prevent or treat infusion-related toxicities.

Dose Modification Criteria

- Myelosuppression: yes

Adverse Reactions

- CV: hypotension, edema/peripheral edema
- DERM: rash, urticaria, pruritus
- GI: N/V (moderate), diarrhea, anorexia, mucositis/stomatitis
- HEMAT: myelosuppression, lymphopenia
- INFUS: rigors, fever, chills, N/V, hypotension, dyspnea, bronchospasm, headache, rash, urticaria
- NEURO: headache, dysthesias, dizziness
- PULM: dyspnea, cough, bronchitis, pneumonia, bronchospasm
- Other: opportunistic infections, sepsis, fatigue, asthenia, pain.

Comments

- Alemtuzumab-treated patients are at risk for opportunistic infections due to profound lymphopenia. Anti-infective prophylaxis is recommended upon initiation of therapy and for a minimum of 2 months following the last dose of alemtuzumab or until the CD4 count is ≥200 cells/μL. Prophylaxis directed against *Pneumocystis* pneumonia (PCP) (e.g., trimethoprim/sulfamethoxazole) and herpesvirus infections (e.g., famciclovir or equivalent) should be utilized.
- Do not administer as an intravenous push or bolus.
- Careful monitoring of blood pressure and hypotension is recommended especially in patients with ischemic heart disease and in patients on antihypertensive medications.
- Patients who have recently received alemtuzumab should not be immunized with live viral vaccines.

ALTRETAMINE (HEXALEN)

Mechanism of Action

- Unknown, but like an alkylating agent in structure

FDA-approved Indications

- Ovarian cancer: second-line, palliative treatment of persistent or recurrent ovarian cancer

FDA-approved Dosage

- 65 mg/m^2 orally four times daily; total daily dose: 260 mg/m^2 for 14 or 21 consecutive days every 28 days.

Dose Modification Criteria

- Myelosuppression: yes
- Nonhematologic toxicity (GI intolerance, progressive neurotoxicity): yes

Adverse Reactions

- GI: N/V (moderate)
- HEMAT: myelosuppression (WBC, RBC, platelets)
- NEURO: peripheral sensory neuropathy, mood disorders, ataxia, dizziness

Comments

- Monitor for neurologic toxicity

ANASTRAZOLE (ARIMIDEX)

Mechanism of Action

- Selective, nonsteroidal aromatase inhibitor

FDA-approved Indications

- Breast cancer
  - Adjuvant treatment: postmenopausal women with hormone receptor positive early breast cancer
  - First-line: postmenopausal women with hormone receptor positive or hormone receptor unknown locally advanced or metastatic breast cancer
  - Second-line therapy (after tamoxifen) in postmenopausal women with advanced breast cancer

FDA-approved Dosage

- 1 mg orally daily (no requirement for glucocorticoid or mineralocorticoid replacement)

Dose Modification Criteria

- Renal: no
- Hepatic (mild to moderate impairment): no
- Hepatic (severe impairment): unknown

Adverse Reactions

- CV: hot flashes/flushing
- GI: N/V (low), diarrhea
- HEPAT: elevated liver function tests (LFTs) (in patients with liver metastases)
- NEURO: headache
- PULM: dyspnea
- Other: asthenia, pain, back pain, vaginal bleeding

Comments

- Patients with estrogen receptor (ER)-negative disease and patients who do not respond to tamoxifen rarely respond to anastrazole

ARSENIC TRIOXIDE (TRISENOX)

Mechanism of Action

- Mechanism is not completely defined.
- Induces apoptosis in NB4 human promyelocytic leukemia cells in vitro and causes damage or degradation of the fusion protein PML/RAR-alpha.

FDA-approved Indications

- Acute promyelocytic leukemia (APL): second-line treatment for the induction of remission and consolidation of APL patients who are refractory to, or have relapsed from, retinoid and anthracycline chemotherapy.

FDA-approved Dosage

- APL induction: 0.15 mg/kg i.v. over 1 to 2 hours daily until bone marrow remission. Total induction dose should not exceed 60 doses.

- APL consolidation: 0.15 mg/kg i.v. over 1 to 2 hours daily $\times$ 25 doses over a period up to 5 weeks. Consolidation treatment should begin 3 to 6 weeks after completion of induction therapy.

Dose Modification Criteria

- Renal: no data, use with caution
- Hepatic: no data

Adverse Reactions

- CV: QT interval prolongation, complete atrioventricular block, torsade de pointes-type ventricular arrhythmia, atrial dysrhythmias, tachycardia, hypotension, edema
- DERM: rash, dermatitis, dry skin, pruritus
- ENDO: hyperglycemia, hypokalemia, hypomagnesemia
- GI: N/V (moderate), diarrhea, abdominal pain, anorexia, constipation
- HEMAT: leukocytosis, myelosuppression
- HEPAT: elevated LFTs
- NEURO: headache, dizziness, paresthesias
- PULM: dyspnea, cough
- Other: fatigue, arthralgia, myalgia, pain, APL differentiation (RA-APL) syndrome (RA-APL syndrome: fever, dyspnea, weight gain, radiographic pulmonary infiltrates, and pleural or pericardial effusion)

Comments

- The APL differentiation syndrome (RA-APL syndrome) has occurred in some patients treated with arsenic trioxide. Early recognition and high-dose corticosteroids (dexamethasone 10 mg i.v. every 12 hours $\times$ 3 days or until the resolution of symptoms) have been used for management.
- Prior to stating arsenic trioxide, a 12-lead ECG should be performed and serum electrolytes (potassium, calcium, magnesium) and creatinine should be assessed; preexisting electrolyte abnormalities should be corrected. Avoid concomitant drugs that may prolong the QT interval. During therapy with arsenic trioxide, monitor and maintain normal potassium and magnesium concentrations (see package insert).
- Risk factors for QT prolongation and subsequent arrhythmias include other QT prolonging drugs, a history of torsade de pointes, preexisting QT prolongation, congestive heart failure, administration of potassium wasting diuretics, or other drugs or conditions that result in hypokalemia or hypomagnesemia.

ASPARAGINASE (ELSPAR)

Mechanism of Action

- Asparaginase depletes asparagine, an amino acid required by some leukemic cells.

FDA-approved Indications

- Acute lymphocytic leukemia (ALL) induction therapy (primarily in combination with other agents)

FDA-approved Dosage

- Consult current literature for doses.
- ALL: Induction in combination with prednisone and vincristine: 1,000 IU/kg i.v. daily $\times$ 10 days starting day 22 *OR* 6,000 IU/m² i.m. every 3 days for nine doses, starting day 4 of induction (day 1 is first day of chemotherapy)

Dose Modification Criteria

- None available

Adverse Reactions

- DERM: skin rash
- ENDO: hyperglycemia
- GI: N/V (low), pancreatitis
- GU: prerenal azotemia
- HEMAT: coagulopathy
- HEPAT: increased LFTs, hyperbilirubinemia, decreased serum albumin
- NEURO: variety of mental status changes
- Other: hypersensitivity, anaphylactic reactions, hyperthermia

Comments

- Contraindicated in patients with active pancreatitis or history of pancreatitis
- Hypersensitivity and anaphylactic reactions can occur.
- Consult package insert regarding test doses and desensitization schedules.
- Intramuscular administration has a lower incidence of hypersensitivity reactions compared to intravenous administration.
- Intravenous infusions should be over at least 30 minutes.

AZACITIDINE (VIDAZA)

Mechanism of Action

- Antimetabolite, a pyrimidine nucleoside analog of cytidine. Azacitidine causes hypomethylation of DNA and direct cytotoxicity on abnormal hematopoietic cells in the bone marrow.

FDA-approved Indications

- Myelodysplastic syndrome (MDS): The specific subtypes of MDS for which azacitidine is indicated include: refractory anemia or refractory anemia with ringed sideroblasts (if accompanied by neutropenia or thrombocytopenia or requiring tranfusions), refractory anemia with excess blasts, refractory anemia with excess blasts in transformation, and chronic myelomonocytic leukemia.

FDA-approved Dosage

- First treatment cycle: The recommended starting dose for all patients regardless of baseline hematology laboratory values, is 75 mg/m^2 subcutaneously or intravenously, daily for 7 days.
- Subsequent treatment cycles: Cycle should be repeated every 4 weeks. The dose may be increased to 100 mg/m^2 if no beneficial effect is seen after two treatment cycles and if no toxicity other than nausea and vomiting has occurred.
- Duration: recommended minimum duration of four treatment cycles; complete or partial response may take more than four treatment cycles; may be continued as long as the patient continues to benefit.

Dose Modification Criteria

- Renal: no data (use with caution)
- Hepatic: no data (use with caution)
- Myelosuppression: yes
- Nonhematologic toxicity (renal tubular acidosis, renal toxicity): yes

Adverse Reactions

- DERM: injection site erythema or pain, ecchymosis, rash, pruritus
- ELECTRO: renal tubular acidosis (alkaline urine, fall in serum bicarbonate, hypokalemia)
- GI: N/V (minimal), diarrhea, constipation, anorexia, abdominal pain, hepatotoxicity
- GU: increased Cr and BUN, renal failure, renal tubular acidosis
- HEMAT: anemia, neutropenia, thrombocytopenia
- NEURO: headache, dizziness
- PULM: cough, dyspnea
- Other: fever, rigors, fatigue, weakness, peripheral edema

Comments

- Teratogenic (pregnancy category D): Women of child-bearing potential should be advised to avoid becoming pregnant while receiving azacitidine. Men should be advised to not father a child while receiving azacitidine.
- Use caution in patients with liver disease. Azacitidine is potentially hepatotoxic in patients with pre-existing hepatic impairment.
- Azacitidine is contraindicated in patients with advanced malignant hepatic tumors.
- Azacitidine and its metabolites are primarily cleared renally. Patients with renal impairment should be closely monitored for toxicity. Renal toxicity has been reported rarely with intravenous azacitidine in combination with other chemotherapeutic agents for non-MDS conditions.

BCG LIVE (INTRAVESICAL), [THERACYS, TICE (BCG)]

Mechanism of Action

- Local inflammatory and immune response

FDA-approved Indications

- Treatment and prophylaxis of carcinoma in situ of the urinary bladder and for the prophylaxis of primary or recurrent stage Ta and/or T1 papillary tumors following transurethal resection (TUR)

FDA-approved Dosage

- TheraCys: vial contains 81 mg (dry weight) or $10.5 \pm 8.7 \times 10^8$ colony-forming units with accompanying 3 mL diluent vial
  - One reconstituted vial (81 mg/3 mL), diluted in 50 mL sterile, preservative-free normal saline (0.9% sodium chloride injection, USP), instilled into bladder for as long as possible (up to 2 hours) once weekly for 6 weeks (induction therapy) followed by one treatment at 3, 6, 12, 18, and 24 months after initial treatment (maintenance therapy).
- Tice bacille Calmette-Guérin (BCG): vial contains 50 mg (wet weight) or 1 to 8×10^8 colony-forming units
  - One reconstituted vial (50 mg/1 mL), diluted in a total volume of 50 mL preservative free normal saline (0.9% sodium chloride injection, USP), instilled into bladder for as long as possible (up to 2 hours) once weekly for 6 weeks followed by once monthly for 6 to 12 months

Dose Modification Criteria

- Withhold on any suspicion of systemic infection

Adverse Reactions

- GU: irritative bladder symptoms
- Other: malaise, fever, chills; infectious complications (uncommon)

Comments

- May complicate tuberculin skin test interpretation
- BCG live products contain live, attenuated mycobacteria. Because of the potential risk of transmission, it should be prepared, handled, and disposed of as a biohazard material.

BENDAMUSTINE HYDROCHLORIDE (TREANDA)

Mechanism of Action

- Alkylating agent

FDA-approved Indications

- Chronic lymphocytic leukemia (CLL)

FDA-approved Dosage

- 100 mg/m^2 by intravenous infusion over 30 minutes on days 1 and 2 of a 28 day cycle, up to six cycles

Dose Modification Criteria

- Myelosuppression: yes
- Nonhematologic toxicity: yes
- Renal: No data, use with caution in patients with mild to moderate renal impairment, avoid in patients with CrCL <40 mL/min
- Hepatic: No data; use with caution in patients with mild hepatic impairment, avoid in patients with moderate to severe hepatic impairment.

Adverse Reactions

- DERM: rash, pruritis, toxic skin reactions, bullous exanthema
- GI: N/V (low), diarrhea, mucositis
- HEMAT: myelosuppression
- INFUS: fever, chills, pruritis, rash, anaphylaxis or anaphylactoid reactions
- PULM: cough
- OTHER: tumor lysis syndrome; asthenia, infections

Comments

- Infusion reactions occurred commonly in clinical trials. Monitor clinically and discontinue drug for severe reactions (grade 3 or worse). Measures to prevent severe reactions (e.g., antihistamines, antipyretics, corticosteroids) should be considered in subsequent cycles in patients who have previously experienced grade 1 or 2 infusion reactions.
- Monitor for tumor lysis syndrome, particularly with the first treatment cycle and utilize allopurinol during the first 1 to 2 weeks of therapy in patients at high risk.
- Severe skin reactions have been reported necessitating drug therapy to be withheld or discontinued.
- Bendamustine hydrochloride is primarily metabolized via hydrolysis to metabolites with low cytotoxic activity. Some metabolism via cytochrome P450 1A2 (CYP1A2) occurs forming active metabolites, thus potential drug interactions with CYP1A2 inhibitors or inducers should be considered.
- Pregnancy category D: bendamustine may cause fetal harm when administered to a pregnant woman.

BEVACIZUMAB (AVASTIN)

Mechanism of Action

- Recombinant humanized monoclonal IgG1 antibody that binds to and inhibits the biologic activity of human vascular endothelial growth factor (VEGF).

FDA-approved Indications

- Metastatic colorectal cancer: First- or second-line treatment of patients with metastatic carcinoma of the colon or rectum; in combination with intravenous 5-fluorouracil-based chemotherapy.
- Nonsquamous, non–small cell lung cancer (NSCLC): First-line treatment of patients with unresectable, locally advanced, recurrent or metastatic nonsquamous NSCLC; in combination with carboplatin and paclitaxel
- Metastatic breast cancer: Treatment of patients who have not received chemotherapy for metastatic HER2 negative breast cancer; in combination with paclitaxel

FDA-approved Dosage

- Metastatic colorectal cancer: administered as an i.v. infusion (5 mg/kg or 10 mg/kg) every 14 days. The recommended dose of bevacizumab when used in combination with bolus irinotecan/5-FU/leucovorin (IFL) is 5 mg/kg. The recommended dose of bevacizumab when used in combination with 5-FU/leucovorin/oxaliplatin (FOLFOX) is 10 mg/kg.
- Nonsquamous NSCLC: 15 mg/kg i.v. infusion every 3 weeks
- Metastatic breast cancer: 10 mg/kg i.v. infusion every 14 days
- Do not administer as an i.v. push or bolus. The initial bevacizumab dose should be delivered over 90 minutes as an i.v. infusion following chemotherapy. If the first infusion is well tolerated, the second infusion may be administered over 60 minutes. If the 60-minute infusion is well tolerated, all subsequent infusions may be administered over 30 minutes.

Dose Modification Criteria

- Renal: no
- Hepatic: no
- Myelosuppression: no
- Nonhematologic toxicity: yes

Adverse Reactions

- CV: hypertension, hypertensive crisis, congestive heart failure
- GI: N/V, diarrhea, abdominal pain, gastrointestinal perforation and wound dehiscence
- GU: proteinuria, nephrotic syndrome
- INFUS: fever, chills, wheezing, stridor
- NEURO: headache
- PULM: dyspnea, wheezing stridor
- Other: epistaxis and other mild to moderate hemorrhagic events; serious hemorrhagic events; wound healing complications; deep vein thrombosis or other thromboembolic events; asthenia

Comments

- Bevacizumab can result in the development of gastrointestinal perforation and wound dehiscence and other wound healing complications. The appropriate interval between termination of bevacizumab and subsequent elective surgery required to avoid the risks of wound healing/wound dehiscence has not been determined. Product labeling suggests that bevacizumab should not be initiated for at least 28 days following major surgery and the surgical incision should be fully healed.

- Bleeding complications secondary to bevacizumab occur in two distinct patterns: minor hemorrhage (most commonly grade 1 epistaxis) and serious, and in some cases, fatal hemorrhagic events. Patients with squamous cell NSCLC appear to be at higher risk for serious hemorrhagic events. The risk of CNS bleeding in patients with CNS metastases receiving bevacizumab has not been evaluated.
- Blood pressure monitoring should be conducted every 2 to 3 weeks during therapy and more frequently in patients who develop hypertension.
- Monitor urinalysis serially for proteinuria; patients with a 2+ or greater urine dipstick reading should undergo further assessment (e.g., a 24-hour urine collection).
- Pregnancy category C: angiogenesis is critical to fetal development and bevacizumab has been shown to be teratogenic in rabbits.

BEXAROTENE (TARGRETIN)

Mechanism of Action
- A retinoid that selectively binds and activates retinoid X receptor subtypes (RXRs).
- Once activated, these receptors function as transcription factors that regulate the expression of genes that control cellular differentiation and proliferation.

FDA-approved Indications
- Cutaneous T-cell lymphoma: second-line treatment of the cutaneous manifestations of cutaneous T-cell lymphoma in patients who are refractory to at least one prior systemic therapy

FDA-approved Dosage
- 300 mg/m^2 orally daily with a meal

Dose Modification Criteria
- Renal: no (caution due to possible protein binding alterations)
- Hepatic: use with caution
- Toxicity: yes

Adverse Reactions
- CV: peripheral edema
- DERM: dry skin, photosensitivity, rash, pruritus
- ENDO: hypothyroidism, hypoglycemia (diabetic patients)
- GI: nausea, pancreatitis, abdominal pain
- HEMAT: leukopenia, anemia
- HEPAT: elevated LFTs
- NEURO: headache
- Ocular: cataracts
- Other: lipid abnormalities (elevated triglycerides, elevated total and LDL cholesterol, and decreased HDL cholesterol), asthenia, infection

Comments
- Monitor fasting blood lipid tests prior to initiation of bexarotene and weekly until the lipid response is established (usually occurs within 2–4 weeks) and then at 8-week intervals thereafter.
- Monitor LFTs prior to initiation of bexarotene and then after 1, 2, and 4 weeks of treatment, and if stable, at least every 8 weeks thereafter during treatment.
- Monitor complete blood count and thyroid function tests at baseline and periodically thereafter.

- Bexarotene is a teratogen (category X) and may cause fetal harm when administered to a pregnant woman. Bexarotene must not be given to a pregnant woman or a woman who intends to become pregnant. A negative pregnancy test in female patients of childbearing potential should be obtained within 1 week prior to starting bexarotene therapy and then repeated at monthly intervals while the patient remains on therapy. Effective contraception (two reliable forms used simultaneously) must be used for 1 month prior to initiation of therapy, during therapy, and for at least 1 month following discontinuation of therapy. Bexarotene may induce the metabolism of hormonal contraceptives and reduce their effectiveness; thus one form of contraception should be nonhormonal.

BICALUTAMIDE (CASODEX)

Mechanism of Action

- Antiandrogen

FDA-approved Indications

- Prostate cancer: palliation of advanced prostate cancer (stage D2) in combination therapy with a luteinizing hormone-releasing hormone (LHRH) agonist

FDA-approved Dosage

- 50 mg orally daily

Dose Modification Criteria

- Renal: no
- Hepatic (mild to moderate impairment): no
- Hepatic (severe impairment): use with caution

Adverse Reactions

- ENDO: loss of libido, hot flashes, gynecomastia
- GI: N/V, diarrhea, constipation
- GU: impotence

Comments

- Monitor LFTs prior to treatment, at regular intervals for the first 4 months, and periodically thereafter.

BLEOMYCIN (BLENOXANE)

Mechanism of Action

- Unknown, but may inhibit DNA and RNA synthesis

FDA-approved Indications

- Squamous cell cancers, non-Hodgkin lymphoma, testicular cancer, Hodgkin disease, malignant pleural effusions

FDA-approved Dosage

- The product labeling recommends a test dose (2 U or less) for the first two doses in lymphoma patients.

- From 0.25 to 0.50 units/kg (10–20 units/m^2) i.v. or i.m. or s.c. weekly or twice weekly
- Malignant pleural effusions: 60 units as single intrapleural bolus dose

Dose Modification Criteria

- Renal: use with caution (dose modification guidelines are not provided within package insert but are available from other references.)

Adverse Reactions

- DERM: erythema, rash, striae, vesiculation, hyperpigmentation, skin tenderness, alopecia, nail changes, pruritus, stomatitis
- PULM: pulmonary fibrosis (increases at cumulative doses >400 units, but can happen at lower total doses), pneumonitis
- Other: fever, chills; idiosyncratic reaction consisting of hypotension, mental confusion, fever, chills, and wheezing has been reported in 1% of lymphoma patients; local pain with intrapleural administration

Comments

- Risk factors for bleomycin-induced pulmonary toxicity include age (>70 years old), underlying emphysema, prior thoracic radiotherapy, high cumulative doses (e.g., >450 units), and high single doses (>30 units).
- Patients who have received bleomycin may be at increased risk of respiratory failure during the postoperative recovery period after surgery. Use the minimal tolerated concentration of inspired oxygen and modest fluid replacement to prevent pulmonary edema.

BORTEZOMIB (VELCADE)

Mechanism of Action

- Bortezomib is a reversible inhibitor of the 26S proteosome, a large protein complex that degrades ubiquinated proteins. Inhibition of the 26S proteosome prevents targeted proteolysis, which can effect multiple signaling cascades within the cell. This disruption of normal homeostatic mechanisms can lead to cell death.

FDA-approved Indications

- Multiple myeloma: first-line therapy in combination with melphalan and prednisone and in relapsed disease as a single agent
- Mantle cell lymphoma: second-line therapy in mantle cell lymphoma patients who have received at least one prior therapy

FDA-approved Dosage

- Multiple myeloma (first-line therapy in combination with melphalan and prednisone): 1.3 mg/m^2 i.v. as a bolus injection twice weekly on a 6-week treatment cycle on days 1, 4, 8, 11, 22, 25, 29, and 32 for cycles 1 to 4. In cycles 5 to 9, bortezomib is administered once weekly on days 1, 8, 22, and 29 of a 6-week treatment cycle (note that week 3 and week 6 of cycle are rest periods).
- Multiple myeloma (relapsed disease) and mantle cell lymphoma: 1.3 mg/m^2 i.v. as a bolus injection administered twice weekly for 2 weeks (days 1, 4, 8, and 11) followed by a 10-day rest period (days 12–21). For extended therapy of more than eight cycles, bortezomib may be administered on the standard schedule or on a maintenance schedule of once weekly for 4 weeks (Days 1,8,15, and 22) followed by a 13-day rest period (Days 23–35). At least 72 hours should elapse between consecutive doses of bortezomib.

Dose Modification Criteria

- Renal: no data (use caution)
- Hepatic: no data (use caution)
- Myelosuppression: yes
- Nonhematologic toxicity (e.g., neuropathy and neuropathic pain): yes

Adverse Reactions

- CV: hypotension (including orthostatic hypotension and syncope), edema
- DERM: rash
- GI: N/V (low), diarrhea, anorexia, constipation
- HEMAT: myelosuppression (thrombocytopenia > anemia > neutropenia)
- NEURO: peripheral neuropathy, neuropathic pain, dizziness, headache
- Ocular: diplopia, blurred vision
- PULM: dyspnea
- Other: asthenia, fatigue, fever, insomnia, arthralgia

BUSULFAN (MYLERAN); BUSULFAN INJECTION (BUSULFEX)

Mechanism of Action

- Alkylating agent

FDA-approved Indications

- Oral busulfan: palliative treatment of chronic myelogenous leukemia (CML)
- Parenteral (i.v.) busulfan: conditioning regimen (in combination with cyclophosphamide) prior to allogeneic hematopoietic progenitor cell transplantation for CML

FDA-approved Dosage

- Oral busulfan: induction, 4 to 8 mg p.o. daily; maintenance, 1 to 3 mg p.o. daily
- Parenteral (i.v.) busulfan
  - Premedicate patients with phenytoin before busulfan administration.
  - For nonobese patients, use ideal body weight (IBW) or actual body weight, whichever is lower.
  - For obese or severely obese patients, use adjusted IBW. Adjusted IBW (AIBW) should be calculated as follows: AIBW = IBW + 0.25 × (actual weight − IBW).
  - 0.8 mg/kg over 2 hours every 6 hours × 16 doses (total course dose: 12.8 mg/kg) with cyclophosphamide.

Dose Modification Criteria

- Myelosuppression: yes.

Adverse Reactions

- DERM: hyperpigmentation
- GI: N/V oral L1, i.v. L4
- HEMAT: severe myelosuppression
- HEPAT: veno-occlusive disease
- NEURO: seizures
- PULM: pulmonary fibrosis

Comments

- Phenytoin reduces busulfan plasma area under the curve (AUC) by 15%. Use of other anticonvulsants may result in higher busulfan plasma AUCs, and an increased risk of veno-occlusive disease or seizures. Monitor plasma busulfan exposure if other anticonvulsants are used.
- High-dose oral busulfan regimens have also been utilized for conditioning regimens in the allogeneic stem cell transplant setting. Consult current literature for dosing regimens.

CAPECITABINE (XELODA)

Mechanism of Action

- Antimetabolite that is enzymatically converted to fluorouracil in tumors

FDA-approved Indications

- Colorectal cancer
  - Adjuvant therapy: indicated as a single agent for adjuvant treatment in patients with Dukes C colon cancer who have undergone complete resection of the primary tumor when treatment with fluoropyrimidine therapy alone is preferred.
  - Metastatic disease: first-line treatment of patients with metastatic colorectal carcinoma when treatment with fluoropyrimidine therapy alone is preferred.
- Breast cancer
  - Combination therapy: capecitabine combined with docetaxel is indicated for the treatment of patients with metastatic breast cancer after failure with prior anthracycline-containing chemotherapy.
  - Breast cancer monotherapy: Third-line therapy for metastatic breast cancer (after paclitaxel and an anthracycline-containing chemotherapy regimen) or second-line (after paclitaxel) if anthracycline is not indicated.

FDA-approved Dosage

- Give 1,250 mg/m^2 p.o. twice daily (total daily dose: 2,500 mg/m^2) at the end of a meal for 2 weeks, followed by a 1-week rest period, given as 3-week cycles. See product labeling for a dosing chart.

Dose Modification Criteria

- Renal (mild impairment; CrCl 51–80 mL/min): no
- Renal (moderate impairment; CrCl 30–50 mL/min): yes
- Hepatic (mild to moderate impairment due to liver metastases): no
- Toxicity (grade 2 toxicity or higher): yes.
- See product labeling for dose modification guidelines.

Adverse Reactions

- DERM: hand and foot syndrome (palmar-plantar erythrodysesthesia), dermatitis
- GI: N/V (low), diarrhea, mucositis, abdominal pain, anorexia, hyperbilirubinemia
- HEMAT: myelosuppression
- NEURO: fatigue/weakness, paresthesia, peripheral sensory neuropathy

Comments

- Altered coagulation parameters and/or bleeding has been reported in patients receiving concomitant capecitabine and oral coumarin-derivative anticoagulation therapy. Anticoagulant response (INR and prothrombin time) should be monitored frequently to adjust anticoagulant dose accordingly.

CARBOPLATIN (PARAPLATIN)

Mechanism of Action

- Alkylating-like agent producing interstrand DNA cross links

FDA-approved Indications

- Advanced ovarian cancer
  - First-line therapy (in combination with other agents)
  - Second-line therapy (including patients who have previously received cisplatin)

FDA-approved Dosage

- With cyclophosphamide: 300 mg/m^2 i.v. $\times$ one dose on day 1 of the cycle; repeat cycles every 4 weeks $\times$ six cycles
- Single agent: 360 mg/m^2 i.v. $\times$ one dose every 4 weeks
- Formula dosing may be used as an alternative to body surface area (BSA)–based dosing.
- Calvert formula for carboplatin dosing:
  Total dose in milligrams = (target AUC) $\times$ [glomerular filtration rate (GFR) + 25]
- The target AUC of 4 to 6 mg/mL/min using single agent carboplatin appears to provide the most appropriate dose range in previously treated patients.
- The Calvert formula was based on studies where GFR was measured by ^{51}Cr-EDTA clearance. Alternatively, many clinicians commonly use estimated CrCl equations to determine GFR.

Dose Modification Criteria

- Renal: yes
- Myelosuppression: yes

Adverse Reactions

- GI: N/V (moderate)
- ELECTRO: Mg, Na, Ca, K alterations
- GU: Inc. Cr and BUN
- HEMAT: myelosuppression (thrombocytopenia > leukopenia and anemia)
- HEPAT: increased LFTs
- NEURO: neuropathy
- Other: anaphylactic reactions, pain, asthenia

Comments

- Do not confuse with cisplatin for dosing or during preparation

CARMUSTINE (BICNU)

Mechanism of Action

- Alkylating agent

FDA-approved Indications

- Indicated as palliative therapy as a single agent or in established combination therapy with other approved chemotherapeutic agents in the following: brain tumors, multiple myeloma, Hodgkin disease, and non-Hodgkin lymphomas.

FDA-approved Dosage

- Single agent in previously untreated patients: 150 to 200 mg/m^2 i.v. $\times$ one dose every 6 weeks *or* 75 to 100 mg/m^2 i.v. daily $\times$ 2 doses every 6 weeks

Dose Modification Criteria

- Myelosuppression: yes

Adverse Reactions

- GI: N/V >250 mg/m^2: (high), $\leq$ 250 mg/m^2: (moderate)
- GU: nephrotoxicity with large cumulative doses
- HEMAT: myelosuppression (can be delayed)
- HEPAT: increased LFTs
- Ocular: retinal hemorrhages
- PULM: pulmonary fibrosis (acute and delayed)

Comments

- Risk of pulmonary toxicity increases with cumulative total doses >1,400 mg/m^2 and in patients with a history of lung disease, radiation therapy, or concomitant bleomycin.

CETUXIMAB (ERBITUX)

Mechanism of Action

- Recombinant chimeric monoclonal antibody that binds to the extracellular domain of the human epidermal growth factor receptor (EGFR) on both normal and tumor cells, and competitively inhibits the binding of epidermal growth factor (EGF) and other ligands, thus blocking phosphorylation and activation of receptor-associated kinases.

FDA-approved Indications

- Head and neck cancer
  - Locally or regionally advanced squamous cell carcinoma of the head and neck in combination with radiation therapy
  - Recurrent or metastatic squamous cell carcinoma of the head and neck progressing after platinum-based therapy.
- Metastatic colorectal carcinoma
  - Monotherapy: indicated as monotherapy for the treatment of EGFR-expressing metastatic colorectal carcinoma after failure of both irinotecan- and oxaliplatin-based regimens or in patients who are intolerant of irinotecan-based chemotherapy.
  - Combination therapy: cetuximab is indicated in combination with irinotecan in EGFR-expressing metastatic colorectal carcinoma in patients who are refractory to irinotecan-based chemotherapy.

FDA-approved Dosage

- Squamous cell carcinoma of the head and neck (with radiation therapy): 400 mg/m^2 i.v. infusion over 120 minutes administered 1 week prior to the first course of radiation therapy followed by subsequent weekly doses of 250 mg/m^2 i.v. infusion over 60 minutes for the duration of radiation therapy (6–7 weeks). Complete cetuximab administration 1 hour prior to radiation therapy.
- Squamous cell carcinoma of the head and neck (monotherapy): the recommended initial dose is 400 mg/m^2 i.v. infusion over 120 minutes followed by subsequent weekly doses of 250 mg/m^2 i.v. infusion over 60 minutes until disease progression or unacceptable toxicity.

- Metastatic colorectal carcinoma (combined with irinotecan or as monotherapy): 400 mg/m² i.v. infusion over 120 minutes as an initial loading dose (first infusion) followed by a weekly maintenance dose of 250 mg/m² i.v. infusion over 60 minutes.
- Premedication with an H₁ antagonist (e.g., 50 mg of diphenhydramine i.v.) is recommended.

Dose Modification Criteria

- Renal: no
- Hepatic: no
- Nonhematologic toxicity (dermatologic toxicity): yes.

Adverse Reactions

- DERM: acneform rash, skin drying and fissuring, nail toxicity
- GI: nausea, constipation, diarrhea
- INFUS: chills, fever, dyspnea, airway obstruction (bronchospasm, stridor, hoarseness), urticaria, hypotension
- PULM: interstitial lung disease
- Other: asthenia, malaise, fever

Comments

- KRAS mutation predicts for a lack of response to cetuximab. Consider evaluating for the KRAS mutation prior to initiating therapy.
- Grade 1 and 2 infusion reactions (chills, fever, dyspnea) are common (16–23%) usually on the first day of initial dosing. Severe infusion reactions have been observed in approximately 3% of patients and are characterized by a rapid onset of airway obstruction, urticaria, and/or hypotension. Severe infusion reactions require immediate interruption of the cetuximab infusion and permanent discontinuation from further treatment.
- Cardiopulmonary arrest and/or sudden death have been reported in patients with squamous cell carcinoma of the head and neck treated with radiation therapy and cetuximab.
- An acneform rash is common (approximately 90% overall, 10% grade 3) with cetuximab therapy and is most commonly observed on the face, upper chest, and back. Skin drying and fissuring were common and can be associated with inflammatory or infections sequelae. Interruption of therapy and dose modification is recommended for severe dermatologic toxicity (see product labeling).
- Interstitial lung disease has been reported with cetuximab therapy rarely. In the event of acute onset or worsening pulmonary symptoms, interrupt cetuximab therapy and promptly investigate symptoms.
- Pregnancy category C: No animal reproduction studies have been conducted and effects in pregnant women are unknown. However, EGFR has been implicated in the control of prenatal development and human IgG1 is known to cross the placental barrier.
- Do not administer as an i.v. push or bolus.

CHLORAMBUCIL (LEUKERAN)

Mechanism of Action

- Alkylating agent

FDA-approved Indications

- Palliation of CLL, Hodgkin disease, non-Hodgkin lymphomas

FDA-approved Dosage

- Initial and short courses of therapy: 0.1 to 0.2 mg/kg p.o. daily for 3 to 6 weeks as required. Usually the 0.1 mg/kg/day dose is used except for Hodgkin disease, in which 0.2 mg/kg/day is used.

- Alternate regimen in CLL (intermittent, biweekly, or once monthly pulses). Initial single dose of 0.4 mg/kg p.o. × one dose. Increase dose by 0.1 mg/kg until control of lymphocytosis.
- Maintenance: not to exceed 0.1 mg/kg/day.

Dose Modification Criteria

- Myelosuppression: yes

Adverse Reactions

- DERM: rash, rare reports of progressive skin hypersensitivity reactions
- GI: N/V (minimal)
- HEMAT: myelosuppression, lymphopenia
- HEPAT: increased LFTs
- NEURO: seizures, confusion, twitching, hallucinations
- PULM: pulmonary fibrosis
- Other: allergic reactions, secondary acute myelomonocytic leukemia (AML) (long-term therapy), sterility

Comments

- Radiation and cytotoxic drugs render the bone marrow more vulnerable to damage; chlorambucil should be used with caution within 4 weeks of a full course of radiation therapy or chemotherapy.

CISPLATIN (PLATINOL)

Mechanism of Action

- Alkylating-like agent producing interstrand DNA cross-links

FDA-approved Indications

- Metastatic testicular tumors (in combination with other agents) in patients who have already received appropriate surgical and/or radiotherapeutic procedures.
- Metastatic ovarian tumors (in combination with other agents) in patients who have already received appropriate surgical and/or radiotherapeutic procedures.
- Metastatic ovarian tumors (as a single agent) as secondary therapy in patients who are refractory to standard chemotherapy and who have not previously received cisplatin.
- Advanced transitional cell bladder cancer, which is no longer amenable to local treatments such as surgery and/or radiotherapy.

FDA-approved Dosage

- Metastatic testicular tumors: 20 mg/m^2 i.v. daily × 5 days every 4 weeks (in combination with other agents)
- Metastatic ovarian tumors: 75 to 100 mg/m^2 i.v. × one dose (in combination with cyclophosphamide) every 4 weeks, OR as single agent therapy: 100 mg/m^2 i.v. × one dose every 4 weeks.
- Advanced bladder cancer: 50 to 70 mg/m^2 i.v. × one dose every 3 to 4 weeks (single-agent therapy)

Dose Modification Criteria

- Renal: yes
- Myelosuppression: yes

Adverse Reactions

- ELECTRO: Mg, Na, Ca, K alterations
- GI: N/V ($\geq$50 mg/m^2: high, $<$50 mg/m^2: moderate)
- GU: increased Cr and BUN (cumulative)
- HEMAT: myelosuppression, anemia
- HEPAT: increased LFTs (especially SGOT, bilirubin)
- NEURO: neuropathy, paresthesia, ototoxicity
- Ocular: optic neuritis, papilledema, cerebral blindness infrequently reportedOther: anaphylactic reactions, rare vascular toxicities

Comments

- Check auditory acuity
- Vigorous hydration recommended before and after cisplatin administration.
- Use other nephrotoxic agents (e.g., aminoglycosides) concomitantly with caution.
- Exercise precaution to prevent inadvertent cisplatin overdose and confusion with carboplatin.

CLADRIBINE (LEUSTATIN)

Mechanism of Action

- Antimetabolite

FDA-approved Indications

- Hairy cell leukemia

FDA-approved Dosage

- 0.09 mg/kg i.v. continuous infusion over 24 hours daily $\times$ 7 days (a single course of therapy)
- Inadequate data on dosing of patients with renal or hepatic insufficiency

Dose Modification Criteria

- Renal: no data
- Hepatic: no data

Adverse Reactions

- DERM: rash
- GI: N/V (minimal)
- HEMAT: myelosuppression, lymphopenia
- NEURO: fatigue, headache, peripheral neuropathy
- OTHER: fever

Comments

- Immunosuppression (lymphopenia) persists for up to 1 year after cladribine therapy.

CLOFARABINE (CLOLAR)

Mechanism of Action

- Antimetabolite.

FDA-approved Indications

- Acute lymphoblastic leukemia (ALL): pediatric patients (age 1–21 years old) with relapsed or refractory ALL after at least two prior regimens

FDA-approved Dosage

- 52 mg/m^2 by intravenous infusion over 2 hours daily for 5 consecutive days.
- Treatment cycles are repeated following recovery or return to baseline organ function, approximately every 2 to 6 weeks.

Dose Modification Criteria

- Renal: no data, use with caution
- Hepatic: no data, use with caution
- Nonhematologic toxicity: yes

Adverse Reactions

- CV: tachycardia, hypotension
- DERM: dermatitis, palmar-plantar erythrodysesthesia syndrome
- GI: N/V (moderate), abdominal pain, diarrhea, gingival bleeding, anorexia
- GU: elevated Cr
- HEMAT: myelosuppression
- HEPATIC: elevated LFTs, hyperbilirubinemia, hepatomegaly
- INFUS: fever, chills, rigors
- NEURO: headache, dizziness
- PULM: dyspnea, respiratory distress, pleural effusion
- Other: tumor lysis syndrome; infections, fatigue, asthenia

Comments

- Prophylaxis for tumor lysis syndrome (hydration, allopurinol) should be considered and patients should be closely monitored during therapy.
- Capillary leak syndrome or systemic inflammatory response syndrome (SIRS) has been reported and patients should be closely monitored. The use of prophylactic corticosteroids (e.g., 100 mg/m^2 hydrocortisone on days 1 through 3) may be of benefit in preventing SIRS or capillary leak.
- Hepatobiliary toxicities were frequently observed in clinical trials.
- Clofarabine is primarily renally cleared; use caution in patients with significant renal impairment and avoid concomitant nephrotoxins.
- Pregnancy category D: Clofarabine may cause fetal harm when administered to a pregnant woman.

CYCLOPHOSPHAMIDE (CYTOXAN)

Mechanism of Action

- Activated by liver to alkylating agent

FDA-approved Indications

- Lymphomas, leukemias, multiple myeloma, mycosis fungoides (advanced disease), neuroblastoma (disseminated disease), adenocarcinoma of the ovary, retinoblastoma, breast cancer

FDA-approved Dosage

- Parenteral (i.v.): many dosing regimens reported; consult current literature
- Oral: 1 to 5 mg/kg/day (many other regimens reported; consult current literature)

Dose Modification Criteria

- Myelosuppression: yes

Adverse Reactions

- DERM: rash, skin and nail pigmentation, alopecia
- GI: N/V ($\geq$1,500 mg/m^2: high, $<$1,500 mg/m^2: moderate), anorexia, diarrhea
- GU: hemorrhagic cystitis, renal tubular necrosis
- HEMAT: myelosuppression (leukopenia $>$ thrombocytopenia and anemia)
- NEURO: syndrome of inappropriate antidiuretic hormone (SIADH)
- PULM: pulmonary fibrosis
- Other: secondary malignancies; sterility, amenorrhea; anaphylactic reactions; cardiac toxicity with high-dose regimens

Comments

- Encourage forced fluid intake and frequent voiding to reduce the risk of hemorrhagic cystitis. Consider using vigorous intravenous hydration and MESNA therapy with high-dose cyclophosphamide.

CYTARABINE (CYTOSAR AND OTHERS)

Mechanism of Action

- Antimetabolite

FDA-approved Indications

- In combination with other agents for induction therapy of acute nonlymphocytic leukemia (ANLL), acute lymphocytic leukemia (ALL), blast-phase chronic myelocytic leukemia (CML), intrathecal prophylaxis, and treatment of meningeal leukemia

FDA-approved Dosage

- ALL: consult current literature for doses
- ANLL induction (in combination with other agents): 100 mg/m^2 i.v. continuous infusion over 24 hours $\times$ 7 days *OR* 100 mg/m^2 i.v. every 12 hours $\times$ 7 days. Consult current literature for alternative dosing regimens (e.g., high-dose regimens such as $\geq$1 gm/m^2/dose).
- Intrathecally: (use preservative-free diluents) 30 mg/m^2 intrathecally every 4 days until cerebrospinal fluid (CSF) clear, and then one additional dose. Other doses and frequency of administration have been utilized.

Dose Modification Criteria

- Hepatic/renal: Use with caution and at possibly reduced dose in patients with poor hepatic or renal function (no specific criteria)
- Neurotoxicity: yes.

Adverse Reactions

- DERM: rash, alopecia
- GI: N/V L1 ($>$1 g/m^2: moderate; $\leq$200 mg/m^2: low), anorexia, diarrhea, mucositis, pancreatitis (in patients who have previously received asparaginase)
- HEMAT: myelosuppression

- HEPAT: increased LFTs
- NEURO: cerebellar dysfunction, somnolence, coma (generally seen with high-dose regimens), chemical arachnoiditis (intrathecal administration)
- OCULAR: conjunctivitis (generally seen with high-dose regimens)
- Other: cytarabine (Ara-C) syndrome (includes: fever, myalgia, bone pain, rash, conjunctivitis, malaise); acute respiratory distress syndrome reported with high-dose regimens

Comments

- Consider appropriate prophylaxis for tumor lysis syndrome when treating acute leukemias.
- Consider local corticosteroid eye drops to provide prophylaxis for conjunctivitis when employing high-dose regimens of cytarabine.
- Withhold therapy if acute CNS toxicity occurs with high-dose regimens.

CYTARABINE LIPOSOME INJECTION (DEPOCYT)

Mechanism of Action

- Antimetabolite

FDA-approved Indications

- Intrathecal treatment of lymphomatous meningitis

FDA-approved Dosage

- Given only by intrathecal route either via an intraventricular reservoir or directly into the lumbar sac over a period of 1 to 5 minutes.
- Patients should be started on dexamethasone, 4 mg p.o. or i.v. twice daily $\times$ 5 days beginning on the day of the cytarabine liposome injection.
- Induction: 50 mg intrathecally every 14 days $\times$ two doses (weeks 1 and 3)
- Consolidation: 50 mg intrathecally every 14 days $\times$ three doses (weeks 5, 7, and 9) followed by an additional dose at week 13
- Maintenance: 50 mg intrathecally every 28 days $\times$ four doses (weeks 17, 21, 25, 29).

Dose Modification Criteria

- Neurotoxicity: yes

Adverse Reactions

- NEURO: Chemical arachnoiditis, headache, asthenia, confusion, somnolence

DACARBAZINE (DTIC-DOME)

Mechanism of Action

- Methylation of nucleic acids, direct DNA damage, and inhibition of purine synthesis

FDA-approved Indications

- Metastatic malignant melanoma
- Hodgkin disease (second-line therapy)

FDA-approved Dosage

- Malignant melanoma: 2 to 4.5 mg/kg i.v. daily $\times$ 10 days; repeat every 4 weeks, *OR* 250 mg/m^2 i.v. daily $\times$ 5 days; repeat every 3 weeks
- Hodgkin disease: 150 mg/m^2 i.v. daily $\times$ 5 days, repeat every 4 weeks (in combination with other agents), *OR* 375 mg/m^2 i.v. on day 1, repeat every 15 days (in combination with other agents)

Adverse Reactions

- DERM: alopecia, rash, facial flushing, facial paresthesia
- GI: N/V (high), anorexia, diarrhea
- HEPAT: increased LFTs, hepatic necrosis
- Other: pain and burning at infusion, anaphylaxis, fever, myalgias, malaise

DACTINOMYCIN (COSMEGEN)

Mechanism of Action

- Intercalating agent

FDA-approved Indications

- Indicated as part of a combination chemotherapy or multimodality treatment regimen for the following malignancies:
  - Wilms' tumor
  - Childhood rhabdomyosarcoma
  - Ewing sarcoma
  - Metastatic, nonseminomatous testicular cancer
  - Indicated as a single agent or as part of a combination regimen for gestational trophoblastic neoplasia.
  - Indicated as a component of regional perfusion in the treatment of locally recurrent or locoregional solid malignancies.

FDA-approved Dosage

- For obese or edematous patients, dose should be based on BSA.
- Dose intensity should not exceed 15 μg/kg i.v. daily $\times$ 5 days *OR* 400 to 600 μg/m^2 i.v. daily $\times$ 5 days, repeated every 3 to 6 weeks.
- Consult with current literature for dosage regimens and guidelines.

Dose Modification Criteria

- Myelosuppression: yes

Adverse Reactions

- DERM: alopecia, erythema, skin eruptions, radiation recall, tissue damage/necrosis with extravasation
- ELECTRO: hypocalcemia
- GI: N/V (moderate), mucositis, anorexia, dysphagia
- HEMAT: myelosuppression
- HEPAT: increased LFTs, hepatotoxicity
- Other: fever, fatigue, myalgia, secondary malignancies

Comments

- Vesicant

DASATINIB (SPRYCEL)

Mechanism of Action

- Tyrosine kinase inhibitor (BCR-ABL, SRC family, c-KIT, EPHA-2, PDGFRβ)

FDA-approved Indications

- Chronic myeloid leukemia (CML): adults with chronic, accelerated, or myeloid or lymphoid blast phase CML with resistance or intolerance to prior therapy including imatinib
- Acute lymphoblastic leukemia (ALL): adults with Philadelphia chromosome–positive (Ph+) ALL with resistance or intolerance to prior therapy

FDA-approved Dosage

- CML, chronic phase: 100 mg orally once daily
- CML, accelerated phase or myeloid or lymphoid blast phase: 70 mg orally twice daily (140 mg/day)
- ALL (Ph+): 70 mg orally twice daily (140 mg/day)

Dose Modification Criteria

- Myelosuppression: yes
- Nonhematologic toxicity: yes; Renal: no data
- Hepatic: no data, use with caution

Adverse Reactions

- CV: fluid retention events (e.g., CHF), QT prolongation
- DERM: skin rash
- GI: N/V (low), diarrhea
- HEMAT: myelosuppression, hemorrhage
- NEURO: headache
- PULM: pleural effusion, pulmonary edema, pericardial effusion, dyspnea
- Other: fluid retention (e.g., edema), fatigue

Comments

- Myelosuppression may require dose interruption or reduction. Monitor closely.
- Severe bleeding-related events, mostly related to thrombocytopenia, have been reported. Use with caution in patients requiring medications that inhibit platelet function or anticoagulants.
- Dasatinib is metabolized through cytochrome P450 3A4 isoenzyme. Screen for drug interactions with CYP 3A4 inhibitors or inducers.
- Use with caution in patients who have or may develop QT prolongation. Correct hypokalemia or hypomagnesemia prior to starting therapy.
- The bioavailability of dasatinib is pH dependent. Long-term suppression of gastric acid secretion by H_2 antagonists or proton pump inhibitors is likely to reduce dasatinib exposure. Administration of antacids should be separated from dasatinib by a minimum of 2 hours.
- Pregnancy category D: Dasatinib may cause fetal harm when administered to a pregnant woman.

DAUNORUBICIN (CERUBIDINE)

Mechanism of Action

- Intercalating agent; topoisomerase-II inhibition

FDA-approved Indications

- In combination with other agents for remission induction in adult ANLL or ALL, children and adults

FDA-approved Dosage

- ANLL: in combination with cytarabine
  - Age <60 years: (first course) 45 mg/m^2 i.v. daily $\times$ 3 days (days 1, 2, and 3); (subsequent course) 45 mg/m^2 i.v. daily $\times$ 2 days (days 1 and 2)
  - Age $\geq$ 60 years: (first course) 30 mg/m^2 i.v. daily $\times$ 3 days (days 1, 2, and 3); (subsequent course) 30 mg/m^2 i.v. daily $\times$ 2 days (days 1 and 2)
- ALL: (combined with vincristine, prednisone, L-asparaginase) 45 mg/m^2 i.v. daily $\times$ 3 days (days 1, 2, and 3)
- Pediatric ALL: (combined with vincristine, prednisone) 25 mg/m^2 i.v. $\times$ one dose weekly $\times$ 4 weeks initially. In children <2 years of age or below 0.5 m^2 BSA, dosage should be based on weight (1 mg/kg) instead of BSA.

Dose Modification Criteria

- Renal: yes
- Hepatic: yes

Adverse Reactions

- CV: congestive heart failure (CHF), (Risk of cardiotoxicity increases rapidly with total lifetime cumulative doses >400 to 550 mg/m^2 in adults or >300 mg/m^2 in children), arrhythmias
- DERM: nail hyperpigmentation, rash, alopecia, tissue damage/necrosis with extravasation
- GI: N/V (moderate), mucositis
- HEMAT: myelosuppression
- OTHER: red-tinged urine, fever, chills, secondary malignancies

Comments

- Vesicant
- Consider appropriate prophylaxis for tumor lysis syndrome when treating acute leukemias.

DAUNORUBICIN CITRATE LIPOSOME INJECTION (DAUNOXOME)

Mechanism of Action

- Intercalating agent; Topoisomerase II inhibition

FDA-approved Indications

- Advanced HIV-associated Kaposi's sarcoma (first-line therapy)

FDA-approved Dosage

- 40 mg/m^2 i.v. over 60 minutes $\times$ one dose every 2 weeks

Dose Modification Criteria

- Hepatic: yes
- Renal: yes
- Myelosuppression: yes

Adverse Reactions

- CV: CHF, arrhythmias
- DERM: nail, alopecia, hyperpigmentation, rash
- GI: N/V (low), mucositis, diarrhea
- HEMAT: myelosuppression
- INFUS: back pain, flushing, chest tightness (Infusion-related reactions usually subside with interruption of the infusion, and generally do not recur if the infusion is then resumed at a slower rate)
- OTHER: red-tinged urine, fever, chills, fatigue

Comments

- Do not confuse with nonliposomal forms of daunorubicin.
- Liposomal formulations of the same drug may not be equivalent.
- Evaluate cardiac function by history and physical examination of each cycle and determine left ventricular ejection fraction (LVEF) function at total cumulative doses of daunorubicin citrate liposome injection of 320 mg/m^2 and every 160 mg/m^2 thereafter in anthracycline-naive patients. In patients with preexisting cardiac disease, a history of radiotherapy encompassing the heart, or those who previously received anthracyclines (doxorubicin >300 mg/m^2 or equivalent) should have cardiac function (LVEF) monitored before daunorubicin citrate liposome injection therapy and every 160 mg/m^2 thereafter.

DECITABINE (DACOGEN)

Mechanism of Action

- Decitabine is an analogue of the natural nucleoside 2'-deoxycytidine. Decitabine's mechanism of action is as a hypomethylating agent of DNA and also via direct incorporation into DNA.

FDA-approved Indications

- Myelodysplastic Syndrome (MDS): previously treated and untreated de novo and secondary MDS of all FAB subtypes and intermediate-1, intermediate-2, and high-risk International Prognostic Scoring System groups

FDA-approved Dosage

- 15 mg/m^2 by i.v. infusion over 3 hours repeated every 8 hours for 3 days. Cycles may be repeated every 6 weeks. It is recommended that patients be treated for a minimum of four cycles; however, a complete or partial response may take longer than four cycles. Treatment may be continued as long as the patient continues to benefit.

Dose Modification Criteria

- Renal: not studied (use with caution)
- Hepatic: not studied (use with caution)
- Myelosuppression: yes
- Nonhematologic toxicity: yes

Adverse Reactions

- CV: edema, peripheral edema
- DERM: rash, erythema, ecchymosis
- ELECTRO: hypomagnesemia, hypokalemia, hyponatremia

- ENDO: hyperglycemia
- GI: N/V (low), diarrhea, constipation, abdominal pain, stomatitis, dyspepsia
- HEMAT: myelosuppresion
- HEPAT: hyperbilirubinemia, increased LFTs
- NEURO: headache, dizziness, insomnia, confusion
- PULM: cough, pharyngitis
- Other: fatigue, fever, rigors, arthralgis, limb or back pain

Comments

- Pregnancy category D: May cause fetal harm if administered to a pregnant woman. Men should not father a child while receiving treatment with decitabine or for 2 months afterward.

DENILEUKIN DIFTITOX (ONTAK)

Mechanism of Action

- Fusion protein composed of diphtheria toxin fragments linked to interleukin-2 (IL-2) sequences; interacts with IL-2 cell surface receptors and inhibits cellular protein synthesis.

FDA-approved Indications

- Treatment of persistent or recurrent cutaneous T cell lymphoma (CTCL) in patients whose malignant cells express the CD25 component of the IL-2 receptor.

FDA-approved Dosage

- Cells should be tested for CD25 before administration.
- 9 or 18 μg/kg i.v. over at least 15 minutes daily × 5 days; repeat cycles every 21 days. Infusion should be stopped or infusion rate should be reduced for severe infusion-related reactions.

Adverse Reactions

- CV: vascular leak syndrome (hypotension, edema hypoalbuminemia), hypotension, thrombotic events
- DERM: rash, pruritis
- GI: N/V (moderate), anorexia, diarrhea
- HEMAT: anemia
- HEPAT: increased LFTs
- INFUS: acute hypersensitivity-type reactions consisting of one or more of the following: hypotension, back pain, dyspnea, vasodilation, rash, chest pain or tightness, tachycardia, dysphagia, syncope, allergic reactions, or anaphylaxis
- NEURO: dizziness
- PULM: dyspnea, cough
- Other: Flulike syndrome consisting of one or more of the following: fever and/or chills, asthenia, digestive symptoms, myalgias, and arthralgias (appears several hours to days after dose infusion)

Comments

- Consider premedication with antipyretics and antihistamines; have emergency medications and resuscitative equipment readily available during administration.
- Monitor weight, blood pressure, and serum albumin for vascular leak syndrome. Patients with preexisting low serum albumin levels may be predisposed to the syndrome.
- Monitor patients carefully for infection.

DOCETAXEL (TAXOTERE)

Mechanism of Action

- Microtubule assembly stabilization

FDA-approved Indications

- Non–small cell lung cancer
  - First-line therapy in combination with cisplatin for unresectable, locally advanced or metastatic NSCLC
  - Second-line therapy as single agent after failure of prior platinum-based chemotherapy
- Breast cancer
  - Locally advanced or metastatic breast cancer (after failure of prior chemotherapy)
  - For the adjuvant treatment of patients with operable node-positive breast cancer (in combination with doxorubicin and cyclophosphamide)
- Prostate cancer: androgen-independent (hormone refractory) metastatic-prostate cancer (in combination with prednisone)
- Gastric cancer: advanced gastric adenocarcinoma, including adenocarcinoma of the gastroesophageal junction (in combination with cisplatin and fluorouracil), first-line therapy in advanced disease
- Head and neck cancer: induction treatment of locally advanced squamous cell carcinoma of the head and neck (in combination with cisplatin and fluorouracil)

FDA-approved Dosage

- Premedication for hypersensitivity reactions and fluid retention: dexamethasone, 8 mg p.o. twice daily for 3 days starting 1 day before docetaxel administration
- Non–small cell lung cancer
  - First-line therapy (combined with cisplatin): 75 mg/m^2 i.v. over 1 hour $\times$ one dose every 3 weeks (administered immediately prior to cisplatin)
  - Second-line therapy (single agent): 75 mg/m^2 i.v. over 1 hour $\times$ one dose every 3 weeks
- Breast cancer:
  - Locally advanced or metastatic breast cancer: 60 to 100 mg/m^2 i.v. over 1 hour $\times$ one dose every 3 weeks
  - In the adjuvant treatment setting: 75 mg/m^2 i.v. over 1 hour after doxorubicin 50 mg/m^2 and cyclophosphamide 500 mg/m^2 every 3 weeks for six courses. Prophylactic filgrastim may be used.
- Prostate cancer: 75 mg/m^2 i.v. over 1 hour $\times$ one dose every 3 weeks; prednisone 5 mg orally twice daily is administered continuously
- Gastric adenocarcinoma: 75 mg/m^2 i.v. over 1 hour on day 1 only every 3 weeks (in a combination regimen with cisplatin and fluorouracil)
- Head and neck cancer
  - Induction chemotherapy followed by radiotherapy (TAX323): 75 mg/m^2 i.v. over 1 hour on day 1 only (in a combination regimen with cisplatin and fluorouracil), repeat cycle every 3 weeks for 4 cycles.
  - Induction chemotherapy followed by chemoradiotherapy (TAX324): 75 mg/m^2 i.v. over 1 hour on day 1 only (in a combination regimen with cisplatin and fluorouracil), repeat cycle every 3 weeks for 3 cycles.
  - All patients in the TAX323 and TAX324 docetaxel study arms received prophylactic antibiotics.

Dose Modification Criteria

- Hepatic: yes
- Myelosuppression: yes
- Nonhematologic toxicity: yes (consult with package labeling for dose modification guidelines)

Adverse Reactions

- DERM: rash with localized skin eruptions, erythema and pruritis, nail changes (pigmentation, onycholysis, pain), alopecia
- GI: N/V (low), diarrhea, mucositis
- HEMAT: myelosuppression
- HEPAT: increased LFTs
- INFUS: acute hypersensitivity-type reactions consist of hypotension and/or bronchospasm or generalized rash/erythema
- NEURO: peripheral neurosensory toxicity (paresthesia, dysesthesia, pain)
- Other: severe fluid retention, myalgia, fever, asthenia

Comments

- Patients with preexisting hepatic dysfunction are at increased risk of severe toxicity.
- Patients with preexisting effusions should be closely monitored from the first dose for the possible exacerbation of the effusions.
- Lower dose, weekly dosage regimens are commonly utilized. Consult current literature for dose guidelines.
- Use non-DEHP plasticized solution containers and administration sets.

DOXORUBICIN (ADRIAMYCIN AND OTHERS)

Mechanism of Action

- Intercalating agent; topoisomerase-II inhibition

FDA-approved Indications

- ALL, acute myeloblastic leukemia, Wilms' tumor, neuroblastoma, soft-tissue and bone sarcoma, breast, ovarian, thyroid, bronchiogenic, gastric cancer, and transitional cell bladder cancer, Hodgkin disease, malignant lymphoma

FDA-approved Dosage

- Many dosing regimens reported; consult current literature; common dose regimens listed below
- Single agent: 60 to 75 mg/m^2 i.v. $\times$ one dose repeated every 3 weeks
- In combination with other agents: 40 to 60 mg/m^2 i.v. $\times$ one dose, repeated every 3 to 4 weeks

Dose Modification Criteria

- Hepatic: yes
- Myelosuppression: yes

Adverse Reactions

- CV: congestive heart failure (CHF) (risk of cardiotoxicity increases rapidly with total lifetime cumulative doses >450 mg/m^2), arrhythmias
- DERM: nail hyperpigmentation, onycholysis, alopecia, radiation recall, tissue damage/necrosis with extravasation
- GI: N/V (moderate), mucositis
- HEMAT: myelosuppression
- Other: red-tinged urine, fever, chills, secondary malignancies

Comments

- Vesicant

DOXORUBICIN HCL LIPOSOME INJECTION (DOXIL)

Mechanism of Action

- Intercalating agent; topoisomerase-II inhibition

FDA-approved Indications

- AIDS-related Kaposi's sarcoma (progressive disease after prior combination chemotherapy or in patients intolerant to such therapy)
- Ovarian cancer (progressive or recurred disease after platinum-based chemotherapy)
- Multiple myeloma: in combination with bortezomib for patients who have not received bortezomib and have received at least one prior therapy.

FDA-approved Dosage

- AIDS-related Kaposi's sarcoma: 20 mg/m^2 i.v. over 30 minutes $\times$ one dose, repeated every 3 weeks
- Ovarian cancer: 50 mg/m^2 i.v. over 60 minutes $\times$ one dose, repeated every 4 weeks
- Multiple myeloma: 30 mg/m^2 i.v. over 60 minutes on day 4 only following bortezomib (bortezomib dose is 1.3 mg/m^2 i.v. bolus on days 1, 4, 8, and 11), every 3 weeks for up to eight cycles until disease progression or unacceptable toxicity.
- Note: Infusion should start at an initial rate of 1 mg/min to minimize the risk of infusion reactions. If no infusion-related adverse events are observed, the rate of infusion can be increased to complete administration of the drug over 1 hour.

Dose Modification Criteria

- Hepatic: yes
- Palmar-plantar erythrodysesthesia: yes
- Myelosuppression: yes
- Stomatitis: yes

Adverse Reactions

- CV: CHF, arrhythmias
- DERM: palmar-plantar erythrodysesthesia, alopecia, rash
- GI: N/V (low), mucositis/stomatitis
- HEMAT: myelosuppression
- INFUS: flushing, shortness of breath, facial swelling, headache, chills, chest pain, back pain, tightness in chest or throat, fever, tachycardia, pruritis, rash, cyanosis, syncope, bronchospasm, asthma, apnea, and/or hypotension
- Other: asthenia, red-tinged urine

Comments

- Do not confuse with nonliposomal forms of doxorubicin.
- Liposomal formulations of the same drug may not be equivalent.
- Irritant
- Mix only with D5W; do not use inline filters
- The majority of infusion-related events occur during the first infusion.

- Experience with large cumulative doses of doxorubicin HCl liposome injection is limited and cumulative dose limits based on cardiotoxicity risk have not been established. It is recommended by the manufacturer that cumulative dose limits established for conventional doxorubicin be followed for the liposomal product (e.g., cumulative doses $\geq$ 400–550 mg/m^2 depending on risk factors).

EPIRUBICIN (ELLENCE)

Mechanism of Action

- Intercalating agent; topoisomerase-II inhibition

FDA-approved Indications

- Adjuvant therapy of axillary node-positive breast cancer

FDA-approved Dosage

- The following dosage regimens were used in the trials supporting use of epirubicin as a component of adjuvant therapy in patients with axillary-node positive breast cancer.
- CEF 120: 60 mg/m^2 i.v. $\times$ one dose on days 1 and 8, (120 mg/m^2 total dose each cycle), repeated every 28 days for six cycles (combined with cyclophosphamide and fluorouracil)
- FEC 100: 100 mg/m^2 i.v. $\times$ one dose on day 1 only, repeated every 21 days for six cycles (combined with cyclophosphamide and fluorouracil)

Dose Modification Criteria

- Renal: yes
- Hepatic: yes
- Myelosuppression: yes

Adverse Reactions

- CV: CHF (risk of cardiotoxicity increases rapidly with total lifetime cumulative doses >900 mg/m^2), arrhythmias
- DERM: alopecia, radiation recall, tissue damage/necrosis with extravasation
- GI: N/V (moderate), mucositis
- HEMAT: myelosuppression
- Other: facial flushing, secondary malignancies

Comments

- Vesicant

ERLOTINIB (TARCEVA)

Mechanism of Action

- Tyrosine kinase inhibitor [epidermal growth factor receptor type 1 (EGFR/HER1)]

FDA-approved Indications

- NSCLC: locally advanced or metastatic disease after failure of at least one prior chemotherapy regimen
- Pancreatic cancer: first-line treatment in combination with gemcitabine in patients with locally advanced, unresectable, or metastatic pancreatic cancer

FDA-approved Dosage

- NSCLC: 150 mg po daily (administer at least 1 hour before or 2 hours after the ingestion of food)
- Pancreatic cancer: 100 mg po daily (administer at least 1 hour before or 2 hours after the ingestion of food) in combination with gemcitabine

Dose Modification Criteria

- Renal: no
- Hepatic: unknown, use with caution
- Myelosuppression: no
- Nonhematologic toxicity: yes

Adverse Reactions

- DERM: rash, pruritis, dry skin
- GI: N/V (low), diarrhea, anorexia
- HEPAT: elevated LFTs
- Ocular: conjunctivitis, keratoconjunctivitis sicca
- PULM: interstitial lung disease
- Other: fatigue

Comments

- KRAS mutation predicts for a lack of response to anti-EGFR agents like erlotinib. Consider evaluating for the KRAS mutation prior to initiating therapy.
- Interrupt therapy in patients who develop an acute onset of new or progressive pulmonary symptoms (e.g., dyspnea, cough, or fever) for diagnostic evaluation. If interstitial lung disease is diagnosed, erlotinib should be discontinued.
- Diarrhea can usually be managed with loperamide. Interruption of therpay or dose reduction may be necessary in patients with severe diarrhea who are unresponsive to loperamide or who become dehydrated.
- Monitor liver transaminases, bilirubin, and alkaline phosphatase during therapy with erlotinib. Therapy with erlotinib should be interrupted if changes in liver function are severe.
- Erlotinib is metabolized through cytochrome P450 3A4 isoenzyme. Screen for drug interactions with CYP 3A4 inhibitors or inducers.
- Pregnancy category D: erlotinib may cause fetal harm when administered to a pregnant woman.

ESTRAMUSTINE (EMCYT)

Mechanism of Action

- Alkylating agent, estrogen, microtubule instability

FDA-approved Indications

- Palliative treatment of metastatic and/or progressive carcinoma of the prostate

FDA-approved Dosage

- 4.67 mg/kg p.o. three times daily (t.i.d.) *OR* 3.5 mg/kg p.o. four times daily (q.i.d); total daily dose: 14 mg/kg
- Administer with water 1 hour before or 2 hours after meals. Avoid the simultaneous administration of milk, milk products, and calcium-rich foods or drugs.

Dose Modification Criteria

- Hepatic: administer with caution, no specific dose modifications

Adverse Reactions

- CV: Edema, fluid retention, venous thromboembolism
- ENDO: hyperglycemia, gynecomastia, impotence
- GI: diarrhea, nausea
- HEPAT: elevated LFTs (especially SGOT or LDH)
- PULM: dyspnea

ETOPOSIDE (VEPESID)

Mechanism of Action

- Topoisomerase-II interaction

FDA-approved Indications

- Refractory testicular cancer; SCLC, first-line therapy in combination with other agents

FDA-approved Dosage

- Testicular cancer: 50 to100 mg/m² i.v. over 30 to 60 min daily × 5 days (days 1–5), repeated every 3 to 4 weeks *OR* 100 mg/m² i.v. over 30 to 60 minutes on days 1, 3, and 5, repeated every 3 to 4 weeks (in combination with other approved agents). Consult current literature for dose recommendations.
- SCLC: 35 to 50 mg/m² i.v. over 30 to 60 min daily × 4 to 5 days, repeated every 3 to 4 weeks (in combination with other agents). Consult current literature for dose recommendations.
- Oral capsules: In SCLC, the recommended dose of etoposide capsules is two times the i.v. dose rounded to the nearest 50 mg.

Dose Modification Criteria

- Renal: yes

Adverse Reactions

- DERM: alopecia, rash, urticaria, pruritis
- GI: N/V (low), mucositis, anorexia
- HEMAT: myelosuppression
- INFUS: hypotension (infusion-rate related), anaphylactic-like reactions (characterized by chills, fever, tachycardia, bronchospasm, dyspnea, and/or hypotension)
- Other: secondary malignancies

ETOPOSIDE PHOSPHATE (ETOPHOS)

Mechanism of Action

- Rapidly and completely converted to etoposide in plasma, leading to topoisomerase-II interaction

FDA-approved Indications

- Refractory testicular cancer; SCLC, first-line therapy in combination with other agents

FDA-approved Dosage

- Testicular cancer: 50 to 100 mg/m^2 i.v. daily $\times$ 5 days (days 1–5), repeated every 3 to 4 weeks *OR* 100 mg/m^2 i.v. on days 1, 3, and 5, repeated every 3 to 4 weeks (in combination with other approved agents). Consult current literature for dose recommendations.
- SCLC: 35 to 50 mg/m^2 i.v. daily $\times$ 4 to 5 days, repeated every 3 to 4 weeks (in combination with other agents). Consult current literature for dose recommendations.
- Higher rates of i.v. administration have been utilized and tolerated by patients with etoposide phosphate compared to etoposide. Etoposide phosphate can be administered at infusion rates from 5 to 210 minutes (generally infusion durations of 5–30 minutes have been utilized).

Dose Modification Criteria

- Renal: yes

Adverse Reactions

- DERM: alopecia, rash, urticaria, pruritis
- GI: N/V (low), mucositis, anorexia
- HEMAT: myelosuppression
- INFUS: hypotension (infusion rate–related), anaphylactic-like reactions (characterized by chills, fever, tachycardia, bronchospasm, dyspnea, and/or hypotension)
- Other: secondary malignancies

Comments

- Etoposide phosphate is a water soluble ester of etoposide. The water solubility of etoposide phosphate lessens the potential for precipitation following dilution and during intravenous administration. Enhanced water solubility also allows for lower dilution volumes and more rapid intravenous administration compared to conventional etoposide.

EXEMESTANE (AROMISAN)

Mechanism of Action

- Irreversible steroidal aromatase inactivator

FDA-approved Indications

- Breast cancer:
  - Adjuvant treatment of ER-positive early breast cancer in postmenopausal women who have received 2 to 3 years of tamoxifen and are switched to exemestane for completion of a total of 5 consecutive years of adjuvant hormonal therapy.
  - Advanced breast cancer after tamoxifen failure in postmenopausal women

FDA-approved Dosage

- 25 mg orally, daily after a meal

Dose Modification Criteria

- Renal: no
- Hepatic: no (Note: drug exposure is increased with hepatic and/or renal insufficiency. The safety of chronic dosing in these settings has not been studied. Based on experience with exemestane at

repeated doses up to 200 mg daily that demonstrated a moderate increase in non–life-threatening adverse effects, dosage adjustment does not appear to be necessary.)

Adverse Reactions

- CV: hot flashes, edema
- GI: nausea, increased appetite
- HEMAT: lymphocytopenia
- NEURO: depression, insomnia, anxiety
- Other: tumor site pain, asthenia, fatigue, increased sweating, fever

FLOXURIDINE

Mechanism of Action

- Antimetabolite (catabolized to fluorouracil)

FDA-approved Indications

- Palliative management of gastrointestinal adenocarcinoma metastatic to the liver when given by continuous regional intra-arterial infusion in carefully selected patients who are considered incurable by surgery or other means.

FDA-approved Dosage

- 0.1 to 0.6 mg/kg/day by continuous arterial infusion. The higher dose ranges (0.4–0.6 mg/kg/day) are usually employed for hepatic artery infusion because the liver metabolizes the drug, thus reducing the potential for systemic toxicity. Therapy may be given until adverse reactions appear; when toxicities have subsided, therapy may be resumed. Patients may be maintained on therapy as long as response to floxuridine continues.

Dose Modification Criteria

- Renal: no
- Hepatic: no
- Myelosuppression: yes
- Nonhematologic toxicity: yes

Adverse Reactions

- CV: myocardial ischemia
- DERM: alopecia, dermatitis, rash
- GI: N/V, stomatitis, diarrhea, enteritis, gastrointestinal ulceration, and bleeding
- HEMAT: myelosuppression, elevated LFTs
- INFUS: procedural complications of regional arterial infusion: arterial aneurysm, arterial ischemia, arterial thrombosis, embolism, fibromyositis, thrombophlebitis, hepatic necrosis, abscesses, infection at catheter site, bleeding at catheter site, catheter blocked, displaced, or leaking
- Other: fever, lethargy, malaise, weakness

FLUDARABINE (FLUDARA)

Mechanism of Action

- Antimetabolite

FDA-approved Indications

- B cell CLL (second-line after alkylating agent therapy)

FDA-approved Dosage

25 mg/m^2 i.v. over 30 minutes daily $\times$ 5 days, repeated every 28 days

Dose Modification Criteria

- Renal: yes

Adverse Reactions

- CV: edema
- DERM: rash
- GI: N/V (minimal), diarrhea, anorexia
- HEMAT: myelosuppression, autoimmune hemolytic anemia, lymphopenia
- NEURO: weakness, agitation, confusion, visual disturbances, coma (severe neurotoxicity generally seen with high-dose regimens but have been reported rarely at recommended doses), peripheral neuropathy
- PULM: pneumonitis, cases of severe pulmonary toxicity have been reported
- Other: myalgia, tumor lysis syndrome, fatigue

Comments

- Monitor for hemolytic anemia
- A high incidence of fatal pulmonary toxicity was seen in a trial investigating the combination of fludarabine with pentostatin. The combined use of fludarabine and pentostatin is not recommended.
- Transfusion-associated graft-versus-host disease has been observed rarely after transfusion of nonirradiated blood in fludarabine treated patients. Consideration should be given to using only irradiated blood products if transfusions are necessary in patients undergoing treatment with fludarabine.
- Monitor for tumor lysis syndrome and consider prophylaxis in CLL patients with a large tumor burden initiated on fludarabine.

FLUOROURACIL (ADRUCIL AND OTHERS)

Mechanism of Action

- Antimetabolite

FDA-approved Indications

- Palliative management of colon, rectal, breast, stomach, and pancreatic cancer

FDA-approved Dosage

- Consult current literature

Adverse Reactions

- CV: angina, ischemia
- DERM: dry skin, photosensitivity, hand-foot syndrome (palmar-plantar erythrodysesthesia), alopecia, dermatitis, thrombophlebitis
- GI: N/V (low), mucositis, diarrhea, anorexia, gastrointestinal ulceration, and bleeding

- HEMAT: myelosuppression
- NEURO: acute cerebellar syndrome, nystagmus, headache, visual changes, photophobia
- Other: anaphylaxis and generalized allergic reactions

Comments

- Fluorouracil may be given as continuous intravenous infusion or by rapid i.v. administration (i.v. bolus or push). The method of administration will change the toxicity profile of fluorouracil (e.g., greater potential for GI toxicities such as mucositis and diarrhea with continuous i.v. infusions and more hematologic toxicity with bolus administration).

FLUTAMIDE (EULEXIN)

Mechanism of Action

- Antiandrogen

FDA-approved Indications

- Stage D2 metastatic prostate carcinoma (in combination with LHRH agonists) or locally confined stage B2-C prostate carcinoma (in combination with LHRH agonists and radiation therapy)

FDA-approved Dosage

- Stage D2 metastatic prostate carcinoma: 250 mg p.o. three times daily (every 8 hours)
- Stage B2-C prostate cancer: 250 mg p.o. three times daily (every 8 hours) beginning 8 weeks before and continuing through radiation

Adverse Reactions

- DERM: rash
- GI: N/V, diarrhea, constipation
- GU: impotence
- ENDO: loss of libido, hot flashes, gynecomastia
- HEPAT: increased LFTs (monitor LFTs periodically because of rare associations with cholestatic jaundice, hepatic necrosis, and encephalopathy)

Comments

- Interacts with warfarin; monitor international normalized ratio (INR) closely

FULVESTRANT (FASLODEX)

Mechanism of Action

- Estrogen receptor antagonist

FDA-approved Indications

- Breast cancer: second-line treatment of hormone receptor positive metastatic breast cancer in post-menopausal women with disease progression following antiestrogen therapy

FDA-approved Dosage

- 250 mg i.m. injection × 1 dose and repeated at 1-month intervals

Dose Modification Criteria

- Renal: no
- Hepatic (mild impairment): no
- Hepatic (moderate to severe impairment): no data, use caution

Adverse Reactions

- CV: peripheral edema
- ENDO: hot flashes
- GI: N/V, constipation, diarrhea, abdominal pain, anorexia
- NEURO: headache
- Other: pain, pharyngitis, injection site reactions, asthenia

GEFITINIB (IRESSA)

Mechanism of Action

- Tyrosine kinase inhibitor (primarily EGFR).

FDA-approved Indications

- NSCLC: monotherapy for the treatment of patients with locally advanced or metastatic NSCLC, after failure of both platinum-based and docetaxel chemotherapies, who are benefitting or who have benefitted from gefitinib

FDA-approved Dosage

- 250 mg orally daily

Dose Modification Criteria

- Renal: no
- Hepatic: no

Adverse Reactions

- DERM: rash, acne, dry skin, pruritus
- GI: N/V (minimal), diarrhea, anorexia, elevated LFTs
- OCULAR: eye pain, corneal erosion/ulcer (sometimes in association with aberrant eyelash growth)
- PULM: interstitial lung disease (interstitial pneumonia, pneumonitis, and alveolitis)
- Other: asthenia, weight loss

Comments

- Access to gefitinib is restricted (via the Iressa Access Program) based on the lack of survival benefit in a placebo controlled trial in advanced recurrent NSCLC and the availability of other drugs that do prolong life.
- In a patient who presents with acute onset or worsening of pulmonary symptoms (dyspnea, cough, fever), gefitinib therapy should be interrupted and a prompt investigation of these symptoms should occur. Fatalities related to interstitial lung disease have been reported.
- Gefitinib is extensively hepatically metabolized, predominantly by cytochrome (CYP) 3A4. Be aware of potential drug interactions with either potent inhibitors or inducers of CYP 3A4. A dose increase of gefitinib to 500 mg/day may be considered when given concomitantly with a potent CYP 3A4 enzyme inducer such as phenytoin or rifampin.

- Gefitinib may potentially interact with warfarin leading to an elevated prothrombin time (PT) and international normalized ratio (INR) and bleeding events; monitor PT/INR regularly with concomitant use.

GEMCITABINE (GEMZAR)

Mechanism of Action

- Antimetabolite

FDA-approved Indications

- Pancreatic cancer: first-line treatment for patients with locally advanced (nonresectable stage II or stage III) or metastatic (stage IV) adenocarcinoma of the pancreas and in pancreatic cancer patients previously treated with fluorouracil.
- NSCLC: first-line treatment (in combination with cisplatin) for patients with inoperable, locally advanced (stage IIIa or IIIb) or metastatic (stage IV) NSCLC.
- Metastatic breast cancer: first-line treatment (in combination with paclitaxel) for patients with metastatic breast cancer after failure of prior anthracycline-containing adjuvant chemotherapy, unless anthracyclines were clinically contraindicated.
- Ovarian cancer: in combination with carboplatin for advanced ovarian cancer that has relapsed at least 6 months after completion of platinum-based therapy.

FDA-approved Dosage

- Pancreatic cancer (single-agent use): 1,000 mg/m^2 i.v. over 30 minutes once weekly for up to 7 weeks, followed by 1 week of rest from treatment. Subsequent cycles should consist of 1,000 mg/m^2 i.v. over 30 minutes once weekly for 3 consecutive weeks out of every 4 weeks.
- NSCLC (combination therapy with cisplatin)
  - 4-week schedule: 1,000 mg/m^2 i.v. over 30 minutes on days 1, 8, and 15 of each 28-day cycle. Cisplatin (100 mg/m^2 i.v. × one dose) should be administered after gemcitabine only on day 1, *OR*
  - 3-week schedule: 1,250 mg/m^2 i.v. over 30 minutes on days 1 and 8 of each 21-day cycle. Cisplatin (100 mg/m^2 i.v. × one dose) should be administered after gemcitabine only on day 1
- Metastatic breast cancer (combination therapy with paclitaxel): 1,250 mg/m^2 i.v. over 30 minutes on days 1 and 8 of each 21-day cycle. Paclitaxel should be administered at 175 mg/m^2 i.v. over 3 hours × one dose (day 1 only) before gemcitabine administration.
- Ovarian cancer: 1,000 mg/m^2 i.v. over 30 minutes on days 1 and 8 of each 21-day cycle. Carboplatin AUC 4 i.v. should be administered on day 1 after gemcitabine administration.

Dose Modification Criteria

- Renal: use with caution
- Hepatic: use with caution
- Myelosuppression: yes
- Nonhematologic toxicity: yes

Adverse Reactions

- DERM: rash, alopecia
- GI: N/V (low), constipation, diarrhea, mucositis
- GU: proteinuria, hematuria, hemolytic-uremic syndrome
- HEMAT: myelosuppression
- HEPAT: increased LFTs and bilirubin, rare reports of sever hepatotoxicity

- PULM: dyspnea, rare reports of severe pulmonary toxicity (pneumonitis, pulmonary fibrosis, pulmonary edema, acute respiratory distress syndrome)
- Other: fever, pain, rare reports of vascular toxicity (vasculitis)

Comments

- Clearance in women and elderly is reduced.
- Intravenous administration rate has been shown to influence both efficacy and toxicity. Refer to the published literature for the appropriate rate of administration for a specific regimen.

GEMTUZUMAB OZOGAMICIN (MYLOTARG)

Mechanism of Action

- A humanized monoclonal antibody directed at the CD33 cell surface antigen conjugated with a cytotoxic antitumor, antibiotic, calicheamicin. Binding of the anti-CD33 antibody portion of gemtuzumab ozogamicin results in internalization and release of the calicheamicin which subsequently causes DNA double strand breaks and cell death.

FDA-approved Indications

- Acute myeloid leukemia (AML): second-line therapy for CD33 positive AML patients in first relapse who are 60 years of age or older and who are not considered candidates for other cytotoxic chemotherapy.

FDA-approved Dosage

- 9 mg/m^2 i.v. over 2 hours $\times$ one dose. The recommended treatment course is a total of two doses with 14 days between the doses.
- Consider leukoreduction with hydroxyurea or leukapheresis to reduce the peripheral white blood cell count to below 30,000/μL prior to administration of gemtuzumab ozogamicin.
- Premedicate patients with diphenhydramine 50 mg p.o., acetaminophen 650 to 1,000 mg p.o. 1 hour prior to the administration of gemtuzumab ozogamicin; thereafter, two additional doses of acetaminophen every 4 hours as needed.
- Consider prophylaxis for tumor lysis syndrome with hydration and allopurinol.

Dose Modification Criteria

- Renal: no data
- Hepatic: no data (use caution)

Adverse Reactions

- CV: hypotension, hypertension
- DERM: rash
- GI: N/V (low to moderate), mucositis, anorexia, constipation, diarrhea
- HEMAT: myelosuppression
- HEPAT: elevated LFTs and/or bilirubin, hepatic veno-occlusive disease (VOD)
- INFUS: fever, chills, nausea, vomiting, headache, hypotension, hypertension, hyperglycemia, hypoxia, dyspnea, anaphylaxis
- NEURO: headache
- PULM: dyspnea, pulmonary infiltrates, pleural effusions, noncardiogenic pulmonary edema, pulmonary insufficiency and hypoxia, and acute respiratory distress syndrome; Other: tumor lysis syndrome, infection, bleeding episodes, asthenia

Comments

- Hepatotoxicity, including severe VOD has been reported with gemtuzumab ozogamicin as a single agent and as part of a combination regimen. Patients who receive gemtuzumab ozogamicin either before or after hematopoietic stem cell transplant, patients with underlying hepatic disease or abnormal liver function, and patients receiving combination regimens containing gemtuzumab ozogamicin may be at increased risk. Monitor for rapid weight gain, right upper quadrant pain, hepatomegaly, ascites, and elevations in bilirubin and/or liver enzymes.
- Severe hypersensitivity reactions and other infusion-related reactions can occur (including severe pulmonary events) and can be fatal. Interrupt infusion for patients experiencing dyspnea or clinically significant hypotension. Discontinue treatment for patients who develop anaphylaxis, pulmonary edema, or acute respiratory distress syndrome.

GOSERELIN ACETATE IMPLANT (ZOLADEX)

Mechanism of Action

- LHRH agonist; chronic administration leads to sustained suppression of pituitary gonadotropins and subsequent suppression of serum testosterone in men and serum estradiol in women.

FDA-approved Indications

- Prostate cancer
  - Palliative treatment of advanced carcinoma of the prostate
  - Stage B2-C prostatic carcinoma: in combination with flutamide and radiation therapy. Goserelin acetate and flutamide treatment should start 8 weeks prior to initiating radiation therapy.
- Breast cancer: palliative treatment of advanced breast cancer in pre- and peri-menopausal women.
- Other indications: endometriosis, endometrial thinning

FDA-approved Dosage

- Advanced carcinoma of the prostate: 3.6 mg s.c. depot monthly, *OR* 10.8 mg s.c. depot every 12 weeks
- Stage B2-C prostatic carcinoma: Start 8 weeks prior to initiating radiotherapy and continue through radiation. A treatment regimen of 3.6 mg s.c. depot, followed in 28 days by 10.8 mg s.c. depot. Alternatively four injections of 3.6 mg s.c. depot can be administered at 28-day intervals, two depots preceding and two during radiotherapy.
- Breast cancer: 3.6 mg s.c. depot every 4 weeks

Dose Modification Criteria

- Renal: no
- Hepatic: no

Adverse Reactions

- CV: transient changes in blood pressure (hypo- or hypertension)
- ENDO: men: hot flashes, gynecomastia, sexual dysfunction, decreased erections, women: hot flashes, headache, vaginal dryness, vaginitis, emotional lability, change in libido, depression, increased sweating, change in breast size
- GU: erectile dysfunction, lower urinary tract symptoms
- NEURO: pain
- Other: tumor flare in the first few weeks of therapy, loss of bone mineral density, osteoporosis, bone fracture, asthenia

Comments

- Use with caution in patients at risk of developing ureteral obstruction or spinal cord compression.

HISTRELIN ACETATE IMPLANT (VANTAS)

Mechanism of Action

- LHRH agonist; chronic administration leads to sustained suppression of pituitary gonadotropins and subsequent suppression of serum testosterone in men and serum estradiol in women.

FDA-approved Indications

- Prostate cancer: palliative treatment of advanced carcinoma of the prostate
- Other indications: central precocious puberty (alternative product: supprelin LA)

FDA-approved Dosage

- Advanced carcinoma of the prostate: 50 mg s.c. depot every 12 months. The once yearly implant is inserted subcutaneously in the inner aspect of the upper arm. The implant must be removed after 12 months of therapy prior to a new implant insertion for continuation of therapy. Implant insertion is a surgical procedure.

Dose Modification Criteria

- Renal: no
- Hepatic: not studied

Adverse Reactions

- ENDO: men: hot flashes, gynecomastia, sexual dysfunction, decreased erections
- DERM: implant site reactions (pain, soreness, tenderness, erythema)
- GU: erectile dysfunction, renal impairment
- Other: tumor flare in the first few weeks of therapy, loss of bone mineral density, osteoporosis, bone fracture, fatigue

Comments

- Use with caution in patients at risk of developing ureteral obstruction or spinal cord compression.

HYDROXYUREA (HYDREA, DROXIA)

Mechanism of Action

- Inhibits DNA synthesis; radiation sensitizer

FDA-approved Indications

- Melanoma; recurrent, metastatic, or inoperable ovarian cancer; resistant chronic myelocytic leukemia (CML); and primary squamous cell carcinomas of the head and neck (excluding the lip) in combination with radiation therapy. Hydroxyurea is also indicated in adult patients with sickle cell anemia with recurrent moderate-to-severe painful crises.

FDA-approved Dosage

- Dose based on actual or ideal body weight, whichever is less
- Solid tumors

- Intermittent therapy: 80 mg/kg p.o. as a single dose every third day
- Continuous therapy: 20 to 30 mg/kg p.o. daily
- In combination with irradiation for head and neck Cancer: 80 mg/kg p.o. as a single dose every third day, beginning 7 days before initiation of irradiation and continued indefinitely thereafter, based on adverse effects and response
- Resistant chronic myelocytic leukemia (CML): 20 to 30 mg/kg p.o. daily

Dose Modification Criteria

- Renal: use with caution
- Hepatic: use with caution
- Myelosuppression: yes.

Adverse Reactions

- DERM: rash, peripheral and facial erythema, skin ulceration, dermatomyositis-like skin changes, hyperpigmentation
- GI: N/V (minimal), diarrhea, anorexia, mucositis, constipation
- HEMAT: myelosuppression (leukopenia, anemia > thrombocytopenia)
- NEURO: drowsiness (large doses)

Comments

- Capsule contents may be emptied into glass of water and taken immediately (some inert particles may float on surface).
- Patients should be counseled about proper handling precautions if they open the capsules.

IDARUBICIN (IDAMYCIN)

Mechanism of Action

- Intercalating agent; topoisomerase-II inhibition

FDA-approved Indications

- In combination with other agents for adult Acute myeloid leukemia (AML; FAB M1 to M7)

FDA-approved Dosage

- AML induction in combination with cytarabine: 12 mg/m^2 slow i.v. injection (over 10–15 minutes) daily for 3 days

Dose Modification Criteria

- Renal: yes
- Hepatic: yes
- Mucositis: yes

Adverse Reactions

- CV: CHF, arrhythmia
- DERM: alopecia, radiation recall, rash
- GI: N/V (moderate), mucositis, abdominal cramps, diarrhea
- HEMAT: myelosuppression

Comments

- Vesicant
- Myocardial toxicity is increased in patients with prior anthracycline therapy or heart disease. Cumulative dose limit not established within package literature.
- Consider appropriate prophylaxis for tumor lysis syndrome when treating acute leukemias.

IFOSFAMIDE (IFEX)

Mechanism of Action

- Alkylating agent

FDA-approved Indications

- Germ cell testicular cancer (third-line therapy in combination with other agents)

FDA-approved Dosage

- 1.2 g/m^2 i.v. daily for 5 days, repeated every 3 weeks. Give MESNA 20% (wt/wt; 240 mg/m^2 per dose for a 1.2 g/m^2 ifosfamide dose) at time of ifosfamide, and then 4 and 8 hours after ifosfamide.

Dose Modification Criteria

- Renal: unknown
- Hepatic: unknown
- Myelosuppression: yes
- Neurotoxicity: yes

Adverse Reactions

- DERM: alopecia
- GI: N/V (moderate)
- GU: hemorrhagic cystitis, Fanconi syndrome (proximal tubular impairment), glomerular or tubular toxicity
- HEMAT: myelosuppression
- HEPAT: increased LFTs
- NEURO: encephalopathy, somnolence, confusion, depressive psychosis, hallucinations, dizziness

Comments

- Ensure adequate hydration; administer MESNA concurrently; monitor for microscopic hematuria
- Discontinue therapy with the occurrence of neurologic toxicity. The incidence of CNS toxicity may be higher in patients with impaired renal function and/or low serum albumin.

IMATINIB MESYLATE (GLEEVEC)

Mechanism of Action

- Inhibitor of multiple tyrosine kinases including the Bcr-Abl tyrosine kinase, which is created by the Philadelphia chromosome abnormality in chronic myeloid leukemia (CML). Imatinib is also an inhibitor of the receptor tyrosine kinases for platelet-derived growth factor (PDGF) and stem cell factor (SCF), c-kit, and inhibits PDGF- and SCF-mediated cellular events.

FDA-approved Indications

- CML:
  - First-line therapy for newly diagnosed adult patients with Philadelphia chromosome positive (Ph+) CML in chronic phase
  - Second-line therapy for patients in blast crisis, accelerated phase, or in chronic phase after failure of interferon-alpha therapy
  - Second-line therapy for pediatric patients with Ph+ chronic phase CML whose disease has recurred after stem cell transplant or who are resistant to interferon alfa therapy
- ALL: adult patients with relapsed or refractory Philadelphia chromosome positive (Ph+) ALL
- Myelodysplastic/myeloproliferative disease (MDS/MPD): adult patients with MDS/MPD associated with platlet-derived growth factor receptor (PDGFR) gene rearrangement
- Adult patients with aggressive systemic mastocytosis (ASM) without the D816V c-Kit mutation or with c-Kit mutational status unknown
- Hypereosinophilic dyndrome (HES) and/or chronic eosinophilic leukemia (CEL): adult patients who have FIP1L1-PDGFR alfa-fusion kinase and patients who are FIP1L1-PDGFR alfa-infusion kinase negative or unknown
- Dermatofibrosarcoma protuberans (DFSP): adult patients with unresectable, recurrent, and/or metastatic DFSP
- Gastrointestinal stromal tumors (GIST): treatment of patients with Kit (CD117)–positive unresectable and/or metastatic malignant GIST

FDA-approved Dosage

- CML
  - Adult patients, chronic phase: 400 mg p.o. daily. Doses may be escalated to 600 mg/day as clinically indicated (see package insert for criteria)
  - Adult patients, accelerated phase: 600 mg p.o. daily. Doses may be escalated to 800 mg/day (400 mg p.o. bid) as clinically indicated (see package insert for criteria)
  - Pediatric patients: 260 mg/m^2 p.o. daily. Doses may be escalated to 340 mg/day as clinically indicated (see package insert for criteria)
- ALL: 600 mg/day for adult patients with relapsed/refractory Ph+ ALL
- MDS/MDP: 400 mg/day for adult patients
- Aggressive systemic mastocytosis (ASM): adult patients with
  - ASM without the D816V c-Kit mutation: 400 mg/day
  - Unknown c-Kit mutation status: 400 mg/day may be considered for patients not responding to satisfactorily to other therapies
  - ASM associated with eosinophilia: starting dose of 100 mg/day is recommended, consider increasing dose from 100 to 400 mg/day in the absence of adverse drug reactions and insufficient response to therapy
- HES and/or CEL: 400 mg/day (adults). For HES/CEL with demonstrated FIP1L1-PDGFR alfa-fusion kinase start with 100 mg/day, may consider increasing dose from 100 to 400 mg/day in the absence of adverse drug reactions and insufficient response to therapy.
- DFSP: 800 mg/day
- GIST: 400 mg or 600 mg p.o. daily
- The prescribed dose should be administered orally, with a meal and a large glass of water. Doses of 400 mg or 600 mg should be administered once daily, whereas a dose of 800 mg should be administered as 400 mg twice a day. In children, imatinib can be given as a once-daily dose or divided into two doses (bid).

Dose Modification Criteria

- Renal: no data
- Hepatic: no data
- Myelosuppression: yes
- Nonhematologic toxicity: yes

Adverse Reactions

- CV: superficial edema (periorbital, lower limb), severe fluid retention (pleural effusion, ascites, pulmonary edema, rapid weight gain)
- DERM: rash
- GI: N/V, diarrhea, GI irritation, dyspepsia, elevated LFTs, severe hepatotoxicity
- HEMAT: myelosuppression, hemorrhage
- NEURO: headache, dizziness
- PULM: cough
- Other: muscle cramps, pain (musculoskeletal, joint, abdominal), myalgia, arthralgia, nasopharyngitis, fatigue, fever

Comments

- The cytochrome p450 (CYP) 3A4 enzyme is the major enzyme responsible for the metabolism of imatinib. Be aware of potential drug interactions with either potent inhibitors or inducers of CYP 3A4. Dosage of imatinib should be increased at least 50% and clinical response carefully monitored, in patients receiving imatinib with a potent CYP3A4 inducer such as rifampin or phenytoin.
- Monitor regularly for weight gain and signs and symptoms of fluid retention. An unexpected rapid weight gain should be carefully investigated and appropriate treatment provided. The probability of edema is increased with higher doses of imatinib and age >65 years.
- Monitor LFTs prior to initiation of imatinib therapy and monthly thereafter or as clinically indicated.
- Monitor complete blood counts prior to initiation of imatinib therapy, weekly for the first month, biweekly for the second month, and periodically thereafter as clinically indicated (e.g., every 2–3 months).

INTERFERON α-2B (INTRON A)

Mechanism of Action

- Cell-proliferation suppression, macrophage phagocytic activity enhancement, lymphocyte cytotoxicity enhancement

FDA-approved Indications

- Oncology indications (adults, ≥ 18 years of age): hairy cell leukemia, malignant melanoma (adjuvant therapy to surgical treatment), AIDS-related Kaposi sarcoma, follicular lymphoma (clinically aggressive disease in conjunction with anthracycline-containing combination chemotherapy)
- Other indications: Condyloma Acuminata, Chronic Hepatitis C, Chronic Hepatitis B.

FDA-approved Dosage

- Hairy cell leukemia: 2 million IU/m^2 i.m. or s.c. three times a week for up to 6 months
- Malignant melanoma: Induction: 20 million IU/m^2 i.v. for 5 consecutive days per week for 4 weeks. Maintenance: 10 million IU/m^2 s.c. three times per week for 48 weeks
- Kaposi sarcoma: 30 million IU/m^2 s.c. or i.m. three times a week
- Follicular lymphoma: (in combination with an anthracycline-containing chemotherapy regimen): 5 million IU s.c. three times a week for up to 18 months

Dose Modification Criteria

- Serious adverse events: yes

Adverse Reactions

- DERM: skin rash, alopecia
- ENDO: thyroid abnormalities
- GI: diarrhea, N/V, anorexia, taste alteration, abdominal pain

- HEMAT: myelosuppression
- HEPAT: increased LFTs
- NEURO: dizziness, depression, suicidal ideation, paresthesias
- PULM: dyspnea, pulmonary infiltrates, pneumonitis, pneumonia
- Other: flulike symtoms (fever, chills, headache, fatigue, malaise, myalgia), hypersensitivity reactions, ophthalmologic disorders, autoimmune disorders

Comments

- Patients with a preexisting psychiatric condition, especially depression, should not be treated.
- Use with caution in patients with pulmonary disease, diabetes mellitus, coagulopathies, cardiac disorders, autoimmune diseases, or ophthalmologic disorders.
- Recommended laboratory monitoring includes complete blood counts (CBC), blood chemistries, LFTs, and thyroid stimulating hormone (TSH) prior to beginning treatment and then periodically thereafter.
- Other recommended baseline studies include a chest x-ray and an ophthalmologic exam.

IRINOTECAN (CAMPTOSAR)

Mechanism of Action

- Topoisomerase-I inhibitor

FDA-approved Indications

- Metastatic colon or rectal cancer
  - First-line therapy in combination with fluorouracil and leucovorin
  - Second-line therapy (single agent) after fluorouracil-based therapy

FDA-approved Dosage

- First-line combination-agent dosing: See product labeling for fluorouracil/leucovorin dosing.
  - Regimen 1: 125 mg/m^2 i.v. over 90 minutes weekly $\times$ four doses (days 1, 8, 15, 22) followed by 2 weeks of rest. Repeat every 6 weeks.
  - Regimen 2: 180 mg/m^2 i.v. over 90 minutes every 2 weeks (days 1, 15, 29) for each cycle. Each cycle is 6 weeks in duration.
- Second-line single-agent dosing
  - Weekly regimen: 125 mg/m^2 i.v. over 90 minutes weekly for 4 doses (days 1, 8, 15, 22) followed by 2 weeks rest. Repeat every 6 weeks, *OR*
  - Once-every-3-weeks regimen: 350 mg/m^2 i.v. over 90 min every 3 weeks

Dose Modification Criteria

- Hepatic: yes
- Pelvic/abdominal irradiation: yes
- Myelosuppression: yes
- Nonhematologic toxicity: yes (see package labeling for dose modifications)

Adverse Reactions

- CV: vasodilation
- DERM: alopecia, sweating, rash
- GI: N/V (moderate), diarrhea (early and late), abdominal pain, mucositis, anorexia, flatulence
- HEMAT: myelosuppression
- HEPAT: increased bilirubin, LFTs

- NEURO: insomnia, dizziness
- PULM: dyspnea, coughing, rhinitis
- Other: asthenia, fevers

Comments

- Can induce both early (within 24 hours of administration) and late forms of diarrhea. The early-onset diarrhea is cholinergic in nature and may be accompanied by symptoms of rhinitis, increased salivation, miosis, lacrimation, diaphoresis, flushing, and abdominal cramping. These early cholinergic symptoms can be treated by administration of atropine. Late onset diarrhea (generally after 24 hours) should be treated aggressively with high-dose loperamide. Each patient should be instructed to have loperamide readily available so that treatment can be initiated at the earliest onset of diarrhea. See package labeling for dosage recommendations for atropine and loperamide.

IXABEPILONE (IXEMPRA)

Mechanism of Action

- Microtubule Inhibitor

FDA-approved Indications

- Breast cancer
    - In combination with capecitabine in patients with metastatic or locally advanced breast cancer after failure of an anthracycline and a taxane.
    - Monotherapy in patients with metastatic or locally advanced breast cancer after failure of an anthracycline, a taxane, and capecitabine.

FDA-approved Dosage

- 40 mg/m^2 IV over 3 hours every 3 weeks

Dose Modification Criteria

- Renal: no
- Hepatic: yes
- Myelosuppression: yes
- Nonhematologic toxicity: yes

Adverse Reactions

- DERM: alopecia
- GI: N/V (low), stomatitis/mucositis, diarrhea
- HEMAT: myelosuppression
- HEPAT: elevated LFTs
- INFUS: hypersensitivity reactions (e.g., flushing, rash, dyspnea, and bronchospasm) NEURO: peripheral neuropathy
- Other: fatigue, asthenia, myalgia/arthralgia, alopecia

Comments

- Patients should be premedicated approximately 1 hour before the infusion of ixabepilone with an H$_1$ antagonist (e.g., diphenhydramine) and an H$_2$ antagonist (ranitidine).

- Ixabepilone is metabolized through cytochrome P450 3A4 isoenzyme. Screen for drug interactions with CYP 3A4 inhibitors or inducers. A dose modification is suggested if concomitantly used with a potent CYP 3A4 inhibitor.
- Pregnancy category D: ixabepilone may cause fetal harm when administered to a pregnant woman.

LAPATINIB (TYKERB)

Mechanism of Action

- Tyrosine kinase inhibitor (EGFR Type 1 (EGFR/HER1) and human epidermal receptor type 2 (HER2/ErbB2)

FDA-approved Indications

- Breast cancer: in combination with capecitabine for the treatment of patients with advanced or metastatic breast cancer who overexpress HER2 and have received prior therapy including an anthracycline, a taxane, and trastuzumab

FDA-approved Dosage

- Breast cancer: 1,250 mg p.o. once daily (administer at least 1 hour before or 1 hour after the ingestion of food) in combination with capecitabine

Dose Modification Criteria

- Renal: no
- Hepatic: yes
- Myelosuppression: no
- Nonhematologic toxicity: yes

Adverse Reactions

- CV: reduced LVEF, QT prolongation
- DERM: palmar-plantar erythrodysesthesia, rash
- GI: N/V (low), diarrhea, stomatitis
- HEMAT: myelosuppression
- HEPAT: elevated LFTs
- PULM: interstitial lung disease, pneumonitis
- OTHER: fatigue

Comments

- Reported adverse reactions are based on clinical trials in combination with capecitabine.
- Product labeling suggests monitoring LVEF at baseline and during therapy. Interrupt therapy for grade 2 or greater reductions in LVEF. Upon recovery, restart at lower dose.
- Monitor patients for interstitial lung disease or pneumonitis. Lapatinib should be discontinued in patients who experience pulmonary symptoms indicative of $\geq$ grade 3 toxicity.
- Lapatinib is metabolized through cytochrome P450 3A4 isoenzyme. Screen for drug interactions with CYP 3A4 inhibitors or inducers. Dose modifications may be necessary if concomitant use is unavoidable with potent inhibitors or inducers.
- Pregnancy category D: lapatinib may cause fetal harm when administered to a pregnant woman.

LENALIDOMIDE (REVLIMID)

Mechanism of Action

- Immunomodulatory agent with antineoplastic and antiangiogenic properties

FDA-approved Indications

- Myelodysplastic syndrome: treatment of patients with transfusion dependent anemia due to low- or intermediate-1 risk MDSs associated with a deletion 5q cytogenetic abnormality with or without additional cytogenetic abnormalities
- Multiple myeloma: second-line therapy of multiple myeloma patients in combination with dexamethasone who have received at least one prior therapy.

FDA-approved Dosage

- Myelodysplastic syndrome: 10 mg orally daily with water
- Multiple myeloma: 25 mg orally daily on days 1 to 21 of a 28-day treatment cycle in combination with dexamethasone. Dexamethasone is dosed at 40 mg orally once daily on days 1 to 4, 9 to 12, and 17 to 20 every 28 days for the first four cycles of therapy. Thereafter, dexamethasone is dosed at 40 mg orally daily on days 1 to 4 every 28 days.

Dose Modification Criteria

- Renal: yes
- Hepatic: no data
- Myelosuppression: yes
- Nonhematologic toxicity: yes

Adverse Reactions

- CV: edema
- DERM: rash, pruritis, dry skin
- ELECTRO: hypokalemia
- GI: diarrhea, constipation, N/V (minimal to low), abdominal pain, anorexia
- HEMAT: myelosuppression
- NEURO: dizziness, headache, insomnia, tremor
- PULM: dyspnea, cough, nasopharyngitis
- Other: thromboembolic events, fatigue, fever, arthralgia, back or limb pain, muscle cramps

Comments

- Revlimid is only available through a restricted distribution program (RevAssist). Only prescribers and pharmacists registered with the program are allowed to prescribe and dispense lenalidomide.
- Pregnancy category X. Lenalidomide is an analog of thalidomide which is a known teratogen. Lenalidomide may cause severe birth defects or death to an unborn baby. Refer to the product labeling for information regarding requirements for patient consent, pregnancy testing, and patient consent as part of the RevAssist program.
- Myelosuppression (particularly neutropenia and thrombocytopenia) is a common and dose-limiting toxicity. Monitor blood counts closely as indicated in the product labeling.
- Lenalidomide may cause venous thromboembolic events. There is an increased risk of thrombotic events when lenalidomide is combined with standard chemotherapeutic agents, including dexamethasone. Consider concurrent prophylactic anticoagulation or aspirin treatment.

LETROZOLE (FEMARA)

Mechanism of Action

- Selective, nonsteroidal aromatase inhibitor

FDA-approved Indications

- Breast cancer
  - For adjuvant treatment of postmenopausal women with hormone receptor positive early breast cancer
  - For the extended adjuvant treatment of early breast cancer in postmenopausal women who have received 5 years of adjuvant tamoxifen therapy
  - First-line treatment of postmenopausal women with hormone receptor positive or hormone receptor unknown locally advanced or metastatic breast cancer
  - Second-line treatment of advanced breast cancer in postmenopausal women with disease progression following antiestrogen therapy

FDA-approved Dosage

- 2.5 mg orally daily

Dose Modification Criteria

- Renal (CrCl $\geq$ 10 mL/min): no
- Hepatic (mild to moderate impairment): no
- Hepatic (severe impairment): yes

Adverse Reactions

- GI: nausea (minimal), constipation, diarrhea
- NEURO: headache
- Other: hot flashes, fatigue, musculoskeletal pain, arthralgia, peripheral edema

LEUPROLIDE ACETATE (LUPRON, LUPRON DEPOT, LUPRON DEPOT-3 MONTH, LUPRON DEPOT-4 MONTH, VIADUR)

Mechanism of Action

- LHRH agonist; chronic administration leads to sustained suppression of pituitary gonadotropins and subsequent suppression of serum testosterone in men and serum estradiol in women.

FDA-approved Indications

- Palliative treatment of advanced prostate cancer
- Other indications: endometriosis, uterine leiomyomata (fibroids), central precocious puberty

FDA-approved Dosage

- Prostate cancer: Lupron: 1 mg s.c. daily; Lupron depot: 7.5 mg i.m. monthly; Lupron depot 3-month: 22.5 mg i.m. every 3 months; Lupron depot 4-month: 30 mg i.m. every 4 months; Viadur implant: one implant (contains 72 mg of leuprolide acetate) every 12 months

Adverse Reactions

- CV: transient changes in blood pressure (hypo- or hypertension)
- ENDO: hot flashes, gynecomastia, sexual dysfunction, decreased erections
- GU: erectile dysfunction, lower urinary tract symptoms, testicular atrophy
- Other: tumor flare in the first few weeks of therapy, bone pain, injection site reactions, loss of bone mineral density, osteoporosis, bone fracture, asthenia

Comments

- Use with caution in patients at risk of developing ureteral obstruction or spinal cord compression.
- Because of different release characteristics, a fractional dose of the 3-month or 4-month lupron depot formulation is not equivalent to the same dose of the monthly formulation and should not be given.

LOMUSTINE, CCNU (CEENU)

Mechanism of Action

- Alkylating agent

FDA-approved Indications

- Primary and metastatic brain tumors; Hodgkin disease (second-line therapy in combination with other agents)

FDA-approved Dosage

- Single-agent therapy: 100 to 130 mg/m^2 as a single oral dose every 6 weeks

Dose Modification Criteria

- Myelosuppression: yes

Adverse Reactions

- GI: N/V (>60 mg/m^2: high, $\leq$ 60 mg/m^2: moderate), mucositis
- GU: increased BUN, Cr
- HEMAT: severe delayed myelosuppression, cumulative myelosuppression
- HEPAT: increased LFTs
- PULM: (cumulative and usually occurs after 6 months of therapy or a cumulative lifetime dose of 1,100 mg/m^2, although it has been reported with total lifetime doses as low as 600 mg), fibrosis, infiltrate
- Other: secondary malignancies

Comments

- A single dose is given every 6 weeks
- Monitor blood counts at least weekly for 6 weeks after a dose

MECHLORETHAMINE (MUSTARGEN)

Mechanism of Action

- Alkylating agent

FDA-approved Indications

- Systemic (intravenous) palliative treatment of: bronchogenic carcinoma, chronic lymphocytic leukemia (CLL), chronic myelocytic leukemia (CML), Hodgkin disease (stage III and IV), lymphosarcoma, malignant effusions, mycosis fungoides, and polycythemia vera
- Palliative treatment of malignant effusions from metastatic carcinoma administered intrapleurally, intraperitoneally, or intrapericardially

FDA-approved Dosage

- Intravenous administration: 0.4 mg/kg i.v. × one dose per course *OR* 0.2 mg/kg i.v. daily × 2 days repeated every 3 to 6 weeks. Dosage should be based on ideal dry body weight. Other dosing regimens are utilized; consult current literature.
- MOPP regimen (Hodgkin Disease): mechlorethamine 6 mg/m^2 i.v. × 1 dose administered on days 1 and 8 of a 28-day cycle (combined with vincristine, prednisone, and procarbazine)
- Intracavitary administration: 0.2 to 0.4 mg/kg for intracavitary injection. Consult current literature for dose and administration technique. The technique and the dose used for the various intracavitary routes (intrapleural, intraperitoneal, intrapericardial) varies.

Dose Modification Criteria

- Myelosuppression: yes

Adverse Reactions

- DERM: alopecia, phlebitis, tissue damage/necrosis with extravasation, rash
- GI: N/V (high), metallic taste in mouth, diarrhea
- HEMAT: myelosuppression
- NEURO: vertigo, tinnitus, diminished hearing
- Other: hyperuricemia, secondary malignancies, infertility, azospermia

Comments

- Vesicant

MEDROXYPROGESTERONE ACETATE (DEPO-PROVERA)

Mechanism of Action

- Derivative of progesterone

FDA-approved Indications

- Adjunctive therapy and palliative treatment of inoperable, recurrent, and metastatic endometrial or renal cancer

FDA-approved Dosage

- 400 to 1,000 mg i.m. injection × one dose. Doses may be repeated weekly initially; if improvement is noted, the dose may be reduced to maintenance doses as low as 400 mg i.m. monthly.

Adverse Reactions

- CV: edema, weight gain, thromboembolic events
- DERM: urticaria, pruritus, rash, acne, alopecia, hirsutism
- ENDO: breast tenderness and galactorrhea
- GI: nausea, cholestatic jaundice
- GU: breakthrough bleeding, spotting, change in menstrual flow, amenorrhea, changes in cervical erosion and secretions
- NEURO: headache, nervousness, dizziness, depression
- OCULAR: neuro-ocular lesions (retinal thrombosis, optic neuritis)
- Other: hypersensitivity reactions, fever, fatigue, insomnia, somnolence, injection site reactions

MEGESTROL (MEGACE AND OTHERS)

Mechanism of Action

- Progestational agent

FDA-approved Indications

- Palliative therapy of advanced breast cancer and endometrial cancer

FDA-approved Dosage

- Breast cancer: 40 mg p.o. q.i.d. (4 times daily; total daily dose: 160 mg/day)
- Endometrial cancer: 10 mg p.o. q.i.d. to 80 mg p.o. q.i.d. (four times daily; total daily dose: 40–320 mg/day)

Adverse Reactions

- CV: deep vein thrombosis
- DERM: alopecia
- ENDO: Cushing-like syndrome, hyperglycemia, glucose intolerance, weight gain, hot flashes
- GU: vaginal bleeding
- NEURO: mood changes
- Other: carpal tunnel syndrome, tumor flare

Comments

- Other indications include cancer and AIDS-related anorexia and cachexia as an appetite stimulant and to promote weight gain. Usual dose range: 160 to 800 mg/day (consult current literature)

MELPHALAN (ALKERAN); MELPHALAN INJECTION

Mechanism of Action

- Alkylating agent

FDA-approved Indications

- Multiple myeloma: palliative treatment (oral tablets and injection)
- Ovarian cancer: palliative treatment of nonresectable epithelial carcinoma of the ovary (oral tablets)

FDA-approved Dosage

- Multiple myeloma
  - Oral administration: 6 mg p.o. daily × 2 to 3 weeks. Wait up to 4 weeks for count recovery, and then a maintenance dose of 2 mg p.o. daily may be initiated to achieve mild myelosuppression. Refer to package insert and current literature for other dosing regimens.
  - Intravenous administration. (if oral therapy not appropriate): 16 mg/m^2 i.v. over 15 to 20 minutes every 2 weeks × four doses, and then after adequate recovery from toxicity, repeat administration at 4-week intervals. Refer to current literature for other dosing regimens.
- Ovarian cancer: 0.2 mg/kg p.o. daily × 5 days, repeated every 4 to 5 weeks depending on hematologic tolerance. Refer to current literature for other dosing regimens.

Dose Modification Criteria

- Renal: yes
- Myelosuppression: yes

Adverse Reactions

- DERM: vasculitis, alopecia, skin ulceration/necrosis at injection site (rare)
- HEMAT: myelosuppression, hemolytic anemia
- GI: N/V (oral: minimal; high dose i.v.: moderate); diarrhea, mucositis, anorexia
- HEPAT: increased LFTs
- PULM: pulmonary toxicity (pulmonary fibrosis, interstitial pneumonitis)
- Other: hypersensitivity reactions, secondary malignancies, infertility

Comments

- Oral absorption is highly variable with considerable patient-to-patient variability in systemic availability. Oral dosages may be adjusted based on the basis of blood counts to achieve some level of myelosuppression to assure that potentially therapeutic levels of the drug have been reached.

MERCAPTOPURINE (PURINETHOL)

Mechanism of Action

- Antimetabolite

FDA-approved Indications

- ALL: indicated in the maintenance therapy of ALL as part of a combination regimen

FDA-approved Dosage

- ALL maintenance therapy: 1.5 to 2.5 mg/kg p.o. once daily

Dose Modification Criteria

- Renal: yes (consider dose reduction)
- Hepatic: yes (consider dose reduction)
- Myelosuppression: yes

Adverse Reactions

- DERM: rash, alopecia; GI: anorexia, N/V (minimal), mucositis
- HEMAT: myelosuppression
- HEPAT: hepatotoxicity
- Other: tumor lysis syndrome

Comments

- Monitor LFTs, bilirubin at weekly intervals initially and then monthly intervals
- Usually there is complete cross-resistance with thioguanine.
- Oral mercaptopurine dose should be reduced to 25% to 33% of usual daily dose in patients receiving allopurinol concomitantly.
- Consider appropriate prophylaxis for tumor lysis syndrome when treating acute leukemias.

METHOTREXATE

Mechanism of Action

- Antimetabolite

FDA-approved Indications

- Neoplastic disease indications: gestational tumors (choriocarcinoma, chorioadenoma destruens, hydatidiform mole), ALL (maintenance therapy in combination with other agents and in the prophylaxis of meningeal leukemia), treatment of meningeal leukemia, breast cancer, epidermoid cancers of the head or neck, advanced mycosis fungoides, lung cancers (particularly squamous cell and small cell types), advanced stage non-Hodgkin lymphoma, lymphosarcoma, and nonmetastatic osteosarcoma (high-dose therapy followed by leucovorin rescue)
- Other indications: psoriasis (severe, recalcitrant, disabling); rheumatoid arthritis (severe)

FDA-approved Dosage

- Choriocarcinoma and similar trophoblastic diseases: 15 to 30 mg p.o. or i.m. daily $\times$ 5 days. Treatment courses are repeated three to five times with rest periods of one or more weeks between courses to allow for toxic symptoms to subside. Refer to current literature.
- ALL maintenance therapy (following induction): 15 mg/m^2 p.o. or i.m. twice weekly (total weekly dose of 30 mg/m^2) *OR* 2.5 mg/kg i.v. every 14 days (in combination with other agents). Refer to current literature for combination regimens for both induction and maintenance regimens in ALL.
- Meningeal leukemia (intrathecal administration): younger than 1 year: 6 mg intrathecally; 1 to younger than 2 years: 8 mg intrathecally; 2 to younger than 3 years: 10 mg intrathecally; older than 3 years: 12 mg intrathecally. Refer to current literature.
- Mycosis fungoides: 2.5 to 10 mg p.o. daily $\times$ weeks to months *OR* 50 mg i.m. weekly *OR* 25 mg i.m. twice weekly. Refer to current literature.
- Nonmetastatic osteosarcoma: 12 g/m^2 i.v. over 4 hours $\times$ one dose (with leucovorin rescue, vigorous hydration, and urinary alkalinization) given weekly (weeks 4, 5, 6, 7 after surgery), and then weeks 11, 12, 15, 16, 29, 30, 44, 45. Leucovorin doses should be adjusted based on methotrexate concentrations. Methotrexate is generally given with other agents. Refer to current literature.
- Other indications: refer to current literature

Dose Modification Criteria

- Renal: yes

Adverse Reactions

- DERM: alopecia, rash, urticaria, telangiectasia, acne, photosensitivity, severe dermatologic reactions
- GI: N/V ($\leq$50 mg/m^2: minimal, >50 to <250 mg/m^2: low, $\geq$250 mg/m^2: moderate), mucositis/stomatitis, diarrhea
- GU: renal failure (high-dose therapy), cystitis
- HEMAT: myelosuppression
- HEPAT: increased LFTs, acute and chronic hepatotoxicity
- NEURO: acute chemical arachnoiditis (intrathecal), subacute myelopathy (intrathecal), chronic leukoencephalopathy (intrathecal), acute neurotoxicity or encephalopathy (high-dose i.v. therapy)
- PULM: interstitial pneumonitis
- Other: fever, malaise, chills, fatigue, teratogenic, tumor lysis syndome

Comments

- Clearance reduced in patients with impaired renal function or third space fluid accumulations (e.g., ascites, pleural effusions). Methotrexate distributes to third space fluid accumulations with subsequent slow and delayed clearance leading to prolonged terminal plasma half life and toxicity.
- Nonsteroidal anti-inflammatory drugs and acidic drugs inhibit methotrexate clearance. Multiple potential drug interactions; review current literature.
- Use vigorous hydration, urinary alkalinization, and leucovorin rescue with high-dose therapy.

- Use preservative-free product and diluents when administering intrathecally or with high-dose i.v. regimens.

MITOMYCIN-C (MUTAMYCIN)

Mechanism of Action

- Induces DNA cross-links through alkylation; inhibits DNA and RNA synthesis

FDA-approved Indications

- Disseminated gastric cancer or pancreatic cancer (in combination with other agents and as palliative treatment when other modalities have failed)

FDA-approved Dosage

- Single-agent therapy: 15 mg/m^2 i.v. $\times$ 1 dose repeated every 6 to 8 weeks
- Refer to current literature for alternative dosing regimens and combination regimens.

Dose Modification Criteria

- Renal: yes
- Myelosuppression: yes

Adverse Reactions

- CV: CHF (patients with prior doxorubicin exposure)
- DERM: alopecia, pruritus, tissue damage/necrosis with extravasation
- GI: anorexia, N/V (low), mucositis, diarrhea
- GU: hemolytic-uremic syndrome, increased Cr
- HEMAT: myelosuppression (may be cumulative)
- PULM: nonproductive cough, dyspnea, interstitial pneumonia
- Other: fever, malaise, weakness

Comments

- Vesicant

MITOTANE (LYSODREN)

Mechanism of Action

- Adrenal cytotoxic agent

FDA-approved Indications

- Inoperable, functional, and nonfunctional adrenal cortical carcinoma

FDA-approved Dosage

- Initial dose: 2 to 6 g p.o. per day in three to four divided doses. Doses are usually increased incrementally to 9 to 10 g/day or until maximum tolerated dose is achieved. Maximum tolerated dose range varies from 2 to 16 g/day but has usually been 9 to 10 g/day. Total daily doses should be administered in three to four divided doses.

Adverse Reactions

- DERM: transient skin rashes
- GI: anorexia, N/V, diarrhea
- NEURO: vertigo, depression, lethargy, somnolence, dizziness
- Other: adrenal insufficiency

Comments

- Institute adrenal insufficiency precautions.
- Patients should be counseled regarding the common CNS side effects and ambulatory patients should be cautioned about driving, operating machinery, and other hazardous pursuits requiring mental and physical alertness.

MITOXANTRONE (NOVANTRONE)

Mechanism of Action

- Interacts with DNA; intercalating agent; topoisomerase-II inhibition

FDA-approved Indications

- ANLL (myelogenous, promyelocytic, monocytic, erythroid acute leukemia) in adults (initial therapy in combination with other agents)
- Advanced hormone-refractory prostate cancer (in combination with corticosteroids)
- Other indications: multiple sclerosis

FDA-approved Dosage

- ANLL: induction, 12 mg/m^2 i.v. daily $\times$ 3 days (days 1, 2, 3) in combination with cytarabine; consolidation, 12 mg/m^2 i.v. daily $\times$ 2 days (days 1, 2) in combination with cytarabine
- Prostate cancer: 12 to 14 mg/m^2 i.v. $\times$ one dose every 21 days with prednisone or hydrocortisone

Dose Modification Criteria

- Renal: no data, unknown
- Hepatic: yes (use with caution; consider dose adjustment)

Adverse Reactions

- CV: congestive heart failure (clinical risk increases after a lifetime cumulative dose of 140 mg/m^2), tachycardia, ECG changes, chest pain
- DERM: rash, alopecia, urticaria, nailbed changes
- GI: N/V (low to moderate), mucositis, constipation, anorexia
- HEMAT: myelosuppression
- HEPAT: increased LFTs
- PULM: dyspnea
- Other: bluish-green urine, sclera may turn bluish, phlebitis (irritant), fatigue, secondary leukemias, tumor lysis syndrome

Comments

- Consider appropriate prophylaxis for tumor lysis syndrome when treating acute leukemias.

NELARABINE (ARRANON)

Mechanism of Action

- Antimetabolite

FDA-approved Indications

- T cell acute lymphoblastic leukemia and T cell lymphoblastic lymphoma: in patients whose disease has not responded to or has relapsed following treatment with at least two chemotherapy regimens.

FDA-approved Dosage

- Adult: 1,500 mg/m^2 i.v. infusion over 2 hours on days 1, 3, and 5 repeated every 21 days
- Pediatric: 650 mg/m^2 i.v. infusion over 1 hour daily for 5 consecutive days repeated every 21 days

Dose Modification Criteria

- Renal: unknown, use with caution in patients with severe renal impairment
- Hepatic: unknown, use with caution in patients with severe hepatic impairment
- Myelosuppression: no
- Nonhematologic toxicity: yes

Adverse Reactions

- GI: N/V (low), diarrhea, constipation
- HEMAT: myelosuppression
- HEPAT: increased LFTs
- NEURO: neurotoxicity (see comments), somnolence, dizziness, headache, peripheral neuropathy
- PULM: cough, dyspnea, pleural effusion
- Other: tumor lysis syndrome, fever, asthenia, fatigue, edema, myalgia/arthralgia

Comments

- Neurotoxicity is the dose-limiting toxicity of nelarabine. Common signs of nelarabine induced neurotoxicity include somnolence, confusion, convulsions, ataxia, paresthesias, and hypoesthesia. Severe neurologic toxicity can manifest as coma, status epilepticus, craniospinal demyelination, or ascending neuropathy similar in presentation to Guillain-Barré syndrome. Patients treated previously or concurrently with intrathecal chemotherapy or previously with craniospinal irradiation may be at increased risk for neurologic adverse events.
- Appropriate prevention measures for tumor lysis syndrome (e.g., intravenous hydration, urinary alkalization, allopurinol) should be initiated prior to nelarabine therapy for patients considered to be at risk.
- Pregnancy category D: nelarabine may cause fetal harm when administered to a pregnant woman.

NILOTINIB (TASIGNA)

Mechanism of Action

- Tyrosine kinase inhibitor (Bcr-Abl, PDGFR, c-KIT)

FDA-approved Indications

- CML: chronic phase and accelerated phase Philadelphia chromosome–positive CML in adult patients resistant to or intolerant to prior therapy that included imatinib.

FDA-approved Dosage

- 400 mg orally twice daily, approximately 12 hours apart on an empty stomach (no food 2 hours before and 1 hour after taking dose)

Dose Modification Criteria

- Renal: no
- Hepatic: unknown, use with caution
- Myelosuppression: yes
- Nonhematologic toxicity: yes

Adverse Reactions

- CV: QT prolongation
- DERM: rash, pruritis
- ELECTRO: hypophosphatemia, hypokalemia, hyperkalemia, hypocalcemia, hyponatremia
- GI: N/V (low), constipation, diarrhea
- HEMAT: myelosuppression
- HEPAT: elevated LFTs
- NEURO: headache
- PULM: cough, dyspnea
- Other: fatigue, elevated lipase, fever, asthenia, peripheral edema, arthralgia/mylagia

Comments

- Myelosuppression common. Monitor CBC every 2 weeks for the first 2 months of therapy and at least monthly thereafter, or as clinically indicated.
- Correct electrolyte abnormalities (e.g., hypokalemia, hypomagnesemia) prior to initiating therapy and monitor periodically during therapy. Obtain an ECG at baseline, 7 days after initiation, and periodically as clinically indicated. Do not use nilotinib concomitantly with other agents that cause QT prolongation. Sudden deaths have been reported on patients treated with nilotinib.
- Nilotinib is metabolized through the cytochrome p450 3A4 isoenzyme. Screen for potential drug interactions with CYP 3A4 inhibitors or inducers. Dose modification may be necessary if concomitant use with a potent CYP 3A4 inducer or inhibitor cannot be avoided. In addition, nilotinib is a competitive inhibitor and inducer or multiple CYP isoenzymes and p-glycoprotein and subsequently may either increase or decrease concentrations of concomitant medications. Refer to product labeling for additional information.
- Pregnancy category D: nilotinib may cause fetal harm when administered to a pregnant woman.

NILUTAMIDE (NILANDRON)

Mechanism of Action

- Antiandrogen

FDA-approved Indications

- Metastatic prostate cancer (stage D2; in combination therapy with surgical castration). Dosing should begin on same day or day after surgical castration.

FDA-approved Dosage

- Give 300 mg p.o. daily × 30 days, and then 150 mg p.o. daily (with or without food)

Adverse Reactions

- CV: hypertension, angina
- ENDO: hot flashes, impotence, decreased libido
- GI: nausea, anorexia, constipation
- HEPAT: increased LFTs (monitor LFTs periodically because of rare associations with cholestatic jaundice, hepatic necrosis, and encephalopathy)
- NEURO: dizziness
- Ocular: visual disturbances, impaired adaptation to dark
- PULM: interstitial pneumonitis, dyspnea

Comments

- Obtain baseline chest x-ray prior to initiating therapy (with consideration of baseline pulmonary function tests). Patients should be instructed to report any new or worsening shortness of breath and if symptoms occur, nilutamide should be immediately discontinued.
- Monitor LFTs at baseline and at regular intervals $\times$ 4 months and then periodically thereafter.

OXALIPLATIN (ELOXATIN)

Mechanism of Action

- Alkylating-like agent producing interstrand DNA cross links

FDA-approved Indications

- Colorectal cancer
  - Adjuvant treatment of stage III colon cancer in patients who have undergone complete resection of the primary tumor in combination with infusional fluorouracil and leucovorin.
  - Treatment of advanced colorectal cancer in combination with infusional fluorouracil and leucovorin

FDA-approved Dosage

- Combined therapy with infusional fluorouracil and leucovorin (FOLFOX regimen)
- **Day 1**: Oxaliplatin 85 mg/m^2 i.v. over 120 minutes $\times$ 1 dose given concurrently with leucovorin 200 mg/m^2 i.v. over 120 minutes $\times$ 1 dose *followed by* fluorouracil 400 mg/m^2 i.v. bolus over 2 to 4 minutes $\times$ 1 dose *followed by* fluorouracil 600 mg/m^2 i.v. continuous infusion over 22 hours
- **Day 2**: Leucovorin 200 mg/m^2 i.v. over 120 minutes $\times$ 1 dose *followed by* fluorouracil 400 mg/m^2 i.v. bolus over 2 to 4 minutes $\times$ 1 dose *followed by* fluorouracil 600 mg/m^2 i.v. continuous infusion over 22 hours
- Cycles are repeated every 2 weeks

Dose Modification Criteria

- Renal: no data (use caution)
- Myelosuppression: yes
- Nonhematologic toxicity: yes

Adverse Reactions

- CNS: peripheral sensory neuropathies (see comments below), headache
- CV: edema, thromboembolic events
- DERM: injection site reactions
- GI: N/V (moderate), diarrhea, mucositis/stomatitis, abdominal pain, anorexia, taste perversion, elevated LFTs

- GU: elevated serum creatinine
- HEMAT: myelosuppression
- PULM: pulmonary fibrosis, dyspnea cough
- OTHER: fatigue, fever, back pain, pain, hypersensitivity reaction.

Comments

- Anaphylactic reactions have been reported, and may occur within minutes of oxaliplatin administration. Epinephrin, corticosteroids, and antihistamines have been used to alleviate symptoms of anaphylaxis.
- Oxaliplatin is associated with two types of peripheral neuropathy:
  1. An acute, reversible, primarily peripheral, sensory neuropathy that is of early onset (within hours to 1–2 days of dosing), that resolves within 14 days, and that frequently recurs with further dosing. The symptoms include transient paresthesia, dysesthesia, and hypoesthesia in the hands, feet, perioral area, or throat. Symptoms may be precipitated or exacerbated by exposure to cold temperature or cold objects. Patients should be instructed to avoid cold drinks, use of ice, and should cover exposed skin prior to exposure to cold temperature or cold objects.
  2. A persistent (>14 days), primarily peripheral, sensory neuropathy usually characterized by paresthesias, dysesthesias, hypoesthesias, but may also include deficits in proprioception that can interfere with daily activities. Dose modifications are recommended for persistent grade 2 neurotoxicity and discontinuation of therapy is recommended for persistent grade 3 neurotoxicity.

PACLITAXEL (TAXOL)

Mechanism of Action

- Microtubule assembly stabilization.

FDA-approved Indications

- Advanced ovarian cancer (first line and subsequent therapy). As first-line therapy, paclitaxel is indicated in combination with cisplatin.
- Breast Cancer.
  - Adjuvant treatment of node-positive breast cancer (administered sequentially to standard doxorubicin-containing combination chemotherapy).
  - Second-line therapy for breast cancer (after failure of combination chemotherapy for metastatic disease or relapse within 6 months of adjuvant therapy).
- NSCLC (first-line therapy in combination with cisplatin) in patients who are not candidates for potentially curative surgery and/or radiation therapy.
- AIDS-related Kaposi's sarcoma (second-line treatment).

FDA-approved Dosage

- Premedicate patients with dexamethasone, diphenhydramine (or its equivalent), and H_2 antagonists (e.g., cimetidine or ranitidine) to prevent severe hypersensitivity reactions. Suggested package literature premedication regimen: dexamethasone 20 mg p.o. $\times$ 2 doses administered approximately 12 and 6 hours before paclitaxel; diphenhydramine 50 mg i.v. 30 to 60 minutes before paclitaxel; and cimetidine 300 mg i.v. OR ranitidine 50 mg i.v. 30 to 60 minutes before paclitaxel. Consult current literature for alternative premedication regimens.
- First-line ovarian cancer: 135 mg/m² i.v. continuous infusion over 24 hours OR 175 mg/m² i.v. over 3 hours (followed by cisplatin 75 mg/m² i.v.) every 3 weeks.
- Second-line ovarian cancer: 135 mg/m² OR 175 mg/m² i.v. over 3 hours every 3 weeks. Consult current literature for alternative regimens.
- Adjuvant therapy of node-positive breast cancer: 175 mg/m² i.v. over 3 hours every 3 weeks $\times$ four cycles (administered sequentially with doxorubicin-containing chemotherapy).

- Second-line breast cancer: 175 mg/m² i.v. over 3 hours every 3 weeks.
- NSCLC: 135 mg/m² i.v. continuous infusion over 24 hours (followed by cisplatin 75 mg/m² i.v.) every 3 weeks.
- AIDS-related Kaposi's sarcoma: 135 mg/m² i.v. over 3 hours every 3 weeks or 100 mg/m² i.v. over 3 hours every 2 weeks. (Note: reduce the dose of dexamethasone premedication dose to 10 mg p.o. per dose (instead of the suggested 20 mg p.o. dose).

Dose Modification Criteria

- Hepatic: yes; Myelosuppression: yes; Nonhematologic toxicity (neuropathy): yes.

Adverse Reactions

- CV: hypotension, bradycardia, ECG changes; DERM: alopecia, onycholysis (more common with weekly dosing), injection site reactions; GI: N/V (low), diarrhea, mucositis; HEMAT: myelosuppression; INFUS: acute hypersensitivity-type reactions; NEURO: peripheral neurosensory toxicity (paresthesia, dysesthesia, pain); OTHER: arthralgia, myalgia.

Comments

- Use non-DEHP plasticized solution containers and administration sets.
- Inline filtration (0.22-μm filter) required during administration.
- Lower dose, weekly dosage regimens are commonly utilized. Consult current literature for dose guidelines.

PANITUMUMAB (VECTIBIX)

Mechanism of Action

- Monoclonal Antibody to the human EGFR.

FDA-approved Indications

- Colorectal Cancer: indicated as a single agent for the treatment of EGFR-expressing, metastatic colorectal carcinoma with disease progression on or following fluoropyrimidine-, oxaliplatin-, and irinotecan-containing chemotherapy regimens.

FDA-approved Dosage

- 6 mg/kg IV infusion over 60 minutes every 14 days. Doses higher than 1,000 mg should be administered over 90 minutes.

Dose Modification Criteria

- Renal: no (not studied in patients with severe impairment); Hepatic: no (not studied in patients with severe impairment); Myelosuppression: no; Nonhematologic toxicity: yes.

Adverse Reactions

- DERM: dermatitis acneiform, pruritis, erythema, rash, skin exfoliation, paronychia, dry skin, skin fissures, photosensitivity; ELECTRO: hypomagnesemia, hypocalcemia; GI: N/V (low), abdominal pain, diarrhea, stomatitis/mucositis; INFUS: infusion reactions may include fever, chills, dyspnea, bronchospasm, hypotension; OCULAR: conjunctivitis, ocular hyperemia, increased lacrimation; PULM: pulmonary fibrosis (rare); OTHER: fatigue.

Comments

- KRAS mutation predicts for a lack of response to anti-EGFR agents like panitumumab. Consider evaluating for the KRAS mutation prior to initiating therapy.
- Patients enrolled in the colorectal cancer clinical studies were required to have immunohistochemical evidence of EGFR expression; these are the only patients studied and for whom benefit has been shown.
- Reduce infusion rate by 50% in patients experiencing a mild or moderate (grade 1 or 2) infusion reaction for the duration of that infusion. Immediately and permanently discontinue panitumumab in patients experiencing a severe (grade 3 or 4) infusion reaction. The use of premedication was not standardized in the clinical trials and thus the utility of premedication is not known.
- Withhold panitumumab for dermatologic toxicities that are grade 3 or higher or considered intolerable. If toxicity does not improve to $\leq$ grade 2 within 1 month, permanently discontinue panitumumab. If dermatologic toxicity does improve to $\leq$ grade 2 after withholding no more than two doses, treatment may be resumed at 50% of the original dose. See product labeling for further information on dose adjustments.

PEGASPARAGASE (ONCASPAR)

Mechanism of Action

- A modified (pegylated) version of the enzyme L-asparaginase. L-asparaginase depletes asparagine, an amino acid required by some leukemic cells.

FDA-approved Indications

- Acute lymphoblastic leukemia in patients hypersensitive to native forms of L-asparaginase.

FDA-approved Dosage

- The preferred route is i.m.; i.v. administration should be over 1 to 2 hours.
- Combination or sole induction therapy: Adults and children, ≥ 0.6 m^2 BSA: 2,500 IU/m^2 i.m. or i.v. $\times$ one dose every 14 days.
- Children <0.6 m^2 BSA: 82.5 IU/kg i.m. or i.v. $\times$ 1 dose every 14 days.

Adverse Reactions

- CV: chest pain, hypertension, hypotension; DERM: alopecia, itching, injection site reactions; ENDO: hyperglycemia; GI: anorexia; N/V (minimal to low), pancreatitis; GU: increased BUN and Cr; HEMAT: hypofibrinogenemia; HEPAT: hepatotoxicity, increased LFTs; NEURO: malaise, confusion, lethargy, depression; PULM: respiratory distress, cough, epistaxis; OTHER: hypersensitivity reaction, fever, arthralgia, musculoskeletal pain, tumor lysis syndrome.

Comments

- Contraindications: active pancreatitis or history of pancreatitis, serious hemorrhagic episode with native L-asparaginase, serious allergic reactions (e.g., bronchospasm) to native L-asparaginase.

PEMETREXED (ALIMTA)

Mechanism of Action

- Antimetabolite. An antifolate that disrupts folate-dependent metabolic process essential for cell replication.

FDA-approved Indications

- Malignant Pleural Mesothelioma: in combination with cisplatin in patients whose disease is unresectable or who are otherwise not candidates for curative surgery.
- NSCLC: second-line therapy as a single agent for the treatment of patients with locally advanced or metastatic NSCLC after prior chemotherapy.

FDA-approved Dosage

- Malignant Pleural Mesothelioma: 500 mg/m^2 i.v. over 10 minutes on day 1 of each 21-day cycle. The recommended dose of cisplatin (in combination with pemetrexed) is 75 mg/m^2 i.v. over 2 hours beginning approximately 30 minutes after the end of pemetrexed. See comments below regarding premedication regimen for pemetrexed.
- NSCLC: 500 mg/m^2 i.v. over 10 minutes on day 1 of each 21-day cycle.

Dose Modification Criteria

- Renal (CrCl >45 mL/min): no, Renal (CrCl <45 mL/min): yes—administration is not recommended; Hepatic: no data; Myelosuppression: yes; Nonhematologic toxicity: yes.

Adverse Reactions

- DERM: rash, desquamation; GI: N/V (low), mucositis, pharyngitis, diarrhea, anorexia; HEMAT: neutropenia, thrombocytopenia, anemia; HEPAT: increased LFTs; OTHER: fatigue, fever.

Comments

- Vitamin Supplementation: Patients treated with pemetrexed must be instructed to take folic acid and vitamin B$_{12}$ as a prophylactic measure to reduce treatment-related hematologic and GI toxicity. Patients should receive at least five daily doses of folic acid (most common daily dose: 400 μg) during the 7-day period prior to the first dose of pemetrexed and dosing should continue during the full course of therapy and for 21 days after the last dose. Patients must also receive one intramuscular dose of vitamin B$_{12}$ (1,000 μg) during the week prior to the first dose of pemetrexed and every 3 cycles (9 weeks) thereafter.
- Corticosteroid premedication: Pretreatment with dexamethasone (or equivalent) reduces the incidence and severity of cutaneous reactions. Recommended regimen (product labeling): dexamethasone 4 mg p.o. bid × 3 days (six doses) beginning the day prior to each dose of pemetrexed (the day before, the day of, and the day after pemetrexed).
- Pregnancy Category D: pemetrexed may cause fetal harm when administered to a pregnant woman. Pemetrexed is fetotoxic and teratogenic in mice; there are no studies of pemetrexed in pregnant women.

PENTOSTATIN (NIPENT)

Mechanism of Action

- Antimetabolite (adenosine deaminase inhibitor).

FDA-approved Indications

- Hairy cell leukemia (first-line and in alpha-interferon-refractory disease).

FDA-approved Dosage

- 4 mg/m^2 i.v. every other week. The optimal treatment duration has not been determined. The package insert suggests continued treatment until a complete response has been achieved followed by two additional doses.

Dose Modification Criteria
• Renal: yes; Myelosuppression: yes.

Adverse Reactions
• DERM: rash; GI: N/V (moderate); GU: mild transient rise in serum creatinine; HEMAT: leukopenia, anemia, thrombocytopenia; HEPAT: elevated LFTs; OTHER: fever, infection, fatigue.

Comments
• A high incidence of fatal pulmonary toxicity was seen in a trial investigating the combination of fludarabine with pentostatin. The combined use of fludarabine and pentostatin is not recommended.
• Patients should receive hydration (500–1,000 mL) before and after each pentostatin dose.

POLIFEPROSAN 20 WITH CARMUSTINE IMPLANT (GLIADEL WAFER)

Mechanism of Action
• The polifeprosan 20 with carmustine implant is designed to deliver carmustine directly into the surgical cavity created when a brain tumor is resected. On exposure to the aqueous environment of the resection cavity, carmustine is released from the copolymer and diffuses into the surrounding brain tissue. Carmustine is an alkylating agent.

FDA-approved Indications
• High-grade malignant glioma (first-line treatment in newly diagnosed patients as an adjunct to surgery and radiation)
• Recurrent glioblastoma multiforme as an adjunct to surgery.

FDA-approved Dosage
• Each wafer contains 7.7 mg of carmustine. Up to eight wafers should be implanted at time of surgery (eight wafers results in a dose of 61.6 mg).

Adverse Reactions
• GI: N/V (low); NEURO: meningitis, abscess, brain edema; OTHER: abnormal healing, pain, fever.

Comments
• Wafers can be broken in half. Proper handling and disposal precautions should be observed.

PORFIMER (PHOTOFRIN)

Mechanism of Action
• Photosensitizing agent.

FDA-approved Indications
• Esophageal cancer (palliation of complete or partial obstruction)
• Endobronchial NSCLC
  – For reduction of obstruction and palliation of symptoms in patients with completely or partially obstructed endobronchial NSCLC.

– For treatment of microinvasive endobronchial NSCLC in patients for whom surgery and radiotherapy are not indicated.
• High-grade dysplasia in Barrett's esophagus (ablation of high-grade dysplasia in patients who do not undergo esophagectomy).

FDA-approved Dosage

• 2 mg/kg i.v. injection over 3 to 5 minutes × one dose followed by photodynamic therapy. For the treatment of esophageal and endobronchial cancer, patients may receive up to three additional courses; each course should be administered no sooner than 30 days after the prior course. For the ablation of high-grade dysplasia in Barrett's esophagus, patients may receive up to three additional courses; each course should be administered no sooner than 90 days after the prior course.

Adverse Reactions

• CV: hypertension, hypotension, heart failure, chest pain, atrial fibrillation, tachycardia; DERM: photosensitivity; HEMAT: anemia; GI: N/V, abdominal pain, anorexia, constipation, dysphagia, esophageal edema, esophageal stricture; NEURO: anxiety, confusion, insomnia; PULM: pleural effusion, dyspnea, pneumonia, pharyngitis, cough, respiratory insufficiency, tracheoesophageal fistula; OTHER: fever.

Comments

• Patients are photosensitive (including eyes) for at least 30 days after administration.

PROCARBAZINE (MATULANE)

Mechanism of Action

• Mechanism unknown. There is evidence that the drug may act by inhibition of protein, RNA and DNA synthesis.

FDA-approved Indications

• Stage III and IV Hodgkin's disease: first-line treatment in combination with other anticancer drugs. (Procarbazine is used as part of the MOPP [mechlorethamine, vincristine, procarbazine, and prednisone] chemotherapy regimen.)

FDA-approved Dosage

• All doses based on actual body weight unless the patient is obese or there has been a spurious weight increase, in which case lean body weight (dry weight) should be used.
• Doses may be given as a single daily dose or divided throughout the day.
• MOPP regimen for Hodgkin's disease: 100 mg/m² p.o. daily × 14 days (in combination with mechlorethamine, vincristine, and prednisone).
• Adult single agent therapy: 2 to 4 mg/kg p.o. daily × 7 days, and then 4 to 6 mg/kg p.o. daily until maximal response is obtained. Maintenance dose: 1 to 2 mg/kg p.o. daily.
• Pediatric single agent therapy: 50 mg/m² p.o. daily × 7 days, and then 100 mg/m² p.o. daily until maximum response is obtained. Maintenance dose: 50 mg/m² p.o. daily.

Adverse Reactions

• DERM: pruritus, hyperpigmentation, alopecia; GI: anorexia, N/V (moderate), stomatitis, xerostomia, diarrhea, constipation; HEMAT: myelosuppression; NEURO: paresthesias, confusion, lethargy, mental depression; OTHER: fever, myalgia.

Comments

- Disulfiram-like (Antabuse) reaction can occur; avoid alcoholic beverages while taking procarbazine.
- Procarbazine is a weak monoamine oxidase (MAO) inhibitor; avoid tyramine-rich foods, sympathomimetic drugs, and tricyclic antidepressants.

RALOXIFENE (EVISTA)

Mechanism of Action

- Estrogen agonist/antagonist (Selective Estrogen Receptor Modulator).

FDA-approved Indications

- Reduction in risk of invasive breast cancer in postmenopausal women with osteoporosis.
- Reduction in risk of invasive breast cancer in postmenopausal women at high risk of invasive breast cancer.
- Treatment and prevention of osteoporosis in postmenopausal women.

FDA-approved Dosage

- 60 mg orally once daily.

Dose Modification Criteria

- Renal: no (use with caution in patients with moderate or severe impairment); Hepatic: no (use with caution in patients with moderate or severe impairment); Myelosuppression: no; Nonhematologic toxicity: no.

Adverse Reactions

- CV: peripheral edema; GI: N/V (minimal); OTHER: hot flashes, leg cramps, venous thromboembolic events (deep venous thrombosis, pulmonary embolism, retinal vein thrombosis, superficial thrombophlebitis).

Comments

- Women with active or past history of venous thromboembolism should not take raloxifene. Raloxifene should be discontinued at least 72 hours prior to and during prolonged immobilization (e.g., postsurgical recovery, prolonged bed rest), and raloxifene should be resumed only after the patient is fully ambulatory. Women should be advised to move about periodically during prolonged travel.
- In a clinical trial of postmenopausal women with documented coronary heart disease or at increased risk of coronary events, an increased risk of death due to stroke was observed after treatment with raloxifene. However, there was no statistically signficant difference between treatment groups in the incidence of stroke.
- Cholestyramine (and other anion exchange resins) should not be used concurrently with raloxifene.
- If used concomitantly with warfarin, monitor prothrombin time when starting or stopping raloxifene.
- Raloxifene is highly protein bound (95%); use with caution with other highly protein bound drugs.

RITUXIMAB (RITUXAN)

Mechanism of Action

- Chimeric (murine, human) monoclonal antibody directed at the CD20 antigen found on the surface of normal and malignant B lymphocytes.

FDA-approved Indications

- Non-Hodgkin's Lymphoma (NHL)
  - Relapsed or refractory low-grade or follicular, CD20-positive, B-cell, non-Hodgkin's lymphoma as a single agent.
  - Previously untreated follicular, CD20-positive, B-cell NHL in combination with CVP chemotherapy.
  - Nonprogressive (including stable disease), low-grade, CD20-positive, B-cell NHL, as a single agent, after first-line CVP chemotherapy.
  - Previously untreated diffuse large B-cell, CD20-positive NHL in combination with CHOP or other anthracycline-based chemotherapy regimens.
- Other: Rheumatoid Arthritis.

FDA-approved Dosage

- Premedication with acetaminophen and/or diphenhydramine should be considered before each infusion.
- If patient experiences an infusion-related reaction, the infusion should be stopped, the patient managed symptomatically, and then the infusion should be restarted at half the rate once the symptoms have resolved.
- 375 mg/m^2 i.v. weekly $\times$ four doses (days 1, 8, 15, 22) or eight doses.
- First infusion: start at 50 mg/hour, and then may increase by 50 mg/hour every 30 minutes up to a maximum of 400 mg/hour. Subsequent infusions if prior infusions tolerated: Start at 100 mg/hour, and then may increase by 100 mg/hour every 30 minutes up to a maximum of 400 mg/hour.

Adverse Reactions

- CV: hypotension, arrhythmias, peripheral edema; DERM: rash, pruritis, urticaria, severe mucocutaneous reactions; GI: N/V (minimal), abdominal pain; HEMAT: angioedema, leukopenia, thrombocytopenia, neutropenia; INFUS: fever, chills, rigors, hypoxia, pulmonary infiltrates, adult respiratory distress syndrome, myocardial infarction, ventricular fibrillation or cardiogenic shock; NEURO: headache, dizziness; OTHER: throat irritation, rhinitis, bronchospasm, hypersensitivity reaction, myalgia, back pain, tumor lysis syndrome.

Comments

- Tumor lysis syndrome has been reported within 12 to 24 hours after the infusion (high-risk: high numbers of circulating malignant cells).
- Mild to moderate infusion reactions consisting of fever, chills, and rigors occur in the majority of patients during the first infusion. The reactions resolve with slowing or interruption of the infusion and with supportive care measures. The incidence of infusion reactions declines with subsequent infusions.
- A more severe infusion-related complex, usually reported with the first infusion (hypoxia, pulmonary infiltrates, adult respiratory distress syndrome, myocardial infarction, ventricular fibrillation, or cardiogenic shock) has resulted in fatalities.
- Severe mucocutaneous reactions, some with fatal outcome, have been reported in association with rituximab treatment.
- Rituximab is commonly combined with cytotoxic chemotherapy agents in various subtypes of B-cell non-Hodgkin's lymphoma. Consult current literature for dosing regimens.

SORAFENINIB (NEXAVAR)

Mechanism of Action

- Tyrosine kinase inhibitor (Raf kinases, VEGFR-2, 3, FLT-3, KIT, PDGFR-β).

FDA-approved Indications

- Advanced Renal Cell Carcinoma
- Unresectable Hepatocellular Carcinoma

FDA-approved Dosage

- 400 mg orally twice daily without food (1 hour before or 2 hours after eating).

Dose Modification Criteria

- Renal: no (not studied in patients with severe renal impairment); Hepatic: no (not studied in patients with severe hepatic impairment); Myelosuppression: no; Nonhematologic toxicity: yes.

Adverse Reactions

- CV: hypertension, cardiac ischemia/infarction (see comments); DERM: palmar-plantar erythrodysesthesia, rash, alopecia, pruritis, dry skin, erythema; ELECTRO: hypophosphatemia; GI: N/V (low), diarrhea, anorexia, abdominal pain, gastrointestinal perforation (rare); HEMAT: myelosuppression; NEURO: peripheral neuropathy (sensory); OTHER: bleeding/hemorrhage, fatigue, asthenia, weight loss, increased lipase/amylase.

Comments

- Hand-foot skin reaction (palmar-plantar erythrodysesthesia) and rash are the most common adverse events with sorafenib. Monitor closely, provide supportive care, and evaluate for dose interruption of modification for severe toxicity (see product labeling).
- Monitor blood pressure weekly during the first 6 weeks of therapy and thereafter monitor and treat according to standard medical practice.
- Sorafenib may impair wound healing. Temporary interruption of sorafenib is recommended in patients undergoing major surgical procedures.
- In a hepatocellular cancer trial, the incidence of cardiac ischemia/infarction was higher in the sorafenib treated patients (2.7%) compared to the placebo group (1.3%).
- Sorafenib is hepatically metabolized undergoing oxidative metabolism through cytochrome p450 (CYP) isoenzyme 3A4 as well as glucuronidation mediated by UGT1A9 and thus drug exposure may be influenced by inhibitors or inducers of CYP3A4 or UGT1A9. Sorafenib is also a competitive inhibitor of multiple cytochrome enzymes (e.g., CYP2B6, CYP2C8) and of glucuronidation by the UGT1A1 and UGT1A9 pathways. Refer to product labeling and other appropriate references to screen for potential drug interactions.
- Pregnancy category D: may cause fetal harm when administered to a pregnant woman.

STREPTOZOTOCIN (ZANOSAR)

Mechanism of Action

- Alkylating agent

FDA-approved Indications

- Metastatic islet cell carcinoma of the pancreas (functional and nonfunctional carcinomas)

FDA-approved Dosage

- Daily schedule
  - 500 mg/m^2 i.v. daily $\times$ 5 days every 6 weeks until maximum benefit or treatment limiting toxicity is observed, *OR*

- Weekly schedule
  - Initial dose: 1 g/m^2 i.v. weekly for the first two courses (weeks). In subsequent courses, drug doses may be escalated in patients who have not achieved a therapeutic response and who have not experienced significant toxicity with the previous course of treatment. However, a single dose should not exceed 1,500 mg/m^2.

Dose Modification Criteria

- Renal: use with caution, consider dose reduction

Adverse Reactions

- DERM: injection site reactions (irritant)
- ELECTRO: hypophosphatemia
- ENDO: dysglycemia, may lead to insulin-dependent diabetes
- GI: N/V (high), increased LFTs, diarrhea
- GU: azotemia, anuria, renal tubular acidosis, increased BUN and serum creatinine, glycosuria
- HEMAT: myelosuppression

Comments

- Renal complications are dose-related and cumulative. Mild proteinuria is usually an early sign of impending renal dysfunction. Serial urinalysis is important for the early detection of proteinuria and should be quantified with a 24-hour collection when proteinuria is detected. Adequate hydration may help reduce the risk of nephrotoxicity. Avoid other nephrotoxic agents.

SUNITINIB MALATE (SUTENT)

Mechanism of Action

- Tyrosine kinase inhibitor (VEGFR-1,2,3, FLT-3, KIT, PDGFR-α, β, CSF-1R, RET)

FDA-approved Indications

- GIST: after disease progression on or intolerance to imatinib mesylate
- Advanced renal cell carcinoma

FDA-approved Dosage

- 50 mg orally once daily on a schedule of 4 weeks on treatment followed by 2 weeks off. Sunitinib may be taken with or without food.

Dose Modification Criteria

- Renal: no (not studied in patients with renal impairment)
- Hepatic: no (not studied in patients with severe hepatic impairment)
- Myelosuppression: no;
- Nonhematologic toxicity: yes

Adverse Reactions

- CV: hypertension, left ventricular dysfunction, QT interval prolongation
- DERM: palmar-plantar erythrodysesthesia, rash, skin discoloration (yellow), dry skin
- ENDO: hypothyroidism

- GI: N/V (low), diarrhea, mucositis/stomatitis, dyspepsia, abdominal pain, constipation, altered taste, anorexia
- HEMAT: myelosuppression
- HEPAT: increased LFTs
- NEURO: peripheral neuropathy (sensory)
- Other: bleeding/hemorrhage, fatigue, asthenia, myalgia/limb pain, increased amylase/lipase

Comments

- Hypertension may occur. Monitor blood pressure and treat as needed.
- Left ventricular ejection declines have occurred. Monitor patients for signs or symptoms of congestive heart failure.
- Prolonged QT intervals and Torsade de Pointes have been observed. Use with cation in patients at higher risk. Consider baseline and on-treatment electrocardiograms and monitor electrolytes.
- Hemorrhagic events including tumor-related hemorrhage have occurred. Perform serial complete blood counts and physical examination.
- Hypothyroidism may occur. Patients with signs or symptoms suggestive of hypothyroidism should have laboratory monitoring of thyroid function and be treated as per standard medical practice.
- Adrenal hemorrhage was observed in animal studies. Monitor adrenal function in case of stress such as surgery, trauma, or severe infection.
- Sunitinib is hepatically metabolized undergoing oxidative metabolism through cytochrome p450 (CYP) isoenzyme 3A4 and thus drug exposure may be influenced by potent inhibitors or inducers of CYP3A4. Refer to product labeling and other appropriate references to screen for potential drug interactions.
- Pregnancy category D: may cause fetal harm when administered to a pregnant woman.

TAMOXIFEN (NOLVADEX)

Mechanism of Action

- Nonsteroidal antiestrogen

FDA-approved Indications

- Breast cancer treatment
  - Treatment of metastatic breast cancer
  - Adjuvant treatment of node-positive and node-negative breast cancer following breast surgery and breast irradiation
  - Reduction in breast cancer incidence
    - Ductal carcinoma in situ (DCIS): to reduce the risk of invasive breast cancer following breast surgery and radiation
    - High-risk women, at least 35 years of age with a 5-year predicted risk of breast cancer $\geq 1.67\%$ as calculated by the Gail Model (see package insert).

FDA-approved Dosage

- Breast cancer treatment: 20 mg p.o. daily or 10 to 20 mg p.o. twice daily (20–40 mg/day). Adjuvant therapy should be continued × 5 years. Doses >20 mg/day should be given in divided doses (morning and evening).
- Breast cancer incidence reduction (DCIS and in high risk women): 20 mg p.o. daily × 5 years

Adverse Reactions

- CV: thromboembolism, stroke, pulmonary embolism

- DERM: skin rash
- ENDO: hot flashes
- GI: N/V (minimal), anorexia
- GU: menstrual irregularities, pruritis vulvae, vaginal discharge or bleeding
- HEMAT: bone marrow depression
- Ocular: vision disturbances, cataracts
- PULM: dyspnea, chest pain, hemoptysis
- Other: dizziness, headaches, tumor or bone pain, pelvic pain, uterine malignancies

Comments

- High risk is defined as women at least 35 years old with a 5-year predicted risk of breast cancer of 1.67%, as predicted by the Gail model. Health care professionals can access a breast cancer risk assessment tool on the NCI website (www.cancer.gov/bcrisktool/).
- Serious and life-threatening events associated with tamoxifen in the risk reduction setting include uterine malignancies, stroke and pulmonary embolism. Consult package insert for additional information.

TEMOZOLOMIDE (TEMODAR)

Mechanism of Action

- Alkylating agent

FDA-approved Indications

- Newly diagnosed glioblastoma multiforme concomitantly with radiotherapy and then as maintenance treatment in adults.
- Refractory anaplastic astrocytoma: Second-line treatment in adults (after a nitrosourea and procarbazine).

FDA-approved Dosage

- Newly diagnosed high-grade glioma: 75 mg/m^2 p.o. daily $\times$ 42 days concomitant with focal radiotherapy followed by maintenance temozolamide for six cycles. The temozolamide dose should be continued throughout the 42-day concomitant period up to 49 days to achieve acceptable hematologic and nonhematologic parameters (see package insert). PCP prophylaxis is required during the concomitant administration of temozolamide and radiotherapy and should be continued in patients who develop lymphocytopenia.
- Maintenance phase
  - Cycle 1: 150 mg/m^2 p.o. daily $\times$ 5 followed by 23 days without treatment starting 4 weeks after the temozolamide + RT phase
  - Cycles 2 to 6: cose is escalated to 200 mg/m^2 if the nonhematologic and hematologic parameters are met (see package insert). The dose remains at 200 mg/m^2 per day for the first 5 days of each subsequent cycle except if toxicity occurs.
- Refractory anaplastic astrocytoma: initial dose: 150 mg/m^2 p.o. daily $\times$ 5 consecutive days every 28 days. If the initial dose leads to acceptable hematologic parameters at the nadir and on day of dosing (see criteria in package insert), the temozolomide dose may be increased to 200 mg/m^2 p.o. daily $\times$ 5 consecutive days per 28-day treatment cycle

Dose Modification Criteria

- Renal (severe impairment): use with caution
- Hepatic (severe impairment): use with caution
- Myelosuppression: yes

Adverse Reactions

- HEMAT: myelosuppression
- GI: N/V (low—reduced by taking on an empty stomach)
- NEURO: headache
- Other: asthenia, fatigue

Comments

- Capsules should be taken with water. Administer consistently with respect to food and to reduce the risk of nausea and vomiting it is recommended that temozoloamide be taken on an empty stomach. Bedtime administration may be advised.
- Myelosuppression occurs late in the treatment cycle. The median nadirs in a study of 158 patients with anaplastic astrocytoma occurred at 26 days for platelets (range 21–40 days) and 28 days for neutrophils (range 1–44 days). The package insert recommends obtaining a complete blood count on day 22 (21 days after the first dose) and then weekly until the ANC is above $1.5 \times 10^9/L$ and the platelet count exceeds $100 \times 10^9/L$. The next cycle of temozolomide should not be started until the ANC and platelet count exceed these levels. See package insert for dose modification guidelines.

TEMSIROLIMUS (TORISEL)

Mechanism of Action

- Inhibitor of mammalian target of rapamycin (mTOR)

FDA-approved Indications

- Advanced renal cell carcinoma

FDA-approved Dosage

- 25 mg infused intravenously over 30 to 60 minutes once a week. Treat until disease progression or unacceptable toxicity. Antihistamine pretreatment is recommended.

Dose Modification Criteria

- Renal: no
- Hepatic: no (not studied in patients with hepatic impairment)
- Myelosuppression: yes
- Nonhematologic toxicity: no

Adverse Reactions

- DERM: rash, pruritis, nail disorder, dry skin
- ENDO: hyperglycemia/glucose intolerance
- ELECTRO: hypophosphatemia, hypokalemia
- GI: N/V (low); mucositis, anorexia, weight loss, diarrhea, constipation, taste loss/perversion, bowel perforation (rare)
- GU: elevated serum creatinine, renal failure
- HEMAT: myelosuppression
- HEPAT: elevated LFTs (AST, alkaline phosphatase)
- INFUS: hypersensitivity reactions (anaphylaxis, dyspnea, flushing, chest pain)
- NEURO: headache, insomnia
- PULM: interstitial lung disease

- Other: asthenia, fever, immunosuppression; hyperlipemia, hypertriglyceridemia, impaired wound healing, bleeding/hemorrhage, edema, back pain/arthralgias

Comments

- To reduce the risk of hypersensitivity reactins, premedicate patients with an H_1 antihistamine prior to the administration of temsirolimus. Interrupt the infusion if a patient develops an infusion reaction for patient observation. At the discretion of the physician, the infusion may be resumed after administration of additional antihistamine therapy (H_1 and/or H_2 receptor antagonists) and with a slower rate of infusion for the temsirolimus.
- Serum glucose should be tested before and during treatment with temsirolimus. Patients may require an increase in the dose of, or initiation of, insulin and/or oral hypoglycemic agent therapy.
- Elevations in triglycerides and/or lipids are common side effects and may require treatment. Monitor lipid profiles.
- Monitor for symptoms or radiographic changes of interstitial lung disease. Therapy with temsirolimus should be discontinued if toxicity occurs and corticosteroid therapy should be considered.
- Bowel perforation may occur. Evaluate fever, abdominal pain, bloody stools, and or acute abdomen promptly.
- Renal failure has occurred; monitor renal function at baseline and while on therapy.
- Due to abnormal wound healing, use temsirolimus with caution in the perioperative period.
- Live vaccinations and close contact with those who received live vaccines should be avoided.
- Temsirolimus is hepatically metabolized undergoing oxidative metabolism through cytochrome p450 (CYP) isoenzyme 3A4 and thus drug exposure may be influenced by potent inhibitors or inducers of CYP3A4. Refer to product labeling and other appropriate references to screen for potential drug interactions.
- Pregnancy category D: may cause fetal harm when administered to a pregnant woman.

TENIPOSIDE (VUMON)

Mechanism of Action

- Topoisomerase-II inhibitor

FDA-approved Indications

- Refractory childhood acute lymphoblastic leukemia: induction therapy as a second-line treatment (in combination with other agents)

FDA-approved Dosage

- Refer to current literature for dosing regimens. The package insert cites two dosage regimens based on two different studies:
  - In combination with cytarabine: 165 mg/m² i.v. over 30 to 60 minutes twice weekly × eight to nine doses
  - In combination with vincristine and prednisone: 250 mg/m² i.v. over 30 to 60 minutes weekly × four to eight doses

Dose Modification Criteria

- Renal: use with caution, no guidelines available
- Hepatic: use with caution, no guidelines available

Adverse Reactions

- CV: hypotension with rapid infusion
- DERM: alopecia, thrombophlebitis, tissue damage secondary to drug extravasation

- GI: diarrhea, N/V (low), mucositis
- HEMAT: myelosuppression
- Other: anaphylaxis, hypersensitivity

Comments

- Observe patient for at least 60 minutes after dose.
- Consider premedication with antihistamines and/or corticosteroids for retreatment (if indicated) after a hypersensitivity reaction.
- Use non-DEHP plasticized solution containers and administration sets.

TESTOLACTONE (TESLAC)

Mechanism of Action

- Synthetic derivative of testosterone that appears to inhibit steroid aromatase activity and consequently cause a reduction in estrone synthesis.

FDA-approved Indications

- Breast cancer: adjunctive therapy in the palliative treatment of advanced or disseminated breast cancer in postmenopausal women when hormonal therapy is indicated or in premenopausal women in whom ovarian function has been terminated.
- Advanced or disseminated mammary cancer.

FDA-approved Dosage

- 250 mg orally four times daily; total daily dose: 1,000 mg/day

Adverse Reactions

- CV: hypertension, peripheral edema
- DERM: maculopapular erythema, alopecia, nail growth disturbance
- GI: anorexia, N/V
- NEURO: paresthesia
- Other: malaise, aches, glossitis

THALIDOMIDE (THALOMID)

Mechanism of Action

- Immunomodulatory agent with antineoplastic and antiangiogenic properties

FDA-approved Indications

- Multiple myeloma: first-line therapy of newly diagnosed multiple myeloma in combination with dexamethasone
- Other indications: erythema nodosum leprosum

FDA-approved Dosage

- Multiple myeloma: 200 mg orally once daily, preferably at bedtime and at least 1 hour after the evening meal. Thalidomide is administered in combination with dexamethasone in 28-day treatment cycles. Dexamethasone is dosed at 40 mg orally once daily on days 1 to 4, 9 to 12, and 17 to 20 every 28 days.

Dose Modification Criteria

- Renal: no (not studied except in patients on dialysis)
- Hepatic: no data
- Myelosuppression: yes
- Nonhematologic toxicity: yes

Adverse Reactions

- CV: edema, orthostatic hypotension, bradycardia
- DERM: rash, desquamation, dry skin
- ELECTRO: hypocalcemia
- GI: constipation, N/V (minimal to low)
- HEMAT: myelosuppression
- NEURO: peripheral neuropathy (sensory and motor), drowsiness, somnolence, dizziness, confusion, tremor
- PULM: dyspnea
- Other: thromboembolic events, hypersensitivity reactions, fatigue

Comments

- Thalidomide is only available through a restricted distribution program (STEPS). Only prescribers and pharmacists registered with the program are allowed to prescribe and dispense thalidomide.
- Pregnancy category X. Thalidomide is a known teratogen and can cause severe birth defects or death to an unborn baby. Refer to the product labeling for information regarding requirements for patient consent, pregnancy testing, and patient consent as part of the STEPS program.
- Thalidomide may cause venous thromboembolic events. There is an increased risk of thrombotic events when thalidomide is combined with standard chemotherapeutic agents, including dexamethasone. Consider concurrent prophylactic anticoagulation or aspirin treatment.
- Peripheral neuropathy is a common, potentially severe toxicity that may be irreversible. Consideration should be given to electrophysiological testing at baseline and periodically thereafter.

THIOGUANINE (TABLOID)

Mechanism of Action

- Antimetabolite

FDA-approved Indications

- ANLL: remission induction, remission consolidation. Thioguanine is not recommended for use during maintenance therapy or similar long-term continuous treatments due to high risk of liver toxicity.

FDA-approved Dosage

- Combination therapy: refer to current literature
- Single-agent therapy: 2 mg/kg p.o. daily as a single daily dose. May increase to 3 mg/kg p.o. daily as a single daily dose after 4 weeks if no clinical improvement.

Adverse Reactions

- GI: anorexia, stomatitis, N/V (minimal)
- HEMAT: myelosuppression
- HEPAT: increased LFTs, increased bilirubin (cases of veno-occlusive hepatic disease have been reported in patients receiving combination chemotherapy for leukemia)
- Other: hyperuricemia, tumor lysis syndrome

Comments

- Cross-resistance with mercaptopurine
- Consider appropriate prophylaxis for tumor lysis syndrome when treating acute leukemias.

THIOTEPA (THIOPLEX)

Mechanism of Action

- Alkylating agent

FDA-approved Indications

- Superficial papillary carcinoma of the bladder, controlling intracavitary effusions secondary to diffuse or localized neoplasms of the serosal cavities, breast cancer, ovarian cancer, Hodgkin disease, lymphosarcoma

FDA-approved Dosage

- Intravenous administration: 0.3 to 0.4 mg/kg i.v. × one dose repeated at 1- to 4-week intervals. Consult current literature for alternative dosing regimens.
- Intravesical administration: Patients with papillary carcinoma of the bladder are dehydrated for 8 to 12 hours before procedure. Then 60 mg of thiotepa in 30 to 60 mL of sodium chloride injection is instilled into the bladder. For maximum effect, the solution should be retained in the bladder for 2 hours. If desired, reposition patient every 15 minutes to maximize contact. Repeat administration weekly × 4 weeks. A course of treatment (four doses) may be repeated for up to two more courses if necessary, but with caution secondary to bone marrow depression.
- Intracavitary administration: 0.6 to 0.8 mg/kg × one dose through tubing used to remove fluid from cavity.

Adverse Reactions

- CNS: dizziness, headache, blurred vision, conjunctivitis
- DERM: alopecia, pain at the injection site
- GI: anorexia, N/V (low), mucositis at high doses
- GU: amenorrhea, reduced spermatogenesis, dysuria, chemical or hemorrhagic cystitis (intravesical)
- HEMAT: myelosuppression
- Other: fever, hypersensitivity reactions, fatigue, weakness, anaphylaxis

TOPOTECAN (HYCAMTIN)

Mechanism of Action

- Topoisomerase-I inhibitor

FDA-approved Indications

- Metastatic ovarian cancer: second-line therapy after failure of initial or subsequent chemotherapy (topotecan injection)
- Small cell lung cancer: second-line therapy in sensitive disease after failure of first-line chemotherapy (topotecan injection and oral capsules)
- Cervical cancer: combination therapy with cisplatin for stage IV-B, recurrent, or persistent carcinoma of the cervix which is not amenable to curative treatment with surgery and/or radiation therapy.

FDA-approved Dosage

- Ovarian cancer: 1.5 mg/m^2 i.v. over 30 minutes daily $\times$ 5 days, starting on day 1 of a 21-day course
- Small cell lung cancer:
  - Injection: 1.5 mg/m^2 i.v. over 30 minutes daily $\times$ 5 days, repeated every 21 days
  - Oral capsules: 2.3 mg/m^2 orally once daily $\times$ 5 days, repeated every 21 days
- Cervical cancer: 0.75 mg/m^2 i.v. over 30 minutes daily $\times$ 3 days (days 1, 2, and 3), followed by cisplatin 50 mg/m^2 by i.v. infusion on day 1 only; repeated every 21 days (21-day cycle)

Dose Modification Criteria

- Renal (mild impairment, CrCl 40–60 mL/min): no
- Renal (moderate impairment, CrCl 20–39 mL/min): yes
- Renal (severe impairment, <20 mL/min): unknown
- Hepatic (bilirubin, mild to moderate elevation): no
- Myelosuppression: yes
- Nonhematologic toxicity: yes

Adverse Reactions

- DERM: alopecia, rash, injection site reactions
- HEMAT: myelosuppression
- GI: N/V (low), diarrhea, constipation, abdominal pain, stomatitis, anorexia
- NEURO: headache, pain
- PULM: dyspnea, coughing
- Other: fatigue, asthenia, fever

Comments

- Bone marrow suppression (primarily neutropenia) is a dose-limiting toxicity of topotecan. Topotecan should be administered only to patients with baseline neutrophil counts of $\geq$1,500 cells/mm^3 and a platelet count $\geq$ 100,000 cells/mm^3.
- Topotecan-induced neutropenia can lead to neutropenic colitis.
- Severe diarrhea requiring hospitalization has been reported with oral topotecan capsules. Dose may need to be adjusted.
- Concomitant filgrastim may worsen neutropenia. If used, start filgrastim at least 24 hours after last topotecan dose.
- P-glycoprotein inhibitors (e.g., cyclosporine, elacridar, ketoconazole, ritonavir, saquinavir) can cause significant increases in topotecan exposure.
- Pregnancy category D: may cause fetal harm if administered to a pregnant woman.

TOREMIFENE (FARNESTON)

Mechanism of Action

- Nonsteroidal antiestrogen

FDA-approved Indications

- Metastatic breast cancer in postmenopausal women with ER-positive or unknown tumors.

FDA-approved Dosage

- 60 mg orally daily

Adverse Reactions

- CV: thromboembolism, stroke, pulmonary embolism
- DERM: skin discoloration, dermatitis
- ELECTRO: hypercalcemia
- ENDO: hot flashes
- GI: N/V (minimal), constipation, elevated LFTs
- GU: vaginal discharge, vaginal bleeding
- NEURO: dizziness, depression
- Ocular: dry eyes, ocular changes, cataracts
- Other: sweating, tumor flare

Comments

- Do not use in patients with a history of thromboembolic disease or endometrial hyperplasia.

TRASTUZUMAB (HERCEPTIN)

Mechanism of Action

- Humanized monoclonal antibody directed at the human epidermal growth factor receptor 2 protein (HER2)

FDA-approved Indications

- Adjuvant breast cancer:
  - For the adjuvant treatment of HER2 overexpressing breast cancer as part of a regimen containing doxorubicin, cyclophosphamide, and paclitaxel.
  - As a single agent for the adjuvant treatment of HER2 overexpressing node-negative (ER/PR negative or with one high-risk feature) or node-positive breast cancer, following multi-modality anthracycline based therapy.
- Metastatic breast cancer in patients in which tumor overexpresses the HER2 protein including:
  - First-line treatment in combination with paclitaxel
  - Second-line treatment as a single agent therapy

FDA-approved Dosage

- Adjuvant breast cancer: Two dosing regimens are described in the product labeling:
  1. Initiate traztuzumab following completion of anthracycline and concurrently with paclitaxel for the first 12 weeks. Start at an initial dose of 4 mg/kg i.v. infused over 90 minutes followed by subsequent once weekly doses of 2 mg/kg i.v. infused over 30 minutes, as tolerated, for a total of 52 doses.
  2. Initiate traztuzumab following completion of all chemotherapy. Start at an initial dose of 8 mg/kg followed by subsequent doses of 6 mg/kg every 3 weeks for a total of 17 doses. Administer all doses of $\geq$ 4 mg/kg over 90 minutes i.v. infusion.
- Metastatic breast cancer: Initial loading dose of 4 mg/kg i.v. infused over 90 minutes. Weekly maintenance dose of 2 mg/kg i.v. infused over 30 minutes (if first dose is tolerated).

Adverse Reactions

- CV: cardiomyopathy, ventricular dysfunction, CHF (incidence higher in patients receiving concurrent chemotherapy), hypotension (infusion reactions)
- DERM: rash
- HEMAT: myelosuppression (anemia and leukopenia with concurrent chemotherapy)
- GI: diarrhea, nausea, vomiting, anorexia
- INFUS: (first infusion) chills, fever, nausea, vomiting, pain (at tumor sites), rigors, headache, dizziness, dyspnea, rash, hypotension, asthenia

- NEURO: headache, dizziness (see infusion reactions)
- PULM: cough, dyspnea, rhinitis, adult respiratory distress syndrome, bronchospasm, angioedema, wheezing, pleural effusions, pulmonary infiltrates, noncardiogenic pulmonary edema, pulmonary insufficiency, hypoxia (some severe pulmonary reactions required supplemental oxygen or ventilatory support)
- Other: infection (higher incidence of mild upper respiratory infections and catheter infections observed in one randomized trial), asthenia, allergic reactions, anaphylaxis

Comments

- Death within 24 hours of a trastuzumab infusion has been reported. The most severe reactions seem to occur in patients with significant preexisting pulmonary compromise secondary to intrinsic lung disease and/or malignant pulmonary involvement.
- Do not administer i.v. push or i.v. bolus.
- May use sterile water for injection for reconstitution if patient is allergic to benzyl alcohol (supplied diluent is bacteriostatic water for injection); product should be used immediately and unused portion discarded.
- Alternative dosing regimens have been studied including dosing at longer dosing intervals; consult current literature.

TRETINOIN (VESANOID)

Mechanism of Action

- Induces maturation, cytodifferentiation, and decreased proliferation of APL cells.

FDA-approved Indications

- APL: Induction of remission in patients with APL FAB M3 (including the M3 variant), characterized by the t(15:17) translocation and/or the presence of the PML/RAR α gene, who are refractory to or relapsed after anthracycline chemotherapy or for whom anthracycline therapy is contraindicated.

FDA-approved Dosage

- 22.5 mg/m^2 p.o. twice daily (total daily dose: 45 mg/m^2) until complete remission is documented. Therapy should be discontinued 30 days after complete remission is obtained or after 90 days of treatment, whichever comes first.

Adverse Reactions

- CV: hypertension, arrhythmias, flushing, hyperlipidemia
- DERM: dry skin/mucous membranes, rash, pruritis, alopecia, mucositis
- GI: N/V, diarrhea, constipation, dyspepsia
- HEMAT: leukocytosis
- NEURO: dizziness, anxiety, insomnia, headache, depression, confusion, intracranial hypertension, agitation, earaches, hearing loss, pseudotumor cerebri
- OCULAR: visual changes
- OTHER: dyspnea, fever, shivering, retinoic acid–APL syndrome (RA-APL syndrome: fever, dyspnea, weight gain, radiographic pulmonary infiltrates, and pleural or pericardial effusion)

Comments

- Teratogenic; women must use effective contraception during and for 1 month after therapy.
- RA-APL syndrome occurs in up to 25% of patients usually within first month. Early recognition and high-dose corticosteroids (dexamethasone 10 mg i.v. every 12 hours $\times$ 3 days or until the resolution of symptoms) have been used for management.

- During tretinoin treatment about 40% of patients will develop rapidly evolving leukocytosis which is associated with a higher risk of life-threatening complications. If signs and symptoms of the RA-APL syndrome are present together with leukocytosis, high-dose corticosteroids should be initiated immediately. Chemotherapy is often combined with tretinoin in patients who present with leukocytosis (WBC count of $>5 \times 10^9$/L) or with rapidly evolving leukocytosis.
- Consult current literature for APL treatment regimens.

TRIPTORELIN (TRELSTAR)

Mechanism of Action

- LHRH agonist; chronic administration leads to sustained suppression of pituitary gonadotropins and subsequent suppression of serum testosterone in men and serum estradiol in women.

FDA-approved Indications

- Palliative treatment of advanced prostate cancer

FDA-approved Dosage

- Trelstar Depot: 3.75 mg i.m. injection monthly
- Trelstar LA: 11.25 mg i.m. injection every 84 days

Adverse Reactions

- CV: hypertension, peripheral edema
- ENDO: hot flashes, gynecomastia, breast pain, sexual dysfunction, decreased erections
- GU: erectile dysfunction, lower urinary tract symptoms, testicular atrophy
- Other: tumor flare in the first few weeks of therapy, bone pain, injection site reactions, loss of bone mineral density, osteoporosis, bone fracture, asthenia

Comments

- Use with caution in patients at risk of developing ureteral obstruction or spinal cord compression.

VALRUBICIN (VALSTAR)

Mechanism of Action

- Intercalating agent; topoisomerase-II inhibition

FDA-approved Indications

- Carcinoma in situ of the urinary bladder: second-line intravesical treatment after BCG therapy in patients for whom immediate cystectomy would be associated with unacceptable morbidity or mortality.

FDA-approved Dosage

- 800 mg intravesically weekly $\times$ 6 weeks. For each instillation, 800 mg of valrubicin is diluted with 0.9% sodium chloride to a total volume of 75 mL. Once instilled into the bladder, the patient should retain drug in bladder for 2 hours before voiding.

Adverse Reactions

- GU: Irritable bladder symptoms: urinary frequency, dysuria, urinary urgency, hematuria, bladder spasm, bladder pain, urinary incontinence, cystitis, local burning symptoms related to the procedure, red-tinged urine

Comments

- Patients should maintain adequate hydration after treatment.
- Irritable bladder symptoms may occur during instillation and retention of valrubicin and for a limited period following voiding. For the first 24 hours following administration, red-tinged urine is typical. Patients should report prolonged irritable bladder symptoms or prolonged passage of red-colored urine immediately to their physician.
- Use non-DEHP plasticized solution containers and administration sets.

VINBLASTINE (VELBAN)

Mechanism of Action

- Inhibits microtubule formation

FDA-approved Indications

- Palliative treatment of the following malignancies:
- Frequently responsive malignancies: testicular cancer, Hodgkin disease, non-Hodgkin lymphoma, mycosis fungoides, Kaposi sarcoma, histiocytic lymphoma, Letterer-Siwe disease (histiocytosis X)
- Less frequently responsive malignancies: breast cancer, resistant choriocarcinoma

FDA-approved Dosage

- Initial (adults): 3.7 mg/m^2 i.v. weekly. May increase weekly dose up to 18.5 mg/m^2 to maintain WBC >3,000 cells/mm^3 (see package insert for schema).
- Initial (pediatric): 2.5 mg/m^2 i.v. weekly. May increase weekly dose up to 12.5 mg/m^2 to maintain WBC >3,000 cells/mm^3 (see package insert for schema)
- Consult current literature for alternative dosing regimens

Dose Modification Criteria

- Renal: no
- Hepatic: yes
- Myelosuppression: yes

Adverse Reactions

- CV: hypertension
- DERM: alopecia, tissue damage/necrosis with extravasation
- GI: N/V (minimal), stomatitis, constipation, ileus
- GU: urinary retention, polyuria
- HEMAT: myelosuppression
- NEURO: peripheral neuropathy, paresthesias, loss of deep tendon reflexes, SIADH
- Other: bone pain, jaw pain, tumor pain, weakness, malaise, Raynaud phenomenon

Comments

- Vesicant
- Administer only by the intravenous route. Fatalities have been reported when other vinca alkaloids have been given intrathecally.

- Label syringe: Administer only i.v. Fatal if given intrathecally. Label outerwrap (if used): "Do not remove covering until moment of injection. Fatal if given intrathecally. For intravenous use only."

VINCRISTINE (ONCOVIN AND OTHERS)

Mechanism of Action

- Inhibits microtubule formation

FDA-approved Indications

- Acute leukemia
- Vincristine has shown to be useful in combination with other agents for Hodgkin disease, non-Hodgkin lymphoma, neuroblastoma, Wilms' tumor, rhabdomyosarcoma.

FDA-approved Dosage

- Adults: 1.4 mg/m^2 i.v. × one dose. Doses may be repeated at weekly intervals. Some clinicians will limit ("cap") individual doses to a maximum of 2 mg.
- Pediatrics: 1.5 to 2 mg/m^2 i.v. × one dose. For pediatric patients weighing 10 kg or less: 0.05 mg/kg i.v. × one dose. Doses may be repeated at weekly intervals. Some clinicians will limit ("cap") individual doses to a maximum of 2 mg.

Dose Modification Criteria

- Renal: no
- Hepatic: yes

Adverse Reactions

- DERM: alopecia, tissue damage/necrosis with extravasation
- GI: N/V L1, stomatitis, anorexia, diarrhea, constipation, ileus
- GU: urinary retention
- NEURO: peripheral neuropathy, paresthesias, numbness, loss of deep tendon reflexes, SIADH
- Ocular: ophthalmoplegia, extraocular muscle paresis
- PULM: pharyngitis
- Other: jaw pain

Comments

- Vesicant
- Administer only by the intravenous route. Fatalities have been reported when other vinca alkaloids have been given intrathecally.
- Label syringe: Administer only i.v.; Fatal if given intrathecally. Label outerwrap (if used): "Do not remove covering until moment of injection. Fatal if given intrathecally. For intravenous use only."
- A routine prophylactic regimen against constipation is recommended for all patients receiving vincristine.

VINORELBINE (NAVELBINE)

Mechanism of Action

- Inhibits microtubule formation

FDA-approved Indications

- NSCLC: First-line treatment as a single agent (stage IV) or in combination with cisplatin (stage III or IV) for ambulatory patients with unresectable, advanced NSCLC.

FDA-approved Dosage

- Single agent: 30 mg/m^2 i.v. over 6 to 10 minutes weekly
- Vinorelbine in combination with cisplatin:
  - Vinorelbine 25 mg/m^2 i.v. over 6 to 10 minutes weekly, *plus*
  - Cisplatin 100 mg/m^2 i.v. every 4 weeks
  OR
  - Vinorelbine 30 mg/m^2 i.v. over 6 to 10 minutes weekly, *plus*
  - Cisplatin 120 mg/m^2 i.v. $\times$ one dose on day 1 and 29, then every 6 weeks
- Flush line with 75 to 125 mL of fluid (e.g., 0.9% sodium chloride) after administration of vinorelbine.

Dose Modification Criteria

- Renal: no
- Hepatic: yes
- Neurotoxicity: yes
- Myelosuppression: yes

Adverse Reactions

- CV: thromboembolic events, chest pain
- DERM: alopecia, vein discoloration, venous pain, chemical phlebitis, tissue damage/necrosis with extravasation
- GI: N/V (low), stomatitis, anorexia, constipation, ileus
- HEMAT: myelosuppression (granulocytopenia > thrombocytopenia or anemia)
- HEPAT: elevated LFTs
- NEURO: peripheral neuropathy, loss of deep tendon reflexes
- PULM: interstitial pulmonary changes, shortness of breath
- Other: jaw pain, tumor pain, fatigue, anaphylaxis

Comments

- Vesicant
- Administer only by the intravenous route. Fatalities have been reported when other vinca alkaloids have been given intrathecally.

VORINOSTAT (ZOLINZA)

Mechanism of Action

- Histone deacetylase inhibitor

FDA-approved Indications

- Cutaneous T cell lymphoma (CTCL): treatment of cutaneous manifestations in patients with CTCL who have progressive, persistent, or recurrent disease on or following two systemic therapies.

FDA-approved Dosage

- 400 mg orally once daily with food

Dose Modification Criteria

- Renal: no
- Hepatic: no data (use caution)
- Myelosuppression: yes
- Nonhematologic toxicity: yes

Adverse Reactions

- CV: QTc prolongation
- DERM: alopecia
- ENDO: hyperglycemia
- GI: N/V (low), diarrhea, anorexia, weight loss, constipation, taste disorders (dysgeusia, dry mouth)
- GU: increased Cr, proteinuria
- HEMAT: myelosuppresion (thrombocytopenia, anemia)
- Other: constitutional symptoms (fatigue, chills), thromboembolic events (including pulmonary embolism), dehydration, muscle spasms

Comments

- Deep venous thrombosis and pulmonary embolism have been reported. Monitor for pertinent signs and symptoms.
- Patients may require antiemetics, antidiarrheals, and fluid and electrolyte replacement to prevent dehydration.
- Hyperglycemia has been commonly reported. Adjustment of diet and/or therapy for increased glucose may be necessary.
- QTc prolongation has been observed. Monitor electrolytes and ECGs at baseline and periodically during treatment.
- Monitor blood counts and chemistry tests every 2 weeks during the first 2 months of therapy and monthly thereafter.
- Severe thrombocytopenia and gastrointestinal bleeding have been reported with concomitant use of vorinostat and other HDAC inhibitors (e.g., valproic acid).
- Pregnancy category D: may cause fetal harm when administered to a pregnant woman.

REFERENCE

1. Kohler DR, Montello MJ, Green L, et al. Standardizing the expression and nomenclature of cancer treatment regimens. *Am J Health Syst Pharm* 1998;55:137–144.

Appendix

PART 1. *Performance status scales/scores: performance status criteria*

ECOG (Zubrod)		Karnofsky		Lansky[a]	
Score	Description	Score	Description	Score	Description
0	Fully active, able to carry on all predisease performance without restriction	100	Normal, no complaints, no evidence of disease	100	Fully active, normal
1	Restricted in physically strenuous activity but ambulatory and able to carry out work of a light or sedentary nature, e.g., light housework/office work	90	Able to carry on normal activity; minor signs or symptoms of disease	90	Minor restrictions in physically strenuous activity
2	Ambulatory and capable of all self-care but unable to carry out any activities related to work. Up and about more than 50% of waking hours	80	Normal activity with effort; some signs or symptoms of disease	80	Active, but tires faster than in previous phase
3	Capable of only limited self-care, confined to bed or chair more than 50% of waking hours	70	Cares for self, unable to carry on normal activity or do active work	70	Both greater restriction of play activity and less time spent in such activity than in previous phase
4	Completely disabled. Cannot carry on any self-care; totally confined to bed or chair	60	Requires occasional assistance, but is able to care for most of his/her needs	60	Up and around, but minimally active in play; keeps busy with quieter activities than in previous phase
		50	Requires considerable assistance and frequent medical care	50	Gets dressed, but lies around much of the day; no active play; able to participate in quiet play and activities
		40	Disabled, requires special care and assistance	40	Mostly in bed; participates in quiet activities
		30	Severely disabled, hospitalization indicated; death not imminent	30	In bed; needs assistance even for quiet play
		20	Very sick, hospitalization indicated; death not imminent	20	Often sleeping; play entirely limited to very passive activities
		10	Moribund, fatal processes progressing rapidly	10	No play; does not even get out of bed

ECOG, Eastern Cooperative Oncology Group.

Karnofsky and Lansky performance scores are intended to be multiples of 10.

[a]The conversion of the Lansky to ECOG scales is intended for National Cancer Institute reporting purposes only.

PART 2. *World Health Organization (WHO) and Response Evaluation Criteria in Solid Tumors (RECIST) criteria for response*

Characteristic	WHO	RECIST
Measurability of lesions at baseline	1. Measurable, two-dimensional (product of LD and greatest perpendicular diameter)[a] 2. Nonmeasurable/evaluable (e.g., lymphangitic pulmonary metastases abdominal masses)	1. Measurable, unidimensional (LD only, size with conventional techniques ≥20 mm; spiral computed tomography ≥10 mm) 2. Nonmeasurable: all other lesions, including small lesions. Evalua is not recommended.
Objective response	1. Measurable disease (change in sum of products of LDs and greatest perpendicular diameters; no maximum number of lesions specified) CR: disappearance of all known disease, confirmed at ≥4 wk PR: ≥50% decrease from baseline, confirmed at ≥4 wk PD: ≥25% increase of one or more lesions, or appearance of new lesions NC: neither PR nor PD criteria met 2. Nonmeasurable disease CR: disappearance of all unknown disease, confirmed at ≥4 wk PR: estimated decrease ≥50%, confirmed at ≥4 wk PD: estimated increase ≥25% in existent lesions or appearance of new lesions NC: neither PR nor PD criteria met	1. Target lesions (change in sum of LDs, maximum of 5 per organ up to 10 totally [more than one organ]) CR: disappearance of all target lesions, confirmed at ≥4 wk PR: ≥30% decrease from baseline, confirmed at 4 wk PD: ≥20% increase over smallest sum of target lesions observed, or appearance of new lesions SD: neither PR nor PD criteria met 1. Nontarget lesions CR: disappearance of all target lesions and normalization of tumor markers, confirmed at ≥4 wk PD: unequivocal progression of nontarget lesions, or appearance of new lesions Non-PD: persistence of one or more nontarget lesions and/or tumor markers above normal limits

Overall response	1. Best response recorded in measurable disease
	2. NC in nonmeasurable lesions will reduce a CR in measurable lesions to an overall PR
	3. NC in nonmeasurable lesions will not reduce a PR in measurable lesions
	1. Best response recorded in measurable disease from treatment start to disease progression or recurrence
	2. Non-PD in nontarget lesions(s) will reduce a CR in target lesions(s) to an overall PR
	3. Non-PD in nontarget lesion(s) will not reduce a PR in target lesions(s)
Duration of response	1. CR
	From: date CR criteria first met
	To: date PD first noted
	2. Overall response
	From: date of start of treatment
	To: date PD first noted
	3. In patients who achieve only a PR, only the period of overall response should be recorded
	1. Overall CR
	From: date CR criteria first met
	To: date recurrent disease first noted
	2. Overall response
	From: date CR or PR criteria first met (whichever status came first)
	To: date recurrent disease or PD first noted
	3. SD
	From: date of start of treatment
	To: date PD first noted

WHO, World Health Organization; RECIST, Response Evaluation Criteria in Solid Tumors; LD, longest diameter; CR, complete response; PR, partial response; PD, progressive disease; NC, no change; SD, stable disease.

[a]Lesions that can only be measured unidimensionally are considered to be measurable (e.g., mediastinal adenopathy, malignant hepatomegaly).

Source: From *J Natl Cancer Inst* 2000;92:179–181, with permission.

Index

Note: Page numbers followed by *f* denote figures; those followed by *t* denote tables.